Cooking For Healthy Healing

A Reference For

HEALING DIETS & RECIPES

by
Linda Rector-Page
N.D., Ph.D.

He who has health has hope.

He who has hope
has everything.

Other Books
by
LINDA RECTOR-PAGE

Healthy Healing

How To Be Your Own Herbal Pharmacist

Party Lights

and the
Library Series Booklets

- *Renewing Female Balance*
- *Do You Have Blood Sugar Blues?*
- *A Fighting Chance for Weight Loss & Cellulite Control*
- *The Energy Crunch & You*
- *Gland & Hormone Health; Taking Care*
- *Heart & Circulation; Controlling Cholesterol*
- *Body Cleansing & Detoxification to Fight Disease*
- *Allergy Control & Management; Overcoming Asthma*
- *Stress, Tension & Pain Relief*
- *Colds & Flu & You - Building Optimum Immunity*
- *Fighting Infections With Herbs; Controlling STDs*
- *Beautiful Skin, Hair & Nails*
- *Menopause & Osteoporosis*
- *Cancer; Can Alternative Therapies Help?*
- *Overcoming Arthritis With Natural Therapies*
- *Today's "Civilization Diseases"; CFS, Candida, & More*
- *Herbal Therapy For Kids*
- *Renewing Male Health & Energy*
- *Power Plants; Building Immunity with Herbs*
- *Don't Let Your Food Go To Waste*
- *Overcoming Arthritis with Natural Therapies*
- *Do You Want To Have A Baby*

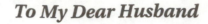

To My Dear Husband

For being the loving life partner that he is.

*For all the lively comments,
and all the hours of proofreading and analysis.*

*For taste-testing his way through all these recipes,
and never getting to have the same thing twice...
even when he liked it.*

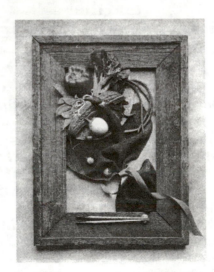

First Edition; November, 1989.
Second Edition: September, 1991./Rev. July, 1995./Rev. October, 1996

ISBN Number 1-884334-56-3

About The Author

Linda Rector-Page has been working in the fields of nutrition and herbal medicine both professionally and as a personal lifestyle choice, since the early seventies. She is a certified Doctor of Naturopathy and Ph.D., with extensive experience in formulating and testing herbal combinations. She received a Doctorate of Naturopathy from the Clayton School of Holistic Healing in 1988, and a Ph.D. in Nutritional Therapy from the American Holistic College of Nutrition in 1989. She is a member of both the American and California Naturopathic Medical Associations.

Linda opened and operated the "Rainbow Kitchen," a natural foods restaurant, then became a working partner in The Country Store Natural Foods company. She has written four successful books and a series of special library booklets in the nutritional healing field. She is the founder and formulator of Crystal Star Herbal Nutrition.

Broad, continuous research in all aspects of alternative healing, from manufacturers, to stores, to consumers has been the cornerstone of success for her reference work "HEALTHY HEALING," now in its ninth edition. Crystal Star Herbal Nutrition products, formulated by Linda, are carried by over three thousand natural food stores nationwide. Feedback from these direct consumer sources provides up-to-the-minute contact with the needs, desires and results being encountered by people taking more responsibility for their own health. Much of the lifestyle information and empirical observation detailed in her books comes from this direct experience - knowledge that is then translated into Crystal Star Herbal Nutrition products, and recorded in every "HEALTHY HEALING" edition.

"COOKING FOR HEALTHY HEALING," now in its second edition, is a companion to "HEALTHY HEALING." It draws on both recipes from the Rainbow Kitchen and the more defined, lifestyle diets that Linda developed from healing results since then. The book contains thirty-three separate diet programs, and over 900 healthy recipes. Every recipe has been taste-tested and time-tested as a part of each recommended diet, so that the suggested healing program can be easily maintained with optimum nutrition.

In "HOW TO BE YOUR OWN HERBAL PHARMACIST," Linda addresses the rising appeal of herbs and herbal healing in America. Many people have expressed an interest in clearly understanding herbal formulation knowledge for personal use. This book is designed for those wishing to take more definitive responsibility for their health through individually developed herbal combinations.

Linda has just completed a new party reference book called "PARTY LIGHTS" in collaboration with restaurateur Doug Vanderberg. This book takes healthy cooking one step further by adding the fun to a good diet. Over sixty party themes are completely planned in "PARTY LIGHTS", all with healthy party food, earthwise decorating, professional garnishing tips, festive napkin folding, interesting games and activities.

TABLE OF CONTENTS

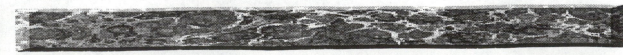

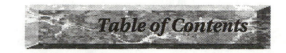

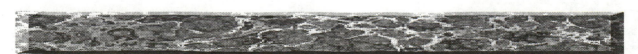

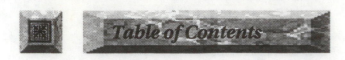

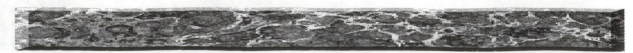

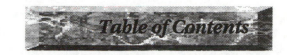

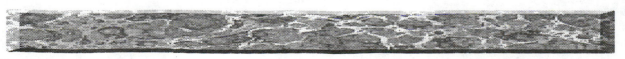

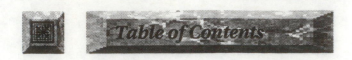
Conditions Effective For: Hyperactivity; Mood & Personality Swings; Gum Disease & Gingivitis; Epilepsy; Schizoprenia; Cataracts & Glaucoma; Diabetic Retinopathy; Drug & Alcohol Addiction/Withdrawal; Male Impotence; Weight Gain; Adrenal Exhaustion.

Diets Included: Colon/Bowel Elimination Diet; Colon Rebuilding Diet; Bladder/Kidney Elimination Diet; Bladder/Kidney Alkalizing and Rebuilding Diet; Prevention Diet for Elimination Problems.
Conditions Effective For: Chronic Constipation; Diarrhea; Irritable Bowel Syndrome; Incontinence; Bladder & Prostate Infections; Cystitis; Kidney Malfunction; Bad Breath & Body Odor; Flatulence; Gas & Bloating; Diverticulitis; Colitis & Spastic Colon; Crohn's Disease; Hemorrhoids.

Diets Included: Liquid Diet for Intense Weight Loss; Eating Light and Low-Fat for Weight Loss; Meal Replacement Diet; Weight Control for Kids.
Conditions Effective For: Weight Loss; Cellulite Control; Energy Improvement; Sluggish Thyroid & Poor Metabolism; High Blood Pressure; Diabetic Weight Gain; Water Retention & Bloating; Poor Circulation; High Cholesterol; Constipation; Liver Malfunction.

Exercise ❦ Bath ❦ Spa Techniques

Section Two   THE HEALING RECIPES

❦ About Red Meats ❦ About Water ❦ About Caffeine ❦ About Salt ❦ About Fats & Oils ❦ Sea Vegetables & Iodine Therapy ❦ Green Superfoods ❦ About Natural Wines ❦ About Fruits ❦ About Therapeutic Herbs ❦ Balancing Your System Type ❦

❦ Whole Foods & the Senses ❦ Avoiding Refined & Processed Foods ❦ Cooking Essentials ❦ The Art of Substituting ❦ Healthy Cooking Techniques ❦ About Culinary Herbs ❦ Glossary of Special Ingredients ❦ About Microwaving ❦

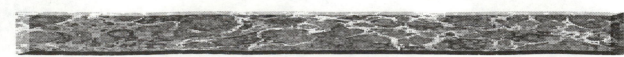

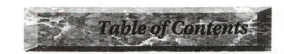

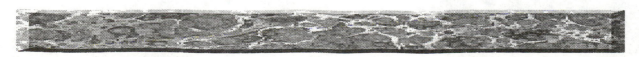

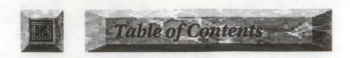

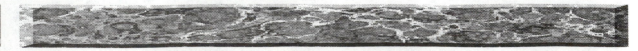

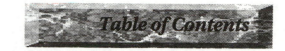

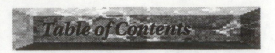

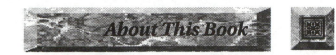
About This Book

Many people are realizing that eating a highly nutritious diet, even eating certain specific foods can help solve health problems. Food can be potent medicine. It can keep energy levels up and stress levels down; skin, hair, and nails healthy; the complexion glowing; the eyes bright; bones and muscles strong; and disease from taking hold.

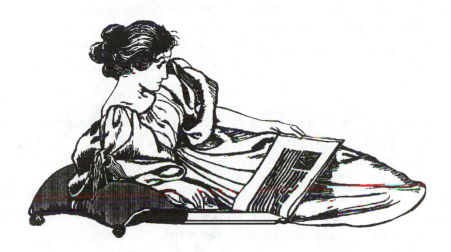

Wholesome food not only fuels the body, but through the mind it can be a key to higher thinking and consciousness. It helps create new balance in a body where there was imbalance, for finer mental tuning and more awareness. A clean, naturally nourished system opens body receivers and transmitters for higher energies.

Good food can be good medicine. It is the primary factor for changing the body chemically and psychologically, and is the foundation element for human life. A clean healthy body allows the beauty of the spirit to begin. Poor diet and junk foods produce lethargy, illness, and indifference.

The food you eat changes your weight, your mood, the texture and look of your body, your outlook on life, indeed the entire universe for you...and therefore your future. Eating right is the first step to the health and balance of your universe.

The history of the world would have been entirely different if the human diet had been different. Our children are literally formed from, and become, the nutrients (or poisons) within us. Not only are <u>we</u> what we eat, our children are as well, before and after birth. The pattern for the immune system and inherited health of your children and grandchildren is laid down by **you**. Healthy parents = healthy children; healthy grandparents = healthy grandchildren, and thus the world.

That's how important diet is!

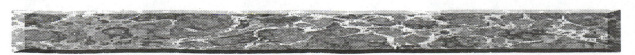

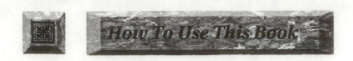

How To Use This Book

This book can lend some help toward using food as a natural pharmacy,
and using your diet and eating habits to change your life and state of health.

It addresses many human health needs with easy-to-follow diets and healing programs, and imaginative, simple, delicious recipes. **The food therapy sections** include cleansing diets, rebuilding diets, maintenance diets, and recipe programs. **The accompanying recipe and menu suggestions** can be used as an initial course, a complete guide, or a jumping off point for individual needs. We recommend that you give your chosen diet program at least four to six weeks to take hold, change body chemistry, and stabilize.

Both the recipes and the diets are tried and true; some in our restaurant, many on family and friends, some at parties, etc. All are low in fats, high in complex carbohydrates and vegetable proteins (you must have protein for healing as well as energy), easy on the digestive system, and non-mucus or acid-forming. This means generally low in pasteurized dairy products, fatty, salty, sugary foods, and fried and refined foods of all kinds. Many of the recipes are followed by a nutritional analysis that includes particular specific nutrients or relevant healing properties.

Good cooking creates health. It can be a source of relaxation, and pleasure rather than a hurried, thoughtless "fueling" process. Good food and good company together can be one of the nicest moments of the day; but increasingly busy lifestyles mean that meals and recipes have to be fast and easy, **and** still be able to keep you healthy. The recipes in this book meet those criteria.

❧ Healthy ❧ Fast ❧ Easy ❧ Delicious

There is a lot of variety, over 900 recipes. Many ailments and problems respond to similar foods and diet. Everything is cross-referenced **in three indexes** so that diet and menu can be expanded as health and balance improve, and the foods and recipes for other health conditions can be included.

This book may also be used as a companion book to **"HEALTHY HEALING," An Alternative Healing Reference,** by Linda Rector-Page. "HEALTHY HEALING" focuses on vitamin, mineral, herbal, and other alternative therapies to supplement and increase healing through diet.

Allergy Control & Management

Allergy problems seem to be increasing every year in our society. Environmental toxins, acid rain, a depleted ozone layer, chemically treated foods, radiation levels, too much anti-biotic and prescription drug use, air and soil pollutants, and stress in our lives, result in lowered immunity and more allergens than our bodies can cope with or neutralize. Cortico-steroid drugs taken over a long period of time for allergy symptoms, greatly reduce immune response, and the ability to overcome allergens permanently.

Most allergens produce clogging and congestion as the body tries to seal them off from its regular processes or tries to work around them. Extra mucous is formed as a shield against these acids, and we get the allergy symptoms of sinus clog, stuffiness, hayfever, headaches and red puffy eyes. Or the body tries to throw the excess acid out, causing the irritation of skin rashes and redness, fever blisters, abscesses or scratchy cough.
There is a growing body of evidence suggesting that some allergies may manifest themselves primarily as changes in personality, emotions, or one's sense of well-being. Allergy reactions are frequently an unrecognized cause of illness.

Allergy origins seem to fall into three main areas:
❦Allergies to environmental pollutants such as asbestos, smoke and fumes.
❦Allergies to seasonal conditions such as dust or pollen, often occurring when the system has an accumulation of mucous or unreleased waste, which then harbors the pollen irritants.
❦Allergies or sensitivities to foods and food additives such as sulfites, nitrates, contaminated seafood, gluten and dairy products. This is the fastest growing allergy group as people are exposed more and longer to chemically altered, processed foods that the body is not equipped to handle. In fact, food allergies are widespread. The most common ones are sensivity to wheat, dairy products, fruits, sugar, yeast, mushrooms, eggs, coffee and greens; all foods that are either heavily treated or sprayed themselves; many animal products we eat are also affected by anti-biotics and hormones. (See Overcoming Food Allergies & Sensitivities in the FOOD COMBINING SECTION, page 85.)

Diet change and supplementation with herbs are the most beneficial and quickest means of controlling allergies. A short three to seven day liquid cleansing diet can rid the body of excess mucous build-up, and pave the way for nutritional changes to have optimal effect. Herbal combinations can work with, or following a mucous cleansing diet to neutralize allergens, increase oxygen uptake, encourage adrenal function, and allow better sleep while therapy on the underlying allergy cause is progressing. Aerobic exercise is important to increase oxygen use in the lungs and tissues. Mental relaxation is also a factor, because stress and tension aggravate allergies.

The following diet will improve several allergy-caused or associated problems:
❧ADRENAL EXHAUSTION ❧ASTHMA ❧HAYFEVER ❧SINUSITIS ❧HEADACHES ❧EPILEPSY ❧EMOTIONAL and PSYCHOLOGICAL DISTURBANCES ❧HYPOGLYCEMIA ❧CANDIDA ALBICANS ❧DIGESTIVE PROBLEMS ❧

Most allergies are not inherited, and can be reduced or curbed. Getting them out of your life will lift an unpleasant burden you have probably been putting up with for years.

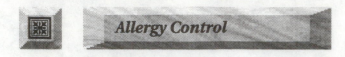

The Three Stage Diet Program For Allergy Control

Allergies can affect any and all parts of the body, and seem to stem from any and all kinds of causes. Coming to grips with allergy origins, and effecting permanent improvement, takes several months, and very conscious effort and attention. But the results are worth it. Getting rid of allergies can totally change your outlook on life. We have found the best way to start is with a short liquid diet.

Allergic rhinitis (congestion and cold symptoms) result from two main areas - allergies to environmental pollutants, such as asbestos, smoke and fumes, and allergies to seasonal conditions, such as dust, pollen or spores. This type of allergic reaction occurs most often when the body has an excess accumulation of mucous, which then harbors the environmental irritants. Common drugstore medications only relieve or mask symptoms. They also have a rebound effect - the more you use them, the more you need them. Cortico-steroid drugs regularly prescribed for rhinitis allergies, and usually taken over a long period of time, do not cure and often make the situation worse by depressing immune response and impeding allergen elimination.

Diet change and cleansing of the internal environment is the single most beneficial thing you can do to control allergic rhinitis reactions.

Buy and use organically grown produce whenever possible. Many allergies are caused by the pesticides, sprays and the chemicals used in agri-business today. It will make a real difference.

Stage One Mucous Elimination Diet; 3 to 7 Days:

On rising: take 2 lemons squeezed in a glass of water; add a packet of chlorella granules if desired.

Breakfast: take a glass of fresh grapefruit or pineapple juice;
or a glass of cranberry/apple juice.
After the third day, fresh fruits may be added.

Mid morning: have a glass of fresh carrot juice; add 1 teasp. Bragg's LIQUID AMINOS if desired;
or a green drink, (pg. 240ff.), **or** Sun CHLORELLA or BARLEY GREEN MAGMA.

Lunch: take a potassium broth drink (pg. 240);
or an alkalizing glass of apple/alfalfa sprout juice;
or a carrot/beet/cucumber juice, if a kidney cleanse is desired.

Mid-afternoon: take another glass of fresh carrot juice;
or a mucous-cleansing herb tea, such as comfrey, comfrey/fenugreek, or wild cherrry bark;
or an herbal blend specifically for mucous cleansing, such as Crystal Star X-PEC TEA™, an expectorant to aid mucous release, or RESPR-TEA™, an antioxidant blend to aid in oxygen uptake.

Dinner: take a glass of pineapple/papaya juice, or apple juice.

Before bed: have a cup of VEGEX yeast broth for relaxation and strength the next day, or a relaxing herb tea, such as scullcap or chamomile.

✓ Drink 6 to 8 glasses of bottled water daily in addition to the juices and other liquids, to thin mucous secretions and aid elimination.

✱ *Supplements & Herbal Aids for the Mucous Elimination Diet:*

❖ Take 10,000mg. of ASCORBATE VITAMIN C crystals daily in your juices or water for the first three days; dissolve 1/4 to 1/2 teasp. at a time every 2 to 3 hours throughout the day until bowel tolerance (a soupy stool) is reached, and tissues are flushed. Then take 5,000mg. daily until the end of the mucous elimination diet.

and, take Natren LIFE START 2, a complex acidophilus culture powder to clean the liver and encourage antihistimine production to combat allergens; $1/4$ to $1/2$ teasp. every 2 to 3 hours with juice.

❖ Add liquid chlorophyll or Sun CHLORELLA or spirulina granules to any juice everyday; $1/2$ to 1 teasp. per drink, for extra blood cleansing and detoxification.

❖ Take 1 teasp. GARLIC/ONION SYRUP 3x daily; mash several garlic cloves and a large slice of onion in a bowl, and stir with 3 TBS. honey. Cover and macerate for 24 hours. Remove garlic and onion. Take only the honey syrup infusion.

✷ *Bodywork Suggestions for the Mucous Elimination Diet:*

✛ Deep breathing exercises are very beneficial during a cleanse. Take 10 deep breaths, with the hands on the rib cage before retiring, and take 10 more each morning. Strong exhalation is very important to expel toxins from the lungs.

✛ Take a brisk walk daily during this diet, breathing deeply, to help lungs and chest eliminate mucous.

✛ Apply warm, wet ginger/cayenne compresses to the chest to increase circulation, and loosen mucous accretions.

✛ Take frequent hot saunas followed by a brisk rubdown to stimulate elimination and circulation.

✛ Relax. Tension and stress reduce the body's ability to deal with allergens.

Stage Two Rebuilding Diet; 1 Month to 6 Weeks:

The second part of the allergy control program is still mildly cleansing, but without the heavy toxin elimination of STAGE 1. It relies on raw fresh foods, adds cultured foods for friendly, immune building intestinal flora and enzymes, and on non-mucous-forming grains and proteins for rebuilding an allergen-free system.
*Make sure that you are avoiding pasteurized dairy products, caffeine, refined foods, canned foods, meats and alcohol during this diet stage. Remember that nicotine **from tobacco or secondary smoke** leaches Vitamin C from the system; lots of this vitamin is necessary for combatting allergens, and building a healthy Ph balanced system.*

On rising: continue with lemon juice and water, adding 1 teasp. honey if desired;
or grapefruit or cranberry juice with honey;
or Crystal Star BIOFLAVONOID, FIBER & C SUPPORT™ DRINK.

Breakfast: take a glass of orange juice with 2 TBS. brewer's yeast and 2 TBS. wheat germ added;
or sprinkle these on fresh fruit and yogurt;
and/or have some oatmeal, muesli or whole grain cereal with apple juice or yogurt.

Mid-morning: take a green drink (pg. 240ff.), Sun CHLORELLA granules, or Crystal Star ENERGY GREEN DRINK™ to flush excess mucous and support clean body energy;
or a glass of fresh carrot juice;
or a cup of miso soup with dried sea vegetables snipped on top.

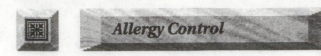

Lunch: have a green salad with baked or simmered tofu and a lemon/oil dressing, and french onion soup with whole grain toast or croutons;
or a whole grain sandwich filled with steamed or fresh veggies and a kefir cheese spread;
or some steamed veggies with soy or kefir cheese topping.

Mid-afternoon: have an apple juice, or an alkalizing herb tea, such as mint or ginger tea, or Crystal Star ALLR-HST TEA™;
or yogurt with fresh fruit, nuts & seeds;
or miso soup with sea veggies and rice noodles.

Dinner: have an onion quiche with a green salad;
or marinated tofu with brown rice or millet;
or a baked potato with yogurt or kefir cheese dressing, and a green salad;
or stir-fried Chinese greens with rice noodles and miso soup;
or a large dinner salad with whole grain bread or muffins;
or a baked veggie casserole with soy cheese, yogurt cheese or kefir cheese.

Before Bed: have a glass of apple juice, or papaya juice;
or a VEGEX yeast broth for relaxation and strength.

✓*Drink and use bottled water whenever possible.*

✓Crystal Star ASTH-AID™ or ALLR-HST TEA™ may be taken daily as needed during allergy season.

✓**Substitute leafy greens and whole grains for dairy foods when you have a choice. They can satisfy the nourishment and nutrient requirements of many dairy products, without forming excess mucous.**

✹ *Supplements for the Rebuilding Diet:*

Natural supplements help reinforce the body's defenses against allergens, and build resistance to further attacks. Take only hypo-allergenic, all natural supplements. Make sure you avoid all foods with sulfites, MSG, preservatives, and colorings; and all refined and fried or fatty foods.

❖ Consider daily bee pollen and/or ginkgo biloba to inactivate bio-allergen substances.

❖ Nourish the adrenal glands with Crystal Star ADR-ACTIVE™ capsules or ADRN™ EXTRACT.

❖ Continue with ascorbate vitamin C, up to 5000mg. daily. Add quercetin plus 1000 to 2000mg., and bromelain 500 to 1000mg. daily for active bioflavonoids and other allergy fighting properties.

❖ Consider a full spectrum digestive enzyme with meals, or take acidophilus, 1/4 teasp. in liquid before each meal.

✹ *Bodywork for the Rebuilding Diet:*

Exercise is important to increase oxygen uptake in the lungs and tissues. Mental relaxation techniques are also a key, since stress and tension aggravate allergies.

✚ Take a daily, brisk aerobic walk, breathing deeply.

✚ Do deep breathing exercises in the morning and before bed for better oxygen use and relaxation.

✚ Avoid smoking and all forms of nicotine. It magnifies allergies more than any other practice.

❋ Sample Recipe Suggestions for the Rebuilding Diet
By section and recipe number:

FASTING & CLEANSING FOODS - 1, 6, 7, 12, 16, 18, 19, 22, 27, 30, 32, 35, 37, 39, 41.

HEALTHY DRINKS, JUICES & WATERS - 44, 46, 47, 49, 51, 52, 53, 54, 58, 61, 65, 66, 71.

BREAKFAST & BRUNCH - 75, 76, 77, 78, 80, 81, 84, 85, 93, 97, 98, 101, 103.

MACROBIOTIC COOKING - 111, 113, 115, 122, 125, 128, 133, 135, 143, 153, 159, 165, 169, 171, 174.

SALADS HOT & COLD - 186, 187, 189, 192, 202, 204, 210, 211, 213, 215, 225, 226, 230, 232, 233, 235.

LOW-FAT & VERY LOW-FAT DISHES - 242, 250, 255, 258, 264, 273, 274, 276, 279, 284, 287, 290, 295.

DAIRY FREE COOKING - 334, 337, 339, 340, 341, 348, 350, 355, 353, 357, 360, 361, 363, 366, 367, 371.

WHEAT FREE BAKING - all

SOUPS - LIQUID SALADS - 447, 448, 451, 452, 453, 455, 456, 457, 458, 459, 460, 462, 463, 466, 467, 472.

TOFU FOR YOU - 571, 574, 573, 576, 577, 579, 580, 583, 585, 587, 592, 593, 597, 598, 600, 601, 602, 603.

❋ Sample Menu Plans
Recipe combinations that work for this diet:

A FAMILY DINNER - 229, 582, 376/388

AN EASY RISING BREAKFAST - 73, 79, 401

A LIGHT SUMMER MEAL - 348, 270, 390, 53

AN EASY WEEKNIGHT MEAL - 332, 224, 610

A SPECIAL DINNER FOR TWO - 262, 153, 271, 371, 192

LUNCH FOR TWO - 248, 189, 380/383

A HEARTY WINTER MEAL - 349, 606, 394

SUNDAY BRUNCH - 399, 49, 92, 261, 222

A WEEKEND PICNIC - 127, 174, 55, 129

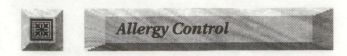
Stage Three; Maintaining an Allergy-free System:

The allergy control maintenance diet continues with some fresh foods every day to keep the body swept clean of pollutants and allergens. It is a light way of eating, low in fats and meats, but still very strengthening and high in energy-enhancing foods. It is a diet you can live with on a long term basis.

On rising: take a high protein vitamin/mineral drink, such as NutriTech ALL 1 or Nature's Plus SPIRU-TEIN in apple juice;
or lemon juice in water to flush excess mucous;
or a green drink, such as Crystal Star ENERGY GREEN™, or Sun CHLORELLA granules in water or juice.

Breakfast: have a poached egg with whole grain muffins and some kefir cheese;
or a hot whole grain cereal with a little maple syrup or yogurt, or apple juice;
or fresh fruit with yogurt or kefir, and a whole grain muesli or cold cereal.
♣ Sprinkle a mix of 2 TBS. brewer's yeast and 2 TBS. toasted wheat germ on any breakfast choice for extra allergy fighting nutrition.

Mid-morning: have some whole grain crackers or crunchy raw veggies with kefir or yogurt cheese or a vegetable dip;
or miso soup with sea veggies snipped on top;
or an energizing no-caffeine herb tea such as Ginseng or Gotu Kola tea, or Crystal Star HIGH ENERGY™ TEA.

Lunch: have a green salad with a yogurt or lemon/oil dressing;
or a fresh fruit salad with cottage or yogurt cheese;
and/or a cup of lentil, black bean or onion soup;
or a seafood and whole grain or veggie pasta salad with a low-fat Italian dressing;
or some baked tofu with brown rice or millet, and a green salad.

Mid-afternoon: have a hard boiled egg with a little sesame salt, and a refreshing herb tea, such as spearmint, alfalfa/mint, or Crystal Star LICORICE MINTS TEA.
or fresh carrot juice;
or a small bottle of mineral water.

Dinner: have a vegetable quiche with whole grain or chapati crust;
or a baked potato with kefir cheese and a large green dinner salad;
or a light Italian whole grain or veggie pasta meal, with minestrone or onion/garlic soup, and polenta;
or an oriental stir-fry with seafood and veggies and brown rice or noodles;
or baked or broiled white fish with steamed veggies and whole grain muffins.

Before bed: have another apple or apple/papaya juice, or a cup of miso soup, or Vegex yeast broth.

✓ Make a mix of equal parts apple cider vinegar and honey. Take 2 TBS. before each meal to acidify saliva, and maximize food assimilation.

✓ Include plenty of cultured foods for friendly G.I. flora.

✓ If you have chronic undiagnosed allergies, avoid common allergens such as pasteurized dairy foods, wheat, eggs, yeasted breads, sugar, corn and nightshade plants.

✓ Drink plenty of bottled or mineral water throughout the day for better assimilation and digestion.

❋ *Supplements for Maintaining an Allergy-Free System:*

✤ Take high Omega-3 flax or fish oils, and/or a germanium-containing supplement such as Solaray TRI-O_2 for better oxygen use and uptake.

✤ Take Evening Primrose oil, 2 to 4 caps daily, or high potency Royal Jelly 2 teasp. daily to neutralize allergens.

✤ Continue to take Vitamin C, about 3000mg. daily for strong immune response and body balance

❋ *Bodywork for Maintaining an Allergy-Free System:*

✤ Keep smoking and nicotine out of your life as much as possible. You need all the oxygen and free arterial activity available.

✤ Continue with deep breathing exercise and regular aerobic walking or workouts. Exercise is a nutrient and energizer in itself.

❋ *Sample Recipe Suggestions for Maintaining Allergy Control By section and number:*

SALADS - HOT & COLD - all.

BREAKFAST & BRUNCH - 73, 75, 77, 80, 83, 87, 92, 94, 96, 100, 107, 108.

DAIRY FREE COOKING - all

WHEAT FREE BAKING - all

SUGAR FREE SPECIALS & SWEET TREATS - 411, 414, 416, 417, 420, 423, 426, 427, 430, 429, 432, 433.

STIR-FRYS - 501, 503, 505, 508, 509, 510, 511, 513, 514, 515, 517,518, 519, 522, 524, 526, 527, 529, 530.

FISH & SEAFOODS - 532, 534, 537, 540, 544, 547, 552, 553, 554, 555, 556, 560, 563, 565, 566, 567, 568.

HIGH MINERAL FOODS - 613, 615, 616, 618, 623, 628, 631, 634, 636, 646, 647, 648, 649, 650, 651, 653.

COMPLEX CARBOHYDRATES FOR ENERGY - 744, 747, 750, 751, 752, 753, 756, 757, 773, 781, 784.

HEALTHY FEASTING - 830, 831, 832, 833, 835, 837, 841, 842, 843, 844, 846, 850, 853, 855, 857, 862.

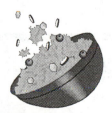

✳ *Sample Menu Plans*
Recipe combinations that work with this diet:

A SPECIAL DINNER FOR TWO - 627, 349, 770, 431

LUNCH FOR TWO - 759, 626, 784

A HEARTY WINTER MEAL - 615, 748, 632, 755

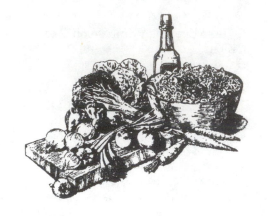

A LIGHT SUMMER MEAL - 744, 237, 438

A WEEKEND PICNIC - 87, 420, 423, 334, 336, 435

SUNDAY BRUNCH - 778, 640, 348, 235, 780

AN EASY RISING BREAKFAST - 73, 93, 80

A FAMILY MEAL - 764, 626, 432

AN EASY WEEKNIGHT DINNER - 743, 628, 658, 190

AN ALL HORS D'OEUVRES PARTY - 636, 429, 646, 334, 337

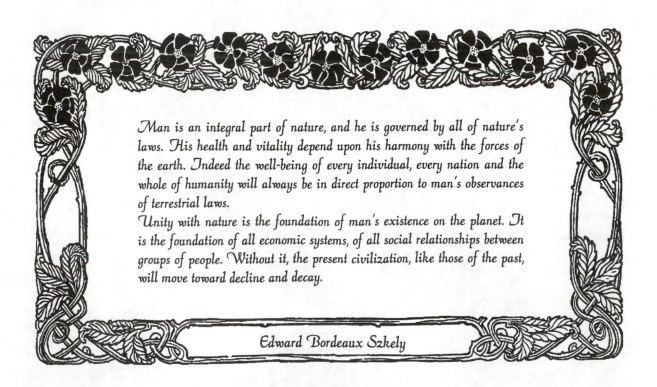

Man is an integral part of nature, and he is governed by all of nature's laws. His health and vitality depend upon his harmony with the forces of the earth. Indeed the well-being of every individual, every nation and the whole of humanity will always be in direct proportion to man's observances of terrestrial laws.

Unity with nature is the foundation of man's existence on the planet. It is the foundation of all economic systems, of all social relationships between groups of people. Without it, the present civilization, like those of the past, will move toward decline and decay.

Edward Bordeaux Szkely

Arthritis;
Changing Your Body Chemistry

Arthritis, and other altered-biochemistry diseases, are some of the most debilitating and widespread today, impairing not only bones and joints, but also blood vessels, kidneys, skin, eyes and brain. Medical science has proven unable to cure these conditions. In fact, not only is there little improvement from current arthritis drugs, most patients who receive drug therapy become progressively worse and often suffer serious side effects.

Much has been written about natural healing methods for arthritic conditions. Since arthritis origins range from metabolic disorders brought on by stress and poor environment, to adrenal exhaustion, faulty elimination, an over-acid system, long emotional resentments and pessimism about life, and overuse of prescription drugs, the common thread of natural treatment has been improved diet and nutrition that can create an environment where the body can support its own healing functions. Even in advanced cases of inflammatory pain, joint degeneration, major digestive problems, and attendant toxic syndromes of depression and fatigue, diet change can effect improvement.

The three stage diet in this chapter promotes body detoxification, dissolves and flushes out inorganic mineral deposits, and helps replace them with non-mucous-forming nutrients. The diet is particularly useful for gland nourishment where extreme inflammation is evidence that the body is not producing enough natural cortisone from adrenal cortex.

The main asset of this diet is that it can change your body chemistry and the way it uses the nutrients you give it. It is alkalizing, anti-inflammatory, and effective for over-acid conditions. It is is free of nightshade plants, such as potatoes, tomatoes, chilies, peppers, eggplant, etc. that impair calcium absorption. It is rich in Vitamin C for connective tissue formation, adrenal health and detoxification. It is full of fiber for digestive/elimination regulation, and free of alcohol, caffeine, sugar and refined foods that aggravate acidity. It is low in fat and meats to reduce pain, and high in whole grains and vegetables for better-formed bone and cartilage.

It is also effective for many other similar acid-caused disorders:
RHEUMATISM •BURSITIS •HEEL & BONE SPURS •CONSTIPATION •NERVES •GOUT •CORNS & CARBUNCLES •OSTEOPOROSIS & POST MENOPAUSAL BONE LOSS •SHINGLES •LUPUS •PROSTATE INFECTION •SOME GUM DISEASES •

Additional beneficial actions you can take for noticeable improvement are seaweed baths (pg. 204ff), hot and cold hydrotherapy (pg. 205), and early morning sunbaths for Vitamin D and better calcium use.

Cortico-steroid drugs, often medically prescribed for arthritic conditions, may depress the immune system so dramatically that even minor infections may become life-threatening. They cause calcium depletion, bone weakening, and adrenal gland depression, a primary cause of arthritis in the first place. Arthritic conditions are degenerative processes that take years to develop. Small or subtle dietary changes will not be successful in reversing them.

Aggressive, vigorous diet therapy is the most beneficial thing you can do to control the causes and improve the symptoms of arthritis.

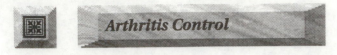

The Three Stage Diet Program for Arthritis Control

The arthritis diet program is in three stages.

The first is a 7 to 10 day liquid diet to cleanse the body of acid wastes and inorganic mineral deposits, and to alkalize the system.

The second stage is a fresh foods, a vegetarian diet, with no animal protein. It should be used for 1 to 2 months, is alkalizing, and will establish body equilibrium, stabilizing the system for a full life-style change.

The third stage is full of complex carbohydrates, vegetable protein and cultured foods; low in fats, acid and mucous-forming foods, and represents continuing diet prevention for arthritis and related conditions.

See also THE FOREVER DIET section for more information.

Stage One Liquid Cleansing Diet; 7 to 10 Days

On rising: take a glass of lemon juice and water;
or a glass of fresh grapefruit juice.

Breakfast: take a glass of potassium broth or essence (pg. 240);
or a glass of carrot/beet/cucumber juice.

Mid-morning: have an apple juice or black cherry juice;
or a green drink such as Sun CHLORELLA, one from page 241ff., or Crystal Star ENERGY GREEN™.

Lunch: have a cup of miso soup with sea veggies snipped on top,
and a glass of fresh carrot juice.

Mid-afternoon: have another green drink;
or a cup of herb tea, such as alfalfa/mint, or Crystal Star AR-EASE TEA™.

Dinner: have a glass of cranberry/apple, or papaya juice, or another glass of black cherry juice.

Before bed: take a glass of celery juice, or a cup of VEGEX yeast extract broth;
or a cup of miso soup.

❊ *Supplements for the Liquid Cleansing Diet:*

❖ While there are many beneficial natural supplements for arthritic conditions, we have found that the body will respond to cleansing faster if only ascorbate Vitamin C powder with bioflavonoids, 1/2 teasp. at a time, in juice or water 4 to 6 times daily, and Omega-3 flax oil, 3 teasp. daily in juice or water are used for this stage.

❊ *Bodywork During the Liquid Cleansing Diet:*

✚ Take alternating hot and cold hydrotherapy (pg. 203ff.) or hot epsom salts baths to relieve pain and loosen joints.

✚ Apply B&T TRI-FLORA ANALGESIC GEL, CAMOCARE CREAM, ginger/cayenne, or cajeput/wintergreen compresses for pain relief.

✚ Get early morning sunlight on the body every day possible.

Stage Two Fresh Foods Diet; 1 to 2 Months

On rising: take a glass of lemon juice and water, or grapefruit juice;
or a glass of apple cider vinegar in water with honey.

Breakfast: have a glass of cranberry, grape or papaya juice, or Crystal Star DAILY BIOFLAVONOID SUPPORT™ DRINK;
and some fresh fruits, especially cherries, bananas, oranges and strawberries.
Make a mix of 2 TBS. **each:** sunflower seeds, lecithin granules, brewer's yeast and wheat germ. Mix 2 teasp. into yogurt, or sprinkle on fresh fruit or greens, but have some every day.

Mid-morning: take a glass of potassium broth (pg. 240) or essence;
and/or more fresh fruit with yogurt;
or a green drink such as Sun CHLORELLA or BARLEY GREEN MAGMA with 1 teasp. Bragg' s LIQUID AMINOS' added.

Lunch: have a large dark green leafy salad with lemon/oil dressing;
and/or a hot veggie broth or onion soup;
and/or some marinated tofu or tempeh in tamari sauce.

Mid-afternoon: have a cup of miso soup with sea veggies on top;
or a green drink, alfalfa/mint tea, or Crystal Star LICORICE MINTS TEA.

Dinner: have a Chinese greens salad with sesame or poppy seed dressing;
or a large dinner salad with soy cheese, nuts, tamari dressing, and a cup of black bean or veggie broth or miso soup;
or some quick steamed vegetables and brown rice for absorbable B vitamins.

Before bed: have a cranberry or apple juice, or black cherry juice;
or a cup of VEGEX yeast extract broth; and/or celery juice.

✓*Make sure you are drinking 6 to 8 glasses of bottled mineral water daily to keep inorganic wastes releasing quickly from the body.*

❋ *Supplements for the Fresh Foods Diet:*
As the body starts to rebuild with a stronger, more alkaline system, additional supplements may be added to speed the process along.

❖ Continue with ascorbate Vitamin C powder in juice ($1/4$ teasp. four times daily) for interstitial tissue and collagen development.

❖ Continue with high Omega-3 flax oil, 3 teasp. daily, and add a complete digestive enzyme for assimilation, and alfalfa tabs, up to 10 daily to help alkalize the system.

❖ Take Crystal Star AR-EASE™ caps as directed, and/or Quercetin Plus with bromelain 500mg. daily to aid release of inorganic calcium and mineral deposits.

❖ Use DLPA 750 to 1000mg. daily, Co Q10, 60mg. twice daily, or highest potency Biotec EXTRA ENERGY ENZYMES for pain relief.

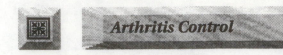

✽ *Bodywork for the Fresh Foods Diet:*

If your arthritic condition is inflammatory, it may be aggravated by eating "nightshade" family plants, such as potatoes, peppers of all kinds, eggplant, tomatoes, etc. This is not the case for most problems, but if it is, the substances in these plants will impair necessary calcium absorption and increase inflammation. Stop smoking and avoid secondary smoke. Tobacco is also a nightshade plant.

✚ Get a good chiropractic adjustment, or Shiatzu treatment for flexibility. Continue with alternating hot and cold hydrotherapy (pg.203).

✚ Cortico-steroid drugs over a long period of time will greatly reduce immunity and weaken the bones. (**Motrin,** a commonly prescribed drug for arthritic symptoms **is a nightshade derivative.** Avoid it if you are nightshade sensitive.)

✚ Avoid aluminum pots, pans, or deodorants with alum or aluminum.

✚ Keep table salt out of your diet during this stage. Use an herbal seasoning instead.

✚ Raise body oxygen with a brisk daily walk and deep breathing exercises every morning and night. Exhale forcefully on your walk to expel toxins from the lungs. Apply H_2O_2 PEROXY GEL to the soles of the feet every 24 hours for additional tissue oxygen.

✽ *Sample Recipes for the Fresh Foods Diet*
By section and number :

FASTING & CLEANSING FOODS - all

HEALTHY DRINKS, JUICES & WATERS - all

BREAKFAST & BRUNCH - all

SALADS HOT & COLD - 186, 187, 188, 189, 191, 193, 196, 197, 198, 199, 200, 201, 202, 203, 210, 211, 213, 215, 216, 218, 220, 221, 222, 224, 225, 226, 230, 231, 232, 233, 236, 237

SOUPS - LIQUID SALADS - all

ORIENTAL & LIGHT MACROBIOTIC EATING - all

Stage Three: Prevention and Maintenance Diet

A prevention diet for arthritis control emphasizes high vitamin C foods for better connective tissue, and adrenal support for cortex production. It features low animal proteins and dairy products to reduce uric acids and mucous formation, and high vegetable fiber to keep the body free flowing and alkaline. Acid-producing foods such as caffeine, refined sugars and flours, fried foods and red meats, should be avoided on a continuing basis, to keep your new alkaline, biochemical changes stable.

On rising: take some lemon juice in water with a little honey;
or a protein drink, such as Nature's Plus SPIRUTEIN in orange or apple juice.

Breakfast: Continue with a mix of 2 TBS. each: toasted wheat germ, sunflower seeds, brewer's yeast, and lecithin granules; sprinkle 2 teasp. on whatever you choose for breakfast, including whole grain toast or pancakes, muffins with yogurt or kefir cheese, whole grain cereal or muesli with apple juice or yogurt;
or some fresh fruits;
or a poached or baked egg with corn bread or whole grain English muffin.

Mid-morning: have some yogurt with fresh fruit;
or a hard boiled egg with sesame salt, mineral water, or an herb tea, such as Crystal Star LICORICE MINTS TEA, or alfalfa/mint tea;
or some crunchy veggies with whole grain crackers, kefir cheese and a green drink such as Sun CHLO-RELLA, Green Foods BARLEY GREEN, or a glass of George's aloe vera juice with herbs.

Lunch: have a large dark green salad with sprouts, cucumbers, celery and lemon/oil dressing, with some baked tofu and brown rice or millet;
or a cup of onion, black bean or lentil soup and a whole grain sandwich with avocados, soy cheese and spicy mayonnaise;
or baked yams with tamari sauce and a small salad;
or a fresh fruit salad with cottage cheese or yogurt cheese;
or a seafood and veggie pasta salad with a light dressing.

Mid-afternoon: have a cup of miso soup, or ramen noodle soup;
or an herb tea, such as Crystal Star FEEL GREAT TEA™, or a small bottle of mineral water;
and/or some fruit juice sweetened cookies or bars.

Dinner: have a Chinese stir-fry with plenty of greens, sprouts, and onions, with a clear soup and brown rice with sea vegetables;
or a baked salmon or seafood dish with basmati rice and peas;
or steamed broccoli with a cup of vegetable or chicken soup;
or a tofu and whole grain casserole and small salad;
or a hearty vegetable stew or seafood paella with a small salad.

Before bed: have a glass of cranberry/apple juice,
or a relaxing herbal mint teat, or Crystal Star RELAX TEA™;
or a cup of VEGEX yeast extract broth for high B Vitamins, strength and relaxation.

✳ *Supplements for the Maintenance & Prevention Diet:*

Continue with the most helpful diet additions you have been using in the STAGE TWO DIET. Others to consider for long range maintenance include:

❖ Antioxidants, such as Solaray TRI-O$_2$ with germanium, Co Q10, 60mg., and Ginkgo Biloba extract drops for more body oxygen.

❖ Quercetin Plus 3x daily, with ascorbate Vitamin C containing high Bioflavonoids for anti-inflammatory activity.

❖ Rainbow Light CALCIUM PLUS, Crystal Star SILICA SOURCE™ extract, or Alta Health SIL-X SILICA for new collagen and tissue formation.

❖ A raw adrenal complex or Crystal Star ADRN-ACTIVE™ caps or ADRN™ extract for better adrenal cortex production.

❋ Bodywork for the Maintenance & Prevention Diet:

✚ Continue with the exercise and aerobic programs you have established.

✚ Occasional pain and stiffness may be eased with a stimulating natural balm, such as Tiger Balm or Chinese White Flower oil.

✚ An occasional Crystal Star ALKALIZING ENZYME HERB WRAP™ to rebalance body chemistry.

❋ Sample Recipes for the Maintenance & Prevention Diet
By section and number:

LOW-FAT & VERY LOW FAT DISHES - all

LOW CHOLESTEROL MEALS - all

SUGAR FREE SWEETS - 411, 415, 416, 419, 420, 422, 424, 425, 426, 427, 430, 432, 435, 437, 438, 439, 441

SANDWICHES - SALADS IN BREAD - 475, 478, 479, 482, 484, 485, 487, 492, 493, 494, 496, 500

STIR-FRYS - all

HIGH MINERAL FOODS - 613, 615, 616, 617, 618, 619, 622, 23, 624, 628, 631, 644, 647, 651, 654, 657

HIGH PROTEIN WITHOUT MEAT - 698, 699, 706, 710, 712, 716, 719, 720, 732, 735, 737, 739, 740, 741

COMPLEX CARBOHYDRATES FOR ENERGY - 743, 745, 750, 755, 765, 767, 769, 772, 773, 774, 777

HIGH FIBER RECIPES - all

GREAT OUTDOORS EATING - all

HEALTHY HOLIDAY FEASTING - 826, 831, 832, 835, 838, 843, 844, 846, 852, 857, 865, 867, 868, 871

❋ Sample Menu Plans
Suggested recipe combinations that work with this diet:

A SPECIAL DINNER FOR TWO - 269, 274, 301, 755, 294

A WEEKEND PICNIC - 489, 257, 795, 249, 423

SUNDAY BRUNCH - 277, 698, 292, 253, 425

A FAMILY MEAL - 259, 753, 313, 443

AN HORS D'OEUVRES PARTY- 695, 319, 877, 239, 475, 244, 250

LUNCH FOR TWO - 260, 306, 418, 240

A HEARTY WINTER MEAL - 321, 329, 299, 310

A LIGHT SUMMER MEAL - 283/286, 905, 241

AN EASY RISING BREAKFAST- 715, 819, 267, 824

AN EASY WEEKNIGHT MEAL - 268, 298, 433, 271

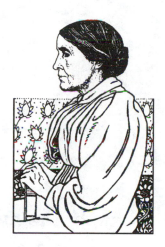

Neither drugs nor herbs nor vitamins are a cure for anything. The body heals itself. The human body is incredibly intelligent. It usually responds to intelligent therapies. The healing professional can help this process along by offering the body intelligent choices.

"The doctor
of the future
will give no medicine
but will interest his patients
in the care of the human
frame, in diet,
and in the cause
and prevention of disease."
-Thomas Edison

Body Cleansing;
Fasting & Detoxification

Environmental toxins, secondary smoke inhalation, alcohol, prescription and pleasure drug abuse, "hidden" chemicals and pollutants in our food that cause allergies and addictions, caffeine overload, poor diet, junk foods, and daily acid-causing stress, are all increasingly a part of our lives. They result in strain and depletion to immune response which eventually results in debilitation and serious disease. Lowered immunity has become a prime factor in today's "civilization, opportunistic diseases," such as Candida Albicans, Chronic Fatigue Syndrome, Cancer, Lupus, and sexually transmitted diseases.

In the past, detoxification was used either clinically for recovering alcoholics/drug addicts, or individually as a once-a-year "spring cleaning" for general health maintenance. Today, detoxification is necessary not only to health, but for the quality of our lives, surrounded as we are by so much involuntary toxicity. Optimally, one should seriously cleanse the system 2 to 3 times a year, especially in the spring, summer and early fall, when the body can get an extra detox boost from sunlight and natural Vitamin D.

A good detoxification program should be in three stages:

❦ CLEANSING ❦ REBUILDING ❦ MAINTAINING

The first step is to clean out waste deposits, so you won't be running with a dirty engine or driving with the brakes on. Years of experience with body cleansing have convinced us that a moderate 3 to 7 day juice fast is the best way to release toxins from the system. Shorter fasts don't get to the root of a chronic or major problem. Longer fasts upset body equilibrium more than most people are ready to deal with except in a controlled, clinical situation.

A well-thought-out moderate fast can bring great advantages to the body by: cleansing it of excess mucous, old fecal matter, trapped cellular and non-food wastes; and by "cleaning the pipes" of uncirculated systemic sludge such as inorganic mineral deposits.

Fasting works by self-digestion. During a cleanse, the body in its infinite wisdom, will decompose and burn only the substances and tissue that are damaged, diseased or unneeded, such as abscesses, tumors, excess fat deposits, and congestive waste. Even a relatively short fast can accelerate elimination from the liver, kidneys, lungs and skin, sometimes causing dramatic changes as masses of accumulated waste are expelled. Live foods and juices literally pick up dead matter from the body and carry it away.

You will be very aware of this if you experience the short period of headaches, fatigue, body odor, bad breath, diarrhea or mouth sores that commonly accompany accelerated elimination. However, digestion usually improves right away and so do many gland and nerve functions. Cleansing also helps release hormone secretions that stimulate the immune system, and encourage a disease-preventing environment. In a couple of weeks the body will start rebalancing, energy levels will rise physically, psychologically and sexually, and creativity will begin to expand. You will begin feeling like a different person, and of course you are. Outlook and attitude have changed, because through cleansing and improved diet, your actual cell make-up has changed.

You really are what you eat.

Even two or three days without solid food can be a refreshing and enlightening experience about your life style. A short fast increases awareness as well as available energy for elimination. Your body becomes easier to "hear." It can tell you what foods and diet are right for your needs, via legitimate cravings such as a desire for protein foods, B vitamins, or minerals, for example. Like a "cellular phone call," this is called natural biofeedback.

All disease, physical and psychological, is created or allowed by the saturation and accumulation of toxic matter in the tissues that throws defense mechanisms off, and vitality out of balance. Detoxification works particularly well when the body shows evidence of the following problems:

❧ALCOHOL and DRUG ABUSE TOXICITY ❧HERPES INFECTION ❧LIVER and SPLEEN DISEASE ❧ACNE ❧MENINGITIS ❧SWOLLEN GLANDS ❧NICOTINE ADDICTION and WITHDRAWAL ❧HEPATITIS ❧HYPOGLYCEMIA ❧ECZEMA and PSORIASIS ❧ INTERNAL PARASITES ❧AIDS and IMMUNE DEFICIENT CONDITIONS ❧MALIGNANT TUMORS ❧KIDNEY STONES and KIDNEY MALFUNCTION ❧EPILEPSY ❧

Getting clean isn't easy. For most people who find themselves in a severe health state, a poor, deficient diet and unwholesome lifestyle has been years in the making. Restoration through lifestyle change and good nutrition takes time. Nature works slowly but surely. Fortunately, our bodies are naturally regenerative. Remember that the pattern for your own health, <u>and</u> the inherited health of your children and your grandchildren, is laid down by you. A clean strong body is necessary for prevention of disease.

Body Cleansing, Fasting & Detoxification Diets

Since the major focus of this section is whole body cleansing, we have included two separate liquid diet programs for this stage. The first is specifically aimed at cleansing excess mucous from the lungs and respiratory system; the second is a colon and bowel cleanser, aimed at removing toxins from the elimination system. Both will help the entire body eliminate trapped and excess waste matter, and alkalize the bloodstream so that more efficient healing can take place.

Cleansing diets may be used before and during any therapeutic program, unless the person is weak and pale, with very low energy, or when immediate emergency measures are indicated. Results are usually well worth the effort.

♣ Have a small fresh salad the night before beginning a liquid fast, with plenty of intestinal "sweepers and scourers," such as beets, celery, cabbage, broccoli, parsley, carrots, etc.
Elimination will begin as soon as the first meal is missed. Use organically grown fresh fruits and vegetables for all juices if possible.

♣ End your fasting period gently, with small simple meals. Have toasted wheat germ or muesli, or whole grain granola for your first morning of solid food, with a little yogurt, apple, or pineapple/ coconut juice. Take a small fresh salad for lunch with Italian or lemon/oil dressing. Have a fresh fruit smoothie during the day. Fix a baked potato with a little butter and a light soup or salad for dinner. Rebuilding starts right away with the nutrition-rich foods you are taking in.

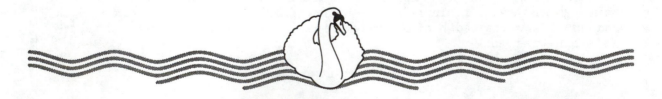

Mucous Cleansing: A 3 to 7 day liquid diet

On rising: take a glass of *fresh-squeezed* lemon juice and water, (add 1 TB. maple syrup if desired).

Breakfast: take a glass of grapefruit juice if the system is over-acid; or cranberry/apple or pineapple juice.

Mid-morning: have a cup of herb tea, such as licorice root, dandelion leaf, or wild cherry bark; <u>or</u> a tea specifically blended to clear mucous congestion, such as Crystal Star X-PECT-T™, an expectorant to aid mucous release, or RSPR TEA™, an aid to oxygen uptake.

Lunch: take a glass of carrot juice, or a potassium broth or essence (page 240).

Mid-afternoon: have a green drink (page 240), or a packet of Chlorella granules in a glass of water; <u>or</u> a greens and sea vegetable mix, such as Crystal Star ENERGY GREEN DRINK™.

Supper: take a glass of apple juice or papaya/pineapple juice.

Before retiring: take a hot broth with 1 teasp. VEGEX extract for relaxation and strength the next day.

♣ Drink 8 glasses of water daily **in addition** to juices, to thin mucous secretions and aid elimination.

♣ **For best results,** break the fast with a small fresh salad on the last night of the cleanse.

✽ *Supplements and Herbal Aids for the Mucous Cleansing Diet:*

❖ Take 10,000mg. of ascorbate vitamin C crystals *with* bioflavonoids daily for the first three days; dissolve $1/4$ - $1/2$ teasp. in water or juice throughout the day until bowel tolerance is reached and tissues are flushed. Take 5,000mg. daily for the next four days.

❖ Take 1 teasp. 3x daily of garlic/onion syrup. Mash several garlic cloves and a large slice of onion in a bowl, and stir with 3 TBS. of honey. Cover, and let macerate for 24 hours; then remove garlic and onion and take only the honey/syrup infusion.

✽ *Bodywork Suggestions for the Mucous Cleansing Diet:*

✚ Take a brisk 1 hour walk each day of the cleanse; breathe deeply to help lungs eliminate mucous.

✚ Take an herbal enema the first and last day of your fasting diet to thoroughly clean out excess mucous. See page for instructions and suggestions.

✚ Apply wet ginger/cayenne compresses to the chest to increase circulation and loosen mucous.

✚ Take a hot sauna, or long warm baths followed by a brisk rubdown, to stimulate circulation.

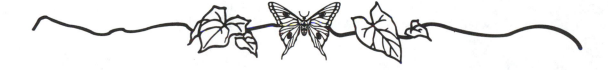

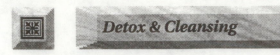

Colon and Bowel Elimination Cleanse: A 3 to 10 day liquid diet

Bowel elimination problems are often chronic, and may require several rounds of cleansing. This fast may be done all at once or in two periods of five days each.

♣ The night before you begin, take a gentle herbal laxative, either in tea or tablet form, such as HER-BALTONE, Wisdom of the Ancients YERBA MATÉ tea, Crystal Star LAXA-TEA™ or FIBER & HERBS COLON CLEANSE™ capsules.

♣ Soak some dried figs, prunes and raisins in water to cover, add 1 TB. unsulphured molasses, and let soak overnight in a covered bowl.

♣ Six to 8 glasses of pure water daily are necessary for the success of this cleanse.

On rising: take 1 teasp. Sonné LIQUID BENTONITE, <u>or</u> 2 teasp. psyllium husks in juice or water;
<u>or</u> 1 heaping teasp. Crystal Star CHO-LO FIBER TONE™ DRINK MIX (either flavor) in water.

Breakfast: discard fruits from their soaking water and take a small glass of the liquid.

Mid-morning: take a glass of George's ALOE VERA JUICE with herbs.

Lunch: take a small glass of potassium broth or essence (page 240); <u>or</u> a glass of fresh carrot juice.

Mid-afternoon: take a large glass of fresh apple juice;
<u>or</u> an herb tea such as alfalfa, fennel, or red clover;
<u>or</u> Crystal Star CLEANSING & PURIFYING™ tea to enhance elimination and provide energy support.

About 5 o' clock: take another small glass of potassium broth or essence; <u>or</u> another fresh carrot juice;
<u>or</u> a green drink (page 54), <u>or</u> Green Foods BARLEY GREEN MAGMA granules, or Crystal Star ENERGY GREEN™ drink in water;

Supper: take a large glass of apple juice or papaya juice.
☙ **Break the fast** with a small raw foods meal on the last night of the cleanse.

Before Bed: repeat the body cleansing liquids that you took on rising, <u>and</u> take a cup of peppermint or spearmint tea.

✻ Supplements and Herbal Aids for the Bowel Elimination Cleanse:

❖ Take 4-6 Crystal Star FIBER & HERBS COLON CLEANSE™ caps, to help increase systol/diastol activity of the colon, and tone bowel tissue during heavy elimination.

❖ Take a catnip or diluted liquid chlorophyll enema every other night during the cleanse. (pg. 244)

✻ Bodywork Suggestions for the Bowel Elimination Cleanse:

✚ Take a brisk daily walk for an hour every day during the fast.

✚ Take several long warm baths during the fast to speed cleansing. A lower back and pelvis massage and dry skin brushing will help release toxins coming out through the skin.

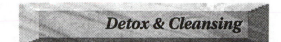
Stage Two: Rebuilding & Restoring the Body: A 2 to 6 week program

The second part of a good cleansing and detoxification program is to rebuild healthy tissue and restore body energy. It is usually begun after 3 to 10 days of waste and toxin elimination from the blood, lungs and bowels. This phase allows the body's regulating powers to become active with obstacles removed, so it can rebuild at optimum levels. A rebuilding/restoring diet emphasizes fresh, and simply prepared foods. It is very low in fat, with little dairy, and no fried foods. Avoid alcohol, caffeine, tobacco, and sugars; avoid meats except fish and sea foods.

On rising: take a vitamin/mineral/protein drink, such as Nutri-Tech ALL 1, Nature's Plus SPIRUTEIN, or Crystal Star SYSTEM STRENGTH™ DRINK with apple or other fruit juice;
or 2 lemons squeezed in water with honey; **or** 2 TBS. apple cider vinegar in water with a little honey.

Breakfast: have some fresh citrus fruit, especially grapefruit or oranges;
or soy milk or low-fat yogurt with fresh fruit; **or** a fresh fruit smoothie with a banana;
or whole grain cereal with a little apple juice.

Mid-morning: take a glass of fresh carrot juice, or potassium broth (pg. 240);
or a cup of Siberian ginseng tea, or Crystal Star FEEL GREAT™ TEA, or chamomile tea;
or a small bottle of mineral water with a packet of CHLORELLA or GREEN MAGMA granules;
or Crystal Star ENERGY GREEN DRINK™ mix in water to deodorize and freshen the GI tract.

Lunch: have a fresh green salad with lemon/oil dressing;
or steamed tofu with fresh greens and dressing;
or steamed veggies such as broccoli, carrots, onions or zucchini with Bragg's LIQUID AMINOS,
or miso, or other Oriental clear soup with Ramen noodles;
and/or a light vegetarian sandwich on whole grain bread.

Mid-afternoon: have a green drink; **or** Crystal Star BIOFLAV., FIBER & C SUPPORT™ drink;
or some raw veggie snacks with kefir cheese or soy cheese and a small bottle of mineral water;
or a cup of herb tea, such as peppermint or red clover, **or** Crystal Star HIGH ENERGY™ TEA.

Dinner: have a baked potato with Bragg's LIQUID AMINOS or soy sauce;
or steamed veggies with brown rice and tofu;
or baked or broiled white fish with a lemon/oil sauce;
or a whole grain vegetarian casserole; **or** a whole grain or vegetable pasta salad, hot or cold.

Before bed: a relaxing cup of herb tea, such as chamomile, or Crystal Star GOOD NIGHT™ TEA.

☙ Continue with plenty of pure water and other fluids to maximize system activity.

✤ *Supplements and Herbal Aids for the Rebuilding Diet:*

❖ Take a potassium broth at least once a week, or Crystal Star SYSTEM STRENGTH™ drink.

❖ Take acidophilus liquid or capsules with meals to encourage friendly bacteria in the GI tract.

❖ Take vitamin B12, either sublingually or internasally, for healthy cell development.

❖ Take ascorbate or Ester vit. C 3-5000mg. with bioflavonoids for interstitial tissue/collagen growth.

❖ Take Crystal Star ADR-ACTIVE™ **with** BODY REBUILDER™ capsules, 2 **each daily**, to encourage healthy gland activity and strength. Take HEARTSEASE/ANEMI-GIZE™ capsules to help build hemoglobin and increase liver, spleen and lymph function. Take FEEL GREAT™ capsules or tea for stamina and endurance. Use HAWTHORN extract, 1 dropperful two times daily as a body tonic.

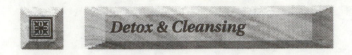

✿ *Bodywork Suggestions for the Rebuilding Diet:*

✚ Get some mild exercise every day.

✚ Get early morning sunlight on the body every day possible. Light builds strength along with food. Eating out of doors is especially beneficial. Consider a short camping trip.

✿ *Sample Recipe Suggestions For Rebuilding & Restoring*
By section and recipe number:

FASTING & CLEANSING FOODS - all.

HEALTHY DRINKS, JUICES AND WATERS - 44, 46, 48, 50, 62, 63, 65, 66, 71.

MACROBIOTIC EATING - 110, 111, 112, 113, 117, 119, 121, 123, 128, 130, 135, 139, 143, 150, 157, 161.

SALADS HOT & COLD - 188, 189, 191, 195, 198, 201, 203, 206, 207, 209, 211, 212, 216, 222, 229, 230.

DAIRY FREE COOKING - all.

HIGH PROTEIN WITHOUT MEAT - 696, 698, 699, 701, 706, 713, 715, 718, 719, 730, 732, 735, 737, 741.

MINERAL RICH FOODS - 612, 614, 615, 619, 621, 622, 623, 631, 635, 638, 640, 648, 643, 656, 657, 658.

FISH & SEAFOODS - 544, 547, 548, 549, 551, 552, 554, 555, 557, 559, 562, 563, 564, 567, 568, 569.

✿ *Sample Meal Planning*
Recipe combinations that work for this diet:

A FAMILY MEAL - 639, 614, 372

AN EASY WEEKNIGHT DINNER - 67, 628, 648, 194

A SPECIAL DINNER FOR TWO - 53, 627, 176, 617, 650, 660

A SUNDAY BRUNCH - 662, 230, 654, 633/638, 123, 199

LUNCH FOR TWO - 16, 637, 369, 228

A HEARTY WINTER MEAL - 64, 641, 612, 652

A LIGHT SUMMER MEAL - 131, 190, 367

AN EASY RISING BREAKFAST - 47, 651, 704, 364

Stage 3: Maintaining A Healthy Immune System:

*The final part of a good cleansing program is keeping your body clean and toxin-free - **very important** after all the hard work of detoxification. Modifying lifestyle habits to include high quality nutrition from both food and supplement sources is the key to a strong resistant body.*

The foods for a good immune defense diet should rely heavily on fresh fruits and vegetables for cleansing and regulating fiber. It should include cooked vegetables, whole grains and seeds for strength, endurance and alkalinity. It should use sea foods, eggs, and low-fat cheeses as alternate sources of quality protein; and lightly cooked sea foods and vegetables with a little dinner wine for circulatory health.

The following *"GOOD PROTECTION TEST"* can help you monitor your support-system health on a regular basis. Essentially it is a fiber check; enough soluble fiber in the diet to make the stool float is the protective level against such problems as colitis, constipation, hemorrhoids, diverticulitis, varicose veins, and bowel cancer.

- ☛ **The bowel movement should be regular and effortless.**
- ☛ **The stool should be almost odorless.**
- ☛ **There should be very little flatulence.**
- ☛ **The stool should float rather than sink.**

✿ *Supplement & Herbal Suggestions For Health Maintenance & Disease Prevention:*

❖ Keep tissue oxygen levels high with 1 to 3000mg. vitamin C with bioflavonoids, vitamin B$_{12}$, internasally or sublingually, and vitamin E 4 to 800IU with selenium daily.

❖ Keep a good level of potassium in the body with high potassium foods, such as broccoli, leafy greens, bananas, and sea vegetables, or a weekly potassium broth or juice; or a potassium supplement such as Twin Lab LIQUID K PLUS, Crystal Star ENERGY GREEN™ drink.

❖ Take unsprayed bee pollen granules, 2 teasp. daily for essential amino acids; and/or high potency royal jelly, 2 teasp. daily for natural pantothenic acid.

❖ Immune enhancing supplements can include bee propolis liquid extract, beta carotene 25,000IU, CoQ10 30 to 60mg., zinc 30 to 50mg., raw thymus extract (during high risk seasons), and Crystal Star HERBAL DEFENSE TEAM™ extract, tea or capsules.

❖ Chlorophyll-rich food supplements fortify immunity, enhance healthy cell development and body balance, and insure alkalinity. Include one or more in your weekly diet. Chlorella, spirulina, Green Foods GREEN MAGMA, Nature's Plus SPIRUTEIN, or Crystal Star ENERGY GREEN™ drink.

❖ Foundation multiple vitamins and minerals should be from food or herbal sources for best absorption. Some of the best are from Living Source, Mezotrace, New Chapter, and Floradix. Crystal Star makes several combinations high in concentrated herbal minerals; IRON SOURCE™, CALCIUM SOURCE™ and MINERAL SOURCE COMPLEX™ extracts and capsules.

❖ Enzymes and lactobacillus acidophilus are important for good assimilation and adequate intestinal flora. The most effective supplements have multiple complex living organisms that can easily unite with the body. Good maintenance products include DR. DOPHILUS or D.D.S. ACIDOPHILUS; for children, Nature's Plus JR. DOPHILUS chewable wafers or DOCTOR DOPHILUS powder. Crystal Star SYSTEM STRENGTH™ instant drink is full of naturally occuring minerals, enzymes, and amino acids.

❖ High soluble fiber supplementation can insure a fully active elimination system, digestive regulation, and cholesterol/blood sugar balance. Some of the most effective and convenient include guar gum capsules before meals, psyllium husks, 2 teasp. in water in the morning and evening, or a high fiber drink such as Yerba Prima COLON CARE, or Crystal Star CHO-LO FIBER TONE™ drink or capsules.

❋ *Bodywork Suggestions For Disease Prevention:*

✚ Daily exercise is one of the most important things to do for your life. It increases oxygen uptake in the body to improve metabolism, circulation, and respiratory activity. Every walk you take, every series of stretches you do, strengthens and lengthens your life and health.

✚ Get early morning sunlight on the body every day possible for regular vitamin D.

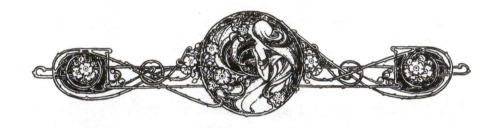

❋ *Sample Recipes for Health Maintenance and Disease Prevention*
By section and recipe number:

BREAKFAST & BRUNCH - 73, 74, 76, 78, 81, 82, 83, 84, 85, 89, 90, 92, 93.

SALADS HOT & COLD - all

LOW-FAT & VERY LOW-FAT RECIPES - all

LOW CHOLESTEROL MEALS - all

FISH & SEAFOODS - all

HIGH MINERAL FOODS - all

HIGH FIBER RECIPES - all

HIGH COMPLEX CARBOHYDRATES FOR ENERGY - all

GREAT OUTDOORS EATING - 875, 877, 879, 880, 882, 887, 888, 893, 895, 896, 908.

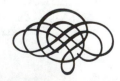

✲ Sample Menu Plans
Recipe combinations that work with this program:

A LIGHT SUMMER MEAL - 894, 189, 906, 294

A SPECIAL DINNER FOR TWO - 193, 291, 613, 258, 301

AN EASY WEEKNIGHT DINNER - 615, 204, 302, 292

A LUNCHEON FOR TWO - 210, 809, 253, 290

AN EASY RISING BREAKFAST - 324, 98, 74, 819

A HEARTY WINTER MEAL - 616, 271, 802, 275, 297

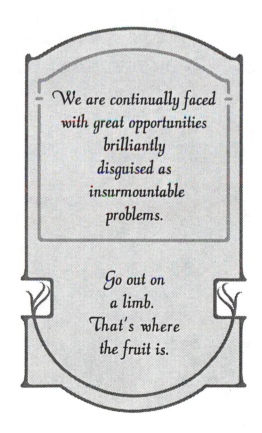

We are continually faced
with great opportunities
brilliantly
disguised as
insurmountable
problems.

Go out on
a limb.
That's where
the fruit is.

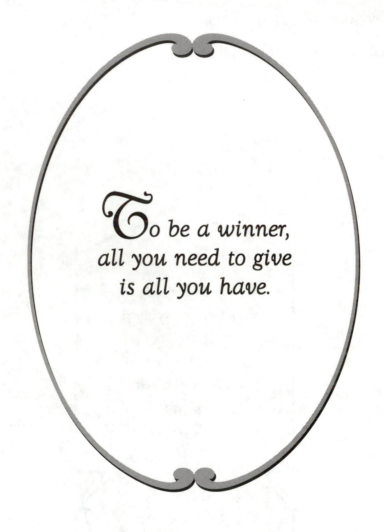

To be a winner,
all you need to give
is all you have.

Bone Building With
Mineral Rich Building Blocks

Bone and cartilage are the ever-changing, ever-growing infrastructure of the body. They need mineral rich nutrients for strength and health. Healthy bones both use and store the body's minerals, acting as reservoirs for its extra mineral needs.

Minerals and trace minerals are the building block of the cells, the most basic elements needed for proper metabolism. They are the bonding agents between the body and food. Without them the body cannot absorb nutrients or utilize them for growth. Minerals regulate acid/alkaline balance, transport body oxygen, and control electrolytic movement between cells, nerves and tissue. They play a key role in heart health, sugar and blood pressure regulation and cancer prevention. Even small mineral deficiencies can produce stress on the body, because imbalances mobilize the needed element(s) out of the various body 'reservoirs' to compensate. We often feel the immediate effects of this process in irritability, nervousness, emotional tension, and depression. A mineral-poor diet can mean osteoporosis, premature aging, hair loss, brittle nails, dry, cracked skin, forgetfulness, food intolerances, back pain, P.M.S., poor motor coordination, joint deformity, difficult pregnancy, taste and smell loss, slow learning, poor attention span, and the inability to heal quickly. And this is only a partial list. MINERALS ARE IMPORTANT!

Minerals are not made by the body, and are not automatically inherent either in kind or quantity. They must be taken in through food, drink or mineral baths. Unfortunately, good mineral quality is not now present in the fruits and vegetables we eat. Years of pesticides, non-organic fertilizers, and chemical sprays used in agri-business have leached them out of the soil. Over a third of our population, and more than 50% of American women, suffer from calcium deficiency alone. Mineral needs increase as the body ages and requires more digestive, hydrochloric acid and enzyme help.

Many factors, including excessive meat consumption, preserved and over-refined foods, lack of vitamin D from sunlight, and too little exercise, are involved in bone porosity and poor mineral absorption. Steroid and excessive anti-biotic use, tobacco, and too much alcohol, all contribute to mineral depletion and weakening of bone structure. Osteoporosis is a far more complex problem than was originally thought, encompassing not only calcium deficiency, but a drop in estrogen levels, a lack of progesterone, thyroid and parathyroid malfunction, and poor collagen protein development. We now know that calcium is not even the main mineral for bone regeneration; silicon is. High stress life styles and habits also inhibit mineral absorption.

But the fact remains that a solid mineral base is of prime importance to bone health. Organically grown foods, sea plants and herbs are becoming the best way to get them. These foods are used by the body's own enzyme action, as a whole, not as an extracted substance, and this is a key to their effectiveness. Vegetarians traditionally have denser and better-formed bones, because the most usable minerals come from green leafy vegetables, sprouts, whole grains, soy foods, eggs, and vegetable complex carbohydrates.

Specific problems that this diet can help include:

OSTEOPOROSIS and BRITTLE BONES BACK, NERVE and MUSCLE PAIN SKIN, HAIR and NAIL HEALTH MENSTRUAL DIFFICULTIES PREVENTING MISCARRIAGE HYPERTHYROIDISM EASY BRUISING MOTION SICKNESS LOW ENERGY HYPERACTIVITY and ATTENTION DEFICIT DISORDER EMOTIONAL INSTABILITY and AGGRESSIVE BEHAVIOR INDIGESTION and BAD BREATH

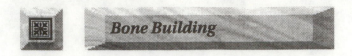

Mineral Rich Strong Bones Diet:

The high mineral diet below is designed to correct many deficiency problems. It includes vitamin C foods to aid mineral absorption, and foods that stimulate HCl and enzyme activity.

On rising: take a high protein drink, such as Nature's Plus SPIRUTEIN in apple or orange juice.

Breakfast: make a mix of 2 TBS <u>each</u>: toasted wheat germ, sesame seeds, brewer's yeast and lecithin granules. Sprinkle 2 teasp. on whatever you have for breakfast every day, such as yogurt with fresh or dried fruits (particularly apricots, figs, dates and raisins);
<u>or</u> poached or baked eggs on whole grain toast;
<u>or</u> whole grain cereal, muesli, granola, or pancakes with apple juice, soy milk, honey or yogurt.

Mid-morning: have a potassium broth (page 240), or Crystal Star SYSTEM STRENGTH DRINK™;
<u>or</u> a green drink (page 240), Sun CHLORELLA, Green Foods BARLEY GREEN MAGMA, or Crystal Star ENERGY GREEN DRINK™;
<u>or</u> fresh carrot juice and miso soup with sea vegetables snipped on top;
<u>and</u> some crunchy veggie sticks with kefir cheese dip.

Lunch: have an omelet with veggies or sprouts, and a carrot/raisin salad;
<u>or</u> a three bean salad, and soup or sandwich on whole grain bread;
<u>or</u> a baked potato with a small shrimp or seafood salad with yogurt or light dressing;
<u>or</u> have a high protein sandwich with avocado, low-fat or soy cheese and light mayonnaise;
<u>or</u> a large green salad with spinach, green peppers, sprouts and a lemon oil dressing.

Mid-afternoon: have a hard boiled egg with yogurt, and a refreshing herb tea, such as rose hips, nettles, dandelion, or Crystal Star BONZ™ TEA;
<u>or</u> have some low-fat cheeses with whole grain crackers, and a small bottle of mineral water.

Dinner: have a mushroom, asparagus, or broccoli quiche;
<u>or</u> a salmon souffle, or baked salmon with brown rice and peas;
<u>or</u> steamed broccoli and cauliflower with brown rice or millet, and baked tofu;
<u>or</u> a light Italian veggie pasta meal with tomatoes and onions;
<u>or</u> a vegetarian pizza on a whole grain crust;
<u>or</u> an oriental stir-fry with veggies and brown rice and miso soup.
Have a glass of wine for extra boron **before** dinner - <u>liquids with meals inhibit mineral absorption</u>.

Before bed: have a glass of apple, pear or papaya juice, <u>or</u> a cup of VEGEX yeast broth.

✳ *Supplements and Herbal Aids for Strong Bones:*

❖ For healthy bone formation, take Alta Health SIL-X Silica capsules or Body Essentials SILICA GEL, and/or MEZOTRACE multimineral capsules; or estrogen balancing herbs such as licorice root, or Crystal Star BONZ™ capsules, or SUPER LICORICE, CALCIUM SOURCE or SILICA SOURCE™ extract.

❖ For better calcium and mineral absorption, take Alta Health CANGEST and Solaray CALCIUM CITRATE with BORON, or Crystal Star MEGA-MINERAL capsules or CALCIUM SOURCE™ extract.

❖ For interstitial tissue and cartilage formation, take ascorbate vitamin C 3000 to 5000mg. daily with bioflavonoids, and vitamin A & D 25,000IU/1000IU, and/or horsetail/comfrey tea.

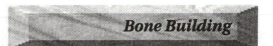

❖ For normal bone-building, and more bone mineral density, take sarsaparilla or ginseng/sarsaparilla capsules.

❖ Phyto-hormone herbal combinations that can help lay down bone: Crystal Star PRO-EST BALANCE GEL, and PSI PROGEST CREAM.

✿ *Bodywork for Strong Bones:*

✚ Exercise has proven to be one of the best ways to build and prevent bone loss. **It is a prime nutrient in itself, actually altering body chemistry and the way the body the body assimilates nutrients.** Walking, jogging, bicycling, swimming and dancing all help maintain bone mass.
Exercise out of doors in the early morning sunlight on the body is the best choice because it also offers the body bone-building, natural vitamin D.

✚ Avoid commercial antacids. These have now been linked to severe bone pain, fractures and bone loss because of aluminum content, suppression of HCl and lack of enzyme production.

✚ Avoid smoking and secondary smoke. Tobacco increases bone brittleness and inhibits bone growth.

✚ Avoid fluorescent lighting, electric blankets, aluminum cookware, non-filtered computer screens, etc. All tend to leach calcium from the body.

✚ Cortico-steroid drugs etc. over a long period of time leach potassium from the system, weaken bones, and deplete immunity.

✿ *Suggested Recipes For Strong Bones*
By section and recipe number:

BREAKFAST & BRUNCH - 74, 75, 76, 77, 78, 80, 81, 86, 93, 96, 97, 101, 103, 105

SALADS HOT & COLD -186, 188, 189, 202, 203, 206, 208, 211, 212, 228, 230, 231, 232, 233, 236, 237

LOW-FAT & VERY LOW-FAT RECIPES - all

SUGAR FREE SWEETS & TREATS - all

STIR-FRIES - ORIENTAL STEAM BRAISING - 502, 504, 505, 506, 510, 511, 512, 515, 517, 519, 520, 524

FISH & SEAFOODS - all

TOFU FOR YOU - all

HIGH MINERAL FOODS - all

HIGH PROTEIN WITHOUT MEAT - 696, 698, 699, 701, 703, 706, 715, 718, 720, 732, 733, 740, 741, 742

HIGH COMPLEX CARBOHYDRATES FOR ENERGY - all

✳ **Sample Menu Plans**
Recipe combinations that build strong bones:

A FAMILY MEAL - 616, 528, 291, 782

AN EASY WEEKNIGHT DINNER - 233, 734, 622, 426

A HEARTY WINTER MEAL - 753, 777, 644, 297, 226

A LIGHT SUMMER MEAL - 299, 776, 221

SUNDAY BRUNCH - 710, 277/276, 267, 590, 436

A WEEKEND PICNIC - 104, 108, 716, 657, 784

AN EASY RISING BREAKFAST - 74, 92, 698

LUNCH FOR TWO - 821, 232

A SPECIAL DINNER FOR TWO - 589, 238, 653, 614, 295

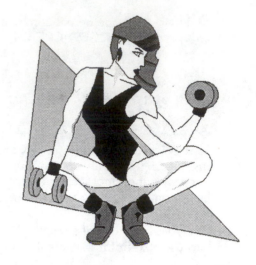

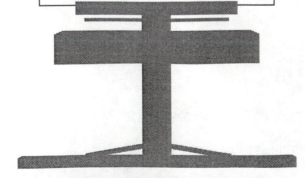

Make no small plans.
They have no magic
to stir the blood,
and they will probably
never be realized.
Always go for the gold.
In great attempts,
it is even glorious
to fail.

Cancer & Degenerative Disease
Rebuilding Healthy Cells & Tissue

The natural healing world has concentrated on cancer and other degenerative diseases in the past few years, and has learned much about how to deal with these often unnecessary killers. Even though today's statistics show that more than a third of all Americans will contract some kind of cancer in their lives, new evidence is indicating that *90% of all cancer is environmentally caused and therefore preventable.* Diet and nutrition are by far the most important of these environmental factors. America's enormous incidence of breast and colon cancer, *500% compared to the rest of the world,* is overwhelmingly felt to be due to poor nutrition and food choices.

Here are some facts we know about cancer:

☛ Cancers are opportunistic, attacking when immune defenses and bloodstream health are low.

☛ Cancerous cells crave dead de-mineralized foods. Starving them out feels like any withdrawal. The fight isn't easy, but as healthy cells rebuild, the cravings subside.

☛ Cancer cells seem to live and grow in unreleased waste and mucous deposits in the body. Avoid red meats, pork, fried foods, refined carbohydrates, sugars, excessive caffeine, preserved or artificially colored foods, and heavy pesticide sprayed foods. These foods clog the system so that the vital organs cannot clean out enough of the waste to maintain health. They deprive the body of oxygen use, and provide little or no usable nutrition for building healthy cells and tissue. Avoid antacids. They interfere with enzyme production, and the body's ability to carry off heavy metal toxins.

☛ Most cancers are caused or aggravated by poor diet and nutrition. Many cancers respond well to diet improvement. Nutritional deficiencies accumulate over a long period of time - too much refined food, fats and red meats; too little fiber and fresh foods; natural vitamin and mineral imbalances. These deficiencies eventually change body chemistry. The immune system cannot defend properly when biochemistry is altered. It can't tell its own cells from invading toxic cells, and sometimes attacks everything or nothing in confusion.

☛ Love your liver! It is the main organ to keep clean and working well. It is a powerful chemical plant in the body that can keep the immune system going, healthy red blood cells forming, and oxygen in the bloodstream and tissues.

☛ Overheating therapy is being brought to the fore in treating cancer. It is an ancient and effective therapy. See Paavo Airola's book HOW TO GET WELL.

☛ New, viable research on colon cancer is showing that plain aspirin *beneficially inhibits* substances that are involved in pathogenic cell proliferation. Other cancers are also expected to respond favorably.

☛ Regular exercise is almost a "cancer defense" in itself. It enhances oxygen use and accelerates passage of material in the colon.

☛ The primary answer to cancer seems to lie in promoting an environment where cancer and degenerative disease can't live - where inherent immunity can remain effective. These diseases don't take hold where oxygen and minerals (particularly potassium) are high in the vital fluids. Vegetable proteins and amino acids in the body allow tmaximum use and assimilation of oxygen and minerals.

☛ It is vitally important to follow a concentrated program incorporating several aspects of natural healing. Diet, exercise, enemas, stress reduction techniques, vitamin therapy and herbs all need to be included for there to be cancer remission.

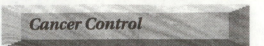

☛ A concerted effort is necessary for at least six months to a year. Don't be discouraged, no matter how many times you have to return to a juice and raw foods diet. Many prople have overcome cancer to lead healthy, productive lives. Success is very possible.

The diets in this chapter are effective for many degenerative diseases, including:
❧SYSTEMIC CANCERS: COLON, BOWEL, STOMACH, ORGAN, & LUNG ❧MALIGNANT TU-MORS ❧MELANOMA ❧LUPUS ❧LEUKEMIA ❧PARKINSON'S DISEASE ❧MULTIPLE SCLER-OSIS ❧LYME DISEASE ❧MUSCULAR DYSTROPHY ❧

Stage One: The Beginning Cleanse For Degenerative Disease

Degenerative disease is often created or allowed by the accumulation and saturation of toxic matter in the body, throwing defense mechanisms and vital body operations out of balance. Some indications that you might benefit from a cleansing fast include chronic constipation or diarrhea, the sudden appearance or enlargement of growths, internal bleeding (especially blood passing in the stool), non-healing wounds and unexplained chronic pain in a specific area. Liquid diets for detoxification are well-documented therapeutic methods that works well in reversing disease symptoms of this kind. The success of cleansing diets acknowledges the intelligence of the human body as a self-healing entity. An elimination fast with alkalizing juices, allows the body in its wisdom to decompose substances and tissue that are damaged, diseased or unneeded, such as abscesses, tumors, and congestive wastes. Fasting also seems to release immune-stimulating hormone secretions which augment the infection and disease-fighting process.

❧ The Liquid Elimination Cleanse; 6 to 10 days:

This cleansing diet may be used as often as necessary during the healing process. Best results are achieved when employed for 6 to 10 days at a time, to allow the body to cleanse and rebuild with the least loss of equilibrium.

On rising: take 2 to 3 teasp. of cranberry concentrate in a glass of water,
or a glass of red grape juice.

Breakfast: take a potassium broth or essence (page 240) with 1 TB. Bragg's LIQUID AMINOS.

Mid-morning: have a mixed raw veggie juice (page 241) with 1 TB. Bragg's LIQUID AMINOS;
or a carrot/beet/cucumber juice for extra cleansing;
and a glass of wheat grass juice, Sun CHLORELLA, Green Foods BARLEY GREEN MAGMA, or Crystal Star ENERGY GREEN DRINK™.

Lunch: take a glass of fresh carrot juice;
then another cranberry juice, as above, if desired.

Mid-afternoon: have another green drink (page 240ff.) with Bragg's LIQUID AMINOS;
and a purifying tea, such as chapparal, red clover, or Crystal Star CLEANSING & FASTING™ TEA.

Dinner: take another fresh carrot juice, potassium broth, green drink, or mixed veggie juice with 1 teasp. Bragg's LIQUID AMINOS;
or a Crystal Star SYSTEM STRENGTH™ DRINK.

Before bed: have another glass of cranberry juice or red grape juice;
and/or a cup of alfalfa/mint or chamomile tea;
or a VEGEX yeast broth for relaxation and strength the next day.

❋ *Supplements & Herbs for the Liquid Elimination Cleanse:*

✤ Take ascorbate vitamin C crystals in each juice or water, $1/2$ teasp. with every drink, until a soupy stool occurs.

✤ Drink distilled water (6 to 8 glasses daily) during the fast to flush out toxins and wastes quickly.

✤ Take Alta Health CANGEST powder, $1/4$ teasp. in juice or water 3x daily, for optimum nutrient assimilation. Do not take commercial antacids. They interfere with enzyme production, and the body's ability to carry off heavy metal toxins.

❋ *Bodywork for the Liquid Elimination Cleanse:*

✤ A coffee enema, wheat grass or chlorella enema or implant, is effective in stimulating the liver to produce bile, and to process metabolic wastes successfully. Any enema choice may be used every other day during this cleanse. (See page 244 for method.)

✤ Get some early morning sunlight on the body every day possible for strengthening vitamin D.

✤ Avoid tobacco, synthetic estrogens, X-Rays, caffeine and caffeine-containing foods, refined sugars, alcohol, and all preserved or chemically treated foods during healing.

✤ Get some mild exercise every day. No healing program will make it without the oxygenating nutrients exercise supplies.

Stage Two; Intensive Macrobiotic Diet For Degenerative Disease

A macrobiotic diet is very effective against degenerative disease, helping to rebuild healthy blood and cells, and preventing diseased tissue from continued growth. This way of eating is non-mucous forming, low in fats that can alter body chemistry and enhance cancer potential in the cells, and high in vegetable fiber and protein. It is stimulating to the heart and circulatory system through its emphasis on oriental foods such as miso, bancha twig tea, and shiitake mushrooms; alkalizing with umeboshi plums, sea vegetables and soy foods, and high in potassium, natural iodine and other minerals and trace elements. Its greatest advantage and benefit is that it is cleansing and strengthening at the same time, and offers a truly balanced way of eating that is easily individualized for one's environment, the seasons, and the constitution of the person using it. The strict form recommended for this stage should be followed for three to six months.

Intensive Building/Balancing Macrobiotic Diet:

On rising: take a potassium broth or essence (page 240) or carrot/beet/cucumber juice;
or cranberry concentrate (2 teasp. in water) or red grape juice;
and a vitamin/mineral drink such as Nutritech ALL 1, or Crystal Star SYSTEM STRENGTH™ DRINK.

Breakfast: make a mixture of 2 TBS. **each:** brewer's yeast, wheat germ, lecithin and bee pollen granules. Sprinkle some on a whole grain cereal, granola or muesli, or mix with yogurt and dried fruit;
and/or use on fresh fruit, such as strawberries or apples with kefir or kefir cheese; add a whole grain breakfast pilaf such as Kashi, bulgar or millet, with apple juice or kefir cheese topping.

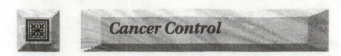

Mid-morning: take a green drink (pg. 240); Sun CHLORELLA, BARLEY GREEN, Crystal Star ENERGY GREEN™, or fresh wheat grass juice. Add 1 teasp. Bragg's LIQUID AMINOS to any choice;
and/or an herb tea, such as Crystal Star CHINESE ROYAL MU, or MEDITATION™ TEA;
or a glass of fresh carrot juice, or Green Foods GREEN ESSENCE DRINK;
or a cup of miso soup with sea vegetables snipped on top. (Take 2 TBS. dry sea vegetables daily.)

Lunch: have some steamed broccoli or cauliflower with brown rice, tofu and a little soy cheese;
or an oriental stir-fry with brown rice and miso sauce;
or a fresh green salad with whole grain pitas or chapatis;
or a black bean, onion or lentil soup, or a 3 bean salad;
or falafels in pita bread with some raw or steamed veggies and a tamari dressing;
or a cabbage or slaw salad with oriental sesame dressing.

Mid-afternoon: have a cup of bancha twig tea, or roasted dandelion tea, or Crystal Star HEARTSEASE-CIRCU-CLEANSE™ TEA or SYSTEM STRENGTH™ DRINK;
and some whole grain crackers with kefir cheese or a soy spread;
or crunchy raw veggies with a little gomashio (sesame salt) sprinkled on top.

Dinner: have a brown rice, millet, bulgar, or kasha casserole with tofu, or tempeh and some steamed vegetables;
or a hearty dinner salad with some sea veggies, nuts and seeds, and whole grain bread or chapatis;
or baked, broiled or steamed fish or seafood with rice and peas or other veggies;
or a baked veggie casserole with mushroom/yogurt or kefir cheese sauce;
or stuffed cabbage rolls with rice, and baked carrots with tamari and a little honey.

Before bed: have a cup of VEGEX yeast paste broth, or a relaxing herb tea, such as alfalfa/mint tea, **or** a glass of organic apple juice.

In order for the macrobiotic balance to be set up, and work correctly with the body in this phase of healing, several foods and food types must be avoided:
  ✦Red meat, poultry, and dairy products
  ✦Coffee, black teas, carbonated drinks, and some stimulant herb teas
  ✦Nightshade plants, such as tomatoes, potatoes, peppers and eggplant
  ✦Sugars, corn syrup and artificial sweeteners; and tropical and sweet fruits
  ✦All refined, frozen, canned and processed foods
  ✦Hot spices, white vinegar, and table salt
(See the **Light Macrobiotic Eating** section for more information.)

❋ *Supplements and Herbal Aids for the Intensive Macrobiotic Diet:*

❖ Siberian ginseng extract or tea several times daily.

❖ Take ascorbate vitamin C crystals in water 3 to 5000mg. daily, <u>with</u> Ginkgo Biloba extract drops.

❖ Mega-potency acidophilus and BARLEY GREEN MAGMA to combat the effects of chemotherapy.

❖ Wheat germ oil, vitamin E 400IU with selenium, or pycnogenol 100 to 200mg. to add tissue oxygen.

❖ Crystal Star PAU D'ARCO/ECHINACEA EXTRACT, REISHI/GINSENG EXTRACT or IODINE THERAPY™ EXTRACT, and high omega-3 flax oil to inhibit tumor growth.

❋ *Bodywork for the Intensive Macrobiotic Diet:*

✚ Get morning sunlight and mild exercise every day possible to accelerate the passage of toxins.

✚ Overheating therapy is effective for degenerative disease. See Paavo Airola, "HOW TO GET WELL," for the proper technique.

❋ *Sample Recipes For the Intensive Macrobiotic Diet*
By section and recipe number:

FASTING & CLEANSING FOODS - all

DRINKS, JUICES & WATERS - 43, 44, 45, 46, 47, 48, 49, 50, 51, 52, 53, 61, 62, 63, 64, 65, 66, 67, 68, 71.

ORIENTAL & LIGHT MACROBIOTIC EATING - all

SALADS HOT & COLD - 186, 187, 189, 190, 191, 195, 200, 202, 204, 206, 207, 209, 211, 212, 213, 215.

SANDWICHES - SALADS IN BREAD - 474, 473, 476, 489.

LOW-FAT & VERY LOW-FAT DISHES - 241, 244, 248, 249, 250, 254, 264, 268, 271, 272, 277, 279, 282.

DAIRY FREE RECIPES - 332, 333, 336, 337, 338, 339, 341, 342, 343, 344, 345, 351, 353, 354, 359, 360.

HIGH PROTEIN MEATLESS COOKING - 715, 719, 720, 724, 734, 735, 737,740, 741, 742.

SOUPS - LIQUID SALADS - 446, 448, 449, 452, 453,454, 455, 463, 469, 470.

HIGH FIBER RECIPES - 785, 789, 791, 799, 802, 815, 816, 817, 818, 819, 820, 823.

❋ *Sample Menu Plans*
Recipe combinations that work with this diet:

AN EASY WEEKNIGHT DINNER - 818, 27, 9, 175

AN EASY RISING BREAKFAST - 819, 35, 820, 11

A HEARTY WINTER MEAL -52, 185, 202, 26

A LIGHT SUMMER MEAL - 186, 448, 130, 53, 151

A FAMILY MEAL - 183, 723, 18, 12

LUNCH FOR TWO -184, 14, 190, 128

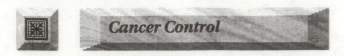

Stage Three; The Modified Macrobiotic Diet:

This way of eating can be lived with in health on a lifetime basis, for resistance to disease recurrence, and good immune strength. It is high in absorbable vitamins and minerals, oxygenating foods, immune and liver stimulating nutrients. It is generally seasonal eating, with a continued emphasis on the body building properties of whole grains and complex carbohydrates.

On rising: take a vitamin/mineral drink such as Nutritech ALL 1 or Nature's Plus SPIRUTEIN in orange juice; or make your own fresh V- 8 juice (page 240) and add 1 TB. Bragg's LIQUID AMINOS.

Breakfast: have a high fiber, whole grain cereal with yogurt, kefir or soy milk, and add your choice of nuts, seeds and dried fruit.
Make a mix of 2 TBS. each: brewer's yeast flakes, lecithin granules, and toasted wheat germ, and sprinkle it every morning over whatever you eat for breakfast; such as some fresh fruit, or yogurt, or a baked or poached egg.

Mid-morning: have some raw crunchy veggies with kefir cheese or a veggie dip, or soy spread;
or a glass of carrot juice (at least once a week);
or an herb tea, or grain coffee substitute, such as ROMA, or Crystal Star MOCHA MOCHA.
or a green drink, such as Sun CHLORELLA, or Crystal Star ENERGY GREEN DRINK'.

Lunch: have a seafood salad, or a large green salad with cucumbers, kiwi, and peas, and yogurt dressing or cottage cheese;
or a cabbage cole slaw salad with yogurt or lemon dressing;
or a quiche with asparagus, broccoli, or artichokes and a whole grain crust;
or a quick veggie pizza with semolina or chapati crust, and soy mozzarella or low-fat cheese;
or a tuna salad sandwich, or tofu burger on whole grain buns;
or a baked potato with a little butter and a mushroom salad side dish;
or a lightly spiced Mexican beans and rice dish.

Mid-afternoon: have a cup of herb tea, or a green drink;
or miso soup with sea vegetables snipped on top;
or some whole grain crackers with a veggie dip or kefir cheese;
or some baked tofu chunks with a little low-fat dressing.

Dinner: have a light Italian whole grain pasta meal, with ricotta cheese or soy mozarella;
or a sweet potato pie, or baked yams and carrots with a little butter and brown rice;
or a zucchini and rice frittata;
or fresh grilled or baked fish with peas and rice;
or a tofu or tempeh casserole with millet or rice;
or a broccoli and cabbage stir-fry with miso soup;
or steam-sautéed broccoli, cauliflower, green beans or zucchini with toasted walnuts and dressing;
or a salmon souffle with rice and green beans.

Before bed: have a cup of relaxing herb tea, or a glass of apple juice.

✱ *Supplements for a Modified Macrobiotic Diet:*

❖ Have a green supplement drink such as Sun CHLORELLA or Crystal Star ENERGY GREEN™ at least twice a week, with drops of Crystal Star PAU D' ARCO/ECHINACEA EXTRACT added.

❖ Take SIBERIAN GINSENG extract, capsules or tea daily, **and** GINKGO BILOBA extract 2x daily.

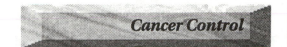

❖ Take beta carotene 50,000IU daily, and ascorbate vitamin C with bio-flavonoids 3-5000mg. daily, or Crystal Star DAILY BIOFLAVONOID SUPPORT™ DRINK.

❖ Take a good multi-mineral such as MEZOTRACE SEA MINERALS, or Crystal Star MEGA-MINERAL CAPS, or MINERAL SOURCE COMPLEX EXTRACT.

❖ Take 1 teasp. Omega-3 flax oil 3x daily, wheat germ oil, or vitamin E 400IU daily for tissue oxygen.

❖ Take Twin Lab LIQUID K PLUS, or Crystal Star IODINE THERAPY™ CAPSULES or EXTRACT daily. Take GINSENG/REISHI EXTRACT if there are tumors or melanoma.

❖ Take a broad spectrum digestive enzyme complex with meals for nutrient assimilation.

✿ *Bodywork for a Modified Macrobiotic Diet:*

✚ Avoid tobacco in all forms. Curtail caffeine intake. Avoid alcohol except for moderate wine.

✚ Be extremely cautious of having X-rays, mammograms, etc. Even small amounts of radiation are sometimes proving to engender cancer growth in delicate tissue. If you feel you are at risk for breast, uterine, ovarian, cervical or prostate cancer, avoid hormone replacement therapy, consciously avoid meats and dairy products that are regularly injected with hormones.

✚ Regular exercise is a healing nutrient in itself. Exercise can actually change body chemistry. No healing program will make it without exercise. Exercise with regular, moderate sunshine is the best choice of all.

✿ *Sample Recipes for the Modified Macrobiotic Diet*
By section and recipe number:

ORIENTAL & LIGHT MACROBIOTIC EATING - all

BREAKFAST & BRUNCH - 73, 74, 75, 76, 77, 78, 81, 82, 83, 84, 85, 86, 87, 91, 92, 93, 94, 95, 96, 97, 105

SALADS HOT & COLD - 188, 193, 196, 198, 199, 201, 203, 205, 214, 222, 223, 228, 233, 234, 235, 237

LOW-FAT & VERY LOW-FAT RECIPES - all

TOFU FOR YOU - 570, 571, 572, 574, 575, 577, 578, 580, 581, 582, 585, 586, 587, 589, 590, 594, 610, 611

SOUPS - LIQUID SALADS - 445, 451, 457, 459, 462, 465, 466, 467, 468, 472

HIGH FIBER RECIPES - 792, 793, 794, 796, 801, 803, 805, 806, 807, 808, 809, 812, 821, 824.

COMPLEX CARBOHYDATES FOR ENERGY - 743, 749, 750, 751, 752, 753, 755, 755, 757, 759, 760, 763, 764, 765, 766, 768, 775, 776, 777, 781, 782

GREAT OUTDOORS EATING - 874, 875, 876, 878, 879, 880, 881, 882, 883, 884, 885, 886, 887, 888, 893

❋ Sample Menu Plans
Some recipe combinations that work with this diet:

A FAMILY MEAL - 792, 582, 176, 791

LUNCH FOR TWO - 131, 188, 133

AN EASY RISING BREAKFAST - 819, 715, 793, 823

A SPECIAL DINNER FOR TWO - 156, 170, 586, 153, 191

A LIGHT SUMMER MEAL - 125, 590, 199, 174

A HEARTY WINTER MEAL - 157, 169, 787, 132, 193, 823

A SUNDAY BRUNCH - 585, 159, 195, 597, 298, 580

HEALTHY FEASTING & ENTERTAINING - 250, 242, 167, 469, 226, 781

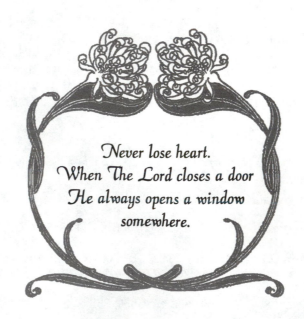

Never lose heart.
When The Lord closes a door
He always opens a window
somewhere.

Defensive Nourishment;
Building Immune Strength

The immune system is the most complex and delicately balanced infrastructure of the body. Its nature and dynamics have been largely a mystery. Yet, because of the devastating rise of opportunistic diseases in the world, the healing community is now being forced to come to terms with its powers and limitations.

Immune response is an individual defense system. It comes charging to the rescue at the first sign of an alien force, such as a harmful viral or bacterial infection. It is also an autonomic, sub-conscious system that can fend off and/or neutralize disease toxins, giving the body the right environment to heal itself. It is this quality of being a part of us, yet not under our conscious control, that is the great power of this system.

But maintaining strong immune defenses in today's world is not easy. Environmental toxins, tobacco and secondary smoke inhalation, overuse of alcohol, prescription and pleasure drugs, hidden chemicals in our foods, caffeine overload, and high stress are all an increasing part of our lives. These things deplete immune strength. Lowered immunity is the prime factor in opportunistic diseases such as candida albicans, chronic fatigue syndrome, lupus, AIDS, mononucleosis, herpes, hepatitis, many sexually transmitted diseases and cancer.

Auto-immune deficiency diseases have become the epidemic of our time, and most of us don't have very much to fight with. An overload of chemical anti-biotics, antacids, vaccinations, immunizations, cortico-steroids, and myriad other drugs can affect immune system balance to the point where it cannot distinguish harmful cells from healthy cells, and attacks everything in confusion. Often, if we can limit over kill from drugs and anti-biotics, and just "get out of the way" by keeping our bodies clean and well-nourished, the immune system will automatically spend its energies rebuilding and strengthening us, instead of fighting, gathering its exhausted resources against disease, or conducting "rear guard" defenses. Giving your body generous, high quality nutrients at the first sign of infection or ill health can swiftly improve your chances of destroying pathogenic bacteria. An immune-enhancing diet is directed at "early warning" problems, and building strength to maintain immune response.

It is effective against:

❧VIRAL and BACTERIAL INFECTIONS ❧STAPH and STREP INFECTIONS ❧EARLY AGING ❧CHRONIC FATIGUE SYNDROME and EBV ❧CANDIDA ALBICANS ❧MONONUCLEOSIS ❧MENINGITIS and RHEUMATIC FEVER ❧COLDS, FLU and PNEUMONIA ❧LUPUS ❧MEASLES ❧PRESCRIPTION or PLEASURE DRUG OVER-USE ❧HERPES ❧ENVIRONMENTAL POLLUTANT and HEAVY METAL POISONING ❧PARASITES and WORMS ❧CYSTS, TUMORS and ABSCESSES ❧TOXIC SHOCK ❧VIRAL WARTS, CERVICAL DYSPLASIA and HPV ❧

Immune restoration is not easy. It takes time and commitment. The immune system is the body system most sensitive to nutritional deficiencies. Good nourishment, and body support with exercise and morning sunlight are the keys to keeping disease resistance high.

Remember that the pattern for your own immunity, and the inherited health
of your children and your grandchildren, is laid down by you.
A strong, clean body for you gives everybody the best chance.

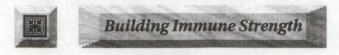

Stage One; Immune Stimulating Diet:

We find that the best way to begin fortifying the immune system, especially after a history of frequent infections and virus invasions, is to go on a simple, cleansing diet for 3 to 7 days, to alkalize the system and reduce the energy it expends on processing and metabolizing cooked or heavy foods. A short term raw foods diet appears to release hormone secretions that stimulate the immune complex and clears the way for its regeneration.

On rising: take 2 lemons in a glass of water, or 2 teasp. cranberry concentrate in water, or 2 TBS. apple cider vinegar in water with honey;
or Crystal Star BITTERS & LEMON EXTRACT™ drops in water.

Breakfast: have some fresh fruit; particularly grapefruit, pineapple, apples or papaya.

Mid-morning: have a green drink, (page 240)such as Sun CHLORELLA or Barley GREEN MAGMA;
or a glass of fresh carrot juice, with 1 TB. Bragg's LIQUID AMINOS added.

Lunch: have a fresh green salad with lemon/oil dressing, and a cup of miso soup with sea veggies.

Mid-afternoon: have another green drink or carrot juice, and crunchy raw veggies, with soy spread;
and/or an immune-enhancing herb tea, such as pau d'arco, or Crystal Star HERBAL DEFENSE TEA™.

Dinner: have a large dinner salad, with tofu, nuts and seeds, and a light dressing,
and a bowl of lentil or black bean soup.

Before bed: have a glass of apple or papaya juice,
or a cup of VEGEX yeast broth.

❋ Supplements and Herbal Aids for the Immune Stimulating Diet:

❖ Take $1/4$ to $1/2$ teasp. vitamin C crystals in juice or water every 2 to 3 hours to flush and alkalize the tissues, (approx. 5000mg. daily).

❖ Add $1/4$ teasp. of a potent lactobacillus or acidophilus complex to each juice during the fast to stimulate friendly G.I. flora, and build enzyme strength, a key factor of strong immunity.

❖ Drink at least 6 glasses of pure water every day.

❋ Bodywork for the Immune Stimulating Diet:

✚ Take a gentle herbal laxative the night before beginning the fast.

✚ Take a daily morning walk with deep breathing to oxygenate the tissues.

✚ Take warm, relaxing baths, and use a gentle dry skin brush daily.

✚ The immune system is stimulated by small amounts of sunlight - not excessive sunlight. Take 15 to 20 minute sunbaths in the <u>early</u> morning every day possible. *Sunburn depresses immunity.*

❋ *Sample Recipes for the Immune Stimulating Diet*
By section and recipe number:

FASTING & CLEANSING FOODS - all

HEALTHY DRINKS, JUICES & WATERS - all

MACROBIOTIC EATING - 109, 110, 119, 120, 121, 123, 124, 131, 132m 139, 142, 145, 165, 169, 170, 172.

SALADS HOT & COLD -186, 187, 195, 198, 200, 202, 204, 206, 210, 211, 217, 226, 229, 232, 233, 236.

❈

Stage Two; Building Immunity Through Diet:

Establishing good enzyme activity is a major part of building high immunity to disease. Much enzyme production comes from mineral and chlorophyll rich, fresh foods. Defense-food families, such as cruciferous vegetables, the anti-body producing onion/garlic foods, anti-oxidant foods, such as wheat germ and leafy greens, and foods high in vitamins A, and C are also important. Disease does not readily overcome a system high in oxygen and minerals. This stage may be used for 1 to 3 months.

On rising: take a sugar-free protein drink such as Nutri-Tech ALL 1 or Nature's Plus SPIRUTEIN.

Breakfast: Make a mix of 2 TBS. <u>each:</u> brewer's yeast, wheat germ, lecithin granules and flax seeds; sprinkle some every morning on your breakfast choice;
some fresh fruit, with yogurt if desired;
or poached or baked eggs with whole grain toast or muffins and kefir cheese;
or whole grain cereal or muesli with apple juice or soy milk or yogurt;

Mid-morning: have a green drink (page 240) or a glass of mineral water with Sun CHLORELLA granules, or Crystal Star ENERGY GREEN DRINK™.
or a cup of herb tea, such as siberian ginseng tea, or Crystal Star FEEL GREAT TEA™.

Lunch: have a large salad or whole grain sandwich with plenty of sprouts, nuts and seeds;
or a light seafood or turkey salad or sandwich with a yogurt cheese dressing;
or some steamed veggies with brown rice and tofu;
or some braised or stir-fried veggies, with plenty of onions, and some miso soup.

Mid-afternoon: have some rice cakes or whole grain crackers with a soy spread or veggie dip;
and/or a refreshing herb tea, such as rose hips, peppermint,or Crystal Star LICORICE MINTS TEA.
or yogurt with fresh fruits and some apple juice.

Dinner: have a high protein soup and sandwich on whole grain bread;
or a light Italian vegetable or whole grain pasta meal;
or an oriental meal with a clear broth soup, stir-fried veggies, and brown rice with sea veggies;
or a tofu and veggie casserole with whole grains and a low-fat yogurt/cheese sauce;
or baked or broiled fish or seafood with brown rice and veggies;

Before bed: take a relaxing cup of herb tea, such as spearmint, or Crystal Star GOODNIGHT™ TEA;
or a VEGEX broth; or miso soup with sea veggies;
or a papaya or apple juice.

✓ **On a continuing basis:** Include some sea vegetables in your diet every day. (See the MACROBIOTIC EATING section for some tasty ways to get them.)

✓ Include some concentrated "green superfoods" several times a week, such as Sun CHLORELLA, Barley GREEN MAGMA, spirulina, Solaray ALFAJUICE, or Crystal Star ENERGY GREEN DRINK™. **The composition of chlorophyll is very similar to that of human plasma, so these foods almost provide a mini-transfusion for the blood.**

✓ Other food immune-enhancers include garlic, onions and papaya.

✓ Include 6 to 8 glasses of bottled water daily to keep the body flushed, hydrated, and lubricated.

❋ *Supplements and Herbal Aids to Strengthen Immunity:*

❖ Take antioxidants such as vitamin C, about 3000mg. daily, beta-carotene, 25,000IU daily, Glutathione 50mg. or TRI-O$_2$ with germanium 50mg. daily to increase oxygen uptake.

❖ Take minerals and trace minerals such as MEZOTRACE SEA MINERAL COMPLEX, or herbal minerals such as Crystal Star MINERAL SPECTRUM (COMPLETE) capsules, or SYSTEM STRENGTH™ DRINK to supplement the mineral supply depleted in our soils and foods.

❖ Take a high potency acidophilus complex, such as Natren LIFE START II, or Solaray MULTIDOPHILUS, or betaine HCl to enhance enzyme production and nutrient assimilation.

❖ Take CoQ 10 30 TO 60MG. as an immuno-stimulating agent, to bring extra energy to rebuilding cells, and increase immuno-competence of existing cells.

❖ Take zinc 30mg. daily to guard against immune dysfunction, promote lymph tissue health, and increase T-Cell generation.

❖ Take a GLA source capsule, such as evening primrose oil or borage seed oil to stimulate *and balance* prostaglandin production.

❖ Crystal Star HERBAL DEFENSE TEAM™ extract, caps, and tea, or Zand IMMUNE HERBAL formulas, combine many of the above properties to cover broad areas of immune enhancing needs.

❋ *Bodywork for the Immune Building Diet:*

✚ Get some outdoor aerobic exercise every day.

✚ Stop smoking. Tobacco and nicotine are immune depressant factors. (Cadmium in tobacco products causes zinc deficiency.) It takes three months to get good immune response even after you quit.

✚ Avoid refined foods, excess caffeine, red meats, and pasteurized dairy products.

✚ Reduce prescription drug use if possible, especially anti-biotics and cortico-steroids that depress immunity.

✱ *Sample Recipes That Strengthen Immune Response:*
By section and recipe number:

SALADS HOT & COLD - all

SOUPS - LIQUID SALADS - all

SANDWICHES - SALADS IN BREAD - 473, 477, 478, 483, 485, 488, 490, 492, 494, 498, 499, 500

FISH & SEAFOODS - 537, 540, 544, 547, 548, 549, 551, 552, 555, 557, 563, 564, 567, 569

TOFU FOR YOU - 570, 572, 578, 580, 582, 583, 588, 589, 592, 594, 598, 599, 601, 603, 604, 608, 609, 610

HIGH MINERAL FOODS - 612, 613, 614, 617, 619, 621, 624, 625, 629, 634, 637, 644, 648, 651, 652, 658

HIGH PROTEIN WITHOUT MEAT - 696, 699, 704, 710, 716, 717, 719, 720, 723, 724, 730, 733, 734, 740

COMPLEX CARBOHYDRATES FOR ENERGY - 743, 746, 748, 752, 753, 757, 759, 762, 770, 791, 796

HIGH FIBER RECIPES - 787, 788, 791, 799, 800, 801, 802, 807, 808, 810, 811, 817, 818, 819, 821, 823, 824

❦ See **The Forever Diet** section (pg. 198) for recipe suggestions and menu planning ideas to maintain a strong immune defense system.

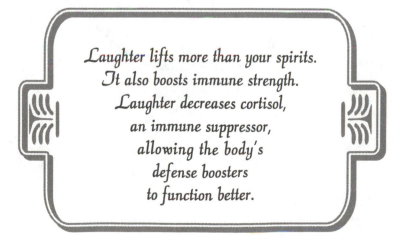

Laughter lifts more than your spirits.
It also boosts immune strength.
Laughter decreases cortisol,
an immune suppressor,
allowing the body's
defense boosters
to function better.

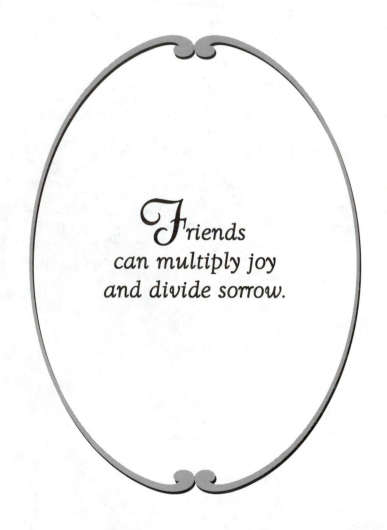

Friends
can multiply joy
and divide sorrow.

Diet Defense Against Opportunistic Disease;
Hepatitis, Herpes, Lupus, M.S., AIDS, & STDs

Many things in today's world serve to depress immunity and make the body vulnerable to disease. We call a virus or bacteria "opportunistic" when it becomes virulent and overwhelms a depressed immune system. This type of infection is usually devastating and difficult to overcome. The harmful organism must be neutralized, while nourishment and vigorous rebuilding of a weakened defense system develops against continuation and recurrence.

Common causes that lower immunity to a drastic level include:

❦ Prolonged use of anti-biotics, prescription or pleasure drugs, infected needles, cortico-steroids, birth control pills, unnecessary childhood vaccinations or travel immunizations. These things may alter thymus gland activity, and its immune-controlling ability.

❦ Sexual contact with infected, contagious persons who pass on opportunistic organisms.

❦ A highly stress lifestyle that depletes basic body reserves.

❦ Poor diet with too many refined and junk foods, causing poor cell health and nutritional deficiencies on a wide scale; too many chemicals in foods that the body cannot use for fuel or replenishment. Poor diet also causes an imbalanced, over-acid system that allows disease elements to exist and grow.

❦ Auto-toxemia through poor waste elimination and constipation.

❦ Exhausted liver and adrenal glands; general gland/hormone depletion and imbalance.

A high resistance, immune-strengthening diet is primary to success over these conditions. Immune compromised diseases are major diseases, and must be approached with vigorous energy, commitment and treatment. Intestinal environment must be improved to create a climate where pathogenic bacteria cannot flourish. The diet programs in this section are for the ill person who needs drastic measures - a great deal of concentrated defense strength in a short time. It represents the first "crash course" stages of the change from cooked to living foods. (Refer to BUILDING IMMUNE POWER in this book for broader building and maintenance, and for gentler progress).

For several months at least, the diet should be vegetarian, low in dairy and gluten foods, and saturated-fat free. This means eliminating all meats, dairy foods except yogurt, fried and fatty foods, with no yeasted breads, coffee, alcohol, salty, sugary or refined foods of any kind; and of course, no drugs, (even prescription ones if possible).

This is essentially a modified macrobiotic diet, emphasizing more fresh than cooked foods, and adding high potency acidophilus powder to the foods that are cooked to convert them to living nourishment with friendly flora. Immune-depressing, pathogenic viruses thrive on dead and waste matter. The ultra purity of this diet controls the multiple allergies and sensitivities that occur in immune deficient diseases, yet still supplies the needs of a body that is suffering primary nutrient depletion. For most people, this way of eating is a radical change, with major limitations, but the success rate has been good. It has been effective in the reversal of HIV positive to HIV negative, in the regeneration efforts of life-threatening cases of hepatitis and M.S., and in improvement of full-blown AIDS cases.

The recipes to go with this diet are still delicious - just simpler in content and preparation.

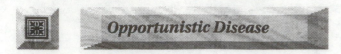

This diet protocol has been found effective for the following opportunistic diseases:
❧AIDS & AIDS RELATED PROBLEMS ❧LUPUS ❧M.S. ❧CANDIDA ALBICANS ❧MUSCULAR DYSTROPHY ❧HERPES ❧RHEUMATIC FEVER ❧MONONUCLEOSIS ❧CHRONIC FATIGUE SYNDROME ❧HPV ❧NEUROLOGICAL LYME DISEASE ❧PARASITE INFECTIONS ❧ECZEMA & PSORIASIS ❧HEPATITIS ❧TOXIC SHOCK SYNDROME ❧

☛Vigorous treatment is recommended on all fronts. See HEALTHY HEALING, 9th EDITION, by Linda Rector-Page for a complete, updated listing of successful holistic therapies.

Stage One; Blood Cleansing Diet for Serious Immune Deficient Diseases:

There is usually severe blood toxicity, fatigue and lack of nutrient assimilation in serious degenerative conditions. A liquid fast is therefore *not recommended*, since it is often too harsh for an already weakened system. The initial diet should, however, be as pure as possible, in order to be as cleansing as possible; totally vegetarian, free of meats, dairy foods, fried, preserved and refined foods, and above all, of saturated fats. The diet may be followed for 1 to 2 months, or longer if the body is still actively cleansing, or needs further alkalizing. The diet may also be returned to when needed, to purify against relapse or additional symptoms.

On rising: take 2 to 3 TBS. cranberry concentrate in 8-oz. water with $1/2$ teasp. ascorbate vitamin C crystals, or use a green tea blood cleansing formula, such as Crystal Star GREEN TEA CLEANSER™;
or cut up $1/2$ lemon (with skin) and blend in the blender w. 1 teasp. honey, and 1 cup distilled water; **and** $1/2$ teasp. Natren LIFE START II lactobacillus complex or Alta Health CANGEST in 8-oz. aloe vera juice.

Take a brisk exercise walk, and get some early morning sunlight every day.

Breakfast: have a glass of fresh carrot juice, with 1 TB. Bragg's LIQUID AMINOS added;
and whole grain muffins or rice cakes with kefir cheese;
or whole grain cereal or pancakes with yogurt and fresh fruit;
or a cup of soy milk or plain yogurt mixed in the blender with a cup of fresh fruit, some walnuts and $1/2$ teasp. Natren LIFE START II lactobacillus complex.

Mid-morning: take a weekly colonic irrigation. On non-colonic days, take a potassium broth or essence (pg. 53) with 1 TB. Bragg's LIQUID AMINOS, and $1/2$ teasp. ascorbate vitamin C crystals;
and another fresh carrot juice, or pau d' arco tea with $1/2$ teasp. Natren LIFE START II added.

Lunch: have a green leafy salad with lemon/flax oil dressing; add sprouts, tofu, avocado, nuts and seeds;
or have an open-face sandwich on rice cakes or a chapati, with soy or yogurt cheese and fresh veggies;
or have a cup of miso soup with rice noodles or brown rice;
or have some steamed vegetables with millet or brown rice and tofu;
and a cup of pau d'arco tea or aloe vera juice with $1/2$ teasp. ascorbate vitamin C and $1/2$ teasp. Natren LIFE START II lactobacillus complex.

Mid-afternoon: have another carrot juice with 1 TB. Bragg's LIQUID AMINOS;
and a green drink (pg. 240), or Sun CHLORELLA, GREEN MAGMA or Crystal Star ENERGY GREEN™.

Dinner: have a baked potato with Bragg's LIQUID AMINOS or lemon/oil dressing and a fresh salad;
and another potassium broth, or black bean or lentil soup;
or fresh spinach or artichoke pasta with steamed vegetables and a lemon/flax oil dressing;
or a Chinese steam/stir-fry with shiitake mushrooms, vegetables and brown rice;
or a tofu and veggie casserole with yogurt or soy cheese.

♣ Sprinkle ¹/₂ teasp. Natren LIFE START II, or Alta Health CANGEST powder over any cooked food at this meal.

Before Bed: take another 8-oz. glass of aloe vera juice with ¹/₂ teasp. ascorbate vitamin C with bioflavs; **and** another carrot juice, or papaya juice with ¹/₂ teasp. Natren LIFE START II lactobacillus powder.

Watchwords for Blood Cleansing and Diet Purification:
   ✓ All produce should be fresh and organically grown when possible.
   ✓ A good juicer is really necessary. The investment is well worth it.
   ✓ Avoid canned, frozen prepackaged foods, and refined foods with colors, preservatives and flavor enhancers. Avoid sodas and artificially flavored drinks.
   ✓ Avoid concentrated sugars, and sweeteners. Keep table salt use to a minimum.
   ✓ No fried foods of any kind.
   ✓ Unsweetened mild herb teas and bottled mineral water (6 to 8 glasses) are recommended throughout each day, to hydrate, alkalize, and keep the body flushed of toxic wastes.
   ✓ One half teasp. ascorbate vitamin C crystals with bioflavonoids may be added to any drink throughout the day to bowel tolerance for optimum results.

Supplements for the Blood Purifying Diet:
Because such vigorous treatment is necessary, supplementation is desirable at all stages of healing.

❖ Antioxidants, such as germanium 100 to 150mg. with astragalus, marine-carotene 100,000IU daily as an anti-infective, Vitamin E 1000IU with selenium 200mcg. to fight cell damage, CoQ 10 60mg. and octacosonal 1000mg. daily can strengthen white blood cell and T-cell activity, and help overcome side effects and nerve damage from many of the drugs prescribed for these conditions. ◆ For best results, take **with** Quercetin Plus and bromelain 500mg. 3x daily, to prevent auto-immune reactions, **and** high potency digestive enzymes, such as Rainbow Light DETOX-ZYME capsules.

❖ Egg yolk lecithin, highest potency, for active lipids that make the cell walls resistant to attack.

❖ Acidophilus culture complex with bifidus - refrigerated, highest potency, 3 teasp. daily, with biotin 1000mcg., and/or ¹/₂ teasp. Lexan B BLEND powder.

❖ Aged aloe vera juice, 2 to 3 glasses daily, to block virus spreading from cell to cell.

❖ Shark liver oil or cartilage, 6 to 10 740mg. capsules, and/or Crystal Star GINSENG/REISHI extract, ¹/₂ dropperful 3x daily, to stimulate production of interferon, interleukin and lymphocytes.

❖ Carnitine 500mg. daily for 3 days. Rest for 7 days, then take 1000mg. for 3 days. Rest for 7 days. Take with high Omega-3 fish or flax oils, 3-6 daily, and evening primrose oil 1000mg. 3x daily.

❖ H_2O_2 - food grade Care Plus OXYGEL, rubbed on the feet morning and evening, or 3% solution taken orally, 1 TB. in 8-oz. water 3 x daily. *Alternate use for best results; one week on and one week off.*
Note: You can take a simple blood-color test to monitor your own blood cleansing improvement. Make a small, quick, sterilized razor cut on your finger, or prick it with a needle. If the blood is a dark, bluish-purplish color it is not healthy. A bright red color indicates healthy blood. H_2O_2 treatment has been successful in this test by oxygenating the blood.

❖ Crystal Star LIV-ALIVE™ capsules and LIV-ALIVE™ tea to detoxify the liver.

❖ St. John's Wort extract or Crystal Star ANTI-VI™ extract for antiviral activity.

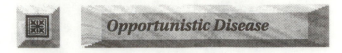
❋ *Bodywork for the Blood Purifying Diet:*

✚ Take a colonic irrigation or a Sonné bentonite clay cleanse once a week to remove lymph congestion infected feces from the intestinal tract.

✚ Overheating therapy has been successful against many of these diseases, by speeding up metabolism, and inhibiting replication of the invading virus. (See HEALTHY HEALING by Linda Rector-Page for technique.)

✚ Exercise daily. The aerobic oxygen intake alone can be a very important nutrient. Get some morning sunlight on the body every day possible.

❋ *Suggested Recipes For The Purifying Diet:*
By section and recipe number:

FASTING & CLEANSING FOODS - all

HEALTHY DRINKS, JUICES & WATERS - all

BREAKFAST & BRUNCH - 73, 76, 77, 81, 83, 85, 87, 89, 91, 92, 93, 94, 99, 100, 101, 102, 103, 104, 106.

SALADS HOT & COLD - 186, 187, 188, 189, 193, 197, 200, 203, 204, 206, 216, 222, 227, 232, 234, 237.

LOW-FAT & VERY LOW-FAT - 41, 245, 254, 260, 268, 269, 270, 272, 274, 280, 282, 284, 295, 296, 300.

DAIRY FREE COOKING - 333, 334, 3338, 342, 345, 348, 350, 352, 354, 356, 364, 366, 69, 370, 371, 374.

WHEAT FREE BAKING - 375, 379, 383, 387, 391, 393, 395, 396, 397, 398, 399, 402, 404, 407, 408, 409.

Stage Two; Rebuilding Diet For Immune Deficient Diseases:
This diet should be used for 6 months to 1 year. It emphasizes changing the intestinal environment to strengthen immunity, provide for good nutrition and fuel assimilation, increase tissue oxygen use, and balance body chemistry.

On rising: take a high vitamin/mineral drink such as Nutritech ALL 1 or Nature's Plus SPIRUTEIN in apple, orange or aloe vera juice.

Breakfast: make a mix of 2 TBS. each: brewer's yeast, wheat germ, and lecithin granules. Sprinkle some on whatever you have for breakfast.
A poached egg on a whole grain muffin with kefir cheese;
or whole grain cereal, granola, muesli or pancakes with apple juice, or yogurt and fresh fruit;
or a mixture of fresh fruits and a whole grain muffin.

Mid-morning: have a cup of miso soup with sea veggies;
or more fresh fruit and an herb tea, such as Crystal Star LICORICE MINTS or mineral water;
or a green drink such as Sun CHLORELLA, or Crystal Star ENERGY GREEN DRINK™ with some raw crunchy veggies and kefir cheese.

Lunch: have a small omelet or baked eggs with a green salad;
or a high protein sandwich on whole grain bread, with lots of sprouts, nuts, seeds and tofu;
or a baked potato with black bean or onion soup and a salad;
or a vegetable soup or potassium broth with brown rice and some steamed veggies.

Mid-afternoon: have some whole grain crackers or cornbread with raw veggies, and kefir cheese;
and an herb tea, such as red clover, or Crystal Star FEEL GREAT TEA™;
or fresh carrot juice, or another green drink and a hard boiled egg with tamari or veggie sauce.

Dinner: have a whole grain or veggie pasta dish with a light sauce and a cup of veggie or onion soup;
or have some marinated, baked tofu with brown rice and steamed veggies;
or have a vegetable stew with cornbread or polenta and a green salad with lemon/oil dressing;
or have a broccoli stir-fry with walnuts and brown rice and miso soup with sea vegetables on top;
or have baked or broiled fish or seafood with brown rice and peas or green beans.

Before bed: have a cup of VEGEX yeast broth, or miso soup;
and/or a glass of apple, papaya, or aloe vera juice.

✓It is absolutely necessary to keep the liver clean and working if healing in these serious conditions is to take place. Avoid caffeine and caffeine-containing foods, hard alcohol, tobacco, junk foods, amphetamines, barbiturates, and other pleasure drugs.

✓Practice careful food combining to maximize digestion and absorption. (page 89).

✱ *Supplements for the Immune Rebuilding Diet:*

❖ Take Sun CHLORELLA, 2 packets in water daily, <u>with</u> Enzymatic Therapy LIQUID LIVER WITH SIBERIAN GINSENG, for continued liver stimulation and support. Continue with beta carotene as an antioxidant and to boost immunity.

❖ Continue with at least 5000 to 10,000mg (1 to 2 teasp. powder) **ascorbate vitamin C with bioflavonoids** daily, or Crystal Star BIOFLAVONOID, FIBER & C SUPPORT™ DRINK, and add carnitine 250mg. 3x daily;
and/or take Quercitin 1000mg. or Pycnogenol 50 to 100mg. as very potent bioflavonoids and antioxidants with definite anti-viral impact.

❖ Continue with Alta Health CANGEST or Natren LIFE START II for good assimilation. You are eating very high nutrition with this diet. Get all the energy you can from it.

❖ Take ENER B12 internasal, germanium 150mg. 3 to 4x daily, and Crystal Star HEARTSEASE-ANEMIGIZE™ capsules to rebuild platelet and red blood cells and supply oxygen.

❖ Take high omega-3 flax oils 3x daily, and Crystal Star ADRN-ACTIVE™ capsules or ADRN™ drops to nourish adrenal glands.

❖ Take a GLA supplement, such as evening primrose oil or borage oil for T-Cell activation.

❖ Take CoQ10, at least 60mg. 3 to 4x daily as an immuno-stimulating agent to bring extra energy to rebuilding cells, and increase the immuno-competence of the existing cells.

❋ *Bodywork for the Immune Rebuilding Diet:*

✚ Get plenty of fresh air, early morning sunshine, exercise and rest every day.

✚ Yoga is very effective for at least 5 minutes in the morning and evening to encourage good venous return, organ mobilization, and lymphatic drainage.

❋ *Sample Recipes for the Immune Rebuilding Diet*
By section and recipe number:

ORIENTAL & LIGHT MACROBIOTIC EATING - all

SALADS HOT & COLD - all

LOW-FAT & VERY LOW-FAT DISHES - all

DAIRY FREE COOKING - all

SUGAR FREE SWEETS - 413, 415, 416, 420, 424, 425, 426, 427, 430, 431, 432, 436,438, 439, 440, 443.

TOFU FOR YOU - 570, 572, 575, 576, 579, 581, 58, 585,590, 592, 596, 598, 601, 603, 604, 606, 608, 610.

FISH & SEAFOODS - all

HIGH MINERAL FOODS - all

HIGH PROTEIN WITHOUT MEAT - 696, 698, 699, 701, 703, 706, 711, 712, 714, 718, 738, 740, 741, 742.

HIGH FIBER FOODS - all

❋ *Suggested Menu Plans*
Recipe combinations that work for this diet:

AN EASY RISING BREAKFAST - 793, 73, 820, 704

AN EASY WEEK NIGHT DINNER - 140, 202, 183, 439

A HEARTY WINTER MEAL - 132, 167, 643, 431, 193

A LIGHT SUMMER MEAL -786, 187, 420, 117

A WEEKEND PICNIC - 663, 114, 421, 129

SUNDAY BRUNCH - 431, 208, 653, 662, 121, 198

A FAMILY MEAL - 135, 204, 218, 418

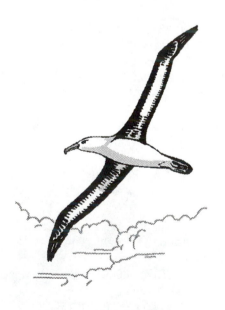

Diet for Longevity;
Health Supportive Anti-Aging

Now the fun begins. . . the golden years, when hectic family life quiets down, financial strains and needs ease, business retirement is here or not far off, and we can do the things we've always wanted to do but never had time for - travel, art, music, a craft, gardening, writing, quiet walks, picnics, more social life, doing what we _want_ to do, not what we _have_ to do. We all look forward to this stress-free time of life, and picture ourselves on that tennis court, bicycle path or cruise ship, healthy and enjoying ourselves. But all this freedom comes in the latter half of life, and many of us don't age gracefully in today's world.

Environmental pollutants, a long standing diet of chemical-laced, refined foods, vitamin and mineral deficiencies, overuse of prescription drugs and anti-biotics, may prevent this dream from becoming a reality. _Age is not the enemy, illness is._

Aging is not the passage of time per se, but the process that reduces the number of healthy and unrestored cells in the body. Cells do not age, but are sloughed off as their efficiency diminishes, to be replaced by new ones. When the body is given the right nutrients, cell restoration may continue for many years past current life expectancy. We know that human life span is at least 20 to 30 years longer than most of us actually live today. Poor nutrition and lack of exercise reduce the capacity of the body to age well. Eighty percent of the population over 65 years old in industrialized nations is chronically ill, usually with arthritis, heart disease, diabetes or high blood pressure. Our seniority is often not very youthful in mind and spirit either. In general, most of us live slightly more than 60% of the years our bodies are capable of.

Our lifespan can be increased. Youth can be rebuilt from the inside. The aging process can be slowed down by maintaining the best internal environment possible; by strengthening lean body mass, metabolism, and immune response with good nutrition, regular exercise and a positive outlook on life. While cell age is largely genetically controlled, disease is usually the result of diet, lifestyle or environment. We can do something about these things.

As we chronologically age, the diet must improve for us to stay youthful, and indeed be optimally nourishing as the years pass. Nutritional _quality_, not quantity, is the key. Eat smaller meals, less volume of food. Fewer calories are needed for good body function as we age. Optimum body weight should be about 10 to 15 pounds less than in the 20's and 30's.

Regular aerobic exercise, such as a brisk daily walk prolongs physical fitness at any age. Exercise helps maintain stamina, strength, agility, circulation and joint mobility. Stretching out every morning limbers the body, oxygenates the tissues, and helps clear it of the previous night's waste and metabolic eliminations. Stretches at night before bed help insure more muscle relaxation and a better night's rest.

Don't worry. Be happy. Clinical studies show that a pessimistic outlook on life depresses your personality, and your immune response. An optimistic, well-rounded, loving life needs friends and family. Regular contact is important for you and for them. Doing for, and giving to others at the stage of your life when there is finally enough time to do it graciously, will make a world of difference to your quality of life.

Youth is not a chronological age. It is a state of good health and optimistic spirit.

One should die young, as late as possible. **Ashley Montague.**

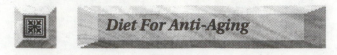

❋ *Diet For a Longer, Healthier Life:*

Longevity and a healthy "seniority" can be greatly enhanced and extended by using a few simple dietary watchwords.

❦ Eat plenty of cultured food; kefir and kefir cheese, yogurt and yogurt cheese, tempeh, relishes and sauerkraut, and a glass or two of wine at the evening meal. All these foods promote nutrient assimilation and friendly flora in the digestive system.

❦ Have some fish and fresh seafoods two to three times a week, to enhance thyroid and metabolic balance with high Omega-3 oils and absorbable iodine.

❦ Get plenty of food source vitamins and minerals for body building blocks and healthy cell replacement, from fruits, leafy greens and root vegetables, onions and cruciferous vegetables. Sea veggies and herbs can insure gland balance and immune stimulation from natural iodine and potassium.

❦ Promote an alkaline system with green drinks, miso, tofu and other macrobiotic foods, which help prevent disease. The use of balancing proteins from vegetable and grain sources instead of meats is better for you and better for the environment.

❦ Include high fiber foods every day from whole grains, fruits and fresh vegetables, to assure regular passing of toxic body wastes and a free-flowing system.

❦ Keep dietary fats and oils low - 2 to 3 tablespoons a day - from unsaturated vegetable sources.

❦ Drink plenty of pure water and/or mineral water every day; and take gentle herbal tonics and green drinks often to keep the system clear and immunity strong.

❦ Avoid fried foods, excess caffeine, red meats, highly seasoned foods, refined and chemically processed foods.

The following diet suggests ways to put it all together.

On rising: take a high protein drink, such as Nature's Plus SPIRUTEIN, or a vitamin/mineral drink such as NutriTech ALL I, in orange or apple juice. **Add 2 teasp. bee pollen granules to either drink.**

Breakfast: Make a mix of 2 TBS. <u>each</u> brewer' s yeast, lecithin granules, toasted wheat germ, bee pollen granules and flax seeds. Sprinkle some on your breakfast choice;
fresh fruits, plain or with yogurt;
or a whole grain muesli or granola with apple juice, yogurt, or soy milk topping;
or whole grain toast or muffins with a little kefir cheese;
or a baked or poached egg or omelet;
and/or a Crystal Star SYSTEM STRENGTH™ DRINK for optimum mineral/amino acid absorption.

Mid-morning: have a green drink (page 240) or Sun CHLORELLA, Green Foods GREEN MAGMA, or Crystal Star ENERGY GREEN™ DRINK in apple juice or mineral water;
and/or a cup of tonifying herb tea, such as Siberian ginseng, red clover, or Crystal Star CHINESE ROYAL MU™ or GINSENG 6 DEFENSE RESTORATIVE™ TEA;
and some more fresh fruit with yogurt;
or a Crystal Star DAILY C & BIOFLAVONOIDS SUPPORT DRINK™.

Lunch: have a leafy green salad with a cup of miso or ramen noodle soup;
or a cup of black bean, lentil, or other protein soup wlth baked potato and kefir cheese or yogurt sauce;
or a fresh fruit salad with cottage cheese or yogurt cheese, and whole grain baked chips or crackers;
or a light seafood or turkey salad;
or a hot or cold vegetable pasta salad.

Mid-afternoon: have some fresh or dried fruits with yogurt;
or some crackers or rice cakes with a vegetable, soy or kefir spread, and a cup of light broth;
or a cup of ginseng tea, mint tea, or Crystal Star FEEL GREAT™ TEA;
and/or some crunchy raw veggies with a yogurt or soy cheese dip;

Dinner: have a hearty high protein vegetable, nut and seed salad with soup and whole grain muffins or cornbread;
or an oriental stir-fry with brown rice and miso soup;
or a baked veggie, tofu and whole grain casserole;
or a vegetable quiche with a whole grain crust, and light yogurt/white wine sauce;
or baked or broiled fish or seafood with a green salad and brown rice or steamed veggies;
or roast turkey with cornbread or rice and a light salad.
Have a glass of white wine for digestion and relaxation.

Before Bed: have a cup of chamomile tea or apple or papaya juice, or a cup of VEGEX broth;
or a glass of aloe vera juice for regularity the next morning.

✓ Drink six to eight glasses of bottled water daily on a regular basis.

✳ *Supplements and Herbal Aids for a Longer Healthier Life:*

The following suggestions are included for their anti-aging activity. The choices you make should reflect individual needs and problems. All recommendations are daily amounts.

❖ Vitamin E 400IU with selenium, and CoQ 10, 30mg., or CHLORELLA daily for better tissue oxygen levels.

❖ Ester C or ascorbate vitamin C with bioflavonoids 1000 to 3000mg. daily, **and** Vit. B12 sub-lingual or inter-nasal for good cell formation and replacement.

❖ Omega-3 rich flax oil, 3 teasp. daily for heart and artery health.

❖ Beta carotene 25,000IU for disease prevention and liver health.

❖ Vitamin D for continued bone growth and strength, and for skin health and tone. Better yet, take an early morning walk every day for sunlight vitamin D.

❖ Alta Health CANGEST caps or Schiff ENZYMALL tabs for digestive and food assimilation help.

❖ Evening primrose oil caps for prostaglandin balance and essential fatty acids.

❖ Ginkgo biloba extract **with** 2 teasp. unsprayed bee pollen granules for circulation stimulation and increased memory retention.

❖ Highest potency royal jelly 2 teasp. daily for pantothenic acid and regenerative activity.

❋ *Bodywork for a Longer Healthier Life:*

✛ *Don't smoke.* In addition to all its other well-documented hazards, smoking uses up available body and tissue oxygen, which feeds the brain and helps prevent disease.

✛ Drink all alcohol in moderation, especially hard and fortified liquors. Tolerance for alcohol decreases as you grow older because of nervous system changes.

✛ Maintain your desired weight. Ten to 30 pounds of extra weight can take two years off your life, 30 to 50 excess pounds takes off four years, and over 50 pounds takes off eight years.

✛ Take a long walk every day, especially after the largest meal of the day, to strengthen heart, lungs, bones and muscles, increase energy and reduce stress, and help you sleep better.

✛ Do deep breathing and mild stretching exercises every morning, (outdoors if possible for early sun-light), to keep tissue oxygen levels high.

✛ Rest and relaxation are essential. Stress ages people more quickly, and as we get older it actually takes years off life expectancy. It is <u>normal to eat and sleep less</u> as metabolism slows, but feeling rested is important.

❈

❋ *Suggested Recipes to Encourage a Longer Healthier Life By section and recipe number:*

BREAKFAST & BRUNCH - 74, 76, 77, 78, 79, 81, 83, 86, 88, 89, 91, 92, 98, 103, 104, 107.

HIGH MINERAL FOODS - 612, 613, 618, 619, 621, 623, 626, 629, 631, 636, 638, 640, 641, 644, 647, 648.

HIGH PROTEIN WITHOUT MEAT - 689, 701, 702, 704, 711, 718, 720, 724, 730, 731, 732, 736, 737, 740.

GREAT OUTDOOR EATING - 875, 878, 880, 881, 882, 884, 888, 886, 891, 893, 895, 899, 903.

FISH & SEAFOODS - 532, 533, 534, 542, 547, 548, 551, 556, 558, 563, 567, 568, 569.

LOW-FAT & VERY LOW-FAT DISHES - all

LOW CHOLESTEROL MEALS - all

SUGAR FREE SPECIALS & TREATS - all

HIGH FIBER RECIPES - all

HEALTHY HOLIDAY FEASTING - 826, 831, 833, 837, 841, 843, 847, 849, 850, 851, 853, 854, 855, 856, 860, 861, 863, 866.

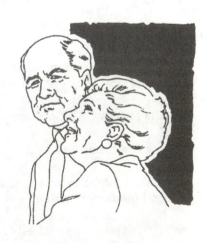

❋ Sample Menu Plans
Some recipe combinations that will work with this diet:

A HEARTY WINTER MEAL - 792, 224, 661, 442

A LIGHT SUMMER MEAL - 626, 787, 427

SUNDAY BRUNCH - 433, 699, 712, 662

A FAMILY MEAL - 621, 644, 426

LUNCH FOR TWO - 808, 737

AN EASY RISING BREAKFAST - 819, 74, 79

AN EASY WEEKNIGHT MEAL - 798, 714, 660

A SPECIAL DINNER FOR TWO - 719A, 613, 441, 545

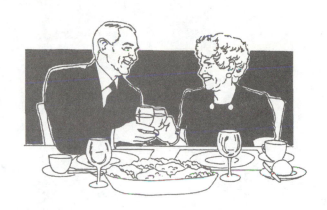

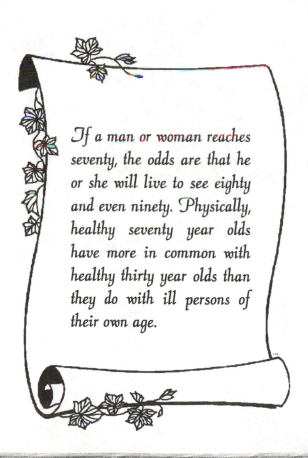

If a man or woman reaches seventy, the odds are that he or she will live to see eighty and even ninety. Physically, healthy seventy year olds have more in common with healthy thirty year olds than they do with ill persons of their own age.

*W*hat you are is
God's gift to you.
What you make of yourself is
your gift to God.

Eating for Good Looks
Diet for Skin, Hair, Nails & Eyes

Radiant skin, lustrous, lively hair, bright eyes and strong pink nails, all mirror the body's good health state. Appearance elements are the surest signs of its nutritional condition. If your "cosmetic elements" need help, feed them the best nutrients. The body beautiful, of course, comes from within. The skin is the largest organ of ingestion and egestion. Good dietary care and habits show quickly. We have found that most people experience noticeable appearance improvement in about 3 weeks.

♣Soft smooth skin depends on a diet rich in fresh fruits and vegetables, and plenty of pure water (at least 6-8 glasses a day; see ABOUT WATER in this book). Water keeps the system flushed, so waste and body toxins will not be dumped out through the skin as blemishes or rashes; or through the eyes as crystalline deposits; or clog hair follicles causing dandruff. Bottled water is best. Fluoridation tends to leach Vitamin E out of the body.

♣Beautiful eyes, skin, and nails need vitamin A, vitamin C, mineral-rich foods, and high vegetable protein foods, for collagen and interstitial tissue health.

♣Vibrant hair needs vegetable/whole grain protein for maximum growth, and high carotene foods like broccoli, carrots and greens for "permanent" appeal. Turn your hair from drab to fab with an improved diet.

♣The healthiest skin needs some fresh air and sunlight every day.

♣All tissues need a rich, high oxygen blood supply, and plenty of mineral building blocks. Plants are the most absorbable way for the body to get them.

♣Poor diet, poor circulation, constipation, harmful bacteria, and lack of tissue oxygen uptake, all contribute to skin, hair and eye problems. But diet is the primary factor, where effective improvements can be made most quickly and easily. The following diet is high in mineral foods containing silica, sulphur, calcium and magnesium, low in fatty and fried foods, low in clogging dairy products, and mucous forming foods. Red meats and refined foods of all kinds are eliminated, so that the body will be cleaner, use its nutrients better, and circulate needed elements to skin, hair, eyes and nails.

Good bodywork to enhance your cosmetic diet should include:
+ Early morning sunlight on the body every day for natural vitamin D;
+ Lots of fresh air, rest and mild exercise to keep the circulation free and flowing;
+ Scalp massage and dry skin brushing once a week to increase circulation and slough dead cells.

This diet is also effective for other "cosmetic element" problems:
CHRONIC ACNE ▪HAIR LOSS ▪DETERIORATING VISION and NIGHT BLINDNESS ▪DANDRUFF ▪FUNGAL INFECTIONS ▪DRY SKIN and WRINKLED SKIN ▪LIVER and AGE SPOTS ▪EASY BRUISING ▪CHRONIC SKIN INFECTIONS and DERMATITIS ▪ECZEMA and PSORIASIS ▪SALLOW SKIN ▪SPLIT, BRITTLE NAIL ▪GLAUCOMA ▪ CONJUNCTIVITIS ▪

Nutrition For Healthy Skin & Hair

This good looks diet program is in two stages - the first is a short 3 day elimination diet to clear the body of waste and toxins. The second is light, low fat eating, with good food sources of minerals, amino acids and trace minerals to lay a solid foundation for skin, hair and nail health.

Stage One; The Three Day Elimination Cleanse:

On rising: take a glass of apple juice, or 2 lemons squeezed in a glass of water with a little honey.

Breakfast: take a potassium broth (page 240) with 2 teasp. brewer's yeast and/or wheat germ added; **or** carrot/cucumber juice.

Mid-morning: have a skin tonic drink (page 242);
or a green drink, such as Sun CHLORELLA in mineral water, or Crystal Star ENERGY GREEN™.

Lunch: have a fresh carrot juice or another green drink (page 240), or another skin tonic;
and another small bottle of mineral water.

Mid-afternoon: take a PERSONAL V-8 JUICE (page 241), or other mixed vegetable juice;
or an herb tea such as nettles, Japanese green tea, or Crystal Star SILICA SOURCE™ drops in water.

Dinner: have an apple juice, or apple/alfalfa sprout juice.

Before Bed: take a pineapple/papaya, papaya or apple juice;
or a VEGEX yeast broth for high B vitamins.

✓Drink at least 6 to 8 glasses of pure bottled or mineral water throughout the day for best results.

✱ *Supplements for the Elimination Cleanse:*

❖ Take $1/4$ to $1/2$ teasp. ascorbate vitamin C crystals with any drink or juice 3 to 4 times daily throughout the elimination diet, for interstitial tissue and collagen formation.

❖ Take liquid acidophilus with any juice or drink - 1 teasp. 3 to 4 times daily throughout the elimination diet, for best assimilation and to keep the system alkaline.

✱ *Bodywork for the Elimination Cleanse:*

✚ Get early morning sunlight on the face and body every day possible, for natural A and D.

✚ Rub the face with insides of the papaya and cucumber skins when you peel them for your juices. They are excellent to alkalize acid waste being released through the skin, and add healing properties during the fast.

✚ Make a strong tea of the following herbs; chamomile and calendula flowers, lemon juice, rosehips and rosewater. Strain, and apply with cotton balls to the skin, or pour as a rinse through the hair, to add minerals, alkaline nutrients, and toning agents.

Stage Two; A Diet For Healthy "Cosmetic Elements":

On rising: take a glass of watermelon juice in the summer, apple/cranberry juice in the winter; **and/or** a high protein drink, such as Nature's Plus SPIRUTEIN, or Crystal Star SYSTEM STRENGTH DRINK™.

Breakfast: have a glass of grapefruit juice, **or** Crystal Star DAILY BIOFLAV. & C SUPPORT™ DRINK; **and** make a mix of 2 TBS. each: lecithin granules, wheat germ, and sesame seeds for the skin, or molasses and cider vinegar for hair. Sprinkle some every morning on whatever you have for breakfast.
such as some whole grain muesli, oatmeal or granola with yogurt and fresh fruit (especially bananas, strawberries, papaya and peaches);
or oatmeal or whole grain pancakes, with a little maple syrup or honey.

Mid-morning: have a cup of miso soup with sea veggies snipped on top;
or some yogurt with fresh fruit;
or a green drink, such as Sun CHLORELLA or Crystal Star ENERGY GREEN™ DRINK.

Lunch: have a green leafy salad, with cucumber, sprouts, bell pepper and lemon/oil dressing;
or have some steamed vegetables with marinated tofu and brown rice or a baked potato;
or have a fresh fruit salad, with peaches, apricots and cottage, kefir or yogurt cheese;
or have a seafood and whole grain pasta salad with peas;
or an avocado and low-fat cheese sandwich on whole grain bread, with lentil, or onion soup.

Mid-afternoon: have a cup of refreshing herb tea, such as comfrey, calendula, or Crystal Star BEAUTI-FUL SKIN™ or HEALTHY HAIR & NAILS™ TEA.
or a cup of ramen soup with noodles, or miso soup;
and/or crunchy raw veggies with kefir cheese.

Dinner: have a large dinner salad with red onions, cucumbers and sprouts, and whole grain muffins with kefir cheese;
or a light mexican beans and rice dish with a small green salad;
or a broccoli, or asparagus quiche with onion soup;
or baked or broiled seafood or fish with veggies and brown rice or millet;
or an oriental stir-fry with chinese greens, rice and a light broth soup.

Before bed: have a glass of papaya or apple juice;
or a VEGEX yeast broth for relaxation and B Complex vitamins.

✓ **Drink plenty of pure bottled or mineral water every day for clear skin.**
Avoid red meats, refined or processed sugars and flour, caffeine and caffeine-containing foods, fried or fatty foods, foods with colorings and preservatives. All cause the body to metabolize slowly, use sugars and fats poorly, and encourage sediment and clogs to form. NO JUNK FOODS.

❋ *Diet Watchwords for Beautiful Skin, Hair & Nails:*
➥Avoid all refined foods. Eat little or no sugar. Limit salty foods.
➥**Avoid fried foods. Maintain a generally low-fat diet.**
➥Eat plenty of green, leafy vegetables. Ad more fresh foods of all kinds to your diet.
➥**Eat high fiber foods, such as fruits, vegetables, and whole grains to maintain regularity, and a clean healthy system. Don't rely exclusively on fiber supplements or drinks for your fiber.**
➥Eat only a moderate amount of protein-rich foods, such as poultry, fish, eggs, nuts, seeds, sprouts, whole grains and beans.

❋ Supplements for Healthy "Cosmetic Elements":

For Skin:

❖ Food nutrients: Jojoba, sesame and wheat germ oil, high potency royal jelly, cucumber and papaya skins, oatmeal baths, honey/almond scrub, olive oil soap.

❖ Important vitamins: B Complex 75 to 100mg. daily, vitamin C 2 to 3000mg. daily for connective tissue health, marine source carotene 50-100,000IU daily.

❖ Important minerals: Mezotrace SEA MINERAL COMPLEX, Crystal Star MEGA-MINERAL caps or SILICA SOURCE' extract drops, Alta Health SIL-X caps 2-3 daily, zinc picolinate 50-75mg. daily.

❖ Important fatty acids: Evening primrose oil 2-3 daily; omega 3 Flax oil 2-3 teasp. daily.

❖ Important herbs: Calendula and chamomile flowers, rose hips, CAMOCARE CONCENTRATE, Crystal Star SKIN THERAPY™ #1 and #2 for cleansing and smoothness, SYSTEM STRENGTH™ DRINK for elasticity and tone.

❖ If there are skin cancers, apply Vital Health PEROXY GEL or tea tree oil for 1 to 2 months. If there is eczema or psoriasis, use Crystal Star THERADERM™ CAPS and TEA, or DAILY BIOFLAVONOID & C SUPPORT™ DRINK.

For Hair:

❖ Food nutrients; Take 2 TBS. dried sea vegetables daily, or Crystal Star SYSTEM STRENGTH™ DRINK; and 2 TBS. blackstrap molasses <u>with</u> 2 teasp. royal jelly, or 2 TBS. bee pollen granules.

❖ Important vitamins: Vitamin B Complex 100mg. daily, with extra biotin 600mcg. and folic acid 800mcg.

❖ Important minerals: Mezotrace SEA MINERAL COMPLEX with extra boron for uptake; Alta Health SIL-X capsules for growth and strength, Crystal Star SILICA SOURCE™ extract for collagen.

❖ Important herbs: CamoCare concentrate or New Moon HAIR RUSH for elasticity and shine; rosemary wine for maximum hair minerals uptake.

❋ Bodywork for Healthy "Cosmetic Elements":

For Skin:

✚ Continue with early morning sunshine for vitamin D, and daily exercise for oxygen and tone.

✚ Use lemon juice or Zia SEA TONIC WITH ALOE for pH-acid balancing.

✚ Use a gentle, balancing mask once a week for tightening and cleansing, such as Zia SUPER HYDRATING MASK, or Crystal Star WHITE CLAY & HERBS TONING MASK.

✚ Use Crystal Star LEMON SALT GLOW™ or a loofa sponge for skin color and tone.

For Hair:

✚ Wash hair in warm water, rinse in cool water for best scalp health.

✤ Effective natural rinses: Nettles to darken; kelp or sea water to strengthen; cider vinegar for acid/alkaline balance; Rosemary/sage for dark hair shine; calendula/lemon juice for blonde highlights; chamomile to brighten; 1 egg yolk with the second shampoo for bounce and protein.

✤ Massage the scalp and head each morning for 5 minutes to stimulate hair growth.

✤ If there is balding, take 2 TBS. blackstrap molasses <u>with</u> PABA 100mg. and pantothenic acid 1000mg. daily for 2 to 3 months; <u>or</u> Alta Health SIL-X or Crystal Star SILICA SOURCE™ extract drops in water 3x daily <u>with</u> HEALTHY HAIR & NAILS TEA™ as a hair rinse for applied minerals.

❈

❧ *Suggested Recipes For the "Cosmetic Elements" Diet*
By section and recipe number:

HEALTHY DRINKS, JUICES & WATERS - 44, 48, 49, 51, 53, 54, 55, 57, 65, 69, 71.

BREAKFAST & BRUNCH - 73, 77, 83, 86, 94, 97, 98, 101, 103, 105, 108.

SALADS HOT & COLD - all

LOW-FAT & VERY LOW-FAT DISHES - all

HIGH FIBER RECIPES - all

SUGAR FREE SPECIALS & SWEET TREATS - 413, 414, 416, 419, 423, 426, 427, 429, 430, 431, 437, 438.

FISH & SEAFOODS - all

HIGH PROTEIN WITHOUT MEAT - 696, 700, 702, 705, 713, 720, 723, 724, 728, 732, 735, 737, 739, 741.

HIGH MINERAL FOODS - all

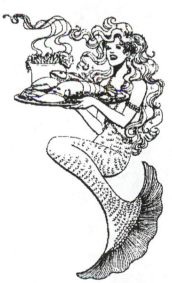

❧ *Sample Menu Plans*
Recipe combinations that work with this diet:

A SPECIAL DINNER FOR TWO - 61, 248, 263, 539, 293, 636

LUNCH FOR TWO - 52, 543, 211, 290

AN EASY RISING BREAKFAST - 48, 75, 77, 76

AN EASY WEEKNIGHT DINNER - 266, 623, 435, 789

A LIGHT SUMMER MEAL - 241, 54, 542, 254, 300

SUNDAY BRUNCH - 47, 79, 89, 101

AN APPETIZERS & HORS D'OEUVRES PARTY - 249, 252, 253, 414, 696, 710

The only way
to see the
incredible power of God,
is to undertake
something so great that you
cannot accomplish it
unaided.

Eating For A Healthy Pregnancy

A woman's body changes so dramatically during pregnancy and childbearing that her normal daily needs change. The body takes care of some of this through cravings - and during this one time of life, the body is so sensitive to its needs, the cravings are usually good for you. We know that every single thing the mother does or takes in, affects the child. The way of eating recommended here will help build a healthy baby with a minimum of discomfort or excess fatty weight build-up that can't be lost after the birth.

Promise yourself and your baby that for at least these few months of your life, during pregnancy and nursing, your diet and lifestyle will be as healthy as you can make it.

❄ Eat a high vegetable protein diet, with plenty of whole grains, seeds, sprouts, and fish or seafood at least twice a week; and/or take a good protein drink several times a week for optimal growth and energy. Protein requirements increase during pregnancy, but studies show that it is the quality of the protein, not the quantity that prevents and cures toxemia.

❄ Have a fresh fruit or green salad every day. Eat lots of high soluble fiber foods like whole grain cereals and vegetables for regularity. Eat complex carbohydrate foods like broccoli and brown rice for strength.

❄ Drink lots of bottled water and juices daily to keep the system free and flowing. Carrot juice twice a week is ideal. Include pineapple and apple juice frequently.

❄ Eat folacin-rich foods, such as raw spinach and asparagus for healthy cell growth.
Eat zinc-rich foods, such as pumpkin and sesame seeds for good body formation.
Eat vitamin C foods - broccoli, bell peppers and fruits for connective tissue formation.
Eat alkalizing foods, such as miso soup and brown rice to prevent and neutralize toxemia.
Eat mineral-rich foods - sea vegetables, greens and whole grains for baby building blocks.

❄ Eat small frequent meals rather than large meals.

❄ Get some mild daily exercise, such as a brisk walk for fresh air, oxygen and circulation. Take an early morning sun bath when possible for vitamin D, calcium absorption and bone growth.

❄ Consciously set aside one stress-free time for relaxation every day. The baby will know, thrive, and be more relaxed itself.

Dietary watchwords to follow for the greatest health of the baby.

❄ Don't diet. Lower calories usually mean lower birth weight. Metabolism becomes deranged during dieting and the baby will receive abnormal nutrition that can impair brain and nerve development. Even if you're gaining too much, this diet is full of nutritious calories, (not empty calories), and you will easily lose the weight after nursing. Until then you are still eating for two.

❄ Don't restrict your food variety. Eat a wide range of healthy foods to assure the baby access to all nutrients. (Avoid cabbages, onions and garlic. They sometimes upset body balance during pregnancy). Particularly avoid red meats. Most are full of nitrates, nitrites and chemical hormones that the baby can't handle. Avoid caffeine and alcohol. Babies can't eliminate it like adults can. Even during breast feeding, toxic concentrations occur easily.

❧ **Don't fast** - even for short periods where fasting would normally be advisable, such as constipation, or to overcome a cold. Food energy supply and nutrient content will be too diminished for healthy pregnancy and nursing.

❧ **Avoid all processed, refined, preserved and colored foods.** Refrain from alcohol, and caffeine. Avoid X-rays, chemical solvents, chloro-fluorocarbons such as hair sprays, and even cat litter. Your system may be able to easily handle all of these things without undue damage; the baby's can't. Even during nursing, toxic concentrations occur easily.

❧ **Don't smoke. Avoid secondary smoke.** The chance of low birth weight and miscarriage is twice as likely if you smoke. Smoker's infants have a mortality rate of 30% higher than non-smoker's. Nursing babies take in small amounts of nicotine with breast milk, and often become prone to chronic respiratory infection.

A highly nutritious diet will help pregnancy be more of a pleasure, with less discomfort or risk of complications. It will aid in instances of:
❧TOXEMIA ❧FLUID RETENTION ❧MISCARRIAGE PREVENTION ❧ANEMIA ❧GAS and HEARTBURN ❧CONSTIPATION ❧HEMORRHOIDS and VARICOSE VEINS ❧HIGH BLOOD PRESSURE ❧MORNING SICKNESS ❧INSUFFICIENT LACTATION ❧POST-PARTUM SWELLING ❧TISSUE TONE and STRETCH MARKS ❧SYSTEM IMBALANCE ❧

Diet for a Healthy Pregnancy: Optimal Eating For Two

A largely vegetarian diet of whole foods provides optimum nutrition for pregnancy. Many staples of a lacto-vegetarian seafood diet are nutritional powerhouses, such as whole grains, leafy greens, fish, eggs, legumes, nuts, seeds, green and yellow vegetables, brewer's yeast, bananas and citrus fruits. You can base your pregnancy diet on these foods with confidence that the baby will be getting the best possible nutrition.

On rising: have some apple juice, pineapple, or pineapple/papaya juice. If there is morning sickness, a few crackers or ice chips, or a little orange juice with 1 teasp. of honey will often neutralize excess acids.

Breakfast: have some fresh fruits;
and make a mix of 1 cup raw milk or soy milk, $^1/_2$ cup yogurt, the juice from one orange, 2 TBS. brewer's yeast, 2 teasp. molasses, 2 TBS. wheat germ, 1 teasp. vanilla, 2 teasp. lecithin granules, and dashes of cinnamon and nutmeg. Drink this every morning. It is the best protein drink we know for health, growth and energy. It is excellent over hot or cold whole grain cereal, such as oatmeal, kashi or millet.

Mid-morning: have some yogurt with fresh fruit:
or a glass of fresh carrot juice with 1 teasp. Bragg's LIQUID AMINOS;
or a green drink (page 240) or Sun CHLORELLA or Barley GREEN MAGMA drink;
or a cup of miso soup with some whole grain crackers and sea vegetables snipped on top.

Lunch: have a green salad with cucumbers, sea veggies and spinach, or a high protein salad with nuts, seeds, sprouts and yogurt;
and/or a vegetable protein sandwich on whole grain or pita bread;
or a seafood and veggie pasta salad with a light lemon dressing;
or an omelet, or baked eggs on whole grain muffins;
or steamed veggies or tofu with brown rice;
or a broccoli quiche with low-fat or soy cheeses;
or a fresh fruit salad with cottage cheese.

Mid-afternoon: take a cup of refreshing herb tea, such as red raspberry, or Crystal Star MOTHERING TEA™ every day;
and have a deviled or hard boiled egg with mayonnaise or vinaigrette;
or some crunchy raw veggies with a vegetable/yogurt or kefir cheese dip;
or a cup of miso soup with sea veggies and noodles;
or some dried fruits and yogurt.

Dinner: have a vegetable quiche, such as asparagus or broccoli, with a small green salad;
or a whole grain or veggie pasta with fresh vegetables and light sauce;
or a brown rice or millet and tofu casserole with a small salad & lemon/oil dressing;
or a baked potato or hot potato salad with light dressing;
or baked or broiled salmon or white fish, or a salmon loaf or souffle, with brown rice and peas;
or a dinner salad and rice pudding or yogurt cheesecake.

Before Bed: have a cup of VEGEX broth, or a kefir drink, or some red raspberry herb tea.

❦ Drink plenty of pure water and mineral water throughout the day to keep the system flushed and flowing. Have frequent small meals, instead of large meals for better balance and assimilation.

✓ **During labor:** Take no solid food. Drink fresh water, or carrot juice; or suck on ice chips
✓ **During lactation:** Add almond milk, brewer's yeast, green drinks and green foods, avocados, carrot juice, goats milk, soy milk and soy foods, and unsulphured molasses, to promote milk quality and richness.
✓ **During weaning:** Drink papaya juice to slow down milk flow.

❋ *Supplements for a Healthy Pregnancy:*

Avoid all drugs during pregnancy and nursing: including alcohol, tobacco, caffeine, MSG, saccharin, valium, librium, tetracycline, and harsh diuretics. Especially keep away from pleasure drugs; cocaine, amphetamines, LSD and all psychedelics. Even the amino acid L-Phenylalanine will affect the nervous system of the unborn child.

✤ Take a good food source pre-natal supplement, such as Rainbow Light PRE-NATAL starting 6 to 8 weeks before expected birth.

✤ Take a food source multi-mineral/trace mineral supplement that will be absorbed well by both you and the baby, such as MEZOTRACE SEA MINERAL COMPLEX or Crystal Star MINERAL SPECTRUM™ CAPSULES.

✤ Take extra folic acid, to prevent neural tube birth defects; vitamin B12 and ascorbate vitamin C with bioflavonoids for cell and tissue development; vitamin B6 for bloating and leg cramps, and vitamin E or wheat germ oil for skin and body elasticity. **Lower dosage to ½ of your usual amount** to avoid toxemia. Mega-doses of <u>anything</u> are not good for a baby's system.

✤ Rub vitamin E oil, wheat germ oil or cocoa butter on the stomach and around the vaginal opening every night to make stretching easier and the skin more elastic.

✓ **During labor:** take vitamin E and calcium/magnesium to relieve pain and aid dilation.
✓ **During nursing:** take calcium lactate with calcium ascorbate vitamin C for collagen development. Apply vitamin E oil to breasts to alleviate crusting.

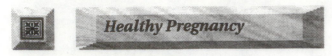

✱ *Herbs for a Healthy Pregnancy:*

♣ Take two cups daily of red raspberry tea, or Crystal Star MOTHERING TEA™, a red raspberry blend. Both are safe, rich in iron and other minerals, strengthening to the uterus and birth canal, effective against birth defects, long labor and afterbirth pain, and elasticizing to the tissues for a faster return to normal.

♣ During the 1st and 2nd trimester, take a mineral-rich pre-natal herbal compound for gentle, absorbable minerals and toning agents to elasticize tissue and ease delivery. Take Crystal Star IRON SOURCE™, SILICA SOURCE™, or CALCIUM SOURCE™ capsules or extracts in water if there is deficiency in these minerals.

♣ Take a naturally-occurring iodine source, such as kelp tabs, MIODIN drops, or Crystal Star IODINE THERAPY™ CAPS against birth defects.

✓ **During labor:** Take Medicine Wheel LABOR TINCTURE drops, or Crystal Star CRAMP CONTROL EXTRACT™ drops to ease contraction pain. Use Crystal Star BACK TO RELIEF™ caps for afterbirth pain.
✓ **During nursing:** Add 2 TBS. brewer's yeast to your diet, along with red raspberry, marshmallow, chaste tree berry extract, or Crystal Star MOTHERING TEA™ to promote and enrich milk. Fennel, alfalfa, and red raspberry tea can help keep the baby colic-free.
✓ **During weaning:** Take parsley/sage tea to dry up milk.

✱ *Bodywork for a Healthy Pregnancy:*

✤ Get some mild exercise every day. The best is a brisk walk for fresh air, oxygen and circulation.

✤ Get some early morning sunlight for half an hour every day possible, for vitamin D, calcium absorption and bone growth.

✤ If you practice reflexology do not press the acupressure point just above the ankle on the inside of the leg. It could start contractions.

✤ Get plenty of rest and adequate sleep. Body energy turns inward during sleep for repair, restoration and fetal growth.

✱ *Suggested Recipes For A Healthy Pregnancy*
By section and recipe number:

HEALTHY DRINKS, JUICES & WATERS - 43, 44, 45, 46, 47, 48, 49, 50, 51, 52, 53, 57, 61, 62, 65, 66, 67

SALADS - HOT & COLD - 186, 187, 188, 189, 190, 191, 193, 195, 198, 199, 204, 205, 206, 207, 208, 212, 213, 214, 215, 216, 217, 220, 222, 224, 225, 226, 227, 230, 231, 232, 233, 236

FISH & SEAFOODS - all

SOUPS - LIQUID SALADS - all

SUGAR-FREE SWEETS - 411, 413, 416, 417, 419, 420, 422, 423, 425, 427, 430, 431, 432, 436, 439, 441

SANDWICHES - SALADS IN BREAD - 473, 475, 477, 481, 483, 488, 489, 492, 494, 496, 497, 499, 500

HIGH PROTEIN WITHOUT MEAT - 696, 698, 699, 702, 705, 706, 711, 712, 717, 718, 720, 735, 737, 740

COMPLEX CARBOHYDRATES FOR ENERGY - 743, 744, 746, 750, 753, 757, 759, 763, 767, 773, 777

HIGH MINERAL FOODS - 613, 615, 616, 617, 618, 620, 622, 623, 624, 626, 627, 628, 629, 633, 638, 641

Sample Meal Planning
Some recipe combinations that go with this diet:

A FAMILY MEAL - 62, 189, 764, 780, 419

A WEEKEND PICNIC -49, 500, 716, 420, 423

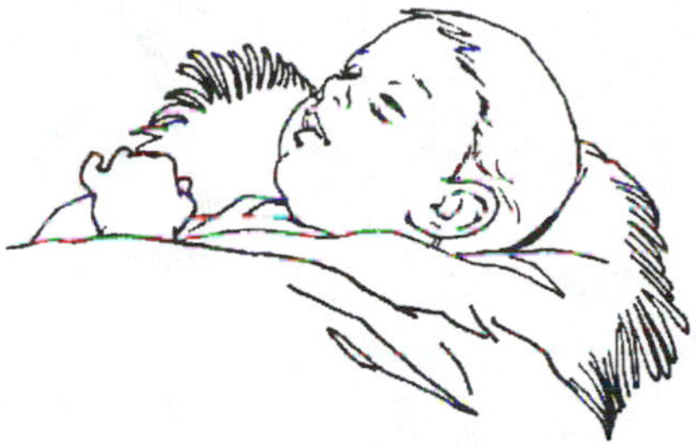

A HEARTY WINTER MEAL - 67, 219, 757, 619, 776

A LIGHT SUMMER MEAL - 51, 783, 414, 221

A SPECIAL DINNER FOR TWO - 627, 53, 554, 453, 238, 430

AN EASY WEEK NIGHT DINNER -765, 219, 743, 52, 781

AN EASY RISING BREAKFAST - 715, 429, 704

Love
is not just a happy moment,
but the journey of a lifetime.
Love changes
everything.

*S*ome people tip-toe
through life so they can
arrive at death safely.
Live life enthusiastically!

Eating for Heart & Circulatory Health

Cardiovascular disease remains the number one killer in civilized nations today. Diet remains its single most influential factor. Not one food, or aspect of diet, but the whole array of high calorie, low nutrient foods and eating habits is the cause. Fried foods, refined low fiber foods, high fats, pasteurized dairy products, too much salt, sugar, coffee, tobacco, alcohol, red meat and processed meats, all contribute to clogged, reduced arteries, high cholesterol, high blood pressure and heart attacks. Fortunately, almost all of these circulatory problems can be treated and prevented with improved diet and nutrition. You can carve a better future with your own knife and fork, than with a lifetime of dependence on drugs, pacemakers, or multiple surgeries.
Life style changes are not easy, and they take time to accomplish, but this choice is infinitely preferable to the quality of life, and must take place for there to be permanent results.

The first diet in this heart health program is for those of you who have survived a heart attack or major heart surgery. Coming back is tough. Sticking to a new lifestyle that changes the way you eat, exercise, handle stress and the details of your life is a challenge. This diet is a rehabilitation outline for a healthier heart and arteries, with reassurance about the fears usually felt in regard to recurrence.

The second diet stage is a low calorie, high nutrition diet, with plenty of complex carbohydrates from grains, vegetables and fresh fruits. It includes some fish, seafoods and poultry instead of red meats. It is low in dairy foods, and avoids refined sugars and flours of all kinds. This diet is beneficial for people with less acute but still serious problems, such as high blood pressure, Alzheimer's disease and hardening of the arteries. It is also excellent for other less-major circulatory malfunctions, such as cold hands and feet, hearing loss, high stress and tension, overweight, high cholesterol and varicose veins.
In general, high calorie fatty, salty, and sugary foods are responsible for cardiovascular problems. A whole foods diet relieves them.
This way of eating will help improve and prevent the following problems:
❧CONGESTIVE HEART FAILURE, ANGINA and OTHER HEART CONDITIONS ❧BLOOD PRESSURE IMBALANCE ❧CHOLESTEROL BUILD-UP ❧ARTERIO and ATHERO-SCLEROSIS ❧EASY BRUISING ❧STRESS and TENSION ❧BLOOD CLOTS, PHLEBITIS, EMBOLISM ❧FIBRILLATION and ARRHYTHMIA ❧ALZHEIMER'S DISEASE ❧EXCESSIVE BLEEDING ❧POOR CIRCULATION ❧HEMORRHOIDS, VARICOSE & SPIDER VEINS ❧

- ❧ Eat plenty of fish. Cold water fish oils have a beneficial effect on blood viscosity and its propensity to clot, with preventive effects on arteriosclerosis and heart attacks.
- ❧ Add exercise as a nutrient to your life; a brisk walk every day possible.
- ❧ Do deep breathing exercises every morning to stimulate the brain, reduce stress, and oxygenate the body for the day.
- ❧ Use dry skin brushing, alternating hot and cold hydrotherapy (page 203), and smaller meals with a little white wine, to increase circulation.
- ❧ Consciously add relaxation and a good daily laugh to your life. A positive mental outlook can do wonders for your heart and your well-being.

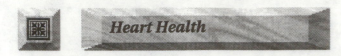

Diet Change and Rehabilitation After a Heart Attack

The following diet program is especially for those of you who have survived a heart attack or major heart surgery. Beginning, and sticking to, a new lifestyle that changes almost everything about the way you eat, exercise, handle stress, down to the smallest details of your life, is a challenge. The mini-rehabilitation program below is a blueprint you can use with confidence. It has proven successful against heart disease recurrence. This way of eating reduces dietary fats at least 30% or more, includes cold water fish and seafood for high Omega-3 oils, emphasizes mineral rich foods, particularly potassium and magnesium for good cardiotonic action, adds plenty of complex carbohydrates from whole grains and vegetables for energy and stamina, has fiber-rich foods for a clean system, and subscribes to a little white wine before dinner for relaxation and digestion.

Note: This diet should be followed for one to three months after an attack or surgery, and may be returned to at any time as needed.

On rising: have some grapefruit, apple or grape juice;
or 2 lemons squeezed in a glass of water with honey.

Breakfast: have some fresh fruit, such as grapes or pears, or tropical fruits for extra potassium. Top with a little yogurt if desired;
and make a mix of 2 TBS. <u>each:</u> lecithin granules, toasted wheat germ, brewer's yeast, sesame seeds, blackstrap molasses and high Omega-3 flax oil. Take 2 teasp. of the mixture every morning. Stir into yogurt, sprinkle on buckwheat pancakes, cereal, or whole grain toast. Add a little maple syrup, honey or apple juice to sweeten if desired.

Mid-morning: have a green drink page 240), or Sun CHLORELLA or Green Foods GREEN ESSENCE, or Crystal Star ENERGY GREEN™ drink with 1 teasp. Bragg's LIQUID AMINOS added;
or a high potassium drink, such as Potassium Broth (page 240), or Vital Health WHITE BIRCH MINERAL WATER or other herbal potassium source drink supplement;
or fresh carrot juice;
and/or an herb tea, such as spearmint or peppermint, or Crystal Star DAILY BIOFLAVONOID & C SUPPORT DRINK™, or HEARTSEASE/ CIRCU-CLEANSE™ TEA.

Lunch: have some steamed or baked onions, **and** a cup of miso soup with sea veggies snipped on top;
or have a fresh green salad with nuts, seeds, sprouts, and a lemon/oil dressing;
or some baked tofu with brown rice or millet and broccoli;
or a baked potato with yogurt or kefir cheese, and a leafy green salad;
or a vegetable/grain or bean soup with a sandwich on whole grain bread;
or a light seafood salad with vegetable pasta.

Mid-afternoon: have a relaxing herb tea such as alfalfa/mint tea, or Crystal Star RELAX TEA™ with some raw crunchy veggies or whole grain crackers and a soy, or veggie and yogurt dip;
or the following circulation stimulating drink: Mix 1 cup tomato juice, 6 TBS. wheat germ oil, 1 cup lemon juice, and 1 TB. brewer's yeast.

Dinner: have a vegetarian casserole with whole grain pasta or brown rice, veggies, and a light sauce;
or baked or broiled fish, (especially salmon and swordfish) or shellfish, (especially oysters and scallops) with brown rice and some steamed veggies;
or have a tofu and whole grain loaf with a green salad;
or some steamed or baked veggies with whole grain muffins or cornbread, and a little butter.

Before bed: have some fresh or dried stewed fruits in a little apple juice;
or a VEGEX yeast paste broth, or a hot Crystal Star SYSTEM STRENGTH DRINK™.

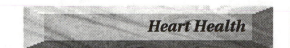

❋ *Supplements and Herbs for the Heart Rehabilitation Diet:*

There are many excellent supplements for cardiovascular improvement. We list the major ones by relevant category. Consider your own individual needs when you choose.

Wheat germ oil 2 to 4 TBS. daily
Vitamin E with selenium, 4 to 800IU daily
CO Q10 30mg. 2x daily   ➤   for energy and tissue oxygenation
Carnitine 250mg. 2x daily
Vitamin C 3 to 5000mg. daily, with bioflavonoids

Niacin 500mg. daily
Chromium picolinate 200mcg. daily
Omega-3 flax or cold water fish oils 3 teasp. daily   ➤   to clean and clear arteries
Oral chelation, 2 packs daily.

Sun CHLORELLA or liquid chlorophyll daily
Hawthorn extract $1/2$ dropperful 2x daily   ➤   to regulate heart and blood pressure
Siberian ginseng extract or tea 2x daily
Cayenne/garlic capsules 4 to 6 daily, as an alternative to the much-touted aspirin therapy. Chronic aspirin use can have side effects, such as stomach irritation, ringing in the ears, and metabolic imbalance. If you choose to take aspirin, take it at low dosage. Small doses are just as effective.

❋ *Body work for Heart Rehabilitation:*

✚ Take <u>regular</u>, not strenuous, exercise every day, such as a brisk half hour walk, or a short swim. Do deep breathing exercises, and set aside a conscious relaxation time every day to lower stress.

✚ Stop smoking. Nicotine can be lethal as a blood vessel constricting agent.

✚ Eat smaller meals more often. NO large heavy meals.

✚ Take alternating warm and cool showers to stimulate circulation. Use a dry skin brush or rough towel afterwards for tissue toner.

Quick Heart Rehabilitation Checkpoints

❤ **Reduce fats to 15% of your diet; less if possible. Limit poly-unsaturates (margarines, oils) to 10%. Add mono-unsaturates, such as olive oil, avocado, nut, and seed oils.**
❤ Have several servings of cold water fish or seafood every week for high Omega-3 oils.
❤ **Have a fresh green salad every day.**
❤ Have a glass of white wine before dinner for relaxation, better digestion and to raise HDLs.
❤ **Add fiber-rich foods for a clean system, such as oat or rice bran, fresh fruits and vegetables.**
❤ Keep the system alkaline with such foods as leafy greens, brown rice, miso and sea vegetables.
❤ **Eat plenty of complex carbohydrates: broccoli, peas, whole grain breads, vegetable pastas, potatoes, sprouts, tofu, brown rice and other whole grains.**

♥ Eat potassium rich foods for cardiotonic activity; fresh spinach and chard, broccoli, bananas, sea vegetables, molasses, papayas, apricots, cantaloupe, mushrooms, tomatoes and yams; or take a high potassium drink regularly, such as Potassium Broth (pg. 240), Crystal Star SYSTEM STRENGTH DRINK™, or Vital Health WHITE BIRCH MINERAL WATER; (a serving of high potassium fruits or vegetables offers about 400mg. of potassium; a serving of one of the above potassium drinks offers approximately 1000-1250mg. of potassium).

♥ Eat copper rich foods for clear arteries; oysters, clams, crab, fish, brewer's yeast, nuts and seeds.

♥ **Choose several of the following supplements as daily micro-nutrients:**
Anti-oxidants: Wheat germ oil (raises body oxygen by 30%), vitamin E with selenium, CoQ 10.
<u>*Cardio-tonics:*</u> Hawthorn extract, cayenne and garlic capsules, Niacin 500mg.
<u>*Anticholesterol:*</u> oral chelation with EDTA, ginger rt., butcher's broom, taurine, guar gum.
<u>*Regulation & stability:*</u> green drinks, evening primrose oil, carnitine 500mg., magnesium.
<u>*Clear arteries:*</u> Solaray CHROMIACIN, selenium, Omega-3 flax or fish oils, oral chelation.
<u>*Balanced blood chemistry:*</u> Chromium picolinate, Ester C 550mg. with bioflavonods.

❋ *Sample Recipes For Heart & Circulation Restoration*
By section and recipe number:

SALADS HOT & COLD - all

LOW-FAT & VERY LOW-FAT DISHES - all

LOW CHOLESTEROL MEALS - all

SUGAR FREE SWEET TREATS - 415, 416, 417, 419, 420, 423, 426, 427, 428, 430, 432, 439, 440, 443, 444

FISH & SEAFOODS - 535, 536, 537, 538, 543, 544, 547, 552, 553, 554, 559, 560, 563, 564, 567, 568, 569

MINERAL RICH RECIPES - 612, 613, 614, 615, 616, 618, 620, 621, 623, 625, 627, 641, 647, 651, 659, 662

HIGH FIBER RECIPES - 785, 789, 791, 792, 794, 796, 799, 801, 802, 806, 807, 817, 818, 819, 820, 823, 824

SOUPS - LIQUID SALADS - all

❋ *Sample Menu Plans*
Some recipe combinations that go with this diet:

A SPECIAL DINNER FOR TWO - 253, 787, 809, 306, 441

AN EASY WEEKNIGHT DINNER - 317, 462, 443

A HEARTY WINTER MEAL - 801, 792, 428, 315

A LIGHT SUMMER MEAL - 303, 459, 264, 420

A FAMILY MEAL - 229, 472, 331, 432

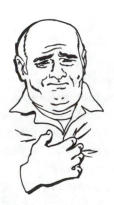

Heart Disease and High Blood Pressure Prevention Diet

The following diet is for long term heart, circulatory and low cholesterol health. It's easy to live with, but has all the necessary elements to keep arteries and veins clear, and heart action regular and strong. It emphasizes fresh (60%), and whole fiber foods; high mineral foods with lots of potassium, magnesium and copper; oxygen rich foods from green vegetables, sprouts and wheat germ (wheat germ oil can raise the oxygen level of the heart as much as 30%), and solid vegetable source protein. Conscious attention must be paid at first to avoid red meats, caffeine, fried and fatty foods, soft drinks, refined pastry, salty foods and prepared meats, but the rewards are high - a longer, healthier life - and control of your life.

On rising: take a high protein or high vitamin/mineral drink such as Nutri-Tech ALL 1 or Nature's Plus SPIRUTEIN in orange or grapefruit juice.

Breakfast: Make a mix of 2 TBS. <u>each</u>; lecithin granules, wheat germ, brewer's yeast, honey, and sesame seeds; sprinkle 2 teasp. every morning on fresh fruits, such as apricots, peaches, apples or nectarines, or mix with yogurt;
and/or have a poached or baked egg with bran muffins or whole grain toast and kefir cheese;
or some whole grain cereal or pancakes with a little maple syrup.

Mid-morning: have a green drink (pg. 240ff.), or Sun CHLORELLA, a potassium drink (pg. 240), Crystal Star SYSTEM STRENGTH DRINK™, or all natural V-8 juice (pg. 242) or Green Foods GREEN ESSENCE drink; **and/or** some crunchy raw veggies with a kefir cheese or yogurt dip;
and/or a cup of miso soup with sea veggies snipped on top.

Lunch: have one cup daily of fenugreek tea with the following additions: 1 teasp. honey, 1 teasp. wheat germ oil, 1 teasp. lecithin granules or liquid;
then have a tofu and spinach salad with some sprouts and bran muffins;
or a high protein salad or sandwich with nuts & seeds and a black bean or lentil soup;
or an avocado, low-fat cheese or soy cheese sandwich on whole grain bread;
or or a seafood and whole grain pasta salad with a light tomato sauce;
or a light veggie omelet and small green salad;
or some grilled or braised vegetables with an olive oil dressing and brown rice.

Mid-afternoon: have a cup of mint tea, or Crystal Star ROYAL MU™ tonic tea;
and/or a cup of miso soup with a hard boiled egg, or whole grain crackers;
or a glass of carrot juice, or Personal V-8 (pg. 242).

Dinner: have a broccoli quiche with a whole grain or chapati crust; and a cup of onion soup;
or a baked seafood dish with brown rice and peas;
or a whole grain and steamed vegetable and tofu casserole;
or an oriental stir-fry with light soup and rice;
or grilled fish or seafood and a small green salad and baked potato;
or a salmon or veggie souffle with a light sauce and salad.

Before bed: have another cup of miso soup, or a cup of VEGEX yeast paste broth;
or some chamomile tea;
or apple or pear juice.

✓ A little white wine before dinner is fine for relaxation, digestion and tension relief.

✓Avoid commercial antacids, that neutralize natural stomach acid, and invite the body to produce even more acid, thus aggravating stress and tension.

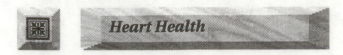

✱ Supplements and Herbal Aids for the Heart Disease Prevention Diet:

❖ Siberian Ginseng extract caps, 2000mg, or extract, $1/2$ dropperful daily.

❖ Vitamin C 3000mg. daily with bioflavonoids, or Crystal Star DAILY BIOFLAVONOID SUPPORT˙.

❖ Evening Primrose oil caps, 2 to 4 daily.

❖ Niacin, 250mg. 2x daily , with PABA 500mg. daily.

❖ High Omega-3 oils, from flax or cold water fish, 1000mg. daily.

❖ Sun CHLORELLA, 1 packet granules, or 15 tabs daily.

❖ Vitamin E with selenium 400IU daily.

✱ Bodywork for long term heart disease prevention:

✜ Regular exercise is a key to heart health. It strengthens the heart and other muscles, and increases aerobic capacity. Beyond these benefits, exercise also improves body chemistry, changing the way the body metabolizes fats. Go dancing, swim, walk, jog, ride a bike cross country ski, etc. The enjoyable sport/exercise list is almost endless.

✱ Sample Recipes for Long Term Heart Health:
By section and recipe number:

BREAKFAST & BRUNCH - all

ORIENTAL & LIGHT MACROBIOTIC EATING - all

LOW-FAT & VERY LOW-FAT DISHES - all

LOW CHOLESTEROL MEALS - all

SOUPS - LIQUID SALADS - all

SANDWICHES - SALADS IN BREAD - 473, 478, 484, 485, 488, 490, 491, 492, 494, 498, 499, 500.

STIR-FRIES - all

HIGH PROTEIN WITHOUT MEAT - 698, 699, 700, 701, 702, 706, 714, 715, 716, 719, 720, 723, 724, 729.

COMPLEX CARBOHYDRATES FOR ENERGY - 743, 744, 747, 749, 751, 760, 763, 766, 780, 782, 783.

✽ ***Sample Menu Plans***
Some recipe combinations that go with this diet:

A SPECIAL DINNER FOR TWO - 252, 269, 185, 267, 290

LUNCH FOR TWO - 504, 283/284, 298

AN EASY RISING BREAKFAST - 75, 96, 98, 261

AN EASY WEEKNIGHT DINNER - 522, 127, 451

A WEEKEND PICNIC - 714, 500, 119, 240

A LIGHT SUMMER MEAL - 515, 263, 450

SUNDAY BRUNCH - 695, 257, 74, 123

A HEARTY WINTER MEAL - 781, 167, 702, 134

AN ALL HORS D'OEUVRES PARTY - 482, 110, 111, 125, 905, 205

GREAT OUTDOOR EATING - 874, 876, 880, 884, 886, 888, 890, 893, 894, 895, 896, 901, 907, 908, 909

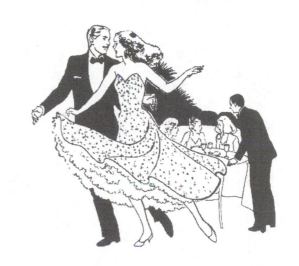

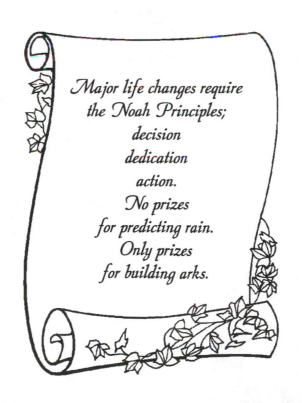

Major life changes require the Noah Principles;
decision
dedication
action.
No prizes
for predicting rain.
Only prizes
for building arks.

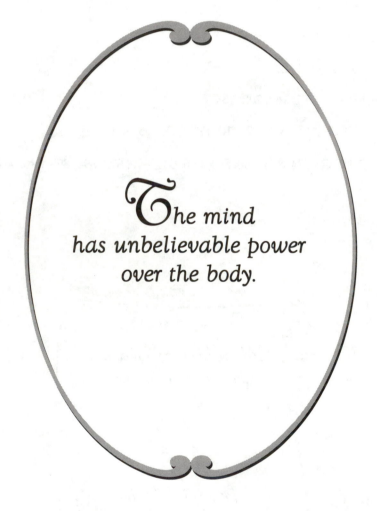

The mind
has unbelievable power
over the body.

Eating With Your Brain In Mind

The brain is an incredibly sensitive organ. Alertness, concentration, memory, and creativity all depend on the quality of nourishment you give your brain. The brain can use nutrients with far more synergistic effects than those same nutrients in other areas of the body; and it is so metabolically active that it needs almost every known nutrient for optimal function. The brain is extremely sensitive to nutritional deficiency, and can noticeably respond to the various nutrients that you take in throughout the day. Some foods cause anger, depression, fear, irritability and irrational emotions. Severe deficiencies can even cause severe mental illness. Clinical tests have shown that two-thirds of mental health problems are physically based, in poor diet.

The brain is also the primary health maintenance organ. When it is well-nourished long enough, even grave mental problems can straighten themselves out. Optimal nutrition can slow and even reverse many aging signs, such as alertness and coordination. The right nutrients stabilize emotional reactions and temperament.

Diet also controls neurotransmitter production, learning, memory, sleep, motor and I.Q. functions. Brain activity is therefore so directly related to the daily nutrients we eat, that sometimes results of a diet improvement can be spectacular.

The following diet to improve mental activity is rich in brain foods - supplying potassium, amino acid protein precursors, B vitamins for choline, and complex carbohydrates for glycogen production. It is low in fats and gooey foods that clog, and free of refined foods that cause blood sugar imbalance. It emphasizes small frequent meals instead of heavy meals that siphon brain fuel and energy away for digestion.

Oxygen is a key nutrient in this diet. The brain uses 20% of the body's oxygen supply. Good red blood flow from the liver and spleen keep brain oxygen high. This diet has plenty of oxygenating foods, like wheat germ, unsaturated oils, fish and soy foods like tofu. The recommended aerobic exercise becomes a nutrient in itself, because it brings oxygen to the brain and relieves mind and body stress. Ten deep "brain breaths" every morning do wonders to start brain activity for the day. An alternating hot and cold shower can bring additional blood to the brain almost immediately.

Consciously try to avoid stress in your life. Stress is one of the most severe deterrents to brain health. We also recommend eliminating tobacco, heavy alcohol and marijuana from your lifestyle because they all inhibit the brain's release of vasopressin, which results in impaired memory, attention, concentration and reaction time.

On the other hand, cheerfulness, optimism and relaxation increase brain function. The brain can actually be expanded with challenging concentration activities such as memory games, chess, and crossword puzzles by promoting new projections from existing nerve cells. Reading, writing and new experiences also stimulate enhanced thought.

This diet has shown encouraging results in improving several areas of poor brain, motor and memory function, including:

STRESS, ANXIETY and DEPRESSION HYPOTHYROIDISM and PARATHYROID DISEASE NERVOUS TENSION MENTAL RETARDATION and DOWNS SYNDROME EXHAUSTION and MENTAL BURNOUT ALZHEIMER'S DISEASE and SENILITY FROM PREMATURE AGING EPILEPSY INSOMNIA AUTISM and HYPERKINESIS SCHIZOPHRENIA, PSYCHOSIS and MENTAL ILLNESS NARCOLEPTIC SLEEP DISORDER

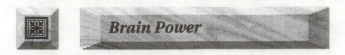
A Diet For More Mental Activity and Capability

The brain responds incredibly quickly to increased nutrition and oxygenating foods. This diet is structured with fast response in mind, and is not in gradual stages. Rather, it immediately offers a long term way of eating for better brain function and permanent help for memory centers.

On rising: take a NutriTech ALL 1, Nature's Plus SPIRUTEIN, Sun CHLORELLA or Crystal Star ENERGY GREEN DRINK™ in juice or water, with 1 teasp. Bragg's LIQUID AMINOS added.
✔Now is a good time to take the supplements you have chosen to increase brain activity. See supplements section at the end of this diet for suggestions.

Breakfast: have some low-fat yogurt with 1 teasp. each wheat germ, lecithin granules, sesame seeds, and brewer's yeast, **and** some fresh fruit in season;
or whole grain cereal or pancakes with a little maple syrup, apple juice, vanilla soy milk, or honey and fresh fruit;
or a poached, baked, or soft boiled egg with whole grain toast or english muffin and a little butter;
or oatmeal with maple syrup and an apple.

Mid-morning: have a green drink (pg. 240) or Sun CHLORELLA or Crystal Star SYSTEM STRENGTH DRINK™;
or a potassium broth or essence (pg. 240);
or an herb tea such as gotu kola or Crystal Star CREATIVI-TEA™, or RAINFOREST ENERGY TEA™;
or low-fat yogurt with nut and seed toppings;
or miso soup with sea vegetables snipped on top and whole grain chips or crackers;
or an apple and a small bottle of mineral water.

Lunch: have a fresh green salad with sprouts and some brown rice, or a baked potato with a light, low-fat sauce;
or baked, broiled seafood or fish with a miso soup or other light broth, or a seafood salad with whole grain pasta;
or roast turkey salad or sandwich on whole grain bread, with a little mayonnaise and low-fat cheese;
or tofu with steamed veggies and brown rice or millet or bulgar;
or any whole grain and veggie sandwich.

Mid-afternoon: This is another good time to take supplementation for brain enhancement - to pick you up from the afternoon blahs and keep you alert for the rest of the day.
Have a refreshing energizing herb tea, such as Crystal Star MEDITATION™ TEA for calm mental energy, or HIGH ENERGY™ TEA for outward energy, or CHINESE ROYAL MU™ TEA for body systems support energy, or a ginseng or rosemary leaf tea;
and/or a low-fat yogurt with fruit or nuts;
or crunchy raw veggies with a low-fat dip and another small bottle of mineral water;
or some fresh fruit with low-fat cheese or soy cheese;

Dinner: steamed veggies with tofu and brown rice or other whole grain, or vegetable pasta;
and baked or broiled seafood if desired, with a fresh green salad or light soup;
or baked, broiled or roasted fish or chicken or turkey with a green salad and light dressing;
or a light vegetable quiche or vegetarian pizza on a chapati or pita crust;
or an oriental stir-fry with brown rice and a light soup.

Before Bed: Brain rest is a big part of brain health. Have a relaxing cup of hot herb tea, such as chamomile, or Crystal Star RELAX™ TEA;
or a cup of hot VEGEX yeast broth for relaxation and B vitamins.

❋ Supplements and Herbal Aids for Better Brain Activity:

Take brain nourishing and stimulating supplements on a regular basis. Don't wait until it really matters, because it always does. In general, brain supplements should be taken on an empty stomach.

❖ Keep brain oxygen levels high with antioxidants: CoQ 10 - 60mg. daily, vitamin E 400IU with selenium, B_{15} (DMG) 2 daily, wheat germ oil (two teasp. daily provide as much available oxygen to the body as an oxygen tent for 30 minutes), germanium 25 to 30mg daily, and carnitine 500mg. daily.

❖ Keep electrical and nerve connections healthy with ginkgo biloba extract, glutamine 500mg, evening primrose oil caps 1000mg. daily, and niacin 250mg twice daily.

❖ Keep circulation free and flowing, and nervous system healthy, with lecithin, choline, high Omega-3 fish or flax oils, and siberian ginseng extract; and a B Complex 100mg. daily.

❖ Feed the brain with minerals; particularly potassium in liquid form, such as Twin Lab LIQUID K, Vital Health WHITE BIRCH MINERAL WATER, or Crystal Star SYSTEM STRENGTH DRINK™; magnesium and zinc; iodine from kelp or Crystal Star IODINE THERAPY™ CAPS or EXTRACT; and trace minerals, such as those from Mezotrace SEA MINERAL COMPLEX .

❖ A rosemary stuffed sleep pillow is excellent for memory center improvement.

❋ Bodywork for Better Brain Activity:

✚ Take some mild exercise every day for oxygen uptake. Practice deep brain breathing every morning. A brisk walk or ocean swim (for high potassium) are particularly good.

✚ Avoid sugar and refined foods. They affect the brain first. Avoid aluminum products, such as deodorants with aluminum chlor-hydrate, and aluminum pots and pans.

❈

❋ Suggested Recipes That Work With This Diet By section and recipe number:

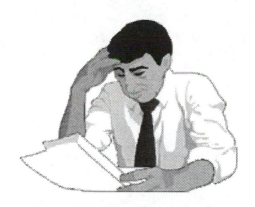

LOW CHOLESTEROL MEALS - all

FISH & SEAFOODS - all

TOFU FOR YOU - all

HIGH MINERAL FOODS - all

PROTEIN WITHOUT MEAT - 698, 700, 699, 701, 704, 706, 710, 713, 715, 717, 718, 719, 733, 738, 742

HIGH COMPLEX CARBOHYDRATES FOR ENERGY - all

HIGH FIBER RECIPES - all

*Authentic power
is built by paying dues.
It's built step by step,
choice by choice.
It cannot be prayed or
meditated into being.
It must be earned.*

Food For Men;
Strengthening the Male Body

Today's fast paced, high stress lifestyle seems to demand that men be Supermen. A man must be strong physically during workouts and sports, supportive emotionally in relationships, balanced under stress, mentally creative and quick, and sexually keen and virile. Diet and exercise are the main pillars supporting a man's health and energy. Both are woefully deficient in the modern American man's life. Poor farming methods and processed foods have made us one of earth's most nutritionally deficient nations. Our hectic, yet sedentary lives don't allow for exercise unless a very conscious effort is made.

Lack of exercise for a man is as great a health risk as high blood pressure, high cholesterol, or even smoking. In fact, regular exercise is a nutrient in itself for the male system. Men need exercise for weight control and general health to a greater degree than women. Heart muscle and tone can be lost if weekly exercise is not included as a regular part of life. To maintain a healthy level of fitness, a man should exercise at least three times a week for 20 to 30 minutes each time. His chosen exercise should raise his heart rate at least 65 to 70% of its capacity - to the point of breathlessness for 5 minutes. A fit male body needs vigorous concentrations of metabolic precursors, such as vitamin, minerals and enzymes for optimum performance. Enhanced nutrition can improve strength, endurance and muscle tissue, and help to maintain low body fat.

An optimal diet for male metabolism requires adequate quantity of food, but not high fats. A man needs more fiber, protein and complex carbohydrates than a woman. His diet should include animal proteins in moderation, like occasional eggs, chicken, turkey, low-fat dairy products, and sea foods. A diet rich in amino acid containing foods provides easily convertible proteins. Zinc-rich foods encourage prostate and reproductive system health. Men also seem to thrive on more cooked than raw foods for the stability of denser, more solid nutrients. Those in whole grains, beans, rice and soy products offer longer endurance and increased sensitivity.

The diet on these pages contains the necessary nutrients that reinforce male energy. (See FOOD, SEX & FERTILITY, page 101, for the differences in male and female dietary needs). The meals are targeted for the strength, vigor and stamina needs of a man's body. They rely in particular on heart and circulatory needs, because arterial clogging often leads to impotence.

This diet is low in fat, high in fiber, strong on exercise. It can be used as a health insurance policy against many health problems facing men today. Its main advantage is that just a little effort and shift in dietary emphasis can definitely change the way a man feel, think and act.

Problems that this diet can help include:
❧COLO-RECTAL and PANCREATIC CANCER ❧IMPOTENCE ❧PARATHYROID DISEASE ❧HIGH BLOOD PRESSURE ❧OVERWEIGHT ❧STRESS ❧PROSTATE INFLAMMATION ❧HEMORRHOIDS ❧ADRENAL EXHAUSTION ❧LOW LIBIDO ❧

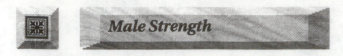

Stage One; A Short Cleansing Diet:

If there are prostate, sexual potency or glandular/hormone problems, a short 3 to 7 day liquid cleansing diet is recommended to clean out sediment or calcification, and to alkalize the bloodstream. If system strength without a beginning cleanse is desired, start with the Stage Two Diet following.

On rising: take 2 lemons **or** 2 teasp. cider vinegar in water with 1 teasp. maple syrup each morning;

Breakfast: take a glass of organic apple juice;
or a potassium broth or essence with 1 teasp. Bragg's LIQUID AMINOS.

Mid-morning: have a glass of fresh carrot juice;
and/or a vegetable mineral drink, such as Green Foods GREEN ESSENCE, or Crystal Star ENERGY GREEN™.

Lunch: have another glass of organic apple juice;
and/or a green drink, such as pineapple/alfalfa sprouts with 1 teasp. spirulina powder.

Mid-afternoon: have another glass of organic apple juice,
and/or a cup of white oak bark tea
or Crystal Star ADR-ACTIVE™ EXTRACT drops in a cup of water.

Dinner: have another glass of organic apple juice;
and/or a cup of Crystal Star CHINESE ROYAL MU™ TEA,

Before bed: have a pineapple/papaya juice, or pineapple/coconut juice;
or a cup of chamomile or alfalfa/mint tea.

❋ *Supplements and Herbs for the Cleansing Diet:*

❖ Take ascorbate vtamin C or Ester C crystals during this cleanse; $1/2$ teasp. in water or juice 4 to 6x daily to bowel tolerance.

❖ Increase circulatory function and activity with niacin 500mg. daily, and CoQ 10 - 30mg. twice daily.

❖ Take a liquid mineral supplement, especially rich in potassium, magnesium and zinc, such as Crystal Star SYSTEM STRENGTH DRINK™, or Twin Lab LIQUID K PLUS for a month.

❖ Avoid chemical anti-histimines and other drugs, alcohol, caffeine, tobacco, and carbonated drinks.

❋ *Bodywork for the Cleansing Diet:*

✚ Get some early morning sunlight on the body and genitals every day possible for general sexual health and to help prevent prostate problems.

✚ Take some mild exercise daily, breathing deeply for aerobic improvement.

Stage Two; Diet to Rebuild the Male System:

This diet should be used for 2 weeks to one month, and is a modified macrobiotic program for adding strength while cleansing. It is very high in vegetable and whole grain fiber for alkalizing, and contains a high percentage of raw foods, essential fatty acids and zinc sources. Use only unsaturated oils in this diet.

On rising: take a glass of cider vinegar and water with 1 teasp. honey, **and** a vitamin/mineral drink, such as ALL 1 or Nature's Plus SPIRUTEIN.

Breakfast: make a mix of 2 TBS. **each:** lecithin granules, wheat germ, brewer's yeast, pumpkin seeds, and oat bran. Sprinkle 1 or 2 TBS. onto a whole grain cereal, or mix into yogurt every morning;
and have some fresh fruit, particularly apples, if desired.

Mid-morning: have an apple or other fresh fruit;
and/or a green drink (page 240) or Sun CHLORELLA, or Crystal Star ENERGY GREEN DRINK™;
and/or a cup of chamomile tea with whole grain crackers or raw vegetables and kefir cheese.

Lunch: have a green leafy salad with a lemon/oil or Italian dressing. Include celery, avocados, nuts and seeds;
and a cup of miso soup, with Chinese rice noodles and sea vegetables, or whole grain crackers;
or a tofu and brown rice casserole with steamed veggies;
or a high protein sandwich with vegetables on whole grain bread;
or a lentil or black bean soup, with a whole grain and vegetable pasta salad.

Mid-afternoon: have a cup of chamomile tea, and/or apples, and **a daily handful of pumpkin seeds**;
or a cup of herb tea, such as Crystal Star CHINESE ROYAL MU™, or MEDITATION TEA™,
and some whole grain crackers with a soy spread or vegetable dip.

Dinner: have some steamed vegetables with brown rice, cous cous or millet.
or a baked or broiled fish or seafood with a small salad;
or a baked potato with an unsaturated oil dressing, and a green leafy salad;
or a vegetable casserole or quiche with whole grain crust;
or a whole grain or vegetable pasta salad, hot or cold;
or a large dinner salad with brown rice, yogurt or vinaigrette dressing, toasted nut/seed toppings.

Before bed: have another cup of chamomile tea, or a cup of VEGEX yeast paste broth (1 teasp. in a cup of hot water);
or a cup of herb tea, such as Crystal Star RELAX TEA™.

❋ *Supplements and Herbs to Rebuild the Male System:*

❖ Take zinc, 75 to 100mg. with vitamin E 400IU daily for reproductive system support.

❖ Take ascorbate vitamin C 3000mg. daily with CoQ 10, 60mg. for antioxidant/immune support.

❖ Take Omega-3 fish oils, 3 daily for unsaturated fatty acids and circulatory health.

❖ Herbs for male vitality include damiana, Siberian ginseng and dandelion; try Crystal Star GINSENG 6 DEFENSE RESTORATIVE TEA™ with SUPER MAN'S ENERGY TONIC™ or MALE PERFORMANCE™ CAPS, for improved gland balance.

❋ *Bodywork for Rebuilding the Male System:*

✚ Take alternating hot and cold hydrotherapy showers each morning for circulatory/organ health.

✚ Add some aerobic exercise to your daily walk. Exercise for the male system is a nutrient in itself.

✚ Get some early morning sunlight on the body every day possible.

✚ Avoid smoking and secondary smoke; it contributes to poor immune response and circulatory disease.

❋ *Sample Recipes For Rebuilding The Male System*
By section and recipe number:

HEALTHY DRINKS, JUICES & WATERS - 43, 55, 60, 61, 63, 65, 66, 68, 71

BREAKFAST & BRUNCH - all

SALADS HOT & COLD - all

SOUPS, LIQUID SALADS - all

LOW CHOLESTEROL MEALS - all

SANDWICHES - SALADS IN BREAD - 4773, 477, 480, 483, 486, 489, 490, 491, 493, 495, 498, 500

HIGH MINERAL FOODS - 612, 613, 614, 618, 622, 624, 629, 631, 638, 639, 643, 646, 647, 653, 656, 661

HIGH PROTEIN WITHOUT MEAT - 695, 697, 704, 708, 712, 715, 719, 722, 726, 727, 730, 732, 738, 740

COMPLEX CARBOHYDRATES FOR ENERGY - 743, 745, 757, 758, 759, 764, 771, 773, 778, 781, 784

HIGH FIBER RECIPES - 789, 793, 795, 797, 800, 802, 806, 808, 809, 810, 811, 816, 817, 818, 820, 822, 824

❋ *Sample Menu Plans*
Some recipe combinations that work with this diet:

A WEEKEND PICNIC - 477, 716, 824, 107

A HEARTY WINTER MEAL - 456, 706, 104

A LIGHT SUMMER MEAL - 454, 818, 660, 53

A SUNDAY BRUNCH - 695, 727, 795, 662, 43 or 48

AN EASY RISING BREAKFAST - 715, 98, 819, 792

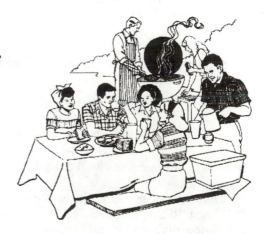

Long Range Optimal Health for the Male Body:

This diet should be used for at least 1 to 3 months. It lays the groundwork for maintaining male system health and good immune response. This third stage remains high in vegetable fiber and grains, adds more proteins, emphasizes low salts and sugars, and avoids refined carbohydrates. It is a strength foundation diet, abundant in complex carbohydrates and high mineral foods.

On rising: take a vitamin/mineral or high protein drink, such as Nutri-Tech ALL 1 or Nature' s Plus SPI-RUTEIN, or make up a soy protein drink in water or juice and add 1 TB. molasses, 1 teasp. spirulina, and 1 teasp. lecithin granules.
✔Now is a good time to take the daily supplements of your choice.

Breakfast: make up a mix of 2 TBS. **each**; bee pollen, sesame seeds, pumpkin seeds, brewer's yeast, wheat germ and oat bran. Sprinkle some daily over a whole grain granola or muesli, or mix into yogurt and top these cereals;
and add fresh fruit if desired.
or poached, baked or soft boiled eggs with whole grain toast;
or whole grain pancakes with maple syrup or a nut butter;
or pineapple/coconut, or pineapple/papaya-juice, and a bowl of fresh fruits.

Mid-morning: have an apple or other fresh fruit;
or some crisp raw veggies with kefir cheese;
or some whole grain crackers or corn chips and a veggie/yogurt dip;
and/or a green drink, or Sun CHLORELLA drink; or a bottle of mineral water, or a cup of herb tea, such as Crystal Star HEARTSEASE HBP TEA™, or HIGH ENERGY TEA™.
✔Now is another good time to take supplements.

Lunch: have some marinated, baked tofu and millet or brown rice, and a light soup;
or a vegetable protein or roast turkey sandwich on whole grain bread with a cup of light soup;
or a hearty but low-fat Mexican beans and rice meal;
or a seafood and shellfish stew or hot salad with pasta;
or a vegetarian pizza on a chapati or whole grain crust.

Mid-afternoon: have a cup of relaxed energy herb tea, such as chamomile or ginseng, or Crystal Star MEDITATION™ TEA or CHINESE ROYAL MU™ TEA;
and some whole grain crackers or chips with a soy or yogurt dip or spread;
or some low-fat cheese and fresh fruit.

Dinner: have an Italian meal with whole grain or vegetable pasta, a light shellfish sauce, and green salad;
or a vegetable or seafood quiche or omelet or frittata with a fresh herb sauce, and green salad;
or a tofu or tempeh casserole with brown rice and vegies;
or a hearty soup or stew with lentils or black beans and whole grain bread with soy or kefir cheese;
or a Chinese stir fry with brown rice and Miso soup with sea vegetables snipped on top.
✔A little white wine at dinner is excellent for digestion and relaxation.

Before bed: have some VEGEX yeast paste broth in a cup of hot water;
or chamomile or other relaxing herb tea, such as Crystal Star RELAX TEA™ or GOODNIGHT TEA™.

✔Avoid excess caffeine, and an overload of caffeine-containing foods such as chocolate; sidestep refined and processed foods like those found in fast food restaurants, stay away from smoking, smokeless tobacco, and secondary smoke.

❋ Supplements and Herbal Aids for Male System Support:

❖ Take Sun CHLORELLA, Green Foods GREEN ESSENCE, or Crystal Star ENERGY GREEN™.

❖ Take ascorbate vitamin C or Ester C, 3000mg., and zinc 50 to 75mg. daily.

❖ Take a B Complex with high potencies of pantothenic acid and B_{12} for stress management.

❖ Take raw adrenal, or Crystal Star ADR-ACTIVE EXTRACT™ for fatigue and endurance, with SUPER MAN'S ENERGY TONIC™ extract for extra male energy.

❖ Take a highly absorbable multiple mineral, such as Mezotrace SEA MINERAL COMPLEX, or Crystal Star MINERAL SPECTRUM™ CAPSULES, or SYSTEMS STRENGTH DRINK™.

❋ Bodywork for Male System Health:

✚ Continue with daily 20 minute aerobic exercise workouts. Each session should raise the heart rate to at least 65% of its capacity. **(You should be able to talk, but not sing, at this exercise level.)** Regular exercise fights against heart disease, high cholesterol levels, high blood pressure, overweight, stress, osteoporosis, constipation, and cancer tendency. Exercise is particularly important if you are dieting, so that muscle (especially heart muscle) is not lost as excess weight is lost.

✚ Add some stretches and deep breathing to your bedtime and rising regimen. Especially with the male body, stretches make a big difference in the quality of sleep and how a man faces the day.

✚ Get some early morning sunlight on the body every day for vitamins A and D, and tonic vigor.

❋ Sample Recipes That Work With This Diet
By section and recipe number:

BREAKFAST & BRUNCH - all

SOUPS - LIQUID SALADS - all

SANDWICHES - SALADS IN BREAD - all

HIGH PROTEIN COOKING WITHOUT MEAT - all

HIGH MINERAL FOODS - all

HIGH COMPLEX CARBOHYDRATES FOR ENERGY - a11

HIGH FIBER RECIPES - all

GREAT OUTDOOR EATING - all

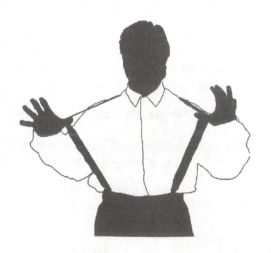

Good Food Combining for
Indigestion & Food Sensitivities

Most digestive problems are long standing, deeply ingrained from family-inherited eating habits and early lifestyle. Digestive disorders and consequent lack of good enzyme activity have far-reaching effects. Poor metabolism is at the root of many serious health problems from over-weight to arthritis to some kinds of cancer. While excess acid, overeating, stress, and overuse of antacids contribute to these problems, a poor diet, that is high in fats and refined carbohydrates, and aggravated by poor food combining, is the primary cause. Food allergies and sensitivities are also increasing in America as more chemicals are added to our food and soil. They are expanding as more foods are refined and processed.

The human digestive system works best when both meals and combinations of different foods are simple. Each category of foods: fruits, starches, proteins, sweets, etc. calls for its own particular digestive juices and enzymes. (See ABOUT FOOD COMBINING in this book.)

Poor food combinations, causing gas and distress, start most of us off "not right" each morning because we eat citrus juice and bread or grain together; it continues through the day, as we drink milk with meals, eat fruits with veggies and grains, and at the end of the day have a heavy, concentrated starch and protein meal that depletes enzyme capacity. A lot of food is only partially digested, or not digested at all, and just sits there in the stomach causing gas, fermentation and other intestinal disorders. Food that remains in the stomach longer than normal because it is highly refined, very heavy or concentrated, or poorly combined, greatly reduces the nutrition the body can receive from it.

Refined, high fat foods with chemical additives, are clearly the most prevalent cause of digestive problems, from gas, to hiatal hernia, to ulcers. Too much meat, especially red meat which stays in the stomach too long, and low fiber which favors constipation, are not far behind. Reduced stomach HCL and bile affects the digestion of acids and proteins, resulting in an over-acid system and fermentation. Many meals in today's busy lifestyles are hurried, eaten under stress, and poorly chewed, all adding to poor digestion. But since life isn't going to slow down, a conscious effort must be made to break the vicious digestive circle. It is never easy to change daily habits. Keep remembering how much better you will feel.

Find a way to relax, especially before you eat; deep breathing, a little mild exercise, some easy listening music, will help. Light meals instead of heavy meals, are another key. Take a teaspoonful, or two capsules of acidophilus before each meal to increase the formation and buildup of friendly bacteria in the G. I. tract.

The causes of poor digestion and assimilation are many; the answer is in simplifying complex meals, and eating lighter, less concentrated foods.

Our "solution diet" can be effective over several extended areas of digestive disorders:
GASTRITIS and GASTRO-ENTERITIS HIATAL HERNIA LIVER MALFUNCTION GALLBLADDER DISEASE and GALLSTONES ULCERS FOOD INTOLERANCES and ALLERGIES GAS and FLATULENCE CROHN'S DISEASE COLITIS and SPASTIC COLON ARTHRITIS DIVERTICULITIS BREATH and BODY ODOR BLOATING HEARTBURN CONSTIPATION DIARRHEA

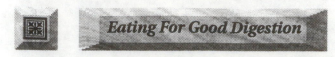

Diet For Good Digestion

The best way to make a major change in eating habits is to ease it into your life. The following diet improves faulty food combining gently and moderately, avoids red meats, sugars, excess caffeine, fatty and fried foods, strong spices and other acid-forming foods, and generally keeps the system alkaline. Since many food intolerances stem from dairy products, the diet largely eliminates these, too, except where they make sense for needed protein and in healthy food combinations. It relies on cultured foods, such as yogurt and tofu, rather than dairy products, for "friendly flora" production.

This good digestion diet is a long range way of eating that you can use for a lifetime. It is varied, yet observes good food combinations for easiest digestion. It features simply and lightly cooked high mineral dishes that are easy on the system. It emphasizes high fiber to give you a feeling of fullness with very little calorie expenditure. It maintains proper acid/alkaline balance and enzyme efficiency with fresh vegetables and whole grains. It is a diet to stimulate and increase your own enzyme production, with absorbable minerals, cultured foods, soluble fiber, and mouth-watering smell and taste.

On rising: have a glass of grapefruit, papaya, or apple juice;
or 2 lemons or 2 TBS. cider vinegar in water with 1 teasp. maple syrup and 1 tsp. acidophilus liquid;
or 10-15 drops Crystal Star BITTERS & LEMON CLEANSE™ EXTRACT in water;
or a glass of aloe vera juice, such as George's ALOE VERA JUICE, with 1 tsp. chlorophyll liquid added.

Breakfast: have a high fiber oat bran, whole grain cereal, or granola with yogurt or apple juice or vanilla soy milk;
and/or have some fresh fruit with yogurt or kefir;
or oatmeal with a little maple syrup or apple juice, kefir, or soy sauce;
or some high fiber buckwheat pancakes with any of these toppings.

Mid-morning: have some whole grain muffins and a green drink, or Green Foods GREEN ESSENCE; **or** carrot juice with 1 teasp. spirulina granules or chlorophyll liquid added, and some whole grain crackers with kefir cheese or a soy or vegetable dip.

Lunch: before eating, have another glass of aloe vera juice, such as Yerba Prima ALOE VERA with HERBS, and add 1 teasp. acidophilus liquid;
then have a green salad with lots of sprouts, green pepper, celery, and carrots, and a cup of miso soup with sea veggies snipped on top;
or a baked potato with kefir cheese or lemon oil topping, and a green salad;
or cole slaw with yogurt dressing and cornbread.
✔Follow any above choice with Crystal Star AFTER MEAL ENZ™ EXTRACT for enzyme stimulation.

Mid-afternoon: have some crunchy raw veggies with kefir or yogurt cheese or a veggie dip, and a mineral drink, such as Crystal Star SYSTEM STRENGTH DRINK™;
or a mild herb tea, such as comfrey, slippery elm or peppermint tea.

Dinner: take another lemon and water drink or aloe vera juice with acidophilus liquid before eating: **then** have some brown rice with tofu and veggies;
or an oriental stir-fry with brown rice and miso soup;
or a grilled fish or seafood dinner with a light vegetable quiche with yogurt sauce
or some millet or bulgar grains with steamed veggies and a soy sauce or light yogurt/chive dressing;
or a hearty veggie stew with whole grain bread.
✔A little white wine at dinner can often help digestion.

Before bed: have some pineapple/papaya juice, or apple juice;
or VEGEX yeast broth; **or** alfalfa/mint tea.

❋ *Supplements and Herbal Aids for Better Digestion:*

There is a wide array of effective natural and herbal digestive aids available for both distinct or overall problems. We only list a few here that work with this diet.

Remember that most commercial antacids neutralize stomach acid, generally making the condition worse, as the stomach produces more acids in an attempt to achieve enzyme rebalance.

Remember that Tagamet and Zantac, both drugs prescribed regularly for ulcers and gastric problems, can be addictive. They also inhibit bone formation and proper liver function. Consider the following natural means instead.

❖ Take a natural or herb source mineral and trace mineral supplement for better food assimilation, such as Mezotrace SEA MINERAL COMPLEX or Crystal Star SYSTEM STRENGTH DRINK™, or MEGA-MINERAL CAPSULES.

❖ Take charcoal tabs or Hyland's Homeopathic *BILIOUSNESS* tabs after meals for flatulence control and heartburn; take 2 ginger caps, or comfrey/pepsin tabs to break up excess acid and prevent gas.

❖ Take HCl tablets after meals for better digestive acid production.

❖ Take a green supplement such as CHLORELLA, spirulina, or liquid chlorophyll daily.

❖ Take alkalizing supplements, such as alfalfa tabs, umeboshi plum balls, peppermint oil drops in a cup of water, or catnip/fennel tea.

❖ Take chewable bromelain or Enzymatic Therapy DGL tablets, or Crystal Star HERBAL ENZ™ caps, or a good double strength enzyme formula for better enzyme production.

❖ Take acidophilus capsules or liquid *before* meals, *or* aloe vera juice with 2 teasp. bee pollen granules *after* meals for best assimilation and enzyme activity.

❖ Take a natural fiber drink in the morning and/or evening, such as Crystal Star CHO-LO FIBER TONE DRINK™ mix or Natrol Grapefruit capsules to keep the stomach "sweet," assure regularity, and friendly G.I. flora formation.

❋ *Bodywork for Better Digestion:*

✚ Eat small meals more frequently; no large meals. Use sesame salt instead of regular table salt.

✚ Chew everything *very* well.

✚ No smoking before meals. Nicotine really affects good digestion.

✚ Avoid caffeine, aspirin, and cortisone drugs. Each of these can damage the stomach and intestinal walls, and cause gastritis and ulcers.

✚ Avoid drinking fluids with meals - especially no sodas or carbonated drinks. Phosphoric acid binds up many digestive enzymes. A little white wine is fine before meals.

✚ Try to eat when relaxed. Take a short walk before and after you eat.

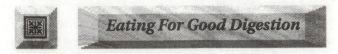

✳ *Sample Recipes For Better Digestion*
By section and recipe number:

HEALTHY DRINKS, JUICES & WATERS - 44, 45, 47, 54, 61, 62, 66, 67, 69, 71

ORIENTAL & LIGHT MACROBIOTIC COOKING - all

SALADS - HOT & COLD - 186, 190, 193, 194, 198, 202, 204, 206, 209, 214, 216, 222, 224, 225, 230, 232

LOW-FAT & VERY LOW-FAT DISHES - all

LOW CHOLESTEROL MEALS - all

DAIRY FREE COOKING - all

SUGAR FREE SPECIALS & SWEET TREATS - all

HIGH MINERAL FOODS - 613, 618, 622, 630, 636, 640, 641, 644, 645, 648, 652

HIGH FIBER RECIPES - all

GREAT OUTDOOR EATING - 874, 876, 879, 880, 883, 884, 888, 890, 893, 894, 895, 901, 908, 909

✳ *Sample Menu Plans*
Some recipe combinations that go with this diet:

LUNCH FOR TWO - 245, 188, 319, 52

A FAMILY MEAL - 213, 270, 289

A SPECIAL DINNER FOR TWO - 195, 154, 181, 295, 67

SUNDAY BRUNCH - 262, 185, 46, 161

A HEARTY WINTER MEAL - 324, 207, 224, 274, 366

A LIGHT SUMMER MEAL - 200, 290, 263, 51

AN EASY RISING BREAKFAST - 97, 83, 71, 73, 96

AN ALL HORS D'OEUVRES PARTY - 252, 121, 122, 114, 123, 241, 125, 369, 191

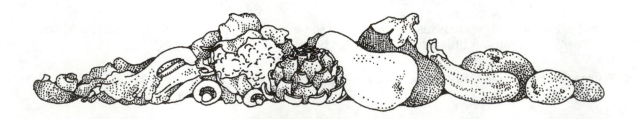

Diet to Overcome Food Allergies & Sensitivities

Food allergies and intolerances are becoming extremely widespread, as people are more and longer exposed to chemically altered and processed foods that the body is not equipped to handle. The fastest growing group of intolerances stems from food additives such as sulfites, nitrates, colorants, preservatives, water pollutants, and heavy metals found in contaminated seafood. Other common sensitivities are to wheat gluten, dairy products, fruits, sugar, yeast, corn, mushrooms, eggs, coffee and greens; all foods that are either heavily treated or sprayed themselves, or in the case of animal products, affected by anti-biotics and hormones.

Other culprits include:

◆ **too much dietary fat, and lack of stomach HCl,** both of which affect the digestion of proteins and acids. When these get into the blood stream undigested, the immune system tries to neutralize them with prostaglandins and histimines, resulting in food allergy symptoms.

◆ **lack of essential fatty acids** for prostaglandin production, causing lowered immunity and glandular function;

◆ **overgrowth of intestinal yeasts,** such as candida albicans, resulting in lowered intestinal flora;

◆ overuse of certain drugs, such as cortico-steroids, anti-biotics, and birth control pills that destroy the body's natural defenses and friendly Gastro-intestinal bacteria;

◆ **too much of too few foods;** (The typical American diet consists of <u>75%</u> dairy, meat and wheat products, <u>15%</u> sugar and fat, and *only 10%* fresh fruits and vegetables;

◆ **pasteurization, homogenization, and the addition of stabilizers and mold inhibitors to all dairy products,** rendering them clogging, mucous-forming, and hard to digest, and depleted of vitamins and absorbable minerals needed for enzyme avtivity.

Diet change and supplementation with herbs is the most beneficial and quickest means of overcoming food intolerances, and restoring digestive tract and immune system integrity.

Minerals and trace minerals are the basic bonding agents between the body and food. Without them, the body cannot absorb nutrients. They are essential to good digestion, keeping the body pH balanced, alkaline instead of acid. Skin pallor, chronic fatigue, and food sensitivities are almost certain signs that the body isn't getting enough minerals, or lacks the ability to absorb them. A high mineral diet can alkalize, balance enzyme activity, and gently build strength to improve digestive chemistry.

Enzyme production is at the heart of good digestion and assimilation. Different foods require different enzymes for proper absorption. Good food combining and relaxed eating bring the right enzymes into play at the right time. Undigested or poorly digested food is a key cause of food intolerances.

Eating fresh, organically grown foods is important in overcoming food sensitivities. When the body consumes processed, refined, enzyme depleted foods, its own enzymatic capacity must assume full responsibility for the digestive procedure. Eventually this capacity becomes weakened, and less and less food is processed correctly. These are then allowed into the blood stream where they are perceived as toxins by the immune system

Four dietary watchwords are important in overcoming food intolerances:

➤ **Get plenty of food and herb source minerals and trace minerals.**

➤ **Practice good food combining habits to increase enzyme production and efficiency.**

➤ **Eat organically grown food whenever possible. Avoid refined, processed foods like the plague.**

➤ **Consciously build immune system strength. Food allergies are caused by a malfunction of the immune system, in which the allergen is mistaken for a harmful invading bacteria and is then attacked, resulting in the runny nose, itchy eyes, headaches, diarrhea and congestion symptoms of food allergies.**

See **The Art Of Substituting** on page 212 for foods you can use in place of those that are making you sick or causing digestive problems.

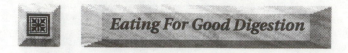

Stage One; Four Day Elimination Cleanse for Food Sensitivities:

This diet is designed to cleanse the body of food allergens. It is dairy and gluten free, and does not include other common allergens, such as corn, yeast, soy products, mushrooms, eggs, refined sweeteners, or sea foods currently at risk of contamination, (tuna, shellfish, etc.) However, identifying specific individual allergens is primary to overcoming them. Suspected foods should be introduced in small amounts, one at a time after this elimination diet, (see CONTROL DIET below) in order to determine personal sensitivity reactions.

On rising: take 2 fresh lemons squeezed in a glass of water with 1 packet of Sun CHLORELLA granules.

Breakfast: take a glass of cranberry/apple juice;
or a glass of papaya juice;
and some citrus or non-sweet fruits such as pineapple or kiwi.

Mid-morning: have a green drink (page 240ff.), or Green Foods GREEN ESSENCE, or Crystal Star ENERGY GREEN DRINK™;
and some fresh raw vegetable snacks with a little sesame salt.

Lunch: have a glass of pineapple/coconut juice for protein and energy;
or a glass of fresh carrot juice, with a small green salad and lemon/olive oil dressing.

Mid-afternoon: take a cup of alkalizing herb tea, such as catnip, alfalfa leaf, peppermint, or Crystal Star LICORICE MINTS TEA.

Dinner: have another small green salad with lemon/olive oil dressing
or a glass of apple/alfalfa sprout juice (recipe #11).

Before bed: have a cup pf relaxing tea, such as chamomile or scullcap tea;
or a glass of pineapple/papaya juice, or apple juice.

✔Drink only bottled water whenever possible.

❋ *Supplements and Herbal Aids for the Food Sensitivity Cleanse:*

❖ Add 1 teasp. liquid chlorophyll, or $1/2$ teasp. spirulina or chlorella granules to any juice or drink throughout the day to neutralize allergens and aid elimination.
Or add a dropperful of Crystal Star PRE-MEAL ENZ™ EXTRACT to water and take before meals; or a dropperful of AFTER MEAL ENZ™ EXTRACT to water after meals.

❖ Take acidophilus capsules or liquid **before** meals, **or** aloe vera juice with 2 teasp. bee pollen granules **after** meals for best assimilation and enzyme activity.

❖ Take HCl tablets after meals for better digestive acid production.

❖ Use Rainbow Light FOOD SENSITIVITY SYSTEM TABLETS as directed.

❋ *Bodywork for the Food Sensitivity Cleanse:*

✤ Consciously minimize stress situations during this cleanse for best results in reducing allergens.

Stage Two; Food Sensitivity Control Diet:

This diet stage should be used for 30 days or more to rebalance, alkalize and energize the system. It is rich in absorbable mineral and enzyme-producing foods, and employs good food combining techniques for optimal absorption. As suspected allergen foods are introduced and identified, they should be completely avoided for one to two months, to allow the body to establish solid immune defense and digestive stability.

Begin testing with the most questionable food substances; foods containing sulfites, nitrates, colorants, preservatives and additives. Then progress to nightshade plants (including tobacco), wheat gluten, pasteurized dairy products, soy foods, refined sweeteners, yeast, corn, mushrooms, eggs, coffee and caffeine-containing foods.

On rising: take a glass of lemon juice with 1 teasp. maple syrup;
or grapefruit or cranberry juice with a little honey.

Breakfast: take a vitamin/mineral drink, such as Nutri-tech ALL 1, or a sugar free protein drink, such as Nature's Plus SPIRUTEIN, in orange or apple juice;
or some oatmeal or wheat free grain cereal with apple juice or yogurt, and 1 TB. maple syrup.

Mid-morning: have a green drink (page 240ff.), or Sun CHLORELLA, or Green Foods GREEN ESSENCE, or a mixed vegetable juice (page 240ff.);
or a glass of fresh carrot juice;
and a cup of light noodle soup with sea vegetables snipped on top.

Lunch: have a green salad with light dressing, and a cup of vegetable or onion soup;
or some steamed vegetables and a baked potato with kefir cheese topping;
or a fruit salad with cottage cheese.

Mid-afternoon: have a glass of apple juice,
or an alkalizing herb tea, such as a hibiscus cooler, comfrey leaf, or alfalfa/mint tea.

Dinner: have a Chinese stir-fry with greens, rice noodles, and a sweet and sour sauce;
or a baked or broiled fish such as salmon or sole with brown rice and peas;
or a large dinner salad with nut and seed toppings and a yogurt or kefir dressing;
or a baked vegetable casserole with a cup of black bean or lentil soup;
or roast turkey slices from free-run organic turkeys, with a salad and baked potato.

Before bed: have a glass of apple or papaya juice;
or a cup of miso soup with sea vegetables.

✔ Drink only bottled water if possible.

❧ Supplements and Herbal Aids to Help Overcome Food Intolerances:

❖ Take only hypoallergenic supplements; free of corn, wheat, yeast, soy, egg, milk and sugar derivatives, with no fillers or additives.

❖ Use Rainbow Light FOOD SENSITIVITY SYSTEM TABLETS. Or add a dropperful of Crystal Star PRE-MEAL ENZ™ EXTRACT to water and take before meals; or a dropperful of AFTER MEAL ENZ™ EXTRACT to water after meals.

❖ Take a natural or herb source mineral and trace mineral supplement for better food assimilation, such as Mezotrace SEA MINERAL COMPLEX or Crystal Star MINERAL SPECTRUM™ CAPSULES.

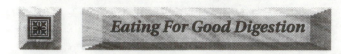

❖ Take HCl tablets after meals for better digestive acid production.

❖ Take a green supplement such as Sun CHLORELLA, spirulina, liquid chlorophyll, or Crystal Star ENERGY GREEN DRINK™ daily.

❖ Take acidophilus capsules or liquid **before** meals, **or** aloe vera juice with 2 teasp. bee pollen granules **after** meals for best assimilation and enzyme activity.

✽ *Bodywork for the Food Sensitivity Diet:*

✚ No smoking before meals. Nicotine magnifies allergies almost more than any other substance.

✚ Avoid caffeine, aspirin, and cortisone drugs. Each of these can damage the stomach and intestinal walls, and cause gastritis and ulcers.

✚ No fluids with meals - especially no sodas or carbonated drinks. Phosphoric acid binds up many digestive enzymes. A little white wine is fine before meals.

✚ Try to eat relaxed. Tension and stress reduce the body's ability to deal with allergens.

✽ *Sample Recipes for the Food Sensitivity Diet*
By section and recipe number:

HEALTHY DRINKS, JUICES & WATERS - 46, 49, 51, 52, 61, 65

MACROBIOTIC EATING - 110, 111, 119, 120, 122, 123, 128, 130, 133, 139, 142, 164, 168, 171, 182, 185

BREAKFAST & BRUNCH - 75, 76, 77, 78, 80, 81, 82, 85, 93, 97, 98, 101, 103, 104, 108

SALADS - HOT & COLD - 187, 188, 189, 195, 196, 199, 211, 212, 213, 217, 218, 226, 229, 231, 236, 237

LOW-FAT & VERY LOW-FAT DISHES - 241, 242, 243, 249, 263, 264, 268, 277, 281, 284, 292, 298, 300

DAIRY FREE COOKING - 334, 335, 337, 340, 342, 351, 352, 355, 357, 360, 361, 366, 369, 370, 371, 373

WHEAT FREE BAKING - 375, 376, 379, 383, 386, 387, 389, 391, 392, 394, 396, 397, 398, 400, 402, 408

HIGH MINERAL FOODS - 615, 616, 619, 621, 626, 629, 631, 634, 647, 649, 651, 656, 659, 662

HIGH COMPLEX CARBOHYDRATES - 743, 744, 747, 750, 759, 760, 761, 764, 765, 772, 773, 777, 781

HIGH FIBER RECIPES - 785, 788, 793, 794, 796, 798, 800, 802, 802, 803, 807, 808, 809, 810, 817, 819, 824

▣ *About Food Combining*

So much confusion surrounds this area of food preparation and eating that a brief discussion about how we see good food combining might be helpful.

We have all suffered indigestion at one time or another, and indeed our society spends over *2 billion dollars a year* on antacids for this problem. Good food combining can help alleviate poor digestion naturally, and return more energy to the body for other needs.

Food combining is only one factor in healthy eating. It will not guarantee good digestion.

Different foods require different acid/alkaline mediums, different enzymes and different digestion times. Eating foods together that have drastically different digestive needs often results in poor or no assimilation. The body simply passes foods through with no digestion, or holds them back to wait for the proper enzyme medium. Sometimes this food decomposes in the digestive tract and then ferments, producing gas and toxins, with resultant heartburn or elimination problems.

Other factors can also reduce digestive capacity, such as overeating, eating under stress or when tired, eating before strenuous exercise, or during strong emotional experiences. Substances such as spicy condiments, vinegars, caffeine and alcohol all irritate and retard digestion considerably. Fever and inflammatory illness also partially suspend digestion to conserve energy.

As the diet incorporates more fresh, unprocessed foods, good food combining naturally becomes part of life style and eating habits. Good food combining rules can become part of meal planning almost subconsciously. You might look back on a particularly good meal and say "Oh yes, the combinations were right."

I have included a very simple chart on the basics of good food combining. (See next page.) In our own everyday use, and in this book, we have found three things to be true:

1) Small amounts of poor combinations don't seem to cause problems, and sometimes really enhance taste and enjoyment, such as a handful of raisins in a cake, or a whole grain cereal with a little apple juice or yogurt.

2) Fruits of all kinds are better eaten fresh, by themselves, in the first half of the day.

3) Don't let food combining rule your life. Most natural food recipes just work out as good combinations automatically.

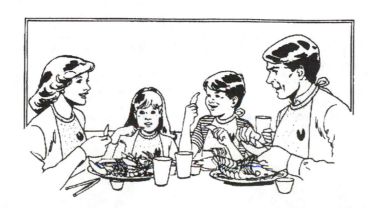

GOOD FOOD COMBINATIONS

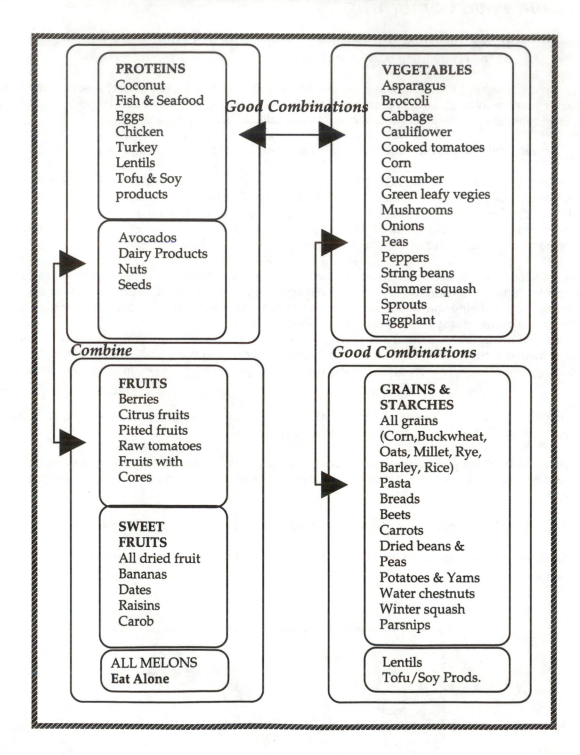

PROTEINS
Coconut
Fish & Seafood
Eggs
Chicken
Turkey
Lentils
Tofu & Soy
products

Avocados
Dairy Products
Nuts
Seeds

Good Combinations

VEGETABLES
Asparagus
Broccoli
Cabbage
Cauliflower
Cooked tomatoes
Corn
Cucumber
Green leafy vegies
Mushrooms
Onions
Peas
Peppers
String beans
Summer squash
Sprouts
Eggplant

Combine

FRUITS
Berries
Citrus fruits
Pitted fruits
Raw tomatoes
Fruits with
Cores

**SWEET
FRUITS**
All dried fruit
Bananas
Dates
Raisins
Carob

ALL MELONS
Eat Alone

Good Combinations

**GRAINS &
STARCHES**
All grains
(Corn,Buckwheat,
Oats, Millet, Rye,
Barley, Rice)
Pasta
Breads
Beets
Carrots
Dried beans &
Peas
Potatoes & Yams
Water chestnuts
Winter squash
Parsnips

Lentils
Tofu/Soy Prods.

✿ Sample Menu Plans
Some recipes combinations that support good food combining:

AN EASY RISING BREAKFAST - 84, 80, 75, 93

LUNCH FOR TWO - 199, 235, 53, 300

AN EASY WEEK NIGHT DINNER - 135, 159, 165, 298

A LIGHT SUMMER MEAL - 110, 219, 50, 338

A HEARTY WINTER MEAL - 142, 167, 307, 299, 131, 61

A SUNDAY BRUNCH - 204, 258, 636, 322, 55

A FAMILY MEAL - 168, 189, 312, 373

A SPECIAL DINNER FOR TWO - 351, 132, 192, 155, 371

AN ALL HORS D'OEUVRES PARTY - 156, 119, 115, 109, 54, 169, 217, 125

HEALTHY FEASTING & ENTERTAINING - 113/112, 197, 314, 349, 374

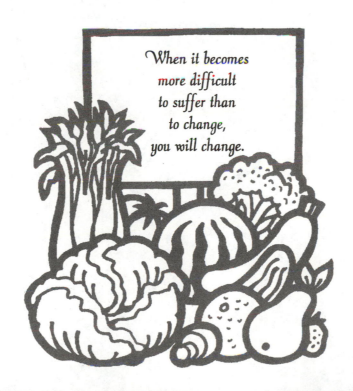

When it becomes
more difficult
to suffer than
to change,
you will change.

*E*verything is
a blessing in disguise.
Even bad news can be
fortuitous from another
vantage point.

Liver & Organ Health

The liver is a key organ of detoxification, and to a large extent the health of the liver determines the health state of the whole body. Many problems can be solved or prevented by a short liver cleanse once or twice a year.

The liver is really a wonderful chemical plant. It filters and rids the bloodstream of toxins and bacterial wastes, helps in the formation of red blood cells, synthesizes and secretes bile, and is the major organ of metabolism for proteins, fats and carbohydrates. It also produces natural antihistimines to keep immunity high.

Liver exhaustion and damage interfere with all of these vital functions. Since the common American diet is high in calories, fats, sugars and alcohol, with unknown amounts of toxic substances in the form of preservatives, pesticides, and nitrates, almost everybody has liver malfunction to some extent.

Slight liver damage appears as low energy, poor digestion, allergies, constipation, age spots, headaches and hair problems.

Major problems occur after many years of abuse, when the liver is so exhausted it loses the ability to detoxify. Fortunately the liver seems to possess almost miraculous powers of recovery. The following emergency diet may be used in extremely toxic situations for rapid improvement, and along with the rest of the healing diet, for eventual long term health. Even in life-threatening situations, such as cirrhosis, hepatitis, acute gallstone attacks, mononucleosis, and pernicious anemia, the liver can be cleansed and rejuvenated, and major surgery or even death averted.

I have personally seen and followed the improvement of several people who have used the emergency liver detoxification program in this chapter. Each had been told by their physicians that they were at terminal status. None were young, and abuse had been going on for years. Each felt he had nothing to lose by commitment to an alternative healing program. As far as I know, all are still walking around today.

Many other organ and glandular imbalances may be remedied by cleansing and keeping a healthy liver, including adrenal, pituitary, kidney, gall bladder, and spleen problems. They include:

WEIGHT & CELLULITE CONTROL ❧**GALLBLADDER HEALTH & GALLSTONES** ❧ **MENSTRUAL AND P.M.S. DIFFICULTIES** ❧**ENDOMETRIOSIS** ❧**BREAST AND UTERINE FIBROIDS** ❧**MALE IMPOTENCE** ❧**FEMALE INFERTILITY** ❧**DRUG & ALCOHOL ABUSE** ❧**TOXIC SHOCK** ❧**HEPATITIS** ❧**SWOLLEN GLANDS** ❧**SHINGLES & NEURITIS** ❧**HERPES** ❧**OSTEOPOROSIS** ❧**SPOTS BEFORE THE EYES** ❧**SPLEEN MALFUNCTION** ❧**KIDNEY DISEASE** ❧**JAUNDICE** ❧

The liver and organ regeneration diet program in this chapter is in three stages. Depending on the status and severity of the problem, an initial emergency cleanse may be used for a few days or for 2 to 3 weeks. Gland function and digestion often improve right away, but effective detoxification takes longer, and is dependent on the general health state of the individual. We recommend close monitoring of the body and its progress for best results.

A permanent diet for continuing liver health should be lacto-vegetarian, low in fats, rich in vegetable proteins, with plenty of vitamin C foods for good iron absorption.

Emergency Liver Cleanse; A Three Day Liquid Diet for Acute Hepatitis or Severely Toxic Liver Conditions:

*It doesn't happen overnight, but you can have every confidence that if there is any chance at all, the liver will find its way to a healthier state, even after severe drug or alcohol abuse. When the crisis has passed, a program of 6 to 9 months on a liver **healing** diet should be undertaken (See Stages 2 and 3 on the following pages).*

On rising: take 1 teasp. acidophilus complex powder such as Natren Life Start II in juice or water; **and** fresh lemon juice or cider vinegar in a glass of water with 1 teasp. honey.

Breakfast: take a glass of carrot/beet/cucumber juice, or a potassium broth (page 240).

Mid-morning: take a glass of potassium juice or broth (page 240) with 1 teasp. of Spirulina or Sun CHLO-RELLA granules **and** $1/2$ teasp. ascorbate vitamin C crystals (about 2500mg.) added;

Lunch: take a green drink (pg. 240ff.), or Sun CHLORELLA drink, or Crystal Star ENERGY GREEN DRINK™ with $1/2$ teasp. acidophilus complex and $1/2$ to 1 teasp. ascorbate vitamin C crystals.

Mid-afternoon: take another glass of lemon juice and water; **or** a glass of papaya juice with $1/2$ teasp. vitamin C crystals added; **and/or** a cup of Crystal Star LIV-FLUSH TEA™.

Dinner: take another green drink with $1/2$ teasp. vitamin C crystals; **and/or** pineapple-papaya juice with $1/2$ teasp. acidophilus powder added.

Before Bed: take another glass of lemon juice and water with 1 teasp. honey added; **or** a cup of Crystal Star LIV-FLUSH TEA™; **and/or** a cup of yeast paste VEGEX broth for B vitamins, body relaxation, and next day strength.

✔ Drink six to eight glasses of bottled water every day, to encourage maximum detoxification.

❧ *Supplements for the Emergency Liver Cleanse:*

✤ We recommend that no supplementation other than those recommended above be taken during this emergency fasting stage.

❧ *Bodywork for the Emergency Liver Cleanse:*

✤ Get plenty of rest all three days.

✤ Take early morning sunbaths every day possible.

✤ A coffee enema (1 cup coffee to 1 qt. water) may be taken to flush released wastes (See page 244 for method.)

✤ Overheating therapy for liver and kidney detoxification is effective. Take a sauna every day of the cleanse to induce sweating and faster toxin elimination.

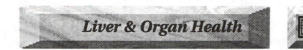

"Spring Cleaning" Liver Cleanse and Detoxification; A 3 Day Diet:

A general spring liver cleanse is excellent once or twice a year for whole body health and tone.

On rising: take 2 TBS. cider vinegar in water with 1 teasp. honey, <u>or</u> 2 TBS. lemon juice in water. Even after this first stage is over, it is often a good idea to continue with one of these drinks.

Breakfast: take a glass of potassium broth or juice, or carrot/beet/cucumber juice, <u>or</u> a glass of organic apple juice.

Mid-morning: take a green drink (page 240ff.), **or** Sun CHLORELLA or Green Foods BARLEY GREEN MAGMA granules, or Crystal Star ENERGY GREEN™ DRINK in a glass of water.

Lunch: have another glass of organic apple juice; <u>and/or</u> fresh carrot juice.

Mid-afternoon: have a cup of peppermint tea, pau d'arco tea, or Crystal Star LIV-FLUSH TEA™; <u>or</u> Crystal Star SYSTEM STRENGTH DRINK™; <u>or</u> another green drink.

Dinner: have another glass of organic apple juice; <u>and/or</u> another potassium broth if cleansing action is not too stressful.

Before bed: take another glass of lemon juice or cider vinegar in water. Add 1 teasp. honey or royal jelly.

❋ *Supplements for the Spring Cleaning Liver Cleanse:*

Except for the following suggestions, supplementation affects the cleansing process, and should not begin until the Stage Two LIVER REBUILDING DIET.

❖ Ascorbate vitamin C crystals, $1/4$ to $1/2$ teasp. at a time.

❖ One teasp. highest quality royal jelly may be added to any of the above liquids for increased cleansing/healing benefit.

❋ *Bodywork for the Spring Cleaning Liver Cleanse:*

✚ Only mild exercise should be undertaken during the fast.

✚ Get plenty of early morning sunlight every day possible.

✚ Drink six to eight glasses of bottled water every day, to encourage maximum flushing of the tissues and organs.

✚ Make a point to get adequate rest and sleep during the cleanse.

✚ Take a hot sauna each day of this cleanse for optimum results.

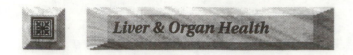

Gallstone Fast and Flush:

The liver and gallbladder are interconnecting and interworking organs. Problems with either affect both. Before undertaking this program to pass gallstones, have a sonogram or low dose X-Ray to determine the size of the stones. If they are too large to pass through the urethral ducts, other methods must be used.

❦ Go on a 3 day Olive Oil and Lemon Juice Flush:

On rising: take 2 TBS. olive oil and the juice of 1 lemon in water;

Breakfast: take a glass of carrot/beet/cucumber juice;
or a potassium juice or broth.

Mid-morning: have 1 to 2 cups of chamomile tea.

Lunch: take another glass of lemon juice in water with 2 TBS. olive oil;
and a glass of black cherry juice, carrot juice or organic apple juice.

Mid-afternoon: have 1 to 2 cups of chamomile tea.

Dinner: have another glass of organic apple, carrot or black cherry juice.

Before bed: take another cup of chamomile tea.

Note: If olive oil is hard for you to take straight, sip it through a straw.

❦ Follow with a 5 day Alkalizing Diet:

On rising: take 2 TBS. cider vinegar in water with 1 teasp. honey;
or 2 TBS. lemon juice in water, or a glass of fresh grapefruit juice.

Breakfast: take glass of carrot/beet/cucumber juice, or a potassium broth or juice.

Mid-morning: have 1 to 2 cups of chamomile tea,
and a glass of organic apple juice.

Lunch: take a green drink of Sun CHLORELLA, Green Foods GREEN MAGMA, or Crystal Star ENERGY GREEN DRINK™;
and a small fresh green salad with lemon/oil dressing. Have a cup of dandelion root tea after lunch.

Mid-afternoon: have 1 to 2 cups of chamomile tea, and another glass of grapefruit juice **or** apple juice.

Dinner; have a small green salad with lemon/oil dressing;
or some steamed veggies with brown rice or millet;
and another glass of organic apple juice.

Before bed: have another cup of chamomile or dandelion tea.
❧ Drink 6-8 glasses of bottled water each day.

Finish with a One Day Intensive Olive Oil Flush:

Starting around 7 P.M. on the evening of the 5th day of the alkalizing diet, make a mix of 1 pint of pure olive oil and 9 or 10 juiced lemons; take $1/4$ cup of this mix every 15 minutes until it is gone, (about 3 or 4 hours). Lie on the right side for better assimilation if desired. Take with a straw if taste and oiliness are unpleasant.

This 9 day program has often been successful in passing gallstones without surgery.
After stones have been passed, the next diet phase should concentrate on healing the liver/gallbladder area, and preventing further stone formation.

Stage Two; Rebuilding Liver Health:
This diet phase is high in alkalizing foods and vegetable proteins, low in fats, and dairy-free with 60% fresh raw foods. Alcohol, caffeine and caffeine-containing foods, saturated fats, and red meats should be avoided while on this diet. Normal duration for this diet stage is about 1 month; less if you only wish a mild cleanse.

On rising: take a glass of lemon juice and water with 1 teasp. honey.

Breakfast: Make a mix of 2 TBS. **each**: brewer's yeast, lecithin, and high Omega-3 flax oil. Take 2 teasp. each morning in prune, organic apple or cranberry juice;
and have some fresh fruits, such as grapefruit or pineapple;
and/or a whole grain cereal or muesli with apple juice or fruit yogurt on top,

Mid-morning: have a green drink (pg. 240ff.), Sun CHLORELLA or Green Foods GREEN MAGMA;
and/or a cup of miso soup with 2 TBS. sea veggies snipped on top,
or a cup of Crystal Star LIV-ALIVE TEA™, or SYSTEM STRENGTH DRINK™.

Lunch: have a large fresh green salad with lemon/olive oil dressing,
and a glass of fresh carrot juice and some whole grain crackers with a yogurt, kefir or soy spread;
or have some marinated, baked tofu with brown rice or millet, and a small spinach/sprout salad with a light olive oil dressing.

Mid-afternoon: have a cup of miso soup, or an alkalizing herb tea, such as chamomile, dandelion root, or milk thistle seed;
and/or a hard boiled egg and cup of yogurt.

Dinner: have a baked potato with kefir cheese or soy cheese dressing, and a large dinner salad with a mayonnaise dressing;
or a light vegetable steam/stir-fry with vegetables, seafood or tofu;
or some steamed veggies with brown rice, millet or bulgar and a light Italian or tofu dressing;
or a vegetable souffle or casserole with a light noodle broth.

Before bed: have an herb tea, such as dandelion root, chamomile or Crystal Star ROYAL MU TEA™;
or a glass of apple juice or prune juice,
or a cup of VEGEX yeast paste broth.

✔ Drink six to eight glasses of bottled mineral water every day to continue cleansing while rebuilding the liver.

✔ Take small meals more frequently all during the day, rather than any large meals.

❋ **Supplements for the Liver Rebuilding Diet:**

❖ Take milk thistle extract in water daily.

❖ Take Floradix LIQUID IRON, and/or Crystal Star HEARTSEASE/ANEMI-GIZE™ CAPS daily.

❖ Take Sun CHLORELLA, Cystal Star ENERGY GREEN DRINK™, or Green Foods GREEN MAGMA daily for chlorophyll and red blood cell formation.

❖ Beta-carotene 100,000IU with ascorbate vitamin C or Ester C, 3000mg., and vitamin E 400IU daily for anti-infective and antioxidant activity.

❖ Take Alta Health CANGEST, or Rainbow Light DETOX-ZYME caps **with** chromium picolinate 200mcg. to rebuild metabolic capability.

❖ Take Enzymatic Therapy LIQUID LIVER caps, and/or vitamin B$_{12}$ sublingual or inter-nasal for red blood formation.

❋ **Bodywork for the Liver Rebuilding Diet:**

✚ Take a brisk walk every day to cleanse the lungs, increase circulation, and oxygenate the blood. Stretching exercises are particularly helpful to organ tissue tone.

❋ **Sample Recipes for the Liver Rebuilding Diet:**
By section and recipe number:

BREAKFAST & BRUNCH - all

SALADS HOT & COLD - 186, 187, 188, 189, 190, 191, 193, 195, 196, 198, 199,
200, 201, 202, 203, 204.

ORIENTAL & LIGHT MACROBIOTIC EATING - all

LOW-FAT & VERY LOW-FAT DISHES - all

LOW CHOLESTEROL MEALS - all

DAIRY FREE COOKING - all

SOUPS - LIQUID SALADS - all

STIR-FRYS - all

FISH & SEAFOODS - all

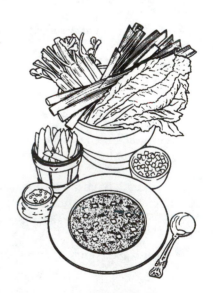

Stage Three; Maintaining Liver & Organ Health

This third diet stage should be used for at least three to six months. It emphasizes permanent support for liver and organ strength - so that problems don't return, and body immunity is fortified. It is high in complex carbohydrates, vegetable proteins and vitamin C foods, with cultured and low-fat dairy foods for good iron absorption. Avoid caffeine, hard alcohol, refined starches, and full fat dairy products on a continuing basis for best liver and organ health.

On rising: take 2 teasp. of cranberry concentrate in 8-oz. water,
or have some apple/cranberry juice.

Breakfast: Make a mix of 2 TBS. **each** brewer's yeast, lecithin, and omega-3 flax oil, and blackstrap molasses. Sprinkle some on your breakfast choice every day.
Have yogurt with fresh fruit, or dried figs and raisins;
and/or a whole grain cereal with some apple juice, or fruit and yogurt topping;
or a baked or poached egg with whole grain muffins and a little kefir cheese.

Mid-morning: have a green drink (page 240ff.), Sun CHLORELLA, Green Foods GREEN ESSENCE, or Crystal Star ENERGY GREEN DRINK™;
or a cup of miso soup with sea veggies;
and some whole grain crackers with garbanzo bean or yogurt vegetable dip;
and/or some crunchy fresh veggies with kefir or yogurt cheese, and roasted dandelion root tea.

Lunch: have an entree size protein salad, or sandwich on whole grain bread, with a low-fat dressing or spread;
or a light vegetable quiche with a low-fat sauce;
or a roast turkey sandwich or salad with a cup of black bean soup;
or an all- greens salad with spinach or chard and brown rice or millet with a light sauce.

Mid-afternoon: have some dried fruit, such as prunes, raisins or figs;
or a refreshing herb drink such as Hibiscus Tea (page 257), or Crystal Star LICORICE MINTS TEA, with some whole grain crackers or muffins and kefir cheese;
or a baked potato with kefir or yogurt cheese;
or a glass of carrot juice.

Dinner: have a whole grain and vegetable casserole with yogurt/chive sauce;
or a light oriental stir-fry with brown rice or crunchy noodles;
or a vegetarian pizza on an omelet 'crust' or a toasted chapati;
or roast turkey with apple/sage stuffing and baked yams;
or baked fish or seafood with rice and peas or green beans;
or a light vegetable or whole grain pasta with a low fat sauce, and green salad.

Before bed: have a cup of miso soup,or Crystal Star SYSTEM STRENGTH DRINK™;
or prune, papaya or apple juice;
or a cup of VEGEX yeast broth.

❖

Liver and Organ Checkpoints:

✔ Keep body minerals, oxygen and iron high with green drinks.

✔ Drink at least 6 to 8 glasses of bottled water daily to keep the organs hydrated, and free of toxic waste accumulation.

✔ Eat smaller, more frequent meals; no large heavy meals.

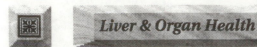

❋ *Supplements for Maintaining Liver & Organ Health:*

❖ Take naturally-occurring iron, such as Crystal Star IRON SOURCE™ CAPS or EXTRACT, or Floradix Herbal Iron extract.

❖ Take ascorbate vitamin C or Ester C, 3000mg. daily with beta carotene 50,000IU daily.

❖ Take carnitine 250-500mg. daily, and a lipotropic complex for better fat metabolism.

❖ Take royal jelly 2 teasp. daily, for liver regeneration.

❋ *Bodywork for Maintaining Liver & Organ Health:*

✛ Continue with daily aerobic exercise, and consciously include some relaxation time in each day.

✺

❋ *Sample Recipes For Maintaining Liver & Organ Health*
By section and recipe number:

LOW-FAT & VERY LOW-FAT DISHES - all

BREAKFAST & BRUNCH - all

FISH & SEAFOODS - all

STIR-FRYS - all

SUGAR FREE TREATS - 422, 413, 415, 416, 417, 420, 422, 426, 427, 429, 430, 431, 432, 433, 436, 440

HIGH MINERAL FOODS - all

HIGH COMPLEX CARBOHYDRATES FOR ENERGY - all

HIGH PROTEIN WITHOUT MEAT - 696, 699, 702, 705, 713, 718, 724, 733, 737, 738, 739, 740, 741, 742

HIGH FIBER RECIPES - all

GREAT OUTDOOR EATING - all

HOLIDAY FEASTING & ENTERTAINING - 826, 831, 832, 833, 838, 841, 843, 849, 858, 865, 867, 870

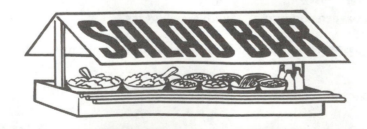

❋ *Sample Menu Plans*
Some recipe combinations that work with this diet:

A FAMILY MEAL - 814, 740, 263, 781, 648

A HEARTY WINTER MEAL - 724, 706, 649, 628, 299

A LIGHT SUMMER MEAL -633/634, 741, 298, 657

A SPECIAL DINNER FOR TWO - 711, 613, 723, 702, 295

LUNCH FOR TWO - 548, 719, 663

AN EASY WEEKNIGHT DINNER - 730, 621, 660

AN EASY RISING BREAKFAST - 77, 97, 78, 89, 74

A SUNDAY BRUNCH - 101, 539, 821, 662, 627

A WEEKEND PICNIC - 824, 259, 239, 260

AN ALL HORS D'OEUVRES PARTY - 710, 534, 646, 899, 907, 414

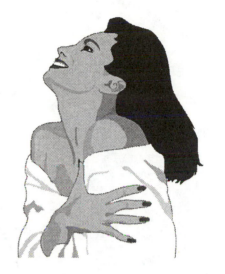

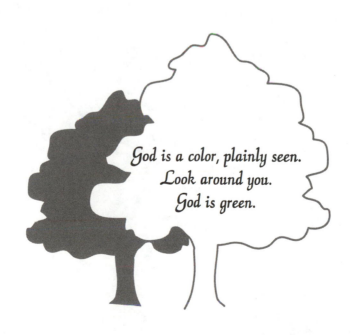

God is a color, plainly seen.
Look around you.
God is green.

*S*trength
is the charm of a man.
*C*harm
is the strength of a woman.

Male & Female Gland Problems
❧ Food ❧ Sex ❧ Impotence ❧ Fertility

Hormone and glandular secretions are the reason for the difference in a man's and a woman's bodies. Glandular functions are at the deepest level of the body processes. They are so potent that it is imperative that they receive optimum nutrition for reproductive success. Sexual vitality for both men and women is based in the health of the sex hormones.

There is metabolic difference, of course, but female hormones, androgens and male hormones are found in both sexes. Women build up tissue; they receive energy, then convert and enrich it to create life. They need fewer proteins and a smaller volume of complex carbohydrates for conception and fertility. Men break down tissue; they expend energy as in the discharge during sex. They need denser foods, more concentrated proteins, and three times the volume of complex carbohydrates as women. However, clinical experience has shown that the sexual vitality of both male and female can be improved with a natural foods diet. The metabolic variations will naturally dictate the diet and choice of foods - for virility or fertility.

An optimum program for a man will usually include a short cleansing diet, then high zinc foods, some fats, some meat and other protein rich foods, some sweets and dairy foods, and lots of whole grain volume. He can usually see improvement the first two weeks in his potency and virility.

A woman uses food more efficiently and so does not usually need an initial cleansing fast. She will benefit more from salads, leafy greens and lighter foods; less fats, no meats except seafoods, very low sugars, and a smaller volume of whole grains and nuts. Fertility rise can take 6 to 18 months after her diet change.

A lower fat, vegetable protein, complex carbohydrate, building diet can improve the nutritional environment in the glands and organs of both sexes. The following way of eating is effective for many conditions that stem from gland and hormone deficiencies.

For male problems: ❧PROSTATE or TESTICULAR INFLAMMATION ❧RECOVERY AFTER PROSTATE SURGERY ❧PARATHYROID DISEASE ❧THYMUS, ADRENAL GLAND & LYMPHATIC IMBALANCE ❧IMPOTENCE ❧DIFFICULT URINATION ❧

For female problems: ❧INFERTILITY ❧PMS SYMPTOMS ❧MENSTRUAL CRAMPS or EXCESSIVE MENSTRUAL BLEEDING ❧THYROID HEALTH, GRAVES DISEASE & HYPOTHYROIDISM ❧ENDOMETRIOSIS ❧MENOPAUSE ❧OSTEOPOROSIS ❧OVARIAN CYSTS ❧BREAST or UTERINE FIBROIDS ❧THYMUS, HYPOTHALAMUS and ADRENAL MALFUNCTION ❧RECOVERY AFTER HYSTERECTOMY or SURGICAL ABORTION ❧POST-NATAL SYSTEM IMBALANCE ❧

There is also a section about EATING FOR LOVE; Diet For Better Relationships. Personal, intimate relationships are at the core of life's happiness. There is a long history of connection between food and libido. The aphrodisiac miracle foods of yesteryear are now seen as part of a valid team effort making up for nutritional deficiencies in the male and female body. Many of us are overfed and undernourished.

It is almost universally recognized today that impotence, frigidity and low libido are overwhelmingly physical, rather than psychological conditions. The main problem is at the dinner table, not in the bedroom. A recent study on male impotence has shown that over 80% of the men involved had atherosclerosis or hardening of the arteries, presumably caused by their high-fat, cholesterol-rich diets. Atherosclerosis had damaged the blood vessels of these men to the extent that the blood vessels of the penis could not sustain an erection.

A high-fat diet may also lead to diabetes or latent diabetes, injuring the nerves that stimulate an erection. Too much fat abnormally elevates prolactin from the pituitary gland, suppressing hormones responsible for good sexual function.

The first step toward a better sex life is to get the fat out of your diet. Low fat, largely vegetarian meals with lots of fresh foods and whole grains provides plenty of complex carbohydrates, proteins and soluble fiber to build and regulate health, while avoiding cholesterol and reducing fat to 20% or less of daily calories.

Physical improvements happen quickly. Within a few hours of eating a low-fat meal, circulation to all organs increases. Prolactin levels fall in just a few days on a low-fat diet. Atherosclerosis begins to reverse. Weight is usually lost and libido rises. Better nutrition can definitely help maximize personal potential for a happier and more rewarding love life. There is no doubt that better sex naturally emerges from a healthier body. A clean, balanced system allows both man and woman to become more aware of each other, and more physically and emotionally sensitive.

The Part One Balancing Diet in this chapter also generates clearer skin, a more even temperament, fewer allergies, sweeter breath, softer hair, brighter eyes and a more pleasing body shape.

The Part Two Diet includes major nutrient sources for renewed libido and sensuality for both men and women. It can be a major factor in overcoming:
IMPOTENCE ❧STERILITY ❧FRIGIDITY ❧INFERTILITY ❧LOW LIBIDO or LACK OF SEXUAL DESIRE ❧PITUITARY and PINEAL GLAND HEALTH ❧

Part One; Balancing Diet for Gland and Hormone Health:

On rising: take a high protein drink such as Nature's Plus SPIRUTEIN;
or lemon juice in water with 1 tsp. honey. Add 2 teasp. brewer's yeast flakes for best results.

Breakfast: for women: make a mix of 2 TBS. **each:** toasted sesame seeds, sunflower seeds, wheat germ and lecithin granules. Sprinkle some each morning on yogurt and/or fresh fruit, or oatmeal or a whole grain cereal. Top with apple juice, 1 TB. maple syrup, or molasses if desired.

     for men: make a mix of 2 TBS. **each:** toasted sunflower and pumpkin seeds, wheat germ and lecithin granules. Sprinkle some each morning on whole grain cereal, muesli or granola. Top with maple syrup, molasses, apple juice or yogurt; add poached or baked eggs with whole grain toast or muffins.

Mid-morning: have a green drink (page 240), Sun CHLORELLA or BARLEY GREEN drink;
and/or a cup of miso or noodle ramen soup with sea veggies snipped on top.

Lunch: for women: have an onion or black bean soup with a carrot and raisin salad;
or baked or broiled seafood with a green leafy salad with sprouts and celery;
or a baked potato or yam with a low-fat dressing and a small green salad.

     for men: have some steamed veggies with brown rice and tofu;
or a chicken, avocado and low-fat cheese sandwich or salad;
or a whole grain protein salad or sandwich with lots of nuts, seeds, tofu or yogurt, and a lentil or black bean soup.

Mid-afternoon: have some low-fat cottage cheese with nuts and seeds and whole grain crackers;
or a dried fruit and nut mix with a bottle of mineral water;
or a hard boiled egg with a refreshing herb drink such as spearmint tea, or hibicus sangria, (pg. 257).

Dinner: for women: have a broccoli or asparagus quiche with a whole grain or chapati crust;
or a stir-fry with Chinese greens and mushrooms, and baked tofu, or miso soup with sea veggies;
or a baked millet and veggie casserole with yogurt sauce.
      for men: have an Italian whole grain pasta or polenta dish with a seafood stew;
or a Mexican beans and rice meal with low fat or soy cheese and a fresh salad;
or fresh baked seafood or salmon with brown rice and peas.
✔A little wine at dinner is nice for relaxation, digestion, and release from stress and inhibitions.

Before bed: men and women: have a cup of VEGEX yeast broth;
or an apple or pineapple/papaya juice.

Watchwords: AVOID ALL JUNK FOODS; particularly sodas, sugary foods, alcohol other than wines, refined, canned foods, fried, fatty and salty foods. Eat small meals more frequently, rather than large meals.

❋ Supplements for Gland & Hormone Balance:

Both men and women need adequate testosterone production for sexual vitality. Essential fatty acids, vitamin E, and B vitamins synthesize this hormone.

For women:

❖ A good multi-mineral such as Mezotrace SEA MINERAL COMPLEX, a good calcium supplement with high magnesium, or Crystal Star MINERAL SPECTRUM™ CAPS or EXTRACT.

❖ Evening primrose oil, 3 daily, or high omega-3 flax oil 3 teasp. daily for essential fatty acids.

❖ Damiana/dong quai capsules or extract, or Crystal Star FEMALE HARMONY™ capsules or CONCEPTIONS TEA™ (for fertility), **and** 2 teasp. high quality royal jelly daily.

❖ Vitamin E 400-800IU daily and B complex 100mg, or 2 teasp. Brewer's yeast daily.

For men:

❖ Vitamin E 400IU daily, with selenium 200mcg, **and** zinc 75-100mg. with vitamin C 3000mg. daily.

❖ B Complex 150mg. or brewer's yeast 2 teasp. daily, Omega-3 fish or flax oil, 3 teasp daily for essential fatty acids, and Crystal Star MALE PERFORMANCE™ capsules for gland rebuilding.

❖ Carnitine 500mg. **with** chromium picolinate for increased sperm count.

❋ Bodywork for Gland & Hormone Balance:

✚ Get some morning sunshine on the body every day possible. Get regular mild exercise every day.

✚ Alternating hot and cold hydrotherapy is excellent for both men and women to stimulate circulation and glandular secretions throughout the body, (see page 205); also alternating hot and cold compresses on the abdomen or scrotum.

✳ Suggested Recipes For Gland & Hormone Health
By section and recipe number:

BREAKFAST & BRUNCH - 73, 77, 84, 87, 93, 101, 103, 107

SALADS HOT & COLD - all

DAIRY FREE COOKING- all

SUGAR FREE SPECIALS & SWEET TREATS - all

SANDWICHES - SALADS IN BREAD - all

FISH & SEAFOODS - 532, 540, 542, 547, 548, 551, 553, 556, 562, 563, 565, 569, 566

HIGH MINERAL FOODS - all

COMPLEX CARBOHYDRATES FOR ENERGY - 743, 745, 751, 752, 759, 761, 764, 765, 770, 773, 780

HIGH PROTEIN WITHOUT MEAT - 696, 701, 703, 707, 710, 75, 717, 723, 724, 732, 738, 740, 741

GREAT OUTDOOR EATING - 874, 876, 879, 883, 884, 887, 888, 890, 894, 895, 896, 898, 908, 909

✳ Sample Menu Plans
Some recipe combinations that work with this diet:

A HEARTY WINTER MEAL - 643, 618, 641, 651

A LIGHT SUMMER MEAL - 373, 657, 232

A SPECIAL DINNER FOR TWO - 756, 189, 650, 373, 777

AN ALL HORS D'OEUVRES PARTY - 879/880, 538, 710, 909, 722, 908

LUNCH FOR TWO - 784, 620, 496

AN EASY WEEKNIGHT DINNER - 714, 633/635, 442

AN EASY RISING BREAKFAST - 73, 97, 86, 77

A SUNDAY BRUNCH - 88, 531, 660, 662, 696

A WEEKEND PICNIC - 652, 904, 53, 487, 104

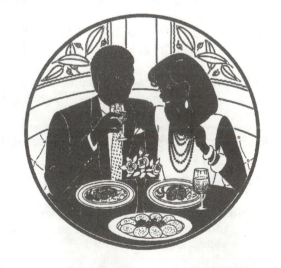

EATING FOR LOVE; A Diet For Better Relationships

This diet is full of key nutrient "superfoods" to rapidly rebuild the body for better sex, vigorous conception, and healthier babies. Remember that good nutrition is a teamwork effort, not one single miracle food or supplement, but the conscious blend of whole and fresh foods that build a foundation for a zestful life.

On rising: take Nutri-Tech ALL 1, or a high protein drink such as Nature's Plus SPIRUTEIN in apple or orange juice; add 1 teasp. brewer's yeast and 1 teasp. wheat germ oil.

Breakfast: for women: make a mix of 2 TBS. **each**: toasted sesame seeds, sunflower seeds, wheat germ and lecithin granules. Sprinkle some each morning on yogurt or fresh fruit, or rice cakes or whole grain cereal. Top with apple juice, 1 TB. maple syrup, molasses, vanilla soy milk or kefir cheese.

        for men: make a mix of 2 TBS. **each**: sunflower seeds, pumpkin seeds, and toasted wheat germ. Sprinkle some each morning on whole grain cereal, pancakes or granola. Top with 1 TB. maple syrup, molasses, apple juice or yogurt; add poached or baked eggs with whole grain toast or muffins.

Mid-morning: have a fresh carrot juice, or a small bottle of mineral water;
or a green drink (pg. 240), Sun CHLORELLA, BARLEY GREEN, or Crystal Star ENERGY GREEN™;
and/or a cup of miso or noodle ramen soup with sea veggies snipped on top.

Lunch: for women: have a leafy green salad with a light soup and corn bread;
or a seafood or broccoli quiche with a green leafy salad;
or a fresh fruit salad with cottage cheese or yogurt.

        for men: have some fish or seafood with brown rice and a small salad;
or a chicken, avocado and low-fat cheese sandwich or salad;
or a whole grain, high protein salad or sandwich with lots of nuts, seeds, tofu or yogurt, and a lentil or black bean soup.

Mid-afternoon: have some low-fat cottage cheese with nuts and seeds and whole grain crackers;
or a dried fruit and nut mix with a bottle of mineral water;
or a hard boiled egg with an herb drink such as ginseng tea (use about 1 dropperful panax ginseng extract in water; or try a ginseng/royal jelly blend in water), or Crystal Star ROYAL MU™ TEA.

Dinner: for women: have a fluffy omelet with vegetables and a green salad;
or a stir-fry with Chinese greens and mushrooms, and baked tofu, or miso soup with sea vesgies;
or a whole grain pasta and vegetable casserole with yogurt/chive sauce.

        for men: have an Italian whole grain pasta or polenta dish with a seafood stew;
or a roast turkey and whole grain stuffing meal, with steamed vegetables and a fresh salad;
or fresh baked seafood or salmon with brown rice and peas.
❧A little wine at dinner is nice for relaxation, digestion, and release from stress and inhibitions.

Before bed: have a cup of VEGEX yeast broth;
or a cup of Crystal Star CUPID'S FLAME TEA™ with honey.

✔ AVOID ALL JUNK FOODS. Particularly avoid sodas, sugary sweets, alcohol, other than wines, refined, chemical and processed foods.

✔ AVOID red meats, saturated fats, fried fatty and salty foods.

✔ Eat small meals more frequently, rather than large meals

✔ Drink plenty of water and mineral water throughout the day to keep the body light and flushed.

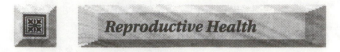

❋ *Supplements for Increased Libido:*

For Women:
❖ Vitamin E 800IU daily with highest potency royal jelly 60,000 to 120,000mg. 1 teasp. daily, or Crystal Star WOMEN'S DRYNESS™ for increased vaginal fluids.

❖ DMG(B15) liquid or sub-lingual tablets, 1 to 2 daily.

❖ Crystal Star LOVE CAPS FEMALE™, 2 daily for a week, and/or DAMIANA/DONG QUAI extract.

❖ Enzymatic Therapy TYROSINE/THYROID capsules, 2 daily.

For Men:
❖ Vitamin E 400IU or lecithin caps with zinc 50mg. 2x daily for healthy seminal fluid.

❖ DMG(B15) liquid or sub-lingual tablets, 2 to3 daily, or Nature's Plus PIZZAZZ (liquid phenylalanine).

❖ BioForce Ginsavena Extract, or SMILAX extract 2x daily for testosterone production.

❖ Yohimbe capsules 500 to 1000mg. as needed for erection help (do **not** take if you have high blood pressure), and testosterone production. Some men have had erection help from liquid niacin before intercourse.

❖ Carnitine 500mg. with chromium picolinate 200mcg daily.

❖ Hghest potency royal jelly, 60,000 to 120,000mg., 1 teasp. daily

❖ Crystal Star LOVE CAPS MALE™ 2 to 4 daily as needed, MALE GINSIAC™ EXTRACT or LOVING MOOD EXTRACT FOR MEN™.

For Both:
❖ Evening primrose oil capsules, as primary essential fatty acids, 2 to 4 daily.

❖ Tyrosine capsules 500mg.

❖ Ginseng/damiana caps, 4 at a time, or Crystal Star CUPID'S FLAME™ TEA.

❖ Avoid tranquilizers, anti-depressants, Aldomet (for high blood pressure), hard alcohol and drugs that suppress hormones. These all suppress desire and sexual ability, too.

❀

❋ *Bodywork for Increased Libido:*

✤ Get regular daily exercise; walking, slow jogging, bicycling, swimming and dancing.

✤ Get plenty of quality rest and sleep. Consciously work to avoid stressful situations. A little vacation together can do wonders, even if it's only a long, quality time weekend doning something you both like.

✽ *Sample Recipes For Increased Libido & Better Relationships*
By section and recipe number:

BREAKFAST & BRUNCH - 74, 75, 76, 82, 83, 86, 96, 98, 102, 104, 107.

SALADS HOT & COLD - all

LOW-FAT & VERY LOW-FAT RECIPES - all

LOW CHOLESTEROL DISHES - all

FISH & SEAFOODS - 524, 538, 541, 546, 550, 552, 554, 558, 567, 568

HIGH MINERAL FOODS - all

HIGH PROTEIN WITHOUT MEAT - 698, 699, 705, 706, 711, 713, 718, 719, 729, 734, 736, 737, 739, 742

COMPLEX CARBOHYDRATES FOR ENERGY - 747, 748, 749, 753, 754, 757, 762, 764, 776, 778, 784

HIGH FIBER RECIPES - 786, 787, 789, 792, 793, 796, 797, 801, 802, 808, 809, 812, 817, 818, 821, 822, 824

GREAT OUTDOOR EATING - all

✽ *Sample Menu Plans*
Some recipe combinations that work with this diet:

AN APPETIZERS & HORS D'OEUVRES PARTY - 533, 909, 906, 882, 904

A SPECIAL DINNER FOR TWO - 563, 539, 795, 811, 289, 812

LUNCH FOR TWO - 657, 561, 616

SUNDAY BRUNCH - 198, 708, 662, 486, 821

A WEEKEND PICNIC - 899, 891, 905, 893

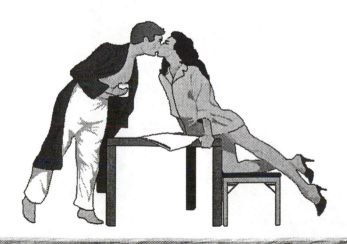

If you don't
change things,
they will stay as they are.
Is that good news?
To change your life,
<u>start immediately.</u>
Give it everything you've got.
It will change
miraculously.

Stress Management & Overcoming Addictions

Most people today seem to be under stress most of the time, depleting energy reserves, and creating over-acid systems that never seem to allow for relaxation. Most of us drive to get as much done as we can in as short a time as possible. Often we try to do as many things as possible at the same time!

A diet high in strengthening, stabilizing minerals and amino acids can go a long way to restoring body and mind energy, and fortifying you for inner calm when the going gets tough.

Chemical overload in our food, pollutants in the air and soil, over use of prescription drugs, too much caffeine, tobacco and alcohol, job pressures, deadlines, unemployment, financial obligations, marital, and family arguments, lack of rest, and fatigue. All cause mental and physiological stress, acid nerve damage, gland imbalance, reduced immune response, mineral and trace mineral deficiencies and changes in normal body chemistry.

Diet improvement can change your life toward better disposition, stability, relaxation, concentration, and gladness instead of sadness at being alive. Correcting nutrient deficiencies is valuable so that prolonged stress won't lead to burn-out or addictions, which eventually intensify the stress, and the problem goes around and around.

Stress is a major factor in reducing immune resistance. A mineral-rich diet affects many stress-related conditions positively. Minerals support and rejuvenate exhausted adrenal glands, the main body resource for tension control and immune stability. During stress-response, the adrenal glands release substances that actually cause the thymus gland to shrink in size and reduce its capacity to stimulate immunity.

In addition to controlling stress & tension, this diet can also benefit:
ANXIETY and DEPRESSION STRESS HEADACHES, MIGRAINES and CLUSTER HEADACHES CHRONIC FATIGUE INSOMNIA COLD SORES and FEVER BLISTERS MENTAL EXHAUSTION LOWER BACK and MUSCLE PAIN NEUR ALGIA, NEURITIS and NERVES DRUG or ALCOHOL ADDICTION and WITHDRAWAL OBSSESSIVE/COMPULSIVE BEHAVIOR SYNDROMES SYSTEM IMBALANCE

Although this program is mainly concerned with diet, there are important bodywork additions to diet improvement that can also alleviate stress.

* Take alternating hot and cold hydrotherapy showers (page 203) to stimulate circulation.

* Take a short get-away vacations. Even a long weekend will do wonders to change your outlook, emotions and body chemistry. You have to unwind before you can unleash.

* Get a massage, full or partial, self-given or by another, to stimulate oxygen uptake and blood flow.

* Get some early morning sunlight on the body every day possible; aerobic exercise 3 to 4 days a week will increase nutrient assimilation, oxygen levels and body balance.

Severe stress and tension often require a reorganization of lifestyle.
Major necessity usually requires major change.

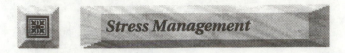

Stage One; A Two Phase Diet For Stress Management

Nearly all stress and nervous tension related problems can benefit from this short cleansing diet; a 3 day liquid fast, followed by a 100% fresh foods diet for 3 more days. This method will gently and steadily alkalize the body, overcoming the acid-producing physiological causes of stress, and infuse the system with concentrated absorbable minerals - especially potassium and magnesium - along with vegetable proteins and complex carbohydrates for energy.

The Three Day Liquid Fast:

On rising: take the juice of 2 lemons or 1 grapefruit in a glass of water with 1teasp. honey.

Breakfast: take a glass of potassium broth or essence (pg. 240).

Mid-morning: have a glass of organic apple juice, or pineapple juice, or a Knudsen "Recharge" electrolyte drink.

Lunch: have a fresh carrot juice every day, and a green drink such as apple/sprout juice, with 1 TB. Bragg's LIQUID AMINOS.

Mid-afternoon: have another organic apple juice, or green drink (pg. 240ff.);
or a refreshing herb tea, such as red clover or gotu kola tea, or Crystal Star CLEANSING & PURIFYING TEA™, RELAX™ TEA or STRESSED OUT™ TEA.

Dinner: have another carrot juice, green drink, or pineapple/coconut juice.

Before bed: have a small apple or papaya juice or relaxing herb tea, such as Crystal Star GOOD NIGHT™ TEA, or chamomile tea,
or a cup of VEGEX broth (1 teasp. yeast paste to 1 cup hot water).

⚜

The Three Day Fresh Foods Diet:

On rising: take 2 lemons squeezed in a glass of water or a glass of grapefruit juice or pineapple/orange juice.

Breakfast: have a potassium broth or essence, with 2 teasp. **each** added: Bragg' s LIQUID AMINOS, unsulphured molasses, and brewer's yeast;
and have some fresh fruit with yogurt.

Mid-morning: have a fresh carrot juice;
and/or a green drink (page240ff.) or Sun CHLORELLA or Barley GREEN MAGMA granules in water;
or Crystal Star ENERGY GREEN™ or SYSTEM STRENGTH™ DRINK.

Lunch: have a leafy green salad with sprouts, carrots, bell peppers, cucumbers, broccoli and lemon/oil dressing. Have celery sticks on the side for cell sodium, with a kefir cheese or fresh yogurt dip.

Mid-afternoon: have a good recharge drink as above for electroytes;
or an herb tea, such as alfalfa/mint, or Crystal Star LICORICE MINTS TEA,
or a fresh fruit smoothie with pineapple, papaya and bananas.

Dinner: have a large dinner salad, with tofu, sprouts, nuts and seeds for protein, and high vitamin C foods, such as bell peppers, broccoli or pea pods,
or a Chinese vegetable salad with tamari dressing.

Before bed: have a VEGEX yeast broth, as above, or a cup of alfalfa/mint tea.

✹ *Supplements for the Cleansing Diet:*
Supplementation should be kept to a minimum during this diet while the body is eliminating stress-causing acids.

❖ Alkalizing/oxygenating food supplements can help: kelp tablets, 8 daily; alfalfa tablets, 8 daily; garlic tablets, 6 daily; acidophilus powder, $1/2$ teasp. before meals; and brewer's yeast, 1 TB. daily.

❖ Make sure you avoid all caffeine containing foods, soft drinks, alcohol, and all acid-forming foods, such as refined sugars and chemically processed foods.

✹ *Bodywork for the Cleansing Diet:*

✚ Relaxing baths with a purpose are excellent at this time, hydrotherapy baths (pg. 203), mineral baths, or herbal baths. Massage feet and legs before bathing to increase circulation.

✚ Do deep breathing exercises followed by a walk around the block to clear the lungs, stimulate circulation, and relieve tension.

✚ Do neck rolls upon rising and at bedtime for stress-free sleep.

Stage Two; Building Body Strength Against Stress And Tension:
This diet is also very alkalizing, and consists of 50% fresh foods. Vitamin B rich foods, and high mineral foods with magnesium and iron are included, to rebuild nerve and muscle systems. Whole grains and vegetable proteins are abundant. Salt and condiments are restricted. All processed and refined foods are omitted because they add to stress, and depletion of the adrenal glands.

On rising: take a glass of lemon/honey/water, or other fresh fruit juice,
and a vitamin/mineral drink such as Nutri-Tech ALL 1 or Crystal Star SYSTEM STRENGTH DRINK™.

Breakfast: have some fresh fruit, such as grapes, papaya, apples or grapefruit;
and yogurt with 1teasp. **each** brewer's yeast, unsulphured molasses and wheat germ;
or have some oatmeal or other whole grain cereal with the above mixture and maple syrup on top.

Mid-morning: have fresh carrot juice with a $1/4$ teasp. sage powder and Bragg's LIQUID AMINOS;
or a potassium broth or refreshing green drink, (pg. 240) with Bragg's LIQUID AMINOS;
or a small bottle of mineral water, or an herb tea, such as red raspberry leaf, or Crystal Star MEDITA-TION™ TEA or CREATIVI-TEA™,
and some crunchy fresh veggies with a vegetable or kefir cheese dip.

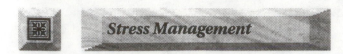

Lunch: have a broccoli quiche with a whole grain crust, or whole grain crepes with broccoli, and lemon sauce;
or a large romaine or other leafy salad, with sprouts, celery, toasted sea vegetables and wheat germ;
or a vegetable sandwich on whole grain bread with avocados;
or marinated, baked tofu with millet or brown rice;
or a tuna or salmon salad or sandwich with green mayonnaise and lemon;
or a whole grain or vegetable pasta salad, hot or cold.

Mid-afternoon: have whole grain crackers, chips or raw vegetables with kefir cheese or a veggie dip;
or some yogurt or kefir with fresh fruit;
and a refreshing herb tea, such as spearmint or lemon grass tea, or Crystal Star RELAX™ TEA`, or LICORICE MINTS TEA.

Dinner: have a baked, broiled, or grilled white fish, such as halibut or sole, with a small green salad;
or a large dinner salad with toasted nuts, seeds, wheat germ and yogurt dressing;
or a seafood salad with baked potato or brown rice;
or some steamed veggies with tofu and brown rice;
or baked salmon with asparagus or peas and rice;
or a little roast turkey with cornbread and herb dressing.
Have a little-white wine before dinner to relax and aid digestion.

Before bed: take 1 teasp. VEGEX yeast paste in a cup of hot water for high B vitamins and relaxation; **or** a relaxing herb tea such as Crystal Star MOONBEAM TEA;
or a glass of carrot, apple or papaya juice.

✳ *Supplements & Herbal Aids for Building a Stress-Free Body:*

❖ Take ascorbate vitamin C 2-3000mg. with bioflavonoids daily as a natural tranquilizer.

❖ Take a Stress B Complex, 100-150mg. daily, <u>with</u> Mezotrace SEA MINERAL COMPLEX 4 daily.

❖ Calcium/magnesium caps 500/500mg. ratio, with B6 100mg if desired, for nerve support.

❖ Crystal Star VALERIAN/WILD LETTUCE or STRESSED OUT™ EXTRACT. Try DLPA 500 to 750mg. capsules or Crystal Star DEPRESS-EX™ EXTRACT for tranquility in depression.

❖ Crystal Star RELAX™ CAPS and ADRN-ALIVE™ caps, 2 daily, and evening primrose oil caps 4 to 6 daily for prostaglandin production and unsaturated fatty acids.

✳ *Bodywork for Building a Stress-Free Body:*

✚ Continue with your exercise program, and deep breathing. Do several neck rolls each morning and at bedtime.

✚ Long weekends are a good stress fighter. Lost time is compensated for by increased productivity.

Diet Help To Overcome Addictions:

Good nutrition is a positive support therapy in the successful recovery from addictions to drugs, alcohol, nicotine or concentrated sugars. The overwhelming majority of habitual drug and addicting substance users suffer from malnutrition, metabolic upset and nutritional imbalances. When these conditions are corrected, the need to get high by artificial means is sharply diminished.

Drug abuse in one form or another has become a fact of modern life. Our high stress lifestyles depletes energy reserves, motivating many people to seek a quick "voltage" fix to overcome fatigue and relieve tension or boredom. Using drugs, sugar, alcohol or caffeine as fuel creates multiple nutritional deficiencies of vitamins, minerals, essential fatty acids, amino acids and enzymes. This depletion sets off a chain reaction which results in stress and craving for nutrients, the process is repeated in a futile effort to satisfy increasing need, and addiction eventually occurs.

For most people, this is just the beginning, because drug-caused malnutrition and reduced immunity swiftly lead to hypothyroidism, Chronic Fatigue Syndrome, and other auto-immune diseases such as Mononucleosis, Hepatitis, M.S. and AIDS Related Syndromes. Even if these serious disorders are avoided, the consequences are high. Drug abusers and potential drug abusers are always either sick or coming down with something. As soon as one cold, sore throat, bout of "flu," or bladder infection is treated, a new one takes its place. Work is impaired, job time is lost, and family and social life greatly affected.

Nutritional support is the essential key to recovery from addictions. The following diet can establish a solid nutrition foundation for rebuilding a depleted system. Regeneration takes time. It often takes up to a year to detoxify and clear drugs from the bloodstream. (See also the DETOXIFICATION & BODY CLEANSING chapter in this book.)

The following diet is designed to establish a solid nutritional base and revitalize metabolic deficiences quickly. It is rich in vegetable proteins, high in minerals (especially magnesium to overcome nerve stress), with Omega-3 oils, vitamin B and C source foods, and antioxidants.

On rising: take a "superfood" drink to give energy and control morning blood sugar drop: 1 teasp. **each** in a glass of apple or orange juice; glycine powder, spirulina **or** chlorella granules, sugar free protein powder, brewer's yeast;
or take a sugar free high protein drink such as Nature's Plus SPIRUTEIN;
or a concentrated mineral drink, such as Crystal Star SYSTEM STRENGTH™ DRINK.

Breakfast: make a concentrated food mineral mix to shore up mineral depletion: 1 teasp. **each:** sesame seeds, toasted wheat germ, unsulphured molasses, bee pollen granules, and brewer's yeast. Sprinkle some on any of the following breakfast choices;
fresh fruit with yogurt or kefir cheese topping;
or oatmeal or hot kashi pilaf with a little yogurt and maple syrup topping;
or a whole grain cereal, muesli or granola with apple juice or fruit yogurt;
or a poached or baked egg on whole grain toast with kefir or yogurt cheese.

Mid-morning: have a green drink (page 240), Sun CHLORELLA or Green Foods GREEN ESSENCE drink, or Crystal Star ENERGY GREEN™ DRINK;
and/or a whole grain muffin or corn bread with a little butter, kefir cheese or yogurt spread;
and/or a small bottle of mineral water.

Lunch: have a fresh veggie salad with cottage cheese, topped with nuts, seeds and crunchy noodles;
and/or a high protein sandwich on whole grain bread, with avocados, low-fat cheese, and greens;
or some oriental fried rice and miso soup with sea vegetables;
or a seafood salad with a black bean or lentil soup;
or a vegetarian pizza on a whole grain or chapati crust.

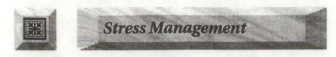

Mid-afternoon: have a hard boiled egg with mayonnaise or yogurt, and some whole grain crackers; **and** another bottle of mineral water, or herb tea, such as Crystal Star HIGH ENERGY' TEA.

Dinner: have a vegetable casserole with tofu, or chicken and brown rice;
or a broccoli or mushroom quiche or whole grain crepes with a light sauce and a green salad;
or a spanish paella with seafoods and rice, or a mexican beans and rice dish;
or an oriental stir-fry with noodles and vegetables, and miso soup;
or a whole grain pasta with steamed vegetables and a green salad.

Before bed: have a cup of VEGEX yeast broth;
or apple or papaya juice.

Dietary Watchwords:
  1) Eat **magnesium-rich foods**, such as green leafy and yellow vegetables, potatoes, citrus fruits, whole grain cereals, fish, eggs, and legumes.
  2) Eat **potassium-rich foods**, such as oranges, broccoli, green peppers, seafoods, sea vegetables, bananas, and tomatoes.
  3) Eat **chromium-rich foods**, such as brewer's yeast, mushroooms, whole grains, sea foods and peas.
  4) Eat some **vegetable protein** at every meal.

✱ *Supplements to Help Overcome Addictions:*

❖ Take ascorbate vitamin C crystals, 1/4 to 1/2 teasp. in water 3 to 4x daily (5 to 10,000mg.), or to bowel tolerance as an antioxidant and detoxifying agent, *with* Solaray CHROMIACIN to restimulate circulation. Take vitamin E as an antioxidant to strengthen adrenals and restore liver function.

❖ Take a full spectrum, pre-digested amino acid compound, 1000mg. daily to rebuild from a low protein diet and poor assimilation.

❖ Take a mega potency Stress B Complex daily, 100-150mg. to overcome deficiencies caused by excess sugar, caffeine or alcohol.

❖ Take glutamine 500mg. and tyrosine 500mg. daily to help reduce drug cravings, or Crystal Star DA-X extract. Use Crystal Star DEPRESS-EX™ extract to help overcome drug-related depression.

❖ Take evening primrose oil or high Omega-3 flax or fish oils for essential fatty acids to stimulate prostaglandin production.

❖ Take a complete herb source multi-mineral/trace mineral, such as Mezotrace SEA MINERAL COMPLEX, or Crystal Star MINERAL SPECTRUM™ capsules, or MINERAL SPECTRUM™ extract.

✱ *Bodywork To Help Overcome Addictions:*

✚ Avoid smoking and secondary smoke. Tobacco increases craving for all drugs. Avoid tobacco, and all drugs, if possible, as major contributors to continued body stress.

✚ Get some exercise every day, to keep body oxygen levels up and blood sugar levels balanced.

✻ Sample Recipes to Help Overcome Addictions
By section and recipe number:

BREAKFAST & BRUNCH - all

SUGAR FREE SWEET TREATS - 413, 415, 416, 420, 422, 423, 425, 426, 430, 433, 438, 440, 441, 443, 444

SANDWICHES - SALADS IN BREAD - 473, 474, 477, 478, 480, 481, 483, 487, 488, 489, 491, 492, 500

STIR-FRYS - 501, 502, 503, 504, 505, 506, 509, 510, 512, 513, 515, 516, 518, 519, 524, 527, 529, 530, 531

FISH & SEAFOODS - all

TOFU FOR YOU - all

HIGH MINERAL FOODS - all

HIGH PROTEIN COOKING WITHOUT MEAT - all

HIGH COMPLEX CARBOHYDRATES FOR ENERGY - all

✻ Sample Menu Palns
Recipe combinations that work with these diets:

AN EASY WEEKNIGHT DINNER - 427, 510, 719A, 579

A HEARTY WINTER MEAL - 426, 649, 612, 652

A LIGHT SUMMER MEAL - 420, 717, 528

A FAMILY MEAL - 727, 443, 579, 719A

LUNCH FOR TWO - 432, 696, 542

SUNDAY BRUNCH - 710, 324, 539, 653, 663

A WEEKEND PICNIC - 712, 412, 331, 621, 487

AN EASY RISING BREAKFAST - 321, 715, 101, 411

A SPECIAL DINNER FOR TWO - 616, 657, 662, 331, 662

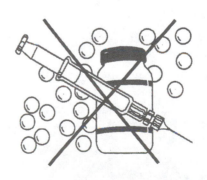

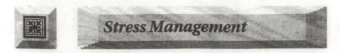

Stage Three; Maintaining a Stress Free Life

The final phase of eating for a stress-less life concentrates on supporting mineral stability in the body with alkalizing foods, high B vitamins, and adrenal nourishment from whole grains and complex carbohydrates. Begin this diet approximately three months after rebuilding on the Stage Two level. You should then feel ready to make permanent changes in your eating habits. Continued avoidance of sugars and other refined carbohydrates needs to become a way of life for adrenal health and body stress control. Several small meals daily instead of large meals will also enhance system equilibrium. As stress increases, calorie and protein needs increase. Stress causes protein to burn up and break down faster, so diet improvement should include foods rich in amino acids and non-meat proteins. Awareness of good food combining is also important in managing stress. (Pg. 89).

On rising: take a glass of fresh citrus juice, and a vitamin/mineral drink such as NutriTech ALL 1:

Breakfast: Make a mix of 2 TBS. each; lecithin granules, toasted wheat germ, brewer's yeast and sesame seeds. Sprinkle some on your breakfast choice each morning; such as fresh fruit with yogurt;
or a whole grain cereal with apple juice or soy milk;
or have oat bran or buckwheat pancakes with a little apple juice or maple syrup;
or a poached egg on whole grain toast or english muffin with a small amount of butter and tamari.

Mid-morning: have some fresh fruit, or a fruit smoothie with a banana;
or some crunchy raw veggies or whole grain chips with kefir cheese or a veggie/yogurt dip;
or Sun CHLORELLA green drink with 1 teasp. Bragg's LIQUID AMINOS;
or an energizing herb tea, such as Siberian ginseng, gotu kola, or Crystal Star HIGH ENERGY TEA™ or FEEL GREAT TEA™.

Lunch: have a salmon patty on whole grain toast with a light sauce, or a salmon salad with brown rice or egg pasta;
or have a high protein salad with dark leafy greens, and toasted nuts, seeds and tofu toppings;
or a vegetable pizza on a whole grain chapati with low-fat cheese;
or a high protein turkey, tuna or chicken salad sandwich with mayonnaise and tamari seasoning;

Mid-afternoon: have some fresh carrot juice once a week, or a good green drink (page 240);
and some fresh raw veggies with a dip or kefir cheese;
or have some fresh fruits and yogurt;
or a bottle of mineral water or herb tea such as Crystal Star LICORICE MINTS or RELAX™ TEA.

Dinner: have baked or grilled halibut, mahi mahi or aji steaks with a green salad, or steamed veggies;
or a light Italian meal with whole grain or veggie pasta, or a deep dish, no-crust pizza;
or a large dinner salad with a light brothy soup;
or an oriental stir-fry with bean sprouts, vegetables, rice stick noodles and miso soup;
or a vegetable quiche and salad meal, with whole grain crust and plenty of greens.
❧ Have a little wine with dinner for digestion and relaxation.

✻ *Supplements & Herbs to Help Maintain a Stress-Free Life:*

❖ Continue with your vitamin C and stress B Complex choices daily. Add CoQ10, 30mg. daily.

❖ Add an herbal tonic, such as Crystal Star HAWTHORN EXTRACT or ADRN ALIVE™ EXTRACT, or ADRN-ALIVE™ CAPSULES with BODY REBUILDER™ CAPSULES to help insure stable and balanced glandular activity.

❖ Take a multi-mineral supplement daily such as MEZOTRACE SEA MINERAL COMPLEX.

✿ *Bodywork to Help Maintain a Stress-Free Life:*

✚ Exercise should be considered a nutrient in itself for stress-free living; there is no substitute for a daily walk, even if it's only around the block.

✚ Use alternating hot and cold hydrotherapy (page 204) several times a week.

✚ Massage tips of fingers and wrists when needed to alleviate body stress.

✿ *Sample Recipes For Maintaining A Stress-Free Life By section and recipe number:*

ORIENTAL & LIGHT MACROBIOTIC EATING - all

SALADS HOT & COLD - all

LOW CHOLESTEROL DISHES - 301, 304, 305, 307, 308, 310, 311, 312, 314, 315, 316, 317, 320, 321, 331

SUGAR FREE SPECIALS & SWEET TREATS - 412, 413, 415, 416, 417, 427, 431, 434, 439, 442, 443, 444

SANDWICHES - SALADS IN BREAD - 473, 474, 477, 481, 483, 485, 488, 489, 491, 492, 494, 498, 500

STIR-FRYS - ORIENTAL STEAM BRAISING - ALL

FISH & SEAFOODS - all

TOFU FOR YOU - all

HIGH MINERAL FOODS - all

HIGH PROTEIN COOKING WITHOUT MEAT - all

HIGH COMPLEX CARBOHYDRATES FOR ENERGY - all

HIGH FIBER RECIPES - all

HEALTHY HOLIDAY FEASTING - 826, 831, 833, 842, 843, 844, 848, 850, 853, 855, 858, 861, 866, 868

GREAT OUTDOOR EATING - 874, 875, 878, 879, 881, 884, 886, 888, 890, 894, 895, 896, 906, 908, 909

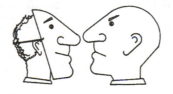

❋ Sample Meal Planning
Recipe combinations that work with this diet:

AN EASY WEEKNIGHT DINNER - 526, 313, 795

A HEARTY WINTER MEAL -315, 628, 525, 823

A LIGHT SUMMER MEAL - 545, 494, 416, 440

A FAMILY MEAL - 134, 511, 325, 418

LUNCH FOR TWO - 615, 549, 414

SUNDAY BRUNCH - 431, 792, 639, 499, 624

A WEEKEND PICNIC - 500, 423, 882, 319, 112/113

AN EASY RISING BREAKFAST - 322, 93, 75, 79

A SPECIAL DINNER FOR TWO - 627, 512, 327, 626, 430

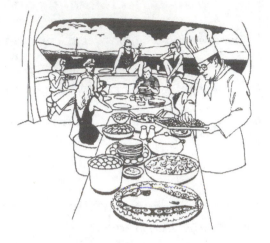

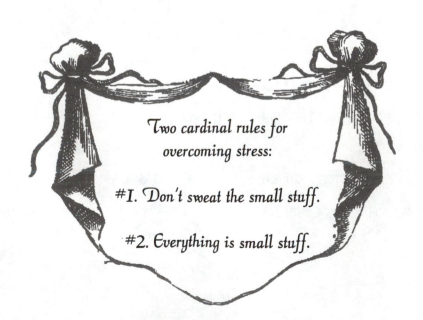

Two cardinal rules for
overcoming stress:

#1. Don't sweat the small stuff.

#2. Everything is small stuff.

Optimal Eating For Childhood Disease Control

Unless unusually or chronically ill, a child is born with a well-developed, powerful immune system, that often needs only the subtle body-strengthening forces that nutritious foods, herbs or homeopathic remedies supply, rather than highly focused drugs that may have drastic side effects on a small body. Unfortunately, however, the undeniable ecological, sociological and diet deterioration in America during the last fifty years has had a marked effect on children's health. Declining educational performance, learning disabilities, mental disorders, drug and alcohol abuse, hypoglycemia, allergies, chronic illness, delinquency and violent behavior are all evidence of declining immune response and general health.

Diet is the most important way to keep a child's immunity and defense mechanisms working. Germs and viruses are everywhere. They are not the major factor in causing disease; the body environment must be suitable for them to flourish. Well-nourished children are usually strong enough to deal with infection in a successful way. They either do not catch the "bugs" that are going around, they contract only a mild case, or they develop strong healthy reactions that are short in duration, and will get the problem over and done with quickly. It is this difference in resistance and inherent immunity that is the key factor in understanding children's diseases.

Kids have extraordinarily sensitive taste buds. Everything they eat is very vivid and important to them. The diet program we offer here has lots of variety, so they can experiment and find out where their own preferences lie. There are plenty of snacks, sandwiches, fresh fruits, and sweet veggies like carrots - all foods children naturally like.

Keep it simple. Let them help prepare their own food, even though they might get in the way and you feel its more trouble than its worth. They will have a better understanding of what good food is, and are more likely to eat things they have a hand in preparing. Keep only good nutritious foods in the house. Your children may be exposed to junk foods and poor foods at school or their friend's houses, but you can build a natural foods foundation diet at home. When they are at home, they should only have good nutrition choices.

Remember: Kids don't want to be sick, they aren't stupid, and they often recognize natural foods and therapies that are good for them. Children are naturally immune to disease. A nutritious diet can help keep them that way.
The diet and therapy suggestions in this chapter are effective for several childhood problems: ❧ACUTE BRONCHITIS ❧CHEST CONGESTION ❧CONSTIPATION ❧INDIGESTION, GAS and FLATULENCE ❧DIARRHEA ❧CHICKENPOX ❧JAUNDICE ❧PARASITES and WORMS ❧EARACHE ❧FEVER ❧MEASLES ❧MUMPS ❧CHILDHOOD ALLERGIES & SENSITIVITIES ❧WHOOPING COUGH ❧HYPERACTIVITY ❧COLDS, FLU, SORE THROAT ❧THRUSH and other FUNGAL INFECTIONS ❧WEAK SYSTEM and LOW IMMUNITY ❧

Four separate diets are included in this chapter: 1) a short liquid cleansing fast for rapid toxin elimination, 2) a raw foods purification diet for body cleansing during the beginning and acute stages of a disease, 3) an optimal whole foods maintenance diet for disease prevention, and 4) a very young child's vegetarian diet that assures adequate protein and nutrition.

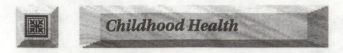

Diet Help For Childhood Diseases

Diet and nutritional therapy for most common childhood diseases, including measles, mumps, chicken pox, strep throat and whooping cough, is fairly simple and basic. A short liquid elimination fast, followed by a fresh light foods diet is the key in the acute stages.

Stage One; A Short Liquid Elimination Fast:

✓ Start the child on cleansing liquids as soon as the disease is diagnosed to clean out harmful bacteria and infection. Give fruit juices such as apple, pineapple, grape, cranberry and citrus juices are all helpful. The juice of 2 lemons in a glass of water with a little honey should be taken once or twice a day to flush the kidneys and alkalize the body.

✓ Alternate fruit juices throughout the day with fresh carrot juice, bottled mineral water, and clear soups. A potassium broth or green drink (page 240ff.) should be taken at least once a day for best results. Encourage the child to drink as many of the healthy cleansing liquids as s/he wants. No dairy products should be given.

Note: This liquid diet may last for 24 hours up to 72 hours, depending on the state of the child and the severity of the disease.

❋ *Supplements for the Child's Liquid Fast*

✤ Herb teas may be taken throughout the fast. Make them about half the strength as that for an adult. Children respond to herb teas quickly, and they like them more than you might think. Just add a little honey if the herbs are bitter. We have found the following teas effective for most childhood diseases; elder flowers with peppermint to induce perspiration; catnip/chamomile/rosemary tea to break out a rash; mullein/lobelia or scullcap as relaxants; catnip, fennel and peppermint for upset stomachs.

✤ Crystal Star COFEX TEA™ for sore throats, X-PEC-TEA™ to help bring up mucous, CHILL CARE™ TEA for warming against chills, and ECHINACEA EXTRACT drops in water every 3 to 4 hours to keep the lymph glands clear and able to process infective toxins.

✤ Acidophilus liquid, such as Natren Life Start, or Lacto-Bifidus are excellent for children to keep friendly bacteria in the G.I. tract (Especially if they are taking anti-biotics). Use 1/4 teasp. at a time in a glass of water or juice three to four times daily.

❋ *Bodywork for the Child's Liquid Fast*

✤ A gentle enema with catnip tea is very effective for clearing the colon of impacted wastes. These hinder the body in its effort to rid itself of diseased bacteria.

✤ Oatmeal baths help neutralize acids and rash coming out on the skin. Hydrotherapy baths (Pg. 205) to induce cleansing perspiration are effective. Use calendula or comfrey tea. A soothing body rub with calendula oil, Tiger Balm or tea tree oil will often loosen congestion after an herbal bath.

✤ Ginger/cayenne compresses applied to affected and sore areas will stimulate circulation and defense mechanisms, to rid the body more quickly of infection.

✤ Herbal steam inhalations, such as eucalyptus or tea tree oil, or Crystal Star RSPR-TEA™ in a vaporizer will help to keep lungs mucous free and improve oxygen uptake.

✤ Goldenseal, myrrh, yellow dock, black walnut, yarrow, or Crystal Star THERADERM™ TEA, may be patted onto sores, scabs and lesions with cotton balls to help heal and soothe.

Stage Two; A Raw Foods Purification Diet For Children's Diseases:

This diet may be used for initial, acute and chronic disease symptoms when a liquid fast is not desired, or to follow a liquid fast when the acute stage has passed. The body will continue cleansing, and the addition of solid foods will start to rebuild strength. Dairy products, except for yogurt should be avoided. This diet should last about 3 days depending on the strength and condition of the child.

On rising: give citrus juice with a teaspoon of acidophilus liquid, or $1/4$ tsp. acidophilus powder;
or a glass of lemon juice and water with honey.

Breakfast: offer fresh fruits, such as apples, pineapple, papaya or oranges. Add some vanilla yogurt or soymilk if desired.

Mid-morning: Give a green drink, a potassium broth, (page 240ff.) or fresh carrot juice. Add $1/4$ teasp. ascorbate vitamin C or Ester C crystals.

Lunch: give some fresh raw crunchy veggies with a little yogurt dip;
or a fresh veggie salad with lemon/oil or yogurt dressing.

Mid-afternoon: offer a refreshing herb tea, such as licorice or peppermint or Crystal Star LICORICE MINTS, or AFTER MEAL EXTRACT™ drops in water to keep stomach settled and calm tension,
or another green drink with $1/4$ teasp. vitamin C added.

Dinner: have a fresh salad, with avocados, carrots, kiwi, romaine and other high vitamin A foods;
and/or a cup of miso soup or other clear broth soup.

Before bed: offer a relaxing herb tea, such as chamomile or scullcap tea, or Crystal Star GOOD NIGHT TEA™. Add $1/4$ teasp. ascorbate vitamin C or Ester C crystals;
or a cup of VEGEX yeast broth for strength and B vitamins.

✳ Supplements for the Raw Food Children's Diet

❖ Continue with your acidophilus choice. Add vitamin A & D in drops if desired, and ascorbate vitamin C crystals in juice as outlined above.

❖ Continue with the therapeutic herbal teas you found effective in the liquid fast.

❖ Use a mild herbal laxative in half dosage if necessary, to keep the child eliminating regularly.

❖ Use garlic oil drops or open garlic capsules into juice or water for natural anti-biotic activity; or give Crystal Star ANTI-BI™ CAPS or EXTRACT in half dosage.

✷ *Bodywork Aids for the Raw Foods Children's Diet*

✚ Continue with herbal baths, washes and compresses to neutralize and cleanse toxins coming out through the skin.

✚ Give a soothing massage before bed.

✚ Get some early morning sunlight on the body every day possible for regenerating vitamin D.

Note: When the crisis has passed, and the child is on the mend with a clean system, it is an excellent time to start them on an optimal nutrition diet for prevention of further problems, and increased general health and energy.

An Optimal Whole Foods Diet For Children

The best health and disease prevention diet for children is high in whole grains and green veggies for minerals, vegetable proteins for growth, and complex carbohydrates for energy. It is low in fats, pasteurized dairy foods and sugars, (sugars inhibit release of growth hormones), and avoids fried foods. It is also very easy on you, the parent. Once children are taught and shown the foods that will give them health and energy they can make a lot of these simply prepared foods on their own. Make sure you tell and graphically show your child what junk and synthetic foods are. We find over and over again that because of beguiling TV advertising and peer pressure, kids often really don't know what wholesome food is, and think they are eating the right way.

On rising: give a vitamin/mineral drink such as NutriTech EARTHSHAKE or Nature's Plus SPIRUTEIN (lots of flavors), or 1 teaspoon liquid multi-vitamin in juice (such as Floradix CHILDREN'S MULTI-VITAMIN/MINERAL).

Breakfast: have a whole grain cereal with apple juice or a little yogurt and fresh fruit;
and, if more is desired, whole grain toast or muffins, with a little butter, kefir cheese or nut butter;
add eggs, scrambled or baked or soft boiled (no fried eggs);
or have some hot oatmeal or kashi with a little maple syrup, and yogurt if desired.

Mid-morning: snacks can be whole grain crackers with kefir cheese or low-fat cheese or dip, and a sugarless juice or sparkling mineral water;
and/or some fresh fruit, dried fruit, or fruit leathers such as apples with yogurt or kefir cheese;
or fresh crunchy veggies with peanut butter or a nut spread;
or a sugar-free dried fruit, nut and seed candy bar (you can easily make your own) or a dried fruit and nut trail mix, stirred into yogurt.

Lunch: have a fresh veggie, turkey, chicken or shrimp salad sandwich on whole grain bread, with low-fat or soy cheese and mayonnaise. Add whole grain or corn chips with a low-fat veggie or cheese dip;
or a hearty bean soup with whole grain toast or crackers, and a small salad or crunchy veggies with garbanzo spread;
or a baked potato with a little butter, kefir cheese, or soy cheese, and a small green salad with Italian dressing;
or a vegetarian pizza on a chapati or whole grain crust;
or whole grain spaghetti or pasta with a light sauce and parmesan cheese;
or a Mexican bean and veggie, or rice burrito (whole grain) with a light natural no-sugar salsa or a small amount of sour cream.

Mid-afternoon: have a sparkling juice and a dried fruit candy bar;
or some fresh fruit or fruit juice, or a kefir drink with whole grain muffins and kefir cheese;
or a hard boiled egg, and some whole grain chips with a veggie or low-fat cheese dip;
or some whole grain toast and peanut butter or other nut butter.

Dinner: have a light pizza on a whole grain, chapati or egg crust, with veggies, shrimp, and soy or low-fat mozarella cheese topping;
or whole grain or egg pasta with vegetables and a light tomato and cheese sauce;
or a baked Mexican quesadilla with soy or low-fat cheese and some steamed veggies or a salad;
or a stir-fry with crunchy noodles, brown rice, baked egg rolls and a light soup;
or some roast turkey with cornbread dressing and a salad;
or a tuna casserole with rice, peas and waterchestnuts and toasted chapatis with a litle butter.

Before bed: a glass of apple juice or a little soy milk or flavored kefir.

Note: A wholesome diet can easily restore a child's natural vitality. Even children who have eaten a junk food diet for years quickly respond to fresh fruits, vegetables, whole grains, and low fats and sugars. We have noted great improvement in only a month's time. Their hair and skin take on new luster, they fill out if they are too skinny, and lose weight if they are fat. They sleep sounder and more regularly. Their attention span markedly increases, and many learning and behavior problems diminish or disappear.

✻ *Supplements for the Optimal Childrens Diet*

Vitamins and minerals are important for a child's physical, emotional and mental growth, and for a healthy immune system. A child's normal immune defenses are strong. If s/he is eating well , with lots of green veggies, and few sugars, refined foods or dairy products, s/he may not need extra supplementation. However, because of depleted soils and sprayed produce, many vitamins, minerals and trace minerals are no longer sufficiently present in our foods, so supplementation is often needed for good body building blocks, and to enable children to think, learn and grow at optimum levels. The most common deficiencies are calcium, iron, B₁, and vitamins A, B-Complex and C.

If your child needs more nutrition than s/he is receiving from diet, daily supplementation might include:

❖ Acidophilus, in liquid or powder; give in juice 2-3x daily for good digestion and assimilation.

❖ Vitamin C in chewable or powder form with bioflavonoids; give in juice $1/4$ teasp. at a time 2 to 3x daily. If chewable wafers are chosen, use 100mg., 250mg., or 500mg. potency according to age and weight of the child, and give 3 to 4 times daily.

❖ Give a sugar-free multi-vitamin and mineral supplement daily, in either liquid or chewable tablet form. Some good choices are from Floradix, Rainbow Light, Solaray and Mezotrace.

❖ Give a protein drink each morning if the child's energy or school performance level is poor, or if a weak system is constantly leading to chronic illness. (The body must have protein to heal.) Good choices are from Nature's Plus SPIRUTEIN, NutriTech EARTHSHAKE, or this book (page 265).

✻ *Bodywork for the Optimal Children's Diet*

Exercise is the key to health, growth and body oxygen. Don't let your kid be a couch potato, or a computer junkie. Encourage outdoor sports and activity every day possible, and make sure s/he is taking P. E. classes in school. Exercise for kids is one of the best nutrients for both body and mind.

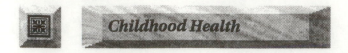
� **Sample Recipes For The Optimal Children's Diet**
By section and recipe number:

BREAKFAST & BRUNCH - 73, 74, 77, 82, 84, 87, 88, 90, 93, 100, 104, 105, 106, 107, 108

LOW CHOLESTEROL RECIPES - 306, 313, 314, 317, 318, 319, 320, 323, 324, 328, 331

SANDWICHES - SALADS IN BREAD - 473, 477, 480, 481, 487, 486, 489, 490, 493, 496, 500

SUGAR FREE SWEET TREATS - 411, 413, 417, 418, 420, 421, 425, 426, 427, 430, 432, 433, 437, 438, 442

HIGH MINERAL FOODS - 614, 618, 620, 623, 638, 639, 641, 643, 646, 650, 652, 653, 656, 658, 659, 663

PROTEIN WITHOUT MEAT - 695, 606, 697, 704, 708, 712, 714, 715, 725, 726, 727, 728, 730, 731, 739

COMPLEX CARBOHYDRATES FOR ENERGY - 743, 745, 760, 764, 771, 773, 778, 779, 780, 781, 784

HIGH FIBRE RECIPES - 786, 788, 792, 793, 794, 795, 796, 802, 804, 806, 809, 811, 814, 817, 818, 819, 820

HOLIDAY FEASTING - 827, 829, 830, 831, 833, 834, 836, 840, 848, 850, 851, 854, 855, 856, 859, 860, 869

GREAT OUTDOOR EATING - 878, 882, 887, 889, 892, 897, 900, 908, 909

Note: ALL of the recipes suggested here have been "kid-tested." They liked 'em, they liked 'em.

✺

A Highly Nutritious Vegan Diet For Very Young Children:

Many parents today feel that it is important to raise a their children as vegetarians, both for the child's health and the health of the planet. Many thoughtful children also understand that a vegetarian diet preserves the earth and its vital diversity. (See ABOUT RED MEAT in this book, page 206). Even if there is no philosophical commitment, a whole foods, vegetarian diet generally provides more vitamins, minerals and trace mineral growth and health factors than the typical American child's diet. Vegetarian children grow up with a proven lower risk of several types of cancer and heart disease, and a history of freedom from chronic colds, allergies and childhood diseases. The following diet suggestions can help assure sufficient, balanced protein, minerals and other nutrients for early growing years.

☺**For the first year** it is important to breastfeed your child. No other foods or formulas, including cow's milk, goat's milk, or soy milk have the right balance of minerals, digestible fats and protein. From birth to six months, *all* of the child's nutritional needs can be met with breast milk. If this is not possible, soy-based infant formula should be used. (Soy **milk alone** is *not* complete enough for infants.) Because of its ideal nutritional profile for infants, breast milk should be a part of the diet for 18 to 24 months. Many allergies and intestinal problems stem from the child's attempt to assimilate solid foods before the digestive system has developed enough to do so.

☺**Around six to eight months,** begin with easily digestible foods. Add more foods one at a time, leaving a day or two in between to check for allergy or indigestibility. When preferences and intolerances are established, foods may be mixed. Encourage variety, but don't force acceptance. If the baby rejects a food, wait and reintroduce the food at a later date. A baby's instincts are often correct about what it wants or shouldn't have.

☺ **Six to Eight Month Foods:** Ripe mashed banana, applesauce, yogurt mixed with applesauce or banana, mashed avocado, mashed peaches, mushy, whole grain cereals, such as oatmeal, mixed with yogurt or breast milk and a little maple syrup, cooked, mashed squash, carrots and yams with a little maple syrup, steamed, pureed peas.

☺ **Add at eight to ten months:** Spinach, romaine, kale and other leafy greens, steamed and pureed in the blender with a little butter or sesame tahini or avocado, boiled and mashed tofu with a little applesauce or maple syrup, steamed, pureed broccoli, cauliflower and green beans.

☺ **Add at ten to twelve months:** Baked potatoes mashed with a little butter or yogurt, dried beans and peas cooked very soft and mashed, chopped ripe fresh *non-citrus* fruits, peanut butter, almond butter, and other nut butters, kefir and kefir cheese.

☺ **Add at twelve to fourteen months:** whole grain bread, toast, pitas and chapatis, with a little butter, nut butter or maple syrup if desired, citrus fruits, cooked pasta, chopped with a little butter, brown rice and other whole grains, such as kashi, bulgar, millet and couscous, celery and other raw or steamed veggies with a little butter or kefir cheese if desired, soy and low-fat *soft* cheeses, baked and scrambled eggs, soaked dried fruits.

☺ **By fourteen to eighteen months:** The child can be eating the same diet you do, including occasional fish, chicken and seafood.

Remember that a child's growth rate is extremely rapid between birth and two years old. Most babies triple their birth weight and double their height by the time they reach their first birthday. Considerable calorie and nutrient intake is necessary. An average of 45-50 calories is required for each pound of weight during the first year. After that growth slows down, but goes through two more major growing spurts from ages five to seven, and twelve to sixteen. Maximum nutrition is obviously necessary at these times, but also during the in-between times, when a child's calorie needs and appetite drop off considerably; everything eaten needs to be nutritious.

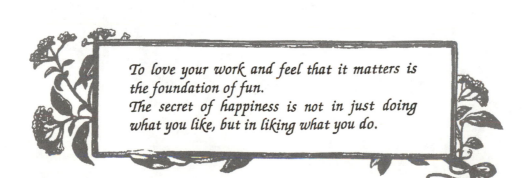

To love your work and feel that it matters is the foundation of fun.
The secret of happiness is not in just doing what you like, but in liking what you do.

Teamwork
is the fuel that allows
common people to attain
uncommon results.

Overcoming Candida Albicans Yeast Overgrowth

Candida Albicans is a strain of yeasts commonly found in the gastro-intestinal and genito-urinary areas of the body. It is normally harmless, but when resistance and immunity are low, Candida is able to multiply rapidly, feeding on the sugar and carbohydrates in these tracts, releasing many toxins into the bloodstream, and causing far-reaching problems for the body. It is a stress-related disease, brought about because the body is severely out of balance; usually either by repeated rounds of anti-biotics, birth control pills, or cortico-steroid drugs, or by a nutritionally poor diet, high in refined sugars, carbohydrates or alcohol, and a hectic life style short on rest. Candida albicans is a modern day opportunistic strain that takes advantage of reduced immune response to overrun the body. Healthy liver function and a strong immune system are the keys to lasting prevention and control of Candida overgrowth.

Diet is the most effective way to rebuild immune and liver strength. The healing/rebuilding process usually takes from 3-6 months or more and is not easy. The necessary changes in diet, habits and life-style are often radical. Some people feel better right away; others go through a rough "healing crisis." (Candida yeasts are living organisms, and part of the body. Killing them off is traumatic.) But most people with Candida are feeling so bad anyway that the treatment and the knowledge that they are getting better pulls them through the hard times. Be as gentle with your body as you can. Give yourself all the time you need, at least 3 to 6 months or more. Of course you want to get better quickly, but doing it all at once can be self-defeating, psychologically upsetting, and too traumatic on the system. Just stick to it and go at your own pace. The following diet program is in several stages, to enhance liver function for detoxification, improve digestion, create an environment for better nutrient assimilation, and build immunity to prevent recurrence.

Candida Albicans healing program stages:

Stage 1: Kill the yeasts by changing the diet. Avoid anti-biotics, immune-suppressing cortico-steroid drugs and birth control pills, unless there is absolute medical need.

Stage 2: Cleanse the dead yeasts and waste cells from the body with a food fiber cleanser.

Stage 3: Strengthen the digestive system by enhancing its ability to assimilate nutrients. Strengthen the afflicted organs and glands, especially the liver. Restore normal metabolism, and promote friendly bacteria in the gastro-intestinal tract.

Stage 4: Rebuild the immune system. Stimulating immune response throughout the healing process speeds results.

◆ Candida Albicans can mimic the symptoms of over 140 different disorders. For instance, chronic fatigue syndrome, salmonella, intestinal parasite infestation and mononucleosis all have similar symptoms, but are treated very differently. Have a test for Candida yeasts before starting a healing program to save time, expense, and for more rapid improvement.

See HEALTHY HEALING, 9th Edition, by Linda Rector-Page for more on causes, symptoms, self-testing, and diagnosis for Candida Albicans.

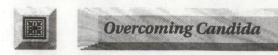

Stage One; Reducing Candida Yeast Proliferation to Normal Levels:

The food recommendations for this initial diet are extremely important; indeed absolutely necessary to control yeast proliferation. Candida yeasts grow on carbohydrates, preserved, processed and refined foods, molds, and gluten breads.

<u>Do not eat</u> the following foods for the first month to 6 weeks: Sugar or sweeteners of any kind, gluten breads or yeasted, baked products, dairy products (except plain kefir or kefir cheese, or yogurt and yogurt cheese), smoked, dried, pickled or cured foods, mushrooms, nuts or nut butters (except almonds and almond butter), fruits, fruit juices, dried or candied fruits, coffee, black tea, caffeine, carbonated drinks, (their phosphoric acid binds up calcium and magnesium), alcohol or vinegar-containing foods. Chemical foods and drugs, such as anti-biotics, steroids, cortico-steroids, and tobacco must be avoided.

This sounds like a long, restrictive list, and it is; but for those first critical weeks, when the energy-sapping Candida yeasts must be deprived of nutrients and killed off, it is the only way.

<u>Acceptable foods</u> during the first stage: Lots of fresh and steamed veggies (especially onions, garlic, ginger root, cabbage, and broccoli), poultry, seafood, fish and sea vegetables, cold pressed olive oil, eggs, mayonnaise, brown rice, amaranth, buckwheat, barley and millet, soy and vegetable pastas, tofu and tempeh, plain yogurt, rice cakes/crackers, some citrus fruit and herb teas. This is a short, limited list; but **diet restriction is the most important way to stop yeast overgrowth.**

❖ Supplementation should be included in the initial diet phase to boost body energy in the yeast reduction and killing process. *See Stage 2 Supplements on the next page.*

✚ Exercise and oxygen are keys to overcoming Candida. *See Stage 2 Bodywork on the next page.*

✴

Stage Two; Cleansing the Body of Dead Yeasts & Cellular Wastes:

The second diet stage concentrates on releasing dead and diseased yeast cells from the body. This phase usually needs from 2 to 4 months to bring about complete cleansing.

On rising: take 2 teasp. cranberry concentrate, or 2 teasp. lemon juice in water to clean the kidneys;
or a glass of cider vinegar, 1 teasp. Sonne #7 powder and water with 1 teasp. honey, if there is flatulence.

Breakfast: take NutriTech ALL 1 vitamin/mineral drink in water;
then take 1 or 2 poached or hard boiled eggs on rice cakes with a little butter;
or almond butter on rice cakes or wheat free bread;
or oatmeal with 1 TB. Bragg's LIQUID AMINOS;
or amaranth or buckwheat pancakes with a little butter and vanilla.

Mid-morning: take a good green drink (page 240ff.) or Sun CHLORELLA or Green Foods BARLEY GREEN or GREEN ESSENCE granules, or Crystal Star ENERGY GREEN™ in a glass of water;
or a cup of pau d' arco tea, or chamomile, barberry, or echinacea extract drops in a cup of water;
or a small bottle of mineral water.

Lunch: have a fresh green salad with lemon/ olive oil dressing;
or open face rice cake or wheat free bread sandwiches, with a little mayonnaise or butter, some veggies, seafood, chicken or turkey;
or a vegetable or miso soup with butter and cornbread;
or steamed veggies with tofu and brown rice;
or chicken, tuna or vegetable pasta salad, with mayonnaise or lemon/oil dressing.

Mid-afternoon: have some rice crackers, or baked corn chips, with a little kefir cheese or butter;
or some raw veggies dipped in lemon/oil dressing or spiced mayonnaise;
or a small mineral water and hard boiled or deviled egg with sesame salt or sea vegetable seasoning.

Dinner: baked, broiled or poached fish or chicken with steamed brown rice or millet and veggies;
or a baked potato with Bragg's LIQUID AMINOS, or a little kefir cheese, or lemon oil dressing;
or an oriental stir-fry with brown rice and a miso or light broth soup;
or a tofu and veggie casserole;
or a vegetarian pizza on a chapati or pita crust;
or a small omelet with veggie filling;
or a hot or cold vegetable pasta salad.

Before bed: have a cup of herb tea such as chamomile, peppermint, or Crystal Star LICORICE MINTS TEA.

✱ *Supplements and Herbs for Stages One & Two Candida Diet Program:*

For best results, rotate anti-yeast and anti-fungal products, so that yeast strains do not build up resistance to any one compound.

✤ **To help kill the yeasts,** take Probiologics CAPRICIN 3x daily with 3 cups pau d' arco tea daily, garlic capsules 6 to 10 daily, or Crystal Star PAU D' ARCO/ECHINACEA EXTRACT, CANDIDEX CAPS™ and CRAN PLUS™ TEA.

✤ **To balance and restore intesinal flora,** take a strong acidophilus culture such as Natren D.F.A (dairy free acidophilus), Women's Health RELEAF, Yerba Prima FIBERDOPHILUS, or Professional Institute Doctor Dophilus.

✤ **To help clean the liver,** take Natren LIFE START II, or Alta Health CANGEST caps.

✤ **For glandular rebalance,** take a raw adrenal complex, Crystal Star ADRN-ALIVE' capsules, or evening primrose oil caps, 4 to 6 daily.

✤ **For bowel regulation,** take Sonne #7 bentonite, psyllium husks each morning and evening, or Crystal Star CHO-LO FIBER TONE™ DRINK or CAPSULES.

✤ **For allergic reactions,** take a good digestive enzyme complex, such as Rainbow Light ALLZYME, Bromelain 500mg. with ascorbate vitamin C 2 to 3000mg daily.

✱ *Bodywork Aids for the Cleansing Candida Diet Stages:*

A positive mind and outlook are essential to overcome this body stress. Relax and have a good laugh every day.

✤ Regular exercise is a key for increased body oxygen use.

✤ Adequate sleep and rest are primary factors in the body's ability to overcome debilitating yeast-induced fatigue.

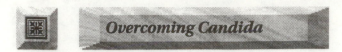

**✻ Sample Recipes for the Stages One & Two Candida Diet
By section and recipe number:**

FASTING & CLEANSING FOODS - 1, 2, 4, 5, 6, 7, 8, 9, 10, 11, 12, 14, 15, 16, 17, 18, 19, 23, 24, 25, 28

HEALTHY DRINKS, JUICES AND WATERS - 46, 48, 49, 50, 61, 62, 63, 64, 65, 66, 67, 68, 69, 71

LIGHT MACROBIOTIC EATING - 111, 112, 113, 114, 118, 119, 130, 132, 140, 142, 145, 146, 147, 150

SALADS HOT & COLD - 186, 187, 188, 192, 196, 198, 200, 201, 220, 229, 231, 232, 235, 236, 237, 238

LOW-FAT & VERY LOW-FAT DISHES - 240, 241, 248, 249, 257, 258, 268, 270, 282, 285, 287, 290, 300

DAIRY FREE COOKING - 333, 338, 340, 341, 343, 346, 351, 355, 356, 357, 358, 359, 361, 363, 365, 370

WHEAT FREE BAKING - 375, 378, 379, 380, 381, 385, 387, 391, 396, 397, 400, 401, 402, 403, 404, 406

FISH & SEAFOODS - 532, 539, 540, 541, 546, 547, 557, 558, 559, 560, 567, 568, 569

SOUPS - LIQUID SALADS - 446, 447, 448, 449, 451, 452, 453, 454, 455, 458, 459, 463, 466, 470, 472

✻

Stage Three; Strengthening the Glands, Organs & Digestive System:

*As you start to see body improvement, and symptoms decrease, usually after three to six months, start adding back some whole grains, fruits, juices, a little white wine, some fresh cheeses, nuts and beans. This third stage of healing takes anywhere from 2 to 6 months. Go slowly, add gradually. Test for food sensitivity until the problem foods stop bothering you. **Remember, eating sugars and refined foods will allow Candida yeasts to grow again.***

On rising: continue with cider vinegar, or lemon juice in water, as in the Stage One diet;
and add NutriTech ALL 1 vitamin/mineral drink in water with 2 teasp. cranberry concentrate.

Breakfast: have a fresh grapefruit, pineapple or papaya, with plain yogurt if desired;
or a poached egg on a rice cake with a little butter;
or oatmeal with Bragg's LIQUID AMINOS;
or amaranth or buckwheat pancakes or a chapati with a little butter or kefir cheese.

Mid-morning: have a small bottle of mineral water;
or some rice or whole grain crackers with kefir cheese;
or a cup of pau d' arco tea or Crystal Star HIGH ENERGY TEA™;
or a green drink, or Sun CHLORELLA, Crystal Star ENERGY GREEN™, or Green Foods BARLEY GREEN granules in water.

Lunch: have a fresh green salad every day with lemon/oil dressing; add an open face whole grain sandwich, with a little mayonnaise or butter, some veggies, seafood, chicken or turkey;
or a light veggie or miso soup with oriental rice noodles, baked chips, or cornbread;
or a small vegetable or whole grain pasta salad with a light oil dressing, and baked or broiled seafood or fish;
or steamed veggies with tofu or tempeh and brown rice;
or a small oven baked frittata or omelet with steamed veggies.

Mid-afternoon: have some raw veggies with a light yogurt or kefir cheese dip;
or a small bottle of mineral water or refreshing herb tea, such as Crystal Star FEEL GREAT™ TEA:
or hard boiled or deviled eggs with some baked chips, and sesame salt;

Dinner: have baked or broiled fish or chicken with steamed veggies and brown rice, millet or bulgur;
or a baked whole grain or vegetable pasta casserole and a green salad;
or a light vegetable or seafood frittata, quiche or souffle. (Substitute yogurt, soy milk or almond milk for dairy products).
or an oriental stir-fry, or light Italian vegetable pasta dish, or a small veggie pizza on a chapati crust;
or a tofu and veggie, whole grain casserole with a light soup and a small salad;
or a large dinner salad, hot or cold with plenty of greens, and Essene bread or corn bread.

✓Add a glass of white wine for relaxation and digestion if desired.

Before bed: take a cup of pau d' arco tea;
or scullcap or chamomile tea, or Crystal Star GOOD NIGHT™ TEA or RELAX™ TEA.

❋ *Supplements and Herbal Help for the Strengthening Diet*

❖ **To maintain healthy bowel flora,** continue with your acidophilus, garlic and bowel cleansing choices from Stage 1 and 2. As the body takes over more of its own work, other supplements may be decreased, such as capricin, Natren LIFE START II, adrenal complex, and primrose oil.

❖ **Immune building herbs to restore homeostasis,** such as Sun CHLORELLA, Crystal Star PAU D' ARCO/ECHINACEA EXTRACT, and CANDID-EX™ caps. Pau d' arco tea should be continued or added during this period.

❖ **For increased tissue oxygen,** add Solaray TRI-O_2 daily, **and** ascorbate vitamin C powder, 2 teasp. daily in $1/4$ teasp. doses in juice or water, **and/or** H_2O_2 PEROXY GEL rubbed daily on the abdomen.

❋ *Bodywork Help for the Strengthening Diet*

✚ Anti-biotics, cortisone drugs, alcohol, tobacco, caffeine, caffeine-containing foods, and sugars must all continue to be avoided.

✚ Regular mild exercise continues in importance for oxygenation.

❋ *Suggested Recipes for the Stage Three Diet*
By section and recipe number:

LIGHT MACROBIOTIC EATING - 115, 116, 120, 134, 136, 138, 139, 141, 143, 179, 180, 181, 184, 185

SALADS HOT & COLD - 189, 191, 195, 199, 202, 204, 207, 208, 209, 211, 212, 213, 214, 215, 216, 217, 218, 222, 226, 234

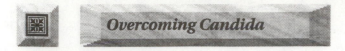

LOW CHOLESTEROL MEALS - 301, 302, 304, 305, 307, 308, 310, 312, 314, 315, 316, 318, 319, 326, 327

DAIRY FREE COOKING - all

SUGAR FREE SPECIALS - 412, 415, 434, 437, 439, 440, 441, 443, 444

SOUPS - LIQUID SALADS - all

STIR-FRYS - 501, 502, 504, 505, 508, 510, 516, 518, 520, 521, 522, 523, 524, 525, 526

FISH & SEAFOODS - 532, 537, 539, 540, 541, 544, 546, 548, 549, 557, 559, 559, 563, 567, 568

TOFU FOR YOU - 572, 574, 577, 579, 580, 582, 585, 589, 591, 598, 599, 600, 606, 609

HIGH FIBER RECIPES - 785, 788, 789, 791, 799, 802, 803, 805, 809, 812, 815, 816, 817, 818, 819, 821

Stage Four; Enhancing Immunity to Control Candida: 6 to 12 months

Diet remains the key to controlling Candida; the fourth stage emphasizes rebuilding immune strength to promote normal metabolism and defense against recurrence. It is along range plan aimed toward prevention and lifestyle stability.

On rising: continue with lemon juice or cranberry concentrate in a glass of water;
and NutriTech ALL 1 vitamin/mineral drink, or Nature's Plus SPIRUTEIN drink.

Breakfast: have a grapefruit, pineapple, papaya or other fresh fruit;
or yogurt with fresh fruit or whole grain granola on top;
or poached, baked or lightly scrambled eggs with tofu or a little cottage cheese, and whole grain toast or muffins with a little butter;
or oatmeal with a little vanilla and butter or Bragg's LIQUID AMINOS;
or whole grain pancakes or granola with apple or pear juice, and yogurt or kefir with fresh fruit.

Mid-morning: have a green or Sun CHLORELLA drink with 1 teasp. Bragg's LIQUID AMINOS;
or a small bottle of mineral water with a piece of fresh fruit;
or pau d' arco or other herb tea, such as Crystal Star HIGH ENERGY™ or FEEL GREAT TEA™;
or some rice crackers or raw veggies with kefir cheese or a soy spread.

Lunch: have a fresh green salad with Italian or other non-dairy light dressing;
and a veggie sandwich on whole grain bread;
or a light oriental soup or ramen noodles and stir-fried vegetables;
or a baked potato with a little butter, and a green salad;
or a small tofu or tempeh casserole with brown rice;
or a seafood and vegetable pasta recipe with a light dressing and a green salad;
or a whole grain chapati or burrito with a bean or veggie filling, and non-dairy sauce.

Mid-afternoon: have a refreshing herb tea such as Crystal Star RELAX™ or LICORICE MINTS TEA;
or a glass of mineral water, green drink, or fresh carrot juice.
and a hard boiled or deviled egg with sesame salt, a non-dairy dip, and baked chips;
or some fresh veggies with a non-dairy dip.
or a cup of miso or other light soup with sea vegetables snipped on top.

Dinner: have baked, broiled, or roasted fish, chicken or turkey, with steamed veggies and rice;
or a whole grain or pasta and veggie casserole;
or an oriental stir-fry with a cup of light soup and sea vegetables;
or a light Italian vegetable meal with whole grain or vegetable pasta, and a light vegetable soup;
or a dinner size salad or whole grain open-face sandwich with favorite ingredients, such as soy cheeses, marinated tofu, toasted nuts and noodles, yogurt, kefir cheese, baked seafood or chicken;
or a light egg dish with white wine and yogurt sauce in place of dairy, and a green salad.

Before bed: have a cup of relaxing herb tea, such as chamomile, or Crystal Star GOOD NIGHT™ TEA or NIGHT ZZZZs EXTRACT™ in water;
or a teasp. of VEGEX yeast paste in a cup hot water, for relaxation and B vitamins.

✱ *Supplements and Herbal Aids for the Candida Immune-Enhancing Diet:*

✤ Continue with acidophilus and garlic choices at least once a day.

✤ **To help rebuild immunity,** take Biotin 1000mcg, zinc picolinate 50mg. and vitamin C ascorbate crystals with bioflavonoids up to 5000mg. daily ($1/4$ teasp. at a time in juice or water).

✤ Continue with green superfoods, such as Sun CHLORELLA, Green Foods GREEN ESSENCE, or Living Foods SUPERFOOD tablets.

✤ Continue with echinacea extract or Crystal Star CANDID-EX™ CAPS for at least 3 months.

✤ Add a good digestive enzyme 2 to 3x a day, such as Alta Health CANGEST, or Rainbow Light DOUBLE STRENGTH ALL-ZYME.

✤ Add a marine carotene source daily, such as Twin Labs marine carotene, or Crystal Star SYSTEM STRENGTH™ DRINK.

✱ *Bodywork Aids for the Candida Immune-Enhancing Diet:*

✛ Continue with an aerobic exercise program on a regular basis.

✛ Avoid antibiotics, birth control pills and cortico-steroid drugs unless absolutely necessary. They set up an easy environment for Candida to flourish.

✱ *Sample Recipes For Candida Control & Prevention Diet*
By section and recipe number:

SALADS HOT & COLD - all

SUGAR FREE SPECIALS - 420, 422, 434, 438, 441, 443, 444

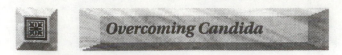

SOUPS - LIQUID SALADS - all

FISH & SEAFOODS - all

HIGH PROTEIN WITHOUT MEAT - 699, 701, 702, 704, 715, 716, 720, 723, 729, 735, 742

HIGH MINERAL FOODS - 613, 615, 616, 617, 618, 620, 621, 623, 624, 625, 629, 630, 644, 646, 647, 651

COMPLEX CARBOHYDRATES FOR ENERGY - 744, 748, 749, 750, 753, 754, 755, 757, 763, 773, 776

GREAT OUTDOOR EATING - 874, 876, 879, 881, 883, 884, 885, 890, 892, 893, 894, 895, 903, 904, 909

HOLIDAY FEASTING & ENTERTAINING - 831, 832, 835, 839, 840, 842, 843, 844, 848, 849, 851, 856

❊ Sample Menu Plans
Some recipe combinations that work with this diet:

A FAMILY MEAL - 451, 618, 637

A LIGHT SUMMER MEAL - 617, 646, 769

AN EASY RISING BREAKFAST - 83, 79, 97, 93

A HEARTY WINTER MEAL - 766, 612, 644, 654

A SPECIAL DINNER FOR TWO - 636, 613, 190, 567, 657, 660

AN EASY WEEKNIGHT DINNER - 453, 621, 647, 629

LUNCHEON FOR TWO - 624, 615, 663

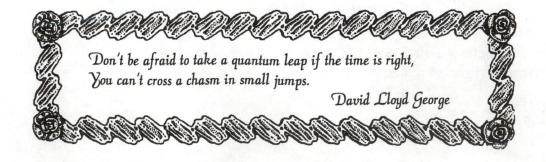

*Don't be afraid to take a quantum leap if the time is right,
You can't cross a chasm in small jumps.*

David Lloyd George

Overcoming Chronic Respiratory Problems
Mucous Cleansing ❧ Asthma ❧ Colds ❧ Flu

Respiratory problems are more than common in our society today. It is estimated that at any one time, over $1/3$ of our America's population has had a cold or flu within the last 2 weeks. It is now generally understood that a common cold is not a disease per se, but an attempt by the body to cleanse itself of excess mucous by opening and draining its channels of elimination, by coughing, sneezing, diarrhea, etc. A cold can be a friendly enemy - the wonderful, complex immune system working against pathogenic overload to rebuild a stronger, cleaner system. Thus, the cure is not really the problem. The cause is. Chronic respiratory diseases stem from several areas of environment and lifestyle, but poor diet is the single most influential cause.

The person who suffers frequently from sinus headaches, bronchitis, chronic colds, flu, sore throat and coughs, is invariably a person whose diet includes many acid and mucous-forming foods, such as red meat, caffeine containing foods, salty, sugary, starchy foods, pasteurized, full-fat dairy products, and refined foods, with few fresh fruits or vegetables.
This way of eating causes excess mucous to form in the system, favoring tissue congestion. Not only is the body full of more mucous than it needs, the mucous is usually filled with toxic impurities and unreleased waste from chemical additives, preservatives, pesticide residues, etc., a perfect breeding ground for unfriendly bacteria and viruses. We are always exposed to a certain amount of these "germs," but poor diet decreases resistance and allows them to gain a disease-strength foothold in the body.

Drugs and over-the-counter medicines only relieve the symptoms of infection. They do not cure, and often make the situation worse by depressing the immune system, drying up neeeded mucous elimination, and keeping the virus or harmful bacteria inside the body. (Another case of 'fooling Mother Nature' that doesn't work). Anti-biotics are not effective against virally caused infections, and aspirin can enhance the reproduction of viral germs. Unfortunately, whatever temporary relief aspirin might afford, it may make it easier for viruses to multiply and spread.
A short liquid mucous elimination fast, diet change, and natural supplementation with herbs and concentrated healing foods, comprise a beneficial, rapid program for overcoming chronic respiratory problems whether they are due to smoking, environmental pollutants, virally related colds, or a habitually poor diet.
Regular exercise encourages immune response. Even just a short walk every day, puts cleansing oxygen into the lungs, restoring vitamin D in the body, and fresh air into the brain.

The following diets will help overcome and prevent:
❧ASTHMA ❧COLDS ❧FLU ❧SEASONAL ALLERGIES ❧PNEUMONIA and PLEURISY ❧BRONCHITIS ❧ADRENAL   EXHAUSTION ❧T.B. ❧EMPHYSEMA ❧COUGH and SORE THROAT ❧SMOKING DISEASES ❧EAR INFECTIONS ❧CYSTIC FIBROSIS ❧SINUSITIS ❧TONSILLITIS ❧TASTE and SMELL LOSS ❧

An ounce of prevention is worth a pound of cure.
Keep your immnne system strong.

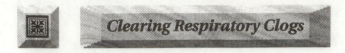

Stage One; Mucous Cleansing and Healing: A 3 to 5 Day Liquid Diet

A program to overcome chronic respiratory problems is usually more successful when it is begun with a short mucous elimination diet. Better and more long lasting results are achieved if you allow your body to rid itself first of toxins and mucous accumulations before attempting to change your eating habits. After your cleanse, avoid the pasteurized dairy products, starches and refined foods that are the breeding ground for congestion. Even though respiratory problems stem from different causes, and need specific treatment, they all benefit from a non-clogging diet. The first stage below is a high vitamin C, liquid diet to follow for 3 to 5 days. It can produce symptomatic relief from many respiratory problems in under 48 hours.

On rising: take a glass of cranberry, apple or grapefruit juice;
or a glass of lemon juice in hot water with 1 teasp. honey;
or a glass of cider vinegar, hot water and honey.

Breakfast: take a hot potassium broth or essence (page 240), or Crystal Star SYSTEM STRENGTH™ DRINK with 1 teasp. liquid chlorophyll, Sun CHLORELLA or Green Foods GREEN MAGMA.
and take 2 or 3 garlic capsules and $1/4$ to $1/2$ teasp. ascorbate vitamin C or Ester C powder in water.

Mid-morning: have a glass of fresh carrot juice;
or a glass of cranberry/apple juice;
and/or a cup of comfrey/fenugreek tea, or Crystal Star RSPR-TEA™ or ASTH-AID TEA™.

Lunch: have a hot vegetable, miso or onion broth, or Crystal Star SYSTEM STRENGTH™;
Take 2 to 3 more garlic capsules and $1/4$ to $1/2$ teasp. ascorbate vitamin C or Ester C powder in water.

Mid-afternoon: have a cleansing herb tea, such as alfalfa/mint or Crystal Star X-PEC™ TEA;
or another green drink such as Sun CHLORELLA, or Crystal Star ENERGY GREEN™.

Dinner: have a hot veggie broth, potassium essence, or miso soup with sea veggies snipped on top;
or another glass of carrot juice.
Take 2 to 3 more garlic capsules, and $1/4$ to $1/2$ teasp. ascorbate vitamin C or Ester C powder in water.

Before bed: take another hot water, lemon and honey drink;
or hot apple or cranberry juice.

✓ Drink six to eight glasses of bottled water or mineral water each day for best cleansing results.

✓ One to 2 teasp. Bragg's LIQUID AMINOS may be added to any broth or juice.

✓ If you have a cold, include even more liquids than described above, such as hot broths, mineral water, fruit and vegetable juices, or a little brandy with lemon.

✱ *Supplements for the Mucous Cleansing Diet*

❖ Add 1 teasp. acidophilus liquid, or $1/4$ to $1/2$ teasp. acidophilus powder to any broth or juice.

❖ Ascorbate vitamin C or Ester C powder may be taken thoughout the day in juice or water, until bowel movement turns soupy, for tissue flushing and detoxification. Take up to 10,000mg. daily for the first three days, then 5,000mg. daily until the end of your cleanse.

✽ *Bodywork for the Mucous Cleansing Diet*

✜ Avoid all tobacco products and secondary smoke. Get plenty of daily fresh air and sunshine, away from environmental pollutants, for vitamin A & D (specifics for lung and respiratory problems).

✜ Exercise encourages immune response. Even just a short walk every day with deep breathing, puts cleansing oxygen into the lungs, vitamin D into the body, and fresh air into the brain.

✜ Take daily hot saunas, and/or oxygen baths if possible, to sweat out toxins quickly (page 203). Get plenty of rest during the cleanse.

✜ Stimulate easier breathing by massaging and gently scratching the lung meridian from the top of the shoulder to the end of the thumb to clear chest mucous.

Stage Two; Mucous-Free Respiratory Rebuilding Diet:
This diet phase should be undertaken after the mucous elimination cleanse. It allows the body's individual elimination powers to become active with excess mucous obstacles removed, so that it can rebuild at optimum levels. Raw, fresh, simply prepared foods are emphasized. Fats, salts and dairy products are reduced or excluded; all fried and sugary foods are omitted. Alcohol, tobacco, caffeine and caffeine-containing foods should be avoided for best results.

On rising: have a glass of grapefruit, pineapple or orange juice juice;
or a protein drink, such as Nature's Plus SPIRUTEIN in pineapple, orange, or apple juice.

Breakfast: have some fresh fruit with low-fat yogurt or vanilla soy milk;
or whole grain pancakes or muffins, with kefir cheese or yogurt and a little maple syrup;
or a fresh fruit smoothie with a banana;
or a whole grain cereal or granola with apple juice or yogurt topping.

Mid-morning: have a fresh apple or glass of apple juice every day;
and/or a green drink (pg. 240), Sun CHLORELLA with 1 TB. Bragg's LIQUID AMINOS, or Crystal Star ENERGY GREEN DRINK™ in a small bottle of mineral water;
or a cup of veggie broth or miso soup with sea vegetables snipped on top;
or a cup of Siberian ginseng tea, or Crystal Star FEEL GREAT™ TEA.

Lunch: have a fresh green salad with lemon/oil dressing;
or a kiwi, strawberry, cucumber salad with cornbread;
or have a baked potato with a spinach and mushroom salad;
or some steamed vegetables, such as broccoli or onions with Bragg's LIQUID AMINOS as dressing;
or some baked tofu or white fish with fresh greens and a light dressing;
or a seafood and whole grain pasta salad with a light sauce;
or a whole grain, high protein sandwich with nuts seeds, tofu, and a kefir cheese spread.

Mid-afternoon: have a cup of cleansing herb tea, such as comfrey/fenugreek, or Crystal Star RSPR-TEA™ or ASTH-AID™ TEA;
or a cup of miso soup with sea vegetables, or Crystal Star SYSTEM STRENGTH™;
and/or some crunchy raw veggies with kefir cheese and a bottle of mineral water.

Dinner: have an oriental stir-fry with miso soup and brown rice or buckwheat noodles (soba);
<u>or</u> a large high protein salad with green pepper, sprouts, nuts, seeds, etc., and whole grain toast;
<u>or</u> some steamed veggies with brown rice and tofu;
<u>or</u> a baked veggie and millet, bulgar or brown rice casserole, and a green salad with yogurt dressing;
<u>or</u> a black bean or lentil soup with fish or seafood, and steamed veggies with a low-fat sauce.

Before bed: take a cup of hot VEGEX yeast broth, or miso soup;
<u>or</u> cranberry juice or celery juice.
<u>or</u> a cup of relaxing herb tea, such as chamomile, passion flower, scullcap, or Crystal Star RELAX TEA™ or GOOD NIGHT TEA™.

✓ Even though the initial mucous elimination period is over, it is often beneficial to go on a short 24 hour liquid diet once a week for a month or more to insure respiratory stability and the success of your new way of eating.

✓ See THE FOREVER DIET (pg. 198) for a diet to maintain a body free of excess mucous.

✱ *Supplements for the Respiratory Rebuilding Diet*

❖ Take Beta carotene 50 to 100,000IU and ascorbate vitamin C or Ester C 3 to 5000mg. with bioflavonoids daily, to maintain anti-infective and oxygen uptake activity.

❖ Take vitamin B$_{12}$, either sub-lingual or internasal for healthy cell development.

❖ Take high potency royal jelly 2 teasp. daily as an exceptionally high source of natural pantothenic acid, <u>and</u> 2 teasp. Bee Pollen granules as a source of amino acids for protein building.

❖ Take Sun CHLORELLA, Green Foods GREEN ESSENCE, or Crystal Star ENERGY GREEN DRINK™ to build healthy blood.

❖ Encourage adrenal gland health and activity with Siberian ginseng, adrenal raw glandular, Tyrosine 500mg. daily, or Crystal Star ADRN ALIVE™ <u>with</u> BODY REBUILDER™ CAPSULES daily.

❖ Take oxygenating, and soothing herb teas to keep respiratoy channels open; such as comfrey/fenugreek, alfalfa/peppermint, or Crystal Star RESPR-TEA™, OPEN UP', DEEP BREATHING™ and ASTH-AID™ TEA.

✱ *Bodywork for the Respiratory Rebuilding Diet*

✚ Get some early morning sunlight on the body every day possible. Sunlight builds strength along with food. Eating out of doors is especially beneficial.

✚ Avoid all tobacco, smoking and secondary smoke.

✚ Aerobic exercise, such as walking and swimming, with lung-cleansing deep breathing exercises are a key factor to keeping lungs open and working well. Exercise is an immune-building nutrient in itself.

A Word About The Chronic Cold

There seem to be almost as many cold "remedies" as there are colds. A cold is usually an attempt by the body to cleanse itself of wastes, toxins and pathogenic bacteria that have built up to the point where natural immunity cannot handle or overcome them. The glands are always affected, and since the endocrine system is on a 6 day cycle, a normal cold usually runs for about a week, as the body works through its detoxification process. Sometimes it is just better to let this happen, so that the body can start fresh with a stronger immune system. But, it is hard to work, sleep, and be around other people with your misery and cold symptoms.

With this in mind, we have developed a QUICK COLD CHECK that has been successful at minimizing misery while your body gets on with its job of cleaning house.

1) Take a brisk walk to rev up the immune system, and get you out of the house into fresh air. A walk puts cleansing oxygen into the lungs, and stops you from feeling sorry for yourself. It works wonders!

2) Take plenty of ascorbate vitamin C or Ester C, preferably in powder form with juice, spread throughout the day. Take zinc lozenges as needed, and other supplements of your choice.

3) No smoking or alcohol (other than a little brandy and lemon). They suppress immunity. Avoid refined flour, sugars, and pasteurized dairy foods. They increase the formation of thick mucous.

4) Drink plenty of liquids; 6 to 8 glasses of water, fresh fruit and vegetable juices, and herb teas every day, to flush toxins through and out of the system.

5) Eat lightly, but with good nutrition. A vegetarian diet is best at this time so your body won't have to work hard at digestion. Remember that sugary, salty junk foods suppress immunity.

6) Keep warm. Don't worry about a fever unless it is prolonged or very high. Take a long hot bath, hot tub, spa or sauna. Lots of toxins can pass out through the skin. **Increase room humidity** so your mucous membranes will remain active against the virus/bacteria.

7) Stay relaxed. Let the body concentrate on overcoming the cold. Go to bed early, and get plenty of rest. Most regeneration of virus-damaged cells occurs between midnight and 4 a.m.

8) Think positively. Optimism is often a self-fulfilling prophecy.

Do You Have A Cold or The Flu? Here are the Differences:

Colds and flu are distinct and separate upper respiratory infections, triggered by different viruses. (Outdoor environment, drafts, wetness, temperature changes, etc. do not cause either of these illnesses.) The flu is more serious, because it can spread to the lungs, and cause sever bronchitis or pneumonia. Beginning stage symptoms for both can be very similar. Both colds and flu begin when viruses, (that unlike bacteria, cannot reproduce outside host cells) penetrate the body's protective barriers. Nose, eyes, and mouth are usually the sites of invasion from cold viruses. The most likely entry target for the flu virus is the respiratory tract. Colds and flu respond to different treatment. The following brief SYMPTOM CHART can help identify you particular condition, and deal with it better.

A Cold Profile Looks Like This:

✚ Slow onset
✚ No prostration
✚ Rarely accompanied by fever and headache
✚ Localized symptoms like runny nose, sneezing
✚ Mild fatigue or weakness from body cleansing
✚ Mild chest discomfort with a hacking cough
✚ Sore throat common

A Flu Profile Looks Like This:

✚ Swift, severe onset
✚ Early prostration with flushed, hot moist skin
✚ High fever usual, headache and sore eyes
✚ General chills, depression and body aches
✚ Extreme fatigue, often for 2 to 3 weeks
✚ Acute chest discomfort, severe hacking cough
✚ Sore throat occasionally

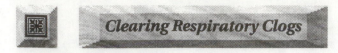
✳ *Sample Recipes for Respiratory Health*
By section and recipe number:

HEALTHY DRINKS, JUICES & WATERS - 44 ,46, 49, 51, 52, 53, 59, 62, 65, 63, 66, 67, 68, 71

ORIENTAL & LIGHT MACROBIOTIC FOODS - all

SALADS HOT & COLD - 186, 187, 188, 189, 190, 193, 195, 198, 199, 200, 202, 203, 204, 206, 210, 229

DAIRY FREE COOKING - all

WHEAT FREE BAKING - all

SUGAR FREE SWEET TREATS - 411, 413, 415, 420, 424, 426, 428, 429, 430, 432, 433, 436, 438, 443, 444

FISH & SEAFOOD - 538, 540, 541, 543, 546, 548, 549, 550, 551, 553, 554, 556, 558, 563, 564, 567, 568

SOUPS - LIQUID SALADS - 445, 446, 447, 449, 450, 451, 452, 453, 454, 455, 456, 458, 459, 468, 470, 472

HIGH PROTEIN WITHOUT MEAT - 697, 699, 701, 714, 716, 719, 720, 723, 724, 729, 733, 734, 737, 740

HIGH FIBER RECIPES - 785, 786, 789, 790, 793, 794, 796, 798, 801, 806, 807, 808, 809, 811, 814, 816, 818

✳ *Sample Menu Plans*
Some recipe combinations that work with this diet:

A FAMILY MEAL - 135, 174, 556, 49, 438

A WEEKEND PICNIC - 114, 55, 728, 116, 126

A LIGHT SUMMER MEAL - 51, 125, 117, 166

A HEARTY WINTER MEAL - 140, 183, 202

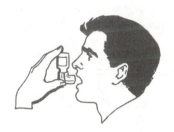

A SPECIAL DINNER FOR TWO - 121, 136, 184, 412, 195, 54

AN EASY RISING BREAKFAST - 48, 819, 823

LUNCH FOR TWO - 162, 138, 369, 50

AN EASY WEEKNIGHT DINNER - 792, 559, 439, 113

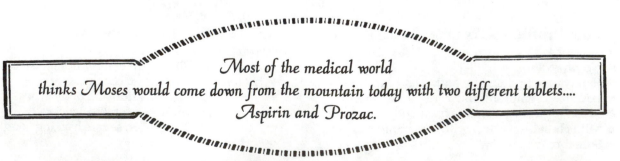

*Most of the medical world
thinks Moses would come down from the mountain today with two different tablets....
Aspirin and Prozac.*

Recuperation & Regeneration
Rebuilding Body Strength
After Illness, Injury or Surgery

Long illness, severe injury, any surgery procedure or hospital stay, puts the body through tremendous physical and psychological trauma. Optimal nourishment at these times is necessary for faster and better healing, for cleaning out drug residues and overcoming their side effects, and for returning the body to health after the poor nutrition of most hospitals. (Why do hospitals have such terrible food!) Hospital meals seem to aggravate illness rather than strengthen for defense against it!

The body has the power to heal itself, but its vital recuperative forces need extra nutritive help after injury or illness to do it; illness, weakness, poor appetite and reduced assimilation call for more concentrated nutrients than a normal diet provides. The emphasis in the recovery diet in this chapter is on rebuilding strength, regenerating healthy new tissue, and replenishing overall vitality. It is very high in protein, which is depleted during trauma and injury. Protein and amino acids are necessary for healing, and for cellular growth.

A healing/mending diet like this gives the body super nutrition for a limited time - temporarily increasing calories, fat, meat and protein, providing concentrated raw materials for serious nutritional deficiencies. Once the system stabilizes and the body begins to supply its own healing powers, this increased support can be moderated to more normal amounts. The body will begin to take over more and more of its own work, and begin replacing the nutrition it has lost.

A restorative diet must be high in vitamin C foods and beta-carotene, as anti-infectives and to supply new collagen and interstitial tissue production. It should be rich in B vitamins to lessen trauma and stress on the body, to build blood and metabolize proteins. And it must be rich in minerals for good digestion and basic body building blocks. Minerals, especially bone minerals are lost when there are long periods of inactivity because of illness; they are also depleted through blood loss, and they are needed for tissue repair. A recuperation diet must be high in oxygenating foods, to create an environment where disease cannot fluorish, and to discourage disease from recurring.

An initial fast for cleansing is _not_ the way to begin when the body is greatly weakened or under acute trauma, even though it will probably be harboring many drug residues. There is often so much depletion and stress, that a rigorous fast is self-defeating. Raw vegetable juices as additions to other foods, however, are an excellent means of purifying and alkalizing the system.

This diet is also effective for other problems where healing-strength nutrition is needed:
❧ANEMIA and PERNICIOUS ANEMIA ❧PARKINSON'S DISEASE ❧MENINGITIS ❧MALNUTRITION FROM EATING DISORDERS such as BULEMIA or ANOREXIA ❧RHEUMATIC FEVER ❧INFERTILITY ❧STERILITY ❧SPORTS INJURIES and MUSCLE ATROPHY ❧WOUND HEALING ❧

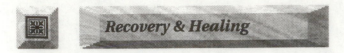

Concentrated, Optimal Nutrition for Recuperation and Regeneration

The object of this diet is to supply an abundance of vitamins, minerals, trace elements, essential fatty acids and proteins to rebuild a weakened body and strengthen overall vitality. It includes generous amounts of fresh fruits, vegetables and juices for gentle cleansing, to encourage the body to release drug residues and toxic wastes while promoting rapid regeneration of healthy tissue. Small, frequent simple meals are recommended instead of large heavy meals, so that the body can assimilate nutritive elements easily and efficiently.

The diet includes plenty of protein-rich foods for tissue repair, complex carbohydrates and unsaturated fats for energy, cultured foods for friendly intestinal flora, and chlorophyll greens for new blood building.

On rising: take a milk/egg protein drink with 1 teasp. spirulina and 1 teasp. Bragg's LIQUID AMINOS;
or Nature's Plus SPIRUTEIN;
or Nutritech ALL 1 vitamin/mineral drink in pineapple/papaya or pineapple/coconut juice.

Breakfast: have some yogurt with fresh fruit;
then a whole grain cereal with wheat germ, sesame seeds and kefir on top;
or baked, poached or scrambled eggs with cottage or kefir cheese and whole grain toast;
or a small omelet with veggies or a low-fat raw cheese filling;
or whole grain buckwheat pancakes or oatmeal with honey, maple syrup or molasses.

Mid-morning: take a potassium broth (page 240) 3 to 4 times a week;
and on alternate days Sun CHLORELLA or Green Foods BARLEY GREEN MAGMA with 1 teasp. each brewer's yeast and wheat germ added, or Crystal Star SYSTEM STRENGTH DRINK™ with 1 teasp. Bragg's LIQUID AMINOS added;
or have some miso soup with sea vegetables snipped on top;
and/or kefir, or kefir cheese with whole grain baked chips;
or some dried fruits, especially raisins and figs, or fresh fruits, especially apples or grapes.

Lunch: have some brown rice with baked tofu and steamed veggies;
or a roast turkey sandwich with mayonnaise, or other high protein sandwich on whole grain bread;
or a light Mexican meal with beans and rice; (easy on the salsa and condiments; use whole grain tortillas or burritos);
or a seafood salad with whole grain or spinach pasta;
or a high protein salad with sprouts, sea vegetables, nuts and seeds;
or a baked potato with a spinach and mushroom salad, and a green dressing.

Mid-afternoon: a cup of strengthening herb tea, such as dandelion root, Siberian ginseng or Crystal Star GINSENG 6 DEFENSE RESTORATIVE SUPER TEA™, FEEL GREAT TEA™, or HIGH ENERGY™ TEA;
or a glass of fresh carrot juice;
or a Knudsen RECHARGE electrolyte replacement drink, or Alacer HIGH K COLA for potassium;
and yogurt with nuts and seeds, or fresh fruit;
or a hard boiled egg with mayonnaise or kefir cheese, or a low-fat cheese with whole grain chips;
or a green drink (page 240) with 2 teasp. unsprayed bee pollen added.

Dinner: have a brown rice casserole with tofu and/or steamed veggies, some baked chicken or fish, and a cup of miso soup;
or roast turkey with baked yams and a green salad with a yogurt dressing;
or a vegetable quiche or pizza on a chapati crust;
or a light Italian whole grain or veggie pasta dish, with a low-fat sauce, and green salad;
or a high protein dinner soup, stew or salad with a baked potato or yam, and a little butter or lemon/yogurt dressing;
or a hearty seafood/vegetable stir-fry with brown rice;
or a large open-face dinner sandwich on whole grain bread or English muffin, and a light soup.

Before bed: have 1 teasp. VEGEX yeast paste extract in hot water;
or a relaxing herb tea, such as chamomile or Crystal Star CHINESE ROYAL MU™ TEA;
or a glass of warm milk with honey;
or a small bowl of oatmeal with maple syrup or honey.

✓Drink plenty of pure water (6 to 8 glasses every day) for good hydration, and to keep drug residues and toxins flushing out of the body.
This diet should be used for approximately 4 to 6 weeks. After the initial period of rebuilding, you might wish to undertake a short elimination fast for further cleansing. (See DETOXIFICATION & CLEANSING DIETS, page 18.)

✹ *Supplements and Herbal Aids for the Recuperation Diet*

Natural supplements may be taken with meals, or throughout the day. The idea is to replace deficiencies and depletion as rapidly as possible.

❖ To clean the body and vital organs, take Sonne´ Liquid Bentonite in the morning, a high potency acidophilus complex 3 times daily with meals, and/or Crystal Star LIVER ALIVE™ CAPS or LIV-ALIVE TEA™.

❖ To rebalance the glandular system, take wild cherry bark or burdock tea, Crystal Star ENDO-BAL™, CAPSULES or ADRN-ALIVE™ EXTRACT, and vitamin B-complex 50mg. 3x daily.

❖ To build healthy body tissue, take vitamin E 400IU 2x daily, Enzymatic Therapy LIQUID LIVER with GINSENG, Alta Health SIL-X CAPS, and vitamin B12 internasal or sublingual;
and/or Crystal Star GINSENG 6 DEFENSE RESTORATIVE SUPER TEA™, BODY RE-BUILDER™ CAPS with ADRN -ALIVE™ caps, or SYSTEM STRENGTH™ DRINK.

❖ To replenish depleted mineral building blocks, take White Birch Mineral Water, (a food source potassium supplement), Crystal Star ENERGY GREEN DRINK™ and MINERAL SPECTRUM™ CAPS, and/or Mezotrace SEA MINERAL COMPLEX tablets.

❖ To encourage wound and body trauma healing, take ascorbate vitamin C with bioflavonoids, up to 5000mg. daily, and/or Crystal Star DAILY BIOFLAVONOID SUPPORT DRINK™, bromelain caps 500mg, and Solaray TRI-O$_2$ tablets 50mg. 2x daily. Apply aloe vera gel on scars and lesions.

❖ To rebuild immunity, take beta-carotene A 25,000IU, Sun Chlorella tabs 15 to 20 daily (or granules), high potency digestive enzymes such as Alta Health CANGEST or Rainbow Light DETOX-ZYME, and immune stimulating herbs such as Crystal Star HERBAL DEFENSE TEAM™ CAPS, TEA or EXTRACT, IRON SOURCE™ CAPS or EXTRACT, and HAWTHORN or ECHINACEA 100% EXTRACT.

✹ *Bodywork for the Recuperation Diet*

✚ Get some early sunlight on the body every day possible for vitamin D and tissue/bone building.

✚ Take some exercise every day during healing; especially a walk with deep breathing.

✚ Avoid all junk foods. They fill you up, but deprive you of much needed nutrition at a critical time.

❋ *Sample Recipes for Recuperation & Regeneration*
By section and recipe number:

HEALTHY DRINKS & JUICES - 46, 48, 49, 52, 54, 61, 63, 66, 70, 71

BREAKFAST & BRUNCH - 73, 76, 80, 86, 92, 93, 94, 98, 101, 105

ORIENTAL & LIGHT MACROBIOTIC EATING - all

SALADS HOT & COLD - all

SOUPS - LIQUID SALADS - all

FISH & SEAFOOD - all

HIGH PROTEIN RECIPES FOR BODY BUILDING - all

HIGH MINERAL FOODS - all

HIGH COMPLEX CARBOHYDRATES FOR ENERGY - all

HIGH FIBER RECIPES - all

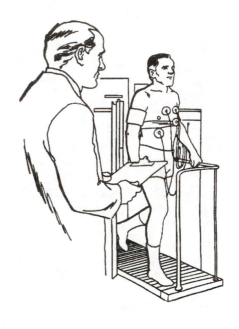

❋ *Sample Menu Plans*
Some recipe combinations that work with this diet:

A HEARTY WINTER MEAL - 67, 447, 764, 823, 747

A LIGHT SUMMER MEAL - 448, 89, 549, 47

A SPECIAL DINNER FOR TWO - 55, 238, 155, 450, 660, 538

A FAMILY MEAL - 756, 190, 652, 787

A SUNDAY BRUNCH - 50, 535, 646, 761, 653, 234

AN EASY RISING BREAKFAST - 97, 80, 48, 821

AN EASY WEEKNIGHT DINNER - 658, 796, 756, 759

LUNCH FOR TWO - 117, 216, 170, 62

> *Complete health and awakening are really the same thing.*
> *We live too short and die too long.*

Normalizing Strength & Immunity After Surgery or Illness

After an initial recovery and rest period, your body may be ready for a short 3 to 7 day elimination fast to clean out drug residues and toxic waste, especially if they are still adversely affecting your well-being. If this is the case, a less intense, but still highly nutritious diet may be followed to continue rebuilding energy and immune defenses.

On rising: continue with your choice of a good high protein or vitamin/mineral drink, as in the initial diet;
and/or take 1 TB. blackstrap molasses in water or juice;
and a Crystal Star DAILY BIOFLAVONOID SUPPORT™ DRINK.

Breakfast: have some plain yogurt with fresh fruit, nuts or seeds;
or granola or muesli with yogurt or kefir topping;
or an omelet, soft boiled or scrambled eggs with whole grain toast or english muffins and butter;
or some oatmeal or whole grain pancakes with maple syrup;
or fresh fruit with vanilla soy milk or kefir or kefir cheese.

Mid-morning: take at least one potassium broth or green drink, or Sun CHLORELLA, Green Foods GREEN ESSENCE, or Crystal Star ENERGY GREEN™ drink every week, with 1 teasp. Bragg's LIQUID AMINOS;
or have an herb tea, such as Crystal Star FEEL GREAT TEA™ or GINSENG 6 DEFENSE RESTORATIVE SUPER TEA™, or ROYAL MU™ TEA; dandelion, licorice root, or Siberian ginseng tea. Add a $1/4$ teasp. royal jelly to any of the recommended teas for an extra healing boost;
or some fresh or dried fruits;
or a cup of instant oriental soup with sea vegetables, and rice or mushroom baked chips.

Lunch: have a tofu and brown rice casserole;
or a veggie pasta and seafood salad;
or a baked yam or potato with a green salad and dressing;
or a light quiche, soufflé, or frittata;
or a high protein salad, or sandwich;
or black bean or lentil soup, or a vegetable stew;
or a large green salad with brewer's yeast and wheat germ sprinkled on top, and a lemon dressing.

Mid-afternoon: have fresh fruit with low-fat cheese or kefir cheese;
and/or a circulatory toning herb tea such as hawthorn berry or ginkgo biloba tea;
or Knudsen RECHARGE electrolyte replacement, or Crystal Star SYSTEM STRENGTH DRINK™;
or deviled eggs with whole grain chips and low-fat raw cheese with a bottle of mineral water.

Dinner: have baked, broiled, or roasted fish, chicken or turkey, with a whole grain dish and green salad;
or an oriental stir-fry with miso soup and brown rice;
or a vegetable or seafood quiche or casserole;
or a low-fat Italian vegetable dish and whole grain pasta with a light vegetable or seafood sauce;
or a hearty vegetable or seafood stew with a green salad.

Before Bed: have a cup of VEGEX broth, or a relaxing herb tea, such as Crystal Star GOOD NIGHT™ or RELAX™ TEA.

➤ *Follow this diet as long as you feel that extra nutrition is needed; then use the THE FOREVER DIET in this book as the basis for health maintenance. (pg. 198)*

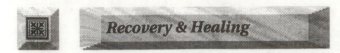
✳ *Supplements and Herbs for Normalizing Strength & Immunity*

As the body takes over its own work and strength returns, decrease the dosage and number of supplements.

❖ Continue with B complex 3x daily, B12 sublingual or internasal, ascorbate vitamin C 2 to 3000mg daily, and vitamin E 800IU daily.

❖ Herbal supplements should include iron and calcium in extract or drink form, Sun CHLORELLA or spirulina granules, minerals and trace minerals such as Mezotrace SEA MINERAL COMPLEX or Crystal Star GINSENG 6 DEFENSE RESTORATIVE SUPER TEA™ or SYSTEM STRENGTH™ DRINK. Take Crystal Star HEARTSEASE ANEMI-GIZE™ CAPS for blood building, FEEL GREAT™ TEA and/or BODY RE-BUILDER™ CAPS for tone.

❖ Take digestive enzymes or acidophilus complex for nutrient assimilation; pre-digested amino acid caps or liquid, or Enzymatic Therapy LIQUID LIVER CAPS with Siberian ginseng for strength.

✳ *Bodywork for Normalizing Strength & Immunity*

✚ Get a massage therapy treatment at least twice a month to align body energy and clear obstructions.

✚ Take a brisk walk every day for circulation and tissue oxygen. Go ocean walking and/or swimming when you can.

✚ Take early morning sun baths every day possible.

✚ Take an oxygen energy bath at least once a week.

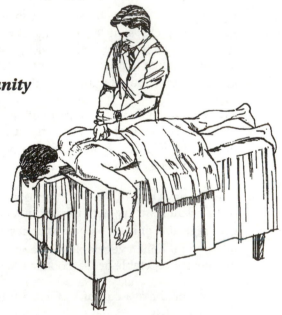

✳ *Sample Recipes for Normalizing Strength & Immunity*
By section and recipe number:

BREAKFAST & BRUNCH - 75, 76, 78, 82, 87, 90, 99, 103, 104

SANDWICHES - SALADS IN BREAD - all

STIR-FRYS - all

FISH & SEAFOODS - all

TOFU FOR YOU - all

HIGH MINERAL FOODS - all

HIGH PROTEIN RECIPES - all

GREAT OUTDOOR EATING - all

COMPLEX CARBOHYDRATES FOR ENERGY - 743, 745, 747, 748, 752, 753, 757, 759, 760, 764, 765, 766, 770, 772, 773, 775, 776, 778, 782, 784

Normalizing the Body After Chemotherapy & Radiation

Chemotherapy and radiation are widely used by the medical community for several types, stages and degrees of cancers and malignant cell growths. While some partial successes have been proven, the after effects are often worse than the disease in terms of healthy cell damage, body imbalances, and lowered immune repsonse. Many doctors and therapists recognize these drawbacks to treatment with chemotherapy, but under current government and insurance restrictions, neither doctors nor patients have any other viable choices.

No treatments except surgery, radiation and chemotherapy have been officially approved by the FDA in the United States for malignant disease. Exorbitantly high costs for major medical treatment have hobbled medical professionals, hospitals and insurance companies in a vicious circle where literally no alternative measures may be used for controlling cancerous growth.

Major medical treatment costs are currently beyond the financial ability of most people, who along with physicians and hospitals must rely on health insurance to pay the expenses. But at the present time, health insurance will only pay for "officially approved" chemotherapy, radiation or surgery. Neither doctors or hospitals are reimbursed if they use alternative therapies, and everyone, including the patient, becomes caught in a political and bureaucratic web that is hardly conducive to confident strides in medicine or healing. In fact, the whole structure and attitude toward major medical care in America today seems to foster greed instead of health.

New testing and alternative research is also incredibly expensive, and lags for lack of funding. Moreover, even when a valid treatment *is* substantiated, the long maze of red tape and political lobbies means that there is no certainty of government (and therefore health insurance) approval for the research company to realize a reasonable return on its effort and investment. This fact is doubly unfortunate as we are see the successful research and alternative therapies used in Europe and other countries to which Americans are denied access.

Fortunately, nutritional counselors, holistic practitioners, therapists and others involved in natural healing have done a great deal of research and work toward minimizing the damage, and rebuilding the body after chemotherapy and radiation. These efforts have had notable success, and may be used with confidence by those recovering from both cancer and its medical treatment.

The following diet is aimed at ridding the body of toxins and residues from these drugs, neutralizing acid/alkaline imbalances, strengthening muscles from wasting, and regenerating healthy tissue.

❋

Diet to Normalize the Body after Chemotherapy or Radiation: a 3-6 week diet

On rising: take a glass of cranberry juice from concentrate with the juice of one fresh lemon;
or apple cide vinegar in water with 1 teasp. honey or maple syrup;
or Crystal Star SYSTEM STRENGTH DRINK™ in apple juice.

Breakfast: have a whole grain cereal with apple juice, vanilla soy milk or yogurt;
or some fresh fruit, or a fresh fruit smoothie with a banana;
or some hot oatmeal with maple syrup and a little butter;
or a high protein drink such as Nature's Plus SPIRUTEIN, or Nutritech ALL 1 DRINK.

Mid-morning: take a glass of fresh carrot juice;
or a potassium broth or essence (page 240);
or a cup of Siberian ginseng tea, chamomile tea, or Crystal Star FEEL GREAT™ TEA;
or a small bottle of mineral water with a packet of Sun CHLORELLA, Green Foods GREEN ESSENCE granules, or Crystal Star ENERGY GREEN™ DRINK.

Lunch: have a fresh green salad with a light dressing, and whole grain muffins with kefir cheese;
or some steamed vegetables with 1 TB. Bragg's LIQUID AMINOS, and a cup of miso soup;
or a baked potato or brown rice with a small salad;
or an open face sandwich with fresh vegetables and a light oil dressing on whole grain bread;
or a seafood pasta salad with a light soup.

Mid-afternoon: raw vegetable snacks with kefir cheese or low-fat cheese, and a glass of mineral water;
or a cup of herb tea, such as peppermint, red clover, or Crystal Star HIGH ENERGY TEA™.

Dinner: have a whole grain and vegetable casserole with a cup of black bean soup;
or a light Italian vegetable and whole grain pasta dinner with a green salad;
or baked or broiled fish or seafood with a green salad and brown rice or millet;
or an oriental stir-fry with plenty of vegetables and seafod or chicken, brown rice and miso soup;
or or a seafood stew with hearty whole grain french bread and some steamed vegetables.

Before Bed: have a hot cup of VEGEX yeast broth for relaxation and B vitamins;
or a cup of herb tea, such as chamomile or Crystal Star LICORICE MINTS TEA.

✽ *Supplements to Normalize After Chemotherapy:* For 3 months take daily

❖ One individual packet of Green Foods BARLEY GREEN MAGMA in water.

❖ Ascorbate vitamin C or Ester C crystals with Bioflavonoids, $1/4$ teasp. in water or juice every 2 hours, to supply approx. 5-10,000mg. daily, and/or Crystal Star DAILY BIOFLAV. & C SUPPORT DRINK.

❖ Germanium 30 to 50mg., **or** dissolve 1 gm. germanium powder in 1-qt. water, and take 3 TBS. daily.

❖ Hawthorn extract 2x daily, with a vitamin E 400IU capsule and one CoQ 10 capsule - 60mg.

❖ Vitamin B$_{12}$, internasal or sublingual, every other day.

❖ Floradix HERBAL IRON liquid, 1 teasp. 3x daily, or Crystal Star GINSENG 6 DEFENSE RESTORATIVE SUPER TEA™.

❖ Crystal Star SYSTEM STRENGTH DRINK™ mix, and/or LIV-ALIVE™ TEA and CAPSULES.

✽ *Bodywork for Normalizing After Chemotherapy*

✤ Get some fresh air and exercise every day with a brisk walk and deep breathing. Exercise is a body chemistry changing nutrient in itself.

✤ Get early morning sunlight on the body every day possible. Light builds strength along with food. Eating outdoors in fresh air is very beneficial. Consider a short camping trip for oxygenating tree and forest energy.

✤ Massage therapy is excellent for releasing drug rsidues, and toning weakened muscle tissue.

✽ *Sample Recipes for Recovery from Chemotherapy & Radiation*
By section and recipe number:

HEALTHY DRINKS, JUICES & WATERS - 45, 47, 49,50, 51, 52, 53, 57, 63, 65, 70, 71
BREAKFAST & BRUNCH - 74, 76, 81, 85, 91, 93, 96, 97, 102, 107, 108

ORIENTAL & LIGHT MACROBIOTIC COOKING - all

SALADS - HOT & COLD - all

SOUPS - LIQUID SALADS - all

FISH & SEAFOODS - 532, 537, 541, 544, 547, 548, 549, 551, 552, 555, 557, 560, 562, 563, 564, 567, 569

HIGH PROTEIN COOKING - 596, 598, 599, 701, 710, 711, 713, 715, 716, 717, 718, 720, 723, 724, 733

HIGH MINERAL RECIPES - all

HIGH COMPLEX CARBOHYDRATES FOR ENERGY - all

GREAT OUTDOOR EATING - 874, 875, 876, 879, 883, 886, 888, 890, 894, 895, 896, 901, 903, 906, 908

✽ *Sample Menu Plans*
Recipe combinations that work for this diet:

A SPECIAL DINNER FOR TWO - 454, 195, 533, 744, 622, 52

A WEEKEND PICNIC - 54, 621, 780, 227, 892

A HEARTY WINTER MEAL - 63, 751, 126, 158

A SUNDAY BRUNCH - 874, 908, 51, 459, 900, 198

A WEEKNIGHT DINNER - 767, 983, 127

LUNCH FOR TWO - 773, 53, 904, 186

A LIGHT SUMMER MEAL - 45, 898, 452

A FAMILY MEAL - 556, 466, 656, 628

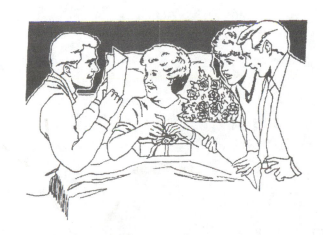

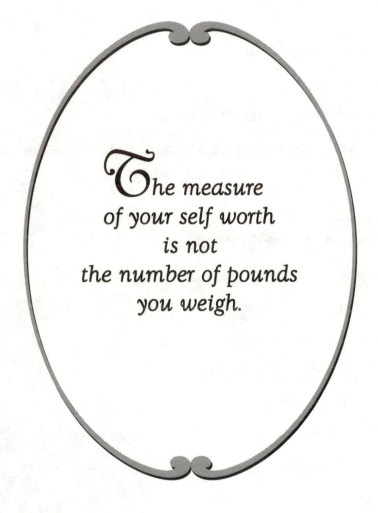

*The measure
of your self worth
is not
the number of pounds
you weigh.*

Renewing Female Balance; Diet Solutions

The female system is an incredibly complex balance...an individual model of the creative universe. A woman is usually a marvelous thing to be, but the intricacies of her body are delicately tuned and easily become unbalanced or obstructed, causing pain and poor function. A woman is such a wholly-bound-together person that imbalances often cause a lack of union between mind and body. She loses the accustomed oneness with herself, resulting in both physiological and emotional problems.

Drugs, chemicals and synthetic medicines, standing as they do outside the natural cycle of things, often do not bring positive results for women. These substances usually try to add something to the body, or act directly on a specific problem area. Whole foods, and herbs as concentrated foods, are identified and used through the body's own enzyme action. They are gentle but effective nutrients that encourage the body to do its own work, recover its own balance. Nutritional therapy nourishes in a broad spectrum, like the female essence itself. A woman's body responds to it easily without side effects. We have found that most women know their own bodies better than anyone else, and can instinctively pinpoint foods within a diet range that are right for their personal renewal and balance. Relief, and response time are often quite gratifying.

Hormones, incredibly important and potent substances, seem to be at the root of most women's problems. They are secreted into the bloodstream by the glands, and carried throughout the body to stimulate specific functions. They are the basis for all metabolic activity. Some have almost immediate effects on the system, some a long-delayed reaction. Even in tiny amounts they have, as any woman can tell you, dramatic effects. A minute imbalance in ratio or deficiency can cause inordinate body malfunction.

Many female problems are caused by too much estrogen production, such as fibrocystic breast disease, endometriosis, pre-menstrual syndrome, and heavy, painful menstrual periods. The growth and function of the breasts and uterus are controlled by estrogens and prolactin which are produced by the ovaries and pituitary gland. A diet too high in fats raises these hormones to disease-forming levels. In women, the whole reproductive system is affected. A healthy endocrine system is a must for solving female problems because the glands are the deepest level of the body processes. Good nutrition and nourishment for the glands can "change the world" for a woman. Many hormones are protein based, so that a diet high in vegetable proteins and whole grains, with some lecithin and brewer's yeast on a regular basis, is very important to effective gland and hormone health.

The diet in this chapter is rich in nourishment for the glands; it is oxygenating, with iodine and mineral-rich foods. It is effective in support for the following conditions:
BREAST and UTERINE FIBROIDS HORMONE and GLAND IMBALANCES INFERTILITY ENDOMETRIOSIS FRIGIDITY PMS, CRAMPS and OTHER MENSTRUAL DIFFICULTIES MENOPAUSAL SYMPTOMS POST-MENOPAUSAL BONE LOSS and OSTEOPOROSIS VAGINAL and BODY DRYNESS CYSTS, POLYPS and BENIGN TUMORS ADRENAL EXHAUSTION

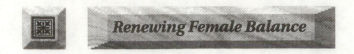

Stage One; A 24 Hour Cleansing Diet:

A short liquid cleanse, followed by a three day fresh foods diet is recommended to clear the system; allowing it a brief digestive rest before beginning a new way of eating that will nourish the body's endocrine and regenerative levels.

On rising: take 2 fresh lemons squeezed in a glass of water with 1 teasp. honey.

Mid-morning: take 2 teasp. of cranberry concentrate in a glass of water with 1 teasp. honey;
or a glass of Crystal Star DAILY BIOFLAVONOID SUPPORT DRINK™.

Mid-day: have a glass of apple juice, with 1 teasp. spirulina, Sun CHLORELLA or Green Foods BARLEY GREEN MAGMA granules.

Mid-afternoon: have a green drink, with 1 teasp. Bragg's LIQUID AMINOS;
and/or another glass of cranberry juice.

Evening: have a glass of apple/strawberry or apple/alfalfa sprout juice.

Before bed: have a glass of papaya or papaya/pineapple juice to enhance enzyme activity;
and/or a cup of VEGEX yeast broth for B vitamins and relaxation.

The Three Day Fresh Foods Diet:

Important note: Drink 6 to 8 glasses of pure water every day of this cleansing diet.

On rising: take a vitamin/mineral drink such as NutriTech ALL 1 or Nature's Plus SPIRUTEIN, with apple or orange juice;
or apple/pineapple, or apple/cranberry juice;
and/or a glass of aloe vera juice with herbs.

Breakfast: have some fresh fruit, mixed with yogurt if desired, with brewer's yeast and toasted wheat germ sprinkled on top.

Mid-morning: have some fresh apple juice or carrot juice;
or V-8 juice (page 241), **or** Knudsen's VERY VEGGIE juice with 1 teasp. Bragg's LIQUID AMINOS;
and some raw celery or cucumber sticks with kefir cheese, and a small bottle of mineral water;
or have a green drink (page 240ff.4), or Sun CHLORELLA, or Green Foods GREEN ESSENCE.

Lunch: Have a green salad with sprouts, carrots and lemon/oil dressing;
and/or a cup of miso soup with sea vegetables snipped on top.

Mid-afternoon: have some raw crunchy veggies (especially broccoli and cauliflower) with an all-vegetable dip or soy spread;
and a balancing herb tea, such as Crystal Star FEMALE HARMONY TEA™, DAILY BIOFLAVONOID SUPPORT DRINK™ or CLEANSING & FASTING TEA™;
or a small bottle of mineral water.

Dinner: have another large salad and cup of miso soup with sea vegetables.

Before bed: have a VEGEX yeast broth;
or an herb tea for relaxation and sleep, such as chamomile tea or Crystal Star RELAX TEA™.

✷ Supplements for the Woman's Cleansing Diet
Take only food source and herbal supplements for easy assimilation during a cleanse.

❖ Include herbal extract drops in water, such as dong quai or sarsaparilla tincture, or Crystal Star ADRN-ALIVE™ EXTRACT, IODINE THERAPY™ EXTRACT, or MIODIN liquid kelp.

❖ Include high potency acidophilus powder or Natren LIFE START II, $1/2$ teasp. 3 times daily, and 1 teasp. lecithin granules with 1 teasp. omega 3 flax oil in water during the cleanse.

❖ Include a green supplement, such as spirulina, Sun CHLORELLA tablets, Green Foods BARLEY GREEN MAGMA, or Crystal Star ENERGY GREEN DRINK™.

❖ Include 1 teasp. ascorbate vitamin C crystals <u>with bioflavonoids</u>, ($1/4$ teasp. doses at a time in water), or Crystal Star DAILY BIOFLAVONOID SUPPORT DRINK™.

✷ Bodywork for the Woman's Cleansing Diet

✚ Take a liquid chlorophyll enema once during the cleansing diet to release old waste.

✚ Do some slow exercise stretches every morning and evening to increase systol/diastol action. Take a short brisk walk every day. Exercise is a cleansing nutrient in itself because it changes body chemistry.

✷ Sample Recipes for the Woman's Cleansing Diet
By section and recipe number:

FASTING & CLEANSING FOODS - 1, 2, 3, 6, 8, 9, 11, 12, 13, 14, 17, 18, 24, 25, 26, 27, 28, 29, 30, 31, 32

SALADS HOT & COLD - 186, 187, 191, 199, 201, 204, 205, 206, 210, 220, 226, 229, 230, 232, 233, 236

HEALTHY DRINKS, JUICES & WATERS - 43, 44, 45, 46, 49, 51, 52, 54, 55, 56, 57, 60, 62, 65, 66, 67, 69

✸

Stage Two; Rebuilding Female Strength and Energy
This diet stage concentrates on nourishing the glands, especially the adrenals, for balanced hormone secretions, on rebuilding energy levels by increasing circulation, and on alkalizing the body through better enzyme activity and nutrient assimilation.

On rising: take a vitamin/mineral drink such as NutriTech ALL 1 or Nature's Plus SPIRUTEIN.

Breakfast: make a mix of 2 TBS. **each** lecithin granules, brewer's yeast, flax seeds, and wheat germ. Sprinkle some daily on whole grain cereal, or fresh fruit, or mix into plain yogurt;
and have poached or baked eggs with whole grain toast or English muffins;
or some tofu scrambled eggs and whole grain muffins with kefir cheese';
or oatmeal with a little maple syrup.
and an herbal digestive tea, such as Crystal Star AFTER MEAL™ extract in water, or alfalfa/mint tea.

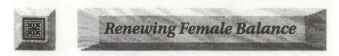

Mid-morning: have some miso soup or a ramen broth with sea veggies;
<u>or</u> some crunchy raw veggies with kefir cheese or low-fat cheese, and an herb tea such as licorice root.

Lunch: have some steamed veggies with rice and tofu;
<u>or</u> a seafood and veggie pasta salad;
<u>or</u> a baked potato with a little butter or kefir cheese and a green salad;
<u>or</u> a light oriental soup and salad, with sea veggies and crunchy noodles;
<u>or</u> a large salad with fresh herbs and lemon/ oil dressing and rice cakes;
✓Have a small bottle of mineral water with any of the above meals.

Mid-afternoon: have a fresh fruit smoothie with a banana;
<u>or</u> some whole grain crackers with kefir cheese, or soy spread, and cottage cheese with a light sauce;
<u>and/or</u> a refreshing herb tea such as Crystal Star FEMALE HARMONY™ or RELAX TEA™.

Dinner: have a vegetable quiche with a whole grain crust;
<u>or</u> have a light protein pasta meal with vegies and a yogurt/chive dressing.
<u>or</u> have a baked potato or some steamed broccoli or cauliflower with low-fat or soy cheese.
<u>or</u> have an oriental vegetable stir-fry with miso soup and brown rice;
<u>or</u> baked or broiled fish or seafood with basmati rice and peas, and a small salad.
✓A light white wine at dinner is good for digestion and relaxation.

Before bed: have a glass of mineral water, or a relaxing herb tea, such as peppermint tea or Crystal Star GOODNIGHT™ TEA.

✓Drink 6 to 8 glasses of water daily to keep the system flowing, and toxins and fats flushed out.
✓The best eating habits work with several small "grazing" meals throughout the day, instead of large meals, giving the body time to use food better without being overloaded or weighed down.

✻ *Supplements for the Woman's Rebuilding Diet*

❖ For blood building and immune enhancement, take extra iron in herbal form, (superior for assimilation and non-constipating) such as Floradix or Crystal Star IRON SOURCE™ caps or extract.

❖ For gland rebuilding and balance, take evening primrose oil caps, with Crystal Star FEMALE HARMONY™ caps and/or DONG QUAI/DAMIANA extract.

❖ For tissue rebuilding, take beta-carotene 25 to 50,000IU daily, or Crystal Star DAILY BIOFLAVONOID SUPPORT DRINK™, and vitamin E 800IU daily.

❖ For adrenal nourishment, take B-complex 100mg. with extra B6, and an adrenal complex such as the capsules from Enzymatic Therapy, or Crystal Star ADRN-ALIVE™ caps or ADRN-ALIVE™ extract.

✻ *Bodywork for the Woman's Rebuilding Diet*

✚ Eliminate caffeine from the diet for the best improvement of female problems; also avoid red meats, carbonated sodas and tobacco.

✚ Take some exercise and/or walking time every day. Get some early sunlight on the body daily.

❈ Sample Recipes For The Female Rebuilding Diet
By section and recipe number:

BREAKFAST & BRUNCH - 73, 74, 75, 76, 77, 78, 80, 82, 84, 86, 87, 92, 93, 95, 96, 97, 101, 103, 105, 108

ORIENTAL & LIGHT MACROBIOTIC COOKING - all

SALADS HOT & COLD - all

LOW-FAT & VERY LOW-FAT DISHES - all

DAIRY FREE COOKING - 333, 334, 335, 337, 338, 340, 342, 346, 348, 351, 352, 354, 355, 357, 359, 361

SOUPS - LIQUID SALADS - all

STIR-FRYS - all

HIGH MINERAL FOODS - 612, 613, 617, 620, 622, 625, 626, 627, 634, 640, 646, 647, 649, 652, 662, 663

HIGH PROTEIN WITHOUT MEAT - 695, 696, 699, 702, 705, 709, 710, 711, 716, 719, 720, 732, 734, 736

COMPLEX CARBOHYDRATES FOR ENERGY - 743, 744, 747, 750, 751, 752, 755, 759, 767, 776, 777

❈ Sample Menu Plans
Some recipe combinations that work with this diet:

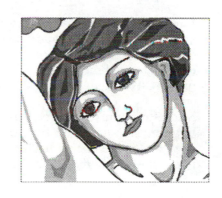

AN EASY WEEKNIGHT DINNER - 350, 187, 158, 374

A HEARTY WINTER MEAL - 333, 167, 643, 781, 767

A LIGHT SUMMER MEAL - 142, 737, 373, 367

A SPECIAL DINNER FOR TWO - 334, 452, 235, 660

A WEEKEND PICNIC - 338, 727, 208, 339

LUNCH FOR TWO - 111, 739, 123, 663

AN EASY RISING BREAKFAST - 74, 75, 78, 81

SUNDAY BRUNCH - 740, 699, 622, 653, 662

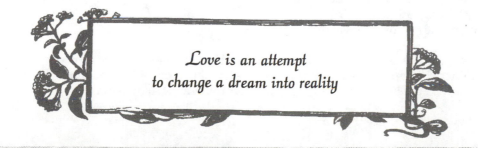

*Love is an attempt
to change a dream into reality*

Stage Three; Long Range Diet Solutions For Women

*A maintenance and disease prevention diet for optimal female nutrition should be low in fats, sweeteners, other refined carbohydrates, and pasteurized dairy products. A woman's system seems to thrive on plenty of fresh foods, fruits and vegetables, rice and other cooked whole grains, with **limited** yeasted breads and beans. Light foods, such as low-fat and raw cheeses, cultured foods, seafoods, whole grains, leafy greens, sprouts and sea vegetables are the basis for a balanced female system. (Men seem to thrive on more root vegetables, beans, breads, whole grains and **some** lean meats).*

Caffeine, and caffeine-containing foods should be limited; red meats, saturated animal fats, tobacco and hard alcohol should be avoided.

On rising: take a vitamin/mineral drink such as Nutri-Tech ALL 1, Nature's Plus SPIRUTEIN, or Crystal Star SYSTEM STRENGTH DRINK™ in juice or mineral water.

Breakfast: Make a mix or 2 TBS. **each:** lecithin granules, brewer's yeast, flax seeds and wheat germ. Sprinkle some daily on whole grain cereal or muesli, fresh fruit or yogurt, poached or baked eggs, or oatmeal with a little maple syrup;
or have a fresh fruit smoothie with prunes and a ripe banana;
or have some tofu scrambled "eggs," or poached eggs with whole grain toast or toasted pita bread.
or some pilaf breakfast grains with Bragg's LIQUID AMINOS or shoyu sauce.

Mid-morning: have some crunchy raw veggies and/or whole grain crackers with a vegetable dip or kefir cheese, and a small bottle of mineral water;
and have a green drink, (page 240ff.) or Sun CHLORELLA, Green Foods BARLEY GREEN MAGMA, or Crystal Star ENERGY GREEN DRINK™ with 1 teasp. Bragg's LIQUID AMINOS;
or a cup of miso or ramen noodle soup with sea veggies snipped on top, and rice cakes.

Lunch: have some steamed veggies with a little butter, or light tamari dressing;
or a salad with boiled/marinated tofu and greens, and a vinaigrette dressing;
or a seafood salad with brown rice or veggie pasta;
or a hot or cold soup with a small green salad and some whole grain muffins or rice cakes;
or a small omelet with a light, low-fat filling and sauce.

Mid-afternoon: have some dried fruits with a little low-fat cheese or cottage cheese dip;
or a fruit smoothie with 1 teasp. spirulina added for energy;
or a hard boiled egg with a little sesame salt, some whole grain crackers and mineral water;
or a refreshing herb tea, such as peppermint, licorice root, or Crystal Star LICORICE MINTS TEA.

Dinner: have some baked, broiled or grilled fish with a light sauce, brown rice, and sautéed veggies;
or an oriental meal, with miso soup and sea vegetables, rice pasta, and Chinese green vegetables;
or a dinner stir-fry with veggies and noodles;
or a light Italian meal with whole grain vegie pasta and baked vegetables;
or a vegetable or seafood quiche with whole grain crust;
or low-fat cheese, vegetable or seafood souffle, with a light white wine for digestion & relaxation.

Before bed: have a cup of VEGEX yeast broth;
or a glass of vanilla soy milk or kefir;
or a glass of organic apple or papaya juice.

✔ A woman's system needs plenty of water to keep it flushed. Even if you don't consciously feel thirsty, keep bottled mineral water handy, and have some every hour or two. Remember that a well-hydrated system actually keeps the body from retaining fluid, a problem for many women.

❊ *Supplements for the Woman's Long Range Maintence Diet*

The following is a list of excellent maintenance supplements for women, to be used as needed or desired.

❖ Nature's Plus vitamin E 800IU, or wheat germ oil 2 teasp. daily, (with Alta Health MAGNESIUM and B$_{12}$ sublingual if there is PMS discomfort).

❖ Ascorbate vitamin C, or Ester C with bioflavonoids, 2 to 3000mg. daily, or Crystal Star DAILY BIO-FLAVONOID SUPPORT DRINK™.

❖ B complex 100mg. daily, with extra B$_6$ 100mg.

❖ Adrenal gland nourishment, such as Crystal Star ADRN-ALIVE™ CAPS or ADRN-ALIVE™ EXTRACT, or Enzymatic Therapy ADRENAL COMPLEX.

❖ Green supplements, such as Spirulina, Sun CHLORELLA, or GREEN FOODS BARLEY GREEN MAGMA tablets or granules daily.

❖ Hormone stability and support from Evening primrose oil capsules 2 to 4 daily for prostaglandin production, and herbal balancers such Crystal Star FEMALE HARMONY™ CAPSULES and DONG QUAI/DAMIANA EXTRACT.

❖ Stress and tension control from licorice root or sarsaparilla teas, Natrol SAF capsules, or Crystal Star RELAX™ CAPS.

❖ P.M.S. relief from burdock tea, Schiff PMS formula, Crystal Star ANTI-SPZ™ CAPS or CRAMP CONTROL™ EXTRACT, or Enzymatic Therapy RAW MAMMARY and RAW OVARY caps. Try FLOW XS TEA™ if periods are excessively heavy.

❖ Mineral and trace mineral support from Mezotrace SEA MINERAL COMPLEX, or Crystal Star CALCIUM SOURCE™, IRON SOURCE™, or MINERAL SPECTRUM™ COMPLEX extracts.

❊ *Bodywork for the Women's Long Range Maintenance Diet*

✛ Regular outdoor exercise when possible, indoor aerobic exercise during bad weather.

✛ Early morning sunlight on the body every day possible.

✛ Small meals throughout the day, rather than large meals.

✛ A massage, shiatzu session, or hot sauna before the menstrual period to loosen and release clogging mucous and fatty deposits, and to improve circulation. Apply ice packs to pelvic area for pain.

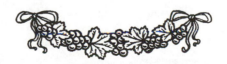

❋ Sample Recipes For A Woman's Long Range Diet
By section and recipe number:

LOW-FAT & VERY LOW-FAT DISHES - all

BREAKFAST & BRUNCH - all

SUGAR FREE SPECIALS & SWEET TREATS - all

STIR-FRYS - all

FISH & SEAFOODS - all

HIGH MINERAL FOODS - all

HIGH PROTEIN WITHOUT MEAT - 696, 698, 699, 700, 701, 720, 723, 735, 736, 737, 738, 740, 741, 742

COMPLEX CARBOHYDRATES FOR ENERGY - all

GREAT OUTDOOR EATING - 874, 875, 877, 880, 881, 883, 884, 888, 890, 893, 894, 895, 896, 899, 901

HOLIDAY FEASTING & ENTERTAINING - 826, 828, 831, 832, 833, 835, 842, 849, 857, 860, 866, 868

❋ Sample Meal Planning
Recipe combinations that work with this diet:

A FAMILY MEAL - 732, 768, 430, 754

A SPECIAL DINNER FOR TWO - 421, 749, 565, 201, 538

SUNDAY BRUNCH - 701, 539, 197, 905, 830

A HEARTY WINTER MEAL - 753, 736, 770, 299

A LIGHT SUMMER MEAL - 542, 283/285, 417

AN ALL HORS D'OEUVRES PARTY - 536, 909, 908, 429, 827, 412

AN EASY RISING BREAKFAST - 819, 822, 74, 75

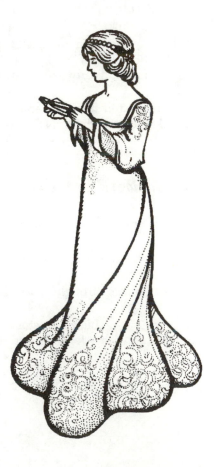

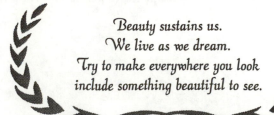

Beauty sustains us.
We live as we dream.
Try to make everywhere you look
include something beautiful to see.

Sports Nutrition
Eating for Energy and Performance

Body building is 85% nutrition. A regular long term, optimally nutritious diet is the basis for high performance - not protein or even carbo-loading before an event. The major body systems involved in energy production are the liver, thyroid, and adrenal glands. Maximum anabolic effect can be achieved through food and herbal sources. Complex carbohydrates such as those from whole grains, pastas, vegetables, rice, beans and fruits are the key to strength and endurance for both the athlete and the casual body builder. They improve performance, promote storage of muscle fuel, and are easily absorbed without excess fats.

Sixty-five to 70% of a high performance diet should be in unrefined complex carbohydrates. Twenty to 25% should be in high grade proteins from whole grains, nuts, beans, raw dairy products, soy foods, yogurt, kefir, eggs, and some occasional poultry, fish and seafood. About 10-15% should be in energy-producing fats and oils necessary for glycogen storage. The best fats are unrefined and mono- or unsaturated -oils, a little pure butter, nuts and seeds, low fat cheeses, and whole grain snacks. The remaining fuel should be liquid nutrients; fruit juices for their natural sugars, mineral waters, electrolyte replacement drinks for lost potassium, magnesium and sodium, and plenty of pure water. When the body senses lack of water, it will naturally start to retain fluid. Waste and body impurities will not be filtered out properly, and the liver will not metabolize stored fats for energy. Six to eight glass of water a day are a must, even if you don't feel thirsty. It takes the sensory system time to catch up with actual body needs. Eating junk foods pays the penalty of poor performance. Athletic excellence cannot be achieved by just adding anabolic steroids to an inferior diet. The only effective action is optimal nutrition.

A WORD ABOUT STEROIDS

As the standards of excellence rise in sports and competition, the use of steroids is increasing. Steroid enhancement has spread beyond the professional and Olympic arenas to dedicated weight lifters, body builders and team players at all levels. The dangers of synthetic steroids far outweigh any advantages. Steroid use leads to wholesale destruction of glandular tissue, stunted growth from bone closure in males, testicle shrinkage, low sperm counts with sterility noticeable after only a few months of use, enlargement and tenderness of the pectorals, weakening of connective tissue, jaundice from liver malfunction, circulation impairment, and adverse side effects of hostile personality behavior and facial changes.

Amino acids from sources such as herbs, and foods high in amino acids, can act as steroid alternatives to help build the body to competitive levels without these consequences. These "natural steroids" help release growth hormone, promote ammonia and acid detoxification, stimulate immunity and encourage liver regeneration. They maximize potential, promote fast recuperation, increase stamina, and support peak performance.

The following diet is rich in amino acids, and is effective for:
&MORE ENERGY, ENDURANCE & STAMINA &OVERCOMING FATIGUE and EX-HAUSTION &IMPROVED PHYSICAL PERFORMANCE &FASTER HEALING OF WOUNDS and INJURIES &HORMONE, GLAND and METABOLIC STIMULA-TION &MUSCLE ACID BUILD-UP &ELECTROLYTE REPLACEMENT &

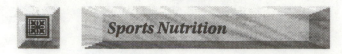

Sports Nutrition, Energy and Performance Diets

This section includes three separate diets. All are strengthening and building, for fuel and energy.

The first is targeted to people who lack consistent daily energy and tire easily, and to those who need more endurance and strength for hard jobs or long hours. It is also for weekend sports enthusiasts who wish to accomplish more than their present level of nutrition allows.

The second is a moderate aerobic diet, for people who work out 3 or 4 times a week. It emphasizes complex carbohydrates for smooth muscle use, and moderate fat and protein amounts. Complex carbohydrates also produce glycogen for the body, resulting in increased energy and endurance.

The third is a training diet, concentrating more on energy for competitive sports participation and long range stamina. For the serious athlete, and for those who are consciously building their bodies for higher workout achievement, this diet can be a good basic foundation for significantly improved performance. Many tests have shown that adjusting the diet before competition can increase endurance 200% or more - well worth consideration. Athletes' nutritional needs are considerably greater than the fuel needs of the average person. Normal recommended daily allowances are far too low for high performance needs, and have no application for competition. Consult with a good sports nutritionist, or knowledgable people at a health food store or gym to determine individual specific supplement requirements. The important consideration is not body <u>weight</u>, but body <u>composition</u>.

Each of the diets in this chapter can be useful to the serious, performing athlete. Competitive training and a training diet alone cannot insure success. Rest time, and building reserves of energy and endurance are also necessary to tune the body for maximum efficiency. When an athlete is not in competition or pre-event training, super high nutritive amounts are not needed, and can be hard for the body to handle. A diet of less concentration is better for basic maintenance tone, and can easily be built up again for competitive performance.

A **Food Exchange List** and a **Chart for Food Amounts by Specific Diet** are included for easy use and adjustment to individual needs.

✦FOOD EXCHANGE LIST

Any food listed in a specific category may be exchanged one-for-one with any other food in that category. Portion amounts are given for a man weighing 170 pounds, and a woman weighing 130 pounds.

❧ GRAINS, BREADS & CEREALS:
One serving is approximately one cup of cooked grains, such as brown rice, millet, barley, bulgur, kashi, couscous, corn, oats, and whole grain pasta;
<u>or</u> one cup of dry cereals, such as bran flakes, Oatios, or Grapenuts;
<u>or</u> three slices of wholegrain bread;
<u>or</u> three six-inch corn tortillas;
<u>or</u> two chapatis or whole wheat pita breads;
<u>or</u> twelve small wholegrain crackers;
<u>or</u> two rice cakes.

❧ VEGETABLES:
Group A: One serving is as much as you want of lettuce (all kinds), Chinese greens and peas, raw spinach and carrots, celery, cucumbers, endive, sea vegetables and watercress, radishes, green onions and chives.
Group B: One serving is approximately two cups of cabbage or alfalfa sprouts;
<u>or</u> one and a half cups cooked bell peppers and mushrooms;
<u>or</u> one cup cooked asparagus, cauliflower, chard, sauerkraut, eggplant, zucchini or summer squash;

or $3/4$ cup cooked broccoli, green beans; onions or mung bean sprouts;
or $1/2$ cup vegetable juice cocktail, or cooked brussels sprouts;
or 8-10 water chestnuts.
Group C: One serving is approximately 1 $1/2$ cups cooked carrots;
or one cup cooked beets, potatoes, or leeks;
or $1/2$ cup cooked peas, corn, artichokes, winter squash or yams;
or one cup fresh carrot or vegetable juice.

⁊ FRUITS:
One serving is approximately one apple, nectarine, mango, pineapple, peach or orange;
or 4 apricots, medjool dates or figs;
or half a honeydew or cantaloupe;
or 20 to 24 cherries or grapes;
or one and a half cups strawberries or other berries.

⁊ DAIRY FOODS:
One serving is approximately one cup of whole milk, buttermilk or full fat yogurt, for 3mg. of fat;
or one cup of low-fat milk or yogurt, for 2gm. of fat;
or one cup of skim milk or non-fat yogurt, for less than 1gm. of fat;
or one ounce of low fat hard cheese, such as swiss or cheddar;
or $1/3$ cup of non-fat dry milk powder.

⁊ POULTRY, FISH & SEAFOOD:
One serving is approximately four ounces of white fish, or fresh salmon, skinned for 3gm. of fat;
or four ounces of chicken or turkey, white meat, no skin for 4gm. of fat;
or one cup of tuna or salmon, water packed for 3gm. of fat;
or one cup of shrimp, scallops, oysters, clams or crab for 3 to 4gm. of fat;

☛WE RECOMMEND AVOIDING RED MEATS. THEY ARE HIGH IN SATURATED FAT AND CHOLESTEROL, AND UNSOUND AS A USE OF PLANETARY RESOURCES.
These include all beef, carved, ground, corned or smoked, such as luncheon meat; veal, lamb, pork, sausage, ham and bacon, and wild game.

⁊ HIGH PROTEIN MEAT & DAIRY SUBSTITUTES:
One serving is approximately four ounces of tofu (one block);
or $1/2$ cup low fat or dry cottage cheese;
or one egg;
or $1/3$ cup ricotta, parmesan or mozzarella;
or $1/2$ cup cooked beans or brown rice.

⁊ FATS & OILS:
One serving is approximately one teaspoon of butter, margarine or shortening for 5gm. of fat;
or one tablespoon of salad dressing or mayonnaise for 5gm. of fat;
or 2 teaspoons of poly-unsaturated or mono-unsaturated vegetable oil for 5gm. of fat.

The following foods are very high in fat and the amounts listed are equivalent to one fat serving on the diet chart. Use sparingly as part of a high fitness diet.
  two tablespoons of light cream, half and half, or sour cream; 1 tablespoon of heavy cream;
$1/8$ slice of avocado;
  ten almonds, cashews or peanuts; twenty pistachios or spanish peanuts; four walnut or pecan halves;
$1/4$ cup of sunflower, sesame, or pumpkin seeds.

❦ CHART FOR FOOD AMOUNTS BY SPECIFIC DIET
Servings should be scaled up or down to fit your individual weight and type of active diet.

Daily Diet for Men			Daily Diet for Women		
High Energy, Active Life Diet Calories 2800 Protein 17% Carbos 70% Fat 13%	**Moderate Aerobic Diet** Calories 3250 Protein 20% Carbos 65% Fat 15%	**Training & Competition Diet** Calories 3950 Protein 23% Carbos 65% Fat 12%	**High Energy, Active Life Diet** Calories 2000 Protein 17% Carbos 70% Fat 13%	**Moderate Aerobic Diet** Calories 2200 Protein 20% Carbos 65% Fat 15%	**Training & Competition Diet** Calories 2750 Protein 23% Carbos 65% Fat 12%
6 whole grain servings	7 whole grain servings	8 whole grain servings	4 whole grain servings	4 whole grain servings	6 whole grain servings
Group A vegetables - all you want	Group A vegetables - all you want	Group A vegetables - all you want	Group A vegetables - all you want	Group A vegetables - all you want	Group A vegetables - all you want
Group B vegetables - 6 servings	Group B vegetables - 6 servings	Group B vegetables - 7 servings	Group B vegetables - 4 servings	Group B vegetables - 4 servings	Group B vegetables - 6 servings
Group C vegetables - 6 servings	Group C vegetables - 6 servings	Group C vegetables - 8 servings	Group C vegetables - 3 servings	Group C vegetables - 4 servings	Group C vegetables - 5 servings
5 fruit servings	5 fruit servings	6 fruit servings	3 fruit servings	`4 fruit servings	4 fruit servings
3 dairy servings	4 dairy servings	4 dairy servings	2 dairy servings	3 dairy servings	3 dairy servings
2 poultry or seafood servings	4 poultry or seafood servings	5 poultry or seafood servings	1 poultry or seafood servings	1 poultry or seafood servings	3 poultry or seafood servings
5 fat servings	5 fat servings	6 fat servings	3 fat servings	3 fat servings	3 fat servings

A High Energy, Active Life Style Diet:
This diet is designed to quickly build up body nutrient content and strength, with several small "refueling" meals throughout the day to regularly support energy with easy assimilation.

On rising: take 1 teasp. molasses and 1 TB. bee pollen granules in apple, or pineapple/coconut juice; **or** 1 TB. NutriTech ALL 1 vitamin/mineral drink mix in juice or water.

Breakfast: take a high protein drink, such as Nature's Plus SPIRUTEIN; **or** make a protein drink with soy protein powder, 1 egg, 2 teasp. brewer's yeast, 1 teasp. spirulina powder, 2 teasp. toasted wheat germ and 1 teasp. sesame seeds; **or** see the suggestions on pages 262 and 263, for good protein energy drinks; **then** have some muesli or whole grain granola, such as coconut/almond granola, with yogurt and fresh fruit, apple juice or soy milk topping;
or hot oatmeal with maple syrup, **or** whole grain (buckwheat) pancakes with maple syrup;
or a poached agg on a whole grain English muffin, with a little butter and Bragg's LIQUID AMINOS; **or** a small plain omelet.

Mid-morning: take a high potency enzyme/mineral drink such as Crystal Star SYSTEM STRENGTH DRINK™;
or Amazake rice drink;
or Crystal Star HIGH ENERGY™ TEA;
or Alacer High K Cola, **and** some fresh fruit such as grapes, figs, or raisins;
or miso soup with sea vegetables snipped on top;
or a green drink or vegetable juice (pg. 240) or Sun CHLORELLA or Green Foods GREEN MAGMA;

Lunch: have a baked potatao, with a little butter and 1 teasp. Bragg's LIQUID AMINOs;
and/or a spinach/endive or other dark green leafy salad;
or a vegetable frittata;
or a seafood salad, whole grain or veggie pasta salad (hot or cold), with whole grain muffins;
or a roast turkey sandwich on whole grain bread with greens and mayonnaise;
or tofu or steamed veggies with brown rice and tamari;
or some low-fat cheeses or cottage cheese with fresh fruit;
or a high protein salad or sandwich with avocados and sprouts.

Mid-afternoon: have some low fat yogurt with nuts, seeds, or fresh fruit;
or a hard boiled or deviled egg with sesame salt for dipping, and a bottle of mineral water;
or a green drink (page 240) with some whole grain crackers and a low-fat dip;
or some dried or fresh fruit with kefir cheese for dipping.

Dinner: have an oriental stir-fry with seafood, or tofu and veggies over rice, and miso or clear soup;
or bulgar, brown rice, or other whole grain pasta and vegetable casserole;
or baked, broiled or grilled poultry or seafood with a salad and whole grain bread;
or a dinner omelet or quiche, with a green leafy salad;
or a hearty vegetable soup or stew with rye or pumpernickel bread.
✓ **A little white wine with dinner is fine for better digestion, raising HDLs, and relaxation.**

Before bed: have a cup of VEGEX yeast extract broth, for B vitamins and relaxation;
or a glass of pineapple/coconut juice, or organic apple juice.
✓ **Drink 6 to 8 glasses of bottled water daily for a clean, hydrated, and well-regulated system.**

❊ Supplements and Herbs for the High Energy Diet

❖ Take a good B complex daily, 100 to 125mg.

❖ Take a green supplement daily; Sun CHLORELLA, Green Foods GREEN MAGMA, or Crystal Star ENERGY GREEN DRINK™.

❖ Take effective herbal energizers, such as Crystal Star ADRN-ALIVE™ CAPS OR EXTRACT **with** BODY REBUILDER™ CAPS, or IRON SOURCE™ CAPS OR EXTRACT, for **women;** and SYSTEM STRENGTH DRINK™, SUPER MAN'S ENERGY TONIC™, SIBERIAN GINSENG EXTRACT or GINSENG 6 SUPER CAPSULES™ for **men.** HIGH ENERGY TEA™ and FEEL GREAT™ CAPS and TEA are effective for **both** sexes.

❖ Take Bioforce GINSAVENA extract tablets for men; Floradix HERBAL IRON LIQUID for women.

❖ Take vitamin B$_{12}$ under the tongue or inter-nasally every other day.

❊ Bodywork for the High Energy Diet

✚ Get some early morning sunlight on the body every day possible.

✚ Take advantage of circulation stimulants regularly, such as a massage, oxygen/energy baths, or hot and cold hydrotherapy in the shower with skin brushing (page 205).

✚ Get regular daily aerobic exercise - a brisk walk after dinner, some swimming or dancing, or a quick series of exercises that you like. (See EXERCISE Chapter, page 202.)

❊ Sample Recipes That Work For The High Energy Diet
By section and recipe number:

SALADS HOT & COLD - 186, 190, 195, 196, 202, 204, 206, 211, 213, 217, 222, 225, 230, 231, 236, 238

BREAKFAST & BRUNCH - 73, 75, 76, 77, 81, 84, 89, 91, 98, 103, 107

SANDWICHES - SALADS IN BREAD - all

STIR-FRIES - all

FISH & SEAFOODS - all

HIGH MINERAL FOODS - all

HIGH PROTEIN COOKING WITHOUT MEAT - all

HIGH COMPLEX CARBOHYURATES FOR ENERGY - all

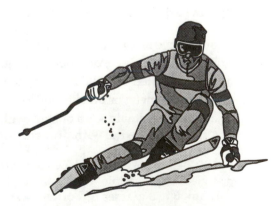

The Moderate Aerobic Diet:

This diet is for the naturally athletic person who works out regularly basis for fitness and muscle tone, but not for competition. It is low in fats, high in complex carbohydrates with moderate protein, and may be used successfully in conjunction with a weight control program.

On rising: take 1 teasp. molasses, 2 teasp. bee pollen granules, and 1 teasp. spirulina in apple, or pineapple juice;
or 1 TB. NutriTech All 1 vitamin/mineral drink mix in juice or water.

Breakfast: take a high protein drink, such as Nature's Plus SPIRUTEIN; **or** make a protein drink with soy protein powder, 1 egg, 2 teasp. brewer's yeast, 1 teasp. spirulina powder, 2 teasp. toasted wheat germ and 1 teasp. sesame seeds; **or** see the suggestions on pages 262 to 263 for good protein energy drinks;
then have some muesli or whole grain granola, such as coconut/almond granola, with yogurt and fresh fruit, apple juice or soy milk topping;
or hot oatmeal with maple syrup, **or** whole grain (buckwheat) pancakes with maple syrup;
or a poached egg on a whole grain English muffin, with a little butter and Bragg's LIQUID AMINOS;
Mid-morning: take a high potency enzyme/mineral drink such as Crystal Star SYSTEM STRENGTH DRINK™;
or Amazake rice drink;
or Crystal Star RAINFOREST ENERGY TEA™ with fresh fruit;
or miso soup with sea vegetables snipped on top;
or a green drink or vegetable juice (pg. 240) or Sun CHLORELLA or Green Foods GREEN MAGMA.

Lunch: have a baked potatao, with a little butter and 1 teasp. Bragg's LIQUID AMINOs;
and/or a spinach/endive or other dark green leafy salad;
or a vegetable frittata or low-fat vegetable pizza;
or a seafood salad, whole grain or veggie pasta salad (hot or cold), with whole grain muffins;
or a roast turkey sandwich on whole grain bread with greens and mayonnaise;
or tofu or steamed veggies with brown rice and tamari;
or some low-fat cheeses or cottage cheese with fresh fruit;
or a high protein salad or sandwich with avocados and sprouts.

Mid-afternoon: have some low-fat yogurt with nuts, seeds, or fresh fruit;
or a hard boiled or deviled egg with sesame salt for dipping, and a bottle of mineral water;
or a Crystal Star FEEL GREAT TEA™ with some whole grain crackers and a low-fat dip;
or some dried or fresh fruit with kefir cheese for dipping.

Dinner: have a low-fat Italian meal with whole grain or vegetable pasta, a soup and antipasto;
or bulgar, brown rice, or other whole grain pasta/vegetable casserole;
or baked, broiled or grilled fish or seafood with a salad and whole grain bread;
or a roast or baked poultry entree with brown rice or other whole grain, and a small salad;
or a dinner omelet or quiche, with a green leafy salad;
or a hearty vegetable soup or stew with rye or pumpernickel bread.
✓ **A little white wine with dinner is fine for better digestion, raising HDLs, and relaxation.**

Before bed: have a cup of VEGEX yeast extract broth, for B vitamins and relaxation;
or a glass of pineapple/coconut juice, or organic apple juice.

✓ **Drink 6 to 8 glasses of bottled water daily for a clean, hydrated, and well-regulated system.**

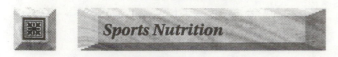

❊ *Supplements for the Moderate Aerobic Diet*

Clearly, vitamin, mineral, and enzyme deficiencies result in strength and energy loss. A fit, actively exercised body requires concentrations of these metabolic presursors for efficiency. During strenuous exercise, proteins and carbohydrates stored in muscle tissue are burned to produce energy. Initially, the body's own reserves are tapped and exhausted, and levels in the blood and tissues drop. Hormone and enzyme activity begins to wane, and fatigue and loss of endurance set in both mentally and physically. If vitamin and mineral depletion continues, normal cell function is disrupted, sometimes with irreversible damage. Supplements can readily overcome depletions, strengthen the body for a fit, athletic life style, and insure that your workout isn't defeating its purpose by burning off muscle tissue.

The following schedule contains effective products in each supplement area:

MINERALS: You need minerals to run - for bone density, speed and endurance; as anabolic enhancers
➡️Potassium/magnesium/bromelain - relieves muscle fatigue/lactic acid buildup.
➡️Cal/mag/zinc with boron - to prevent muscle cramping and maintain bone integrity.
➡️Chromium picolinate, 200mg. - for sugar regulation and glucose energy use.
➡️Zinc picolinate, 30-50mg. daily for athletes - for immunity, healing of epithelial injuries.
➡️MEZOTRACE - sea bottom mineral and trace mineral complex.
➡️Crystal Star MINERAL SPECTRUM™ EXTRACT and CAPSULES, IRON and CALCIUM SOURCE™ CAPSULES - for body building blocks, nutrient absorption, and bone density.

VITAMINS: Anti-stress factors for muscles, nerves and heart.
➡️B Complex, 100mg. or more - for nerve health, muscle cramping, carbohydrate metabolism.
➡️Vitamin C, 3000mg. daily w/bioflavonoids and rutin for connective tissue strength. Take about 5 minutes before exercise to help put the vitamin into resistant areas.
➡️Bioflavonoids - antioxidants to strengthen cell membranes and prevent swelling and bruising.
➡️Dibencozide - active co-enzyme of B_{12} for athlete's absorbability needs.
➡️Lewis Labs BREWER'S YEAST - chromium fortified, to simulate protein synthesis.

ANTIOXIDANTS: To increase oxygen use in blood, tissues and brain.
➡️Vitamin E, 400IU with Selenium - for circulatory health, and protection against free radicals.
➡️Co Q 10 - a catalyst co-emzyme factor to produce and release energy.
➡️B_{15}- DiMethylglycine - to boost oxygen delivery; see Muscle Masters SMILAX + DMG.
➡️Strength Systems ANTIOXIDANT COMPOUND and AMMONIA SCAVENGERS.
➡️Crystal Star ANTI-OXIDANT HERBS - phyto-antioxidants for long range resistance support.

GLANDULARS: Growth gland and hormone stimulation
➡️Pituitary, 200mg. - the master gland, for upper body development.
➡️Adrenal, 500mg.; see Country Life ADRENAL w/ TYROSINE - for adrenal and cortex support.
➡️Liver, 400mg. - for fat metabolism and detox. activity. Enzymatic Therapy LIQUID LIVER w/ SIBERIAN GINSENG for additional blood support. Country Life LIVER BOOSTER.
➡️Orchic - liquid extract best, approx 6 to 10x strength, or 1000mg. - for male testosterone support.
➡️Crystal Star ENDO-BAL™ and ADRN-ALIVE™ CAPSULES AND EXTRACT - phyto-glandulars for gland and hormone stimulation and growth.

TESTOSTERONE SUPPORT: part of a natural anabolic program for increased male performance
➡️Source Naturals YOHIMBE 1000mg. capsules, Strength Systems YOHIMBE extract 1000mg.
➡️Smilax, liquid - strength stamina and energy.
➡️Muira Pauma Bark (potency wood).
➡️Nature Health RAW TESTOSTEROL DROPS.

FREE FORM AMINO ACIDS: Hormone activators to increase body structure and strength.
➡️Arginine/Ornithine/Lysine, 750mg. - to help burn fats for energy, natural growth stimulant.
➡️Anabol Naturals GH RELEASERS and MUSCLE OCTANE, AMINO BALANCE.
➡️Carnitine, 500mg. - to strengthen heart and circulatory system during long exercise bouts.
➡️Inosine, 1000mg. - to reduce workout stress and kick in glycogen use for extra edge performance.
➡️Branched Chain Complex, BCAAs - for ATP energy conversion, endurance improvement.
➡️Strength Systems CHROMAX 1000 - for fat loss and energy (the serious athlete).
➡️Pre-digested amino acids - easily absorbed liquids for better performance, especially in women.
➡️Strength Systems WOMEN'S FITNESS PAKS - 22 day cycle and 8 day menstrual cycle.

ENZYMES: To process fuel nutrients for most efficient body use.
➡Pancreatin, 1400mg. - to metabolize fats, oils and carbohydrates correctly.
➡Bromelain/Papain, 500mg. - for muscle and ligament repair and strength.
➡Proteolytic Enzymes - break down scar tissue build-up and shortens recovery time after injury.

LIPIDS: Liver cleansers to metabolize fats and help form strong red blood cells.
➡Choline/Methionine/Inositol - a basic liver lipid.
➡Methionine/Lysine/Ornithine - with extra fat metabolizing agents.

FAT BURNERS: Metabolize blood and body fats, and enhance muscle growth
➡Strength Systems MCT (medium chain triglycerides); Bricker Labs EN-DURO.
➡Advanced Research FAT BURNERS with L-Carnitine.

PROTEIN/AMINO DRINKS: Mainstays for muscle building, weight gain, energy and endurance
➡Nature's Plus SPIRUTEIN - a maintenance drink with added body cleansers.
➡Natrol VEGETABLE PROTEIN POWDER - an energy drink for vegetarians.
➡Twin Lab AMINO FUEL - effective twice daily for endurance energy.
➡Twin Lab GAINERS FUEL 1000 - for maximum weight gain.
➡Nature's Life SUPER PRO 96.
➡Champion Nutrition 900 - low-fat weight gainer.

SPORTS BARS: Rich sources of various nutrients, especially carbohydrates, protein and fiber
➡Power Foods POWER BARS.
➡Strength Systems BULK UP BARS.
➡Nature's plus SPIRUTEIN ENERGY BARS.
➡Nature's Plus SOURCE OF LIFE ENERGY BARS.

SPORTSDRINKS/ELECTROLYTE REPLACEMENTS: USE After exertion to replace body minerals
➡Twin Lab ULTRA FUEL or Champion Nutrition CYTOMAX.
➡Alacer MIRACLE WATER .
➡Knudsens RECHARGE.
➡Twin Lab ULTRA FUEL.
➡Anabol Naturals CARBO SURGE.
➡Crystal Star GINSENG 6 DEFENSE RESTORATIVE SUPER TEA™, ENERGY GREEN™, and SYSTEM STRENGTH™ - rejuvenating drinks with natural source amino acids, proteins, chlorophyll, bioflavonoids, enzymes and vitamins.

RECOVERY ACCELERATION
➡Strength Systems FIRST AID CAPSULES - anti-inflammatory and muscle tissue repair.
➡Crystal Star BODY REBUILDER™ CAPSULES.

STIMULANTS: For quick, temporary, energy.
➡Excel slow release ginseng/ephedra formulas.
➡Siberian ginseng extract.
➡Crystal Star SUPERMAX™ and HIGH PERFORMANCE™ CAPSULES, HIGH ENERGY™ and RAINFOREST ENERGY™ TEAS and SUPERMAN'S ENERGY TONIC™ and GINSENG ACTIVE PHYSICAL ENERGY™ EXTRACTS; concentrated nutrients for extra endurance.

✻ *Bodywork for the Moderate Aerobic Diet*

✚ Besides your major sport or activity, supplement and strengthen it with auxiliary exercise such as dancing, bicycling, jogging, walking, swimming or aerobics; this balances muscle use and keep heart and lungs strong.

✚ Recuperation time is essential for optimum growth and strength. Muscles do not grow during exercise. They grow during rest periods. Alternate muscle workouts and training days with rest days, or exercise different muscle sets on different days, resting each set in between.

✚ Deep breathing is important. Muscles and tissues must have enough oxygen for endurance and stamina. Breathe in during exertion, out as you relax for the next rep.

✤ Take your pulse during a workout to determine if it is demanding enough to strengthen your heart, but not too demanding. Place the first two fingers on your carotid artery just below the jaw line. Use a watch or clock to count the **number of beats** for six seconds **while you are moving,** then add a zero to that number. This gives you heartbeats per minute. A heart rate between 70 and 85% of your age-range maximum is an ideal workout zone. Examples: 30 to 35 years - 133 to 157 beats per minute: 35 to 40 years - 130 to 153 beats per minute; 40 to 45 years - 126 to 149 beats per minute. **A resting heart rate for a fit adult is normally 65 to 80 beats per minute.**

❋ *Sample Recipes That Work For A Moderate Aerobic Diet*
By section and recipe number:

HEALTHY DRINKS, JUICES & WATERS - 45, 46, 49, 52, 53, 54, 57, 60, 69, 72

BREAKFAST & BRUNCH - 74, 76, 77, 82, 84, 87, 92, 94, 96, 97, 101, 102, 105, 108

SALADS HOT & COLD - 188, 192, 194, 198, 200, 203, 207, 210, 213, 216, 219, 220, 224, 226, 230, 235

LOW-FAT & VERY LOW-FAT RECIPES - all

SANDWICHES - SALADS IN BREAD - all

TOFU FOR YOU - all

FISH & SEAFOODS - all

HIGH MINERAL FOODS - all

HIGH COMPLEX CARBOHYDRATES FOR ENERGY - all

GREAT OUTDOOR EATING - 874, 875, 877, 879, 882, 890, 893, 888, 894, 896, 898, 904, 908, 909

❋ *Sample Menu Plans*
Some Recipe Combinations that Work for this Diet:

A FAMILY MEAL - 569, 654, 204, 612

AN EASY RISING BREAKFAST - 73, 84, 93, 79

A LIGHT SUMMER MEAL - 52, 186, 582

A HEARTY WINTER MEAL - 192, 607, 270, 658, 656

A WEEKEND PICNIC - 298, 580, 487, 53

AN EASY WEEKNIGHT DINNER - 743, 757, 200, 610

SUNDAY BRUNCH - 640, 905, 54, 660, 534, 475

A SPECIAL DINNER FOR TWO - 191, 241, 600, 630, 75, 291

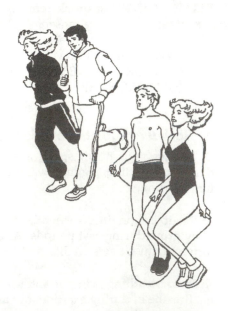

High Performance/Training Diet

This diet has concentrated nutrition for long range energy reserves. Athletics are about body/energy efficiency, so this diet is high in complex carbohydrates for maximum fuel use for muscles. It has plenty of amino acid precursors to enhance the body's own growth hormone production; it is vitamin and mineral rich for solid building blocks. The old watchword of great protein increase for performance has changed as athletes realize the undesirable effects overconsumption of protein can cause; particularly in excess uric acid and its burden on the kidneys and liver. Muscle mass is not increased by excess protein.

Some supplement guidelines are also given in this diet, since **how and when** *supplements are taken during training is as important as* **which** *ones are taken. Additional suggestions are listed in the supplement and herb section following the diet.*

On rising: take a nutrient, such as ALL 1 vitamin/mineral drink in pineapple/coconut juice;
or vanilla soy milk with 2 teasp. bee pollen and 1 teasp. barley green or spirulina granules;
or Crystal Star SYSTEM STRENGTH™ high mineral drink mix in water.
If this is a rest day, now is a good time to take the following nutritional supplementation:
❖ B complex 150mg.
❖ A high potency multi vitamin such as Weider MEGABOLIC PAK or Energen STRESS PAK.
❖ Ascorbate vitamin C 1 to 2000mg. with bioflavonoids and rutin; or ESTER-C with extra minerals and electrolytes.
❖ Bromelain 500mg. for muscle/ligament repair, **or** 2 bromelain/potassium/magnesium capsules.
❖ Methionine/lysine/ornithine capsules or milk thistle seed caps or extract for liver detox.
❖ An herbal mineral supplement, such as Mezotrace SEA MINERAL COMPLEX or Crystal Star MINERAL SPECTRUM EXTRACT.
See supplements section after this diet for additional suggestions.

Breakfast: take more liquid nutrition, in a high-powered protein drink, such as Twin Lab DIET FUEL or Strength Systems 100% EGG PROTEIN for off days, and Twin Lab AMINO FUEL or Strength Systems BULK UP OCTANE for workout days;
or make your own drink from soy protein powder, an egg, 2 teasp. brewer's yeast, 2 teasp. toasted wheat germ, 1 teasp. spirulina granules, and 1 teasp. sesame seed;
or see the suggestions on page 262 and 559 for for high protein energy drinks.
then, have some muesli or whole grain granola with yogurt and fresh fruit, or soy milk topping;
or hot oatmeal with maple syrup, or whole grain pancakes with maple syrup or honey;
or a poached egg on a whole grain English muffin, with a butter and Bragg's LIQUID AMINOS;
or a hot, whole grain breakfast pilaf such as KASHI;
or an omelet with veggie filling, or tofu "scrambled eggs" with vegetables.
If this is a training day, take amino acid, herbal or protein supplements now and/or 25 minutes before your workout:
❖ Chromium picolinate 250-500mcg.or Strength Systems CHROMAX 2 to increase muscle mass and reduce body fat.
❖ CoQ 10, 60mg., or DMG (Di-Methylglycine) to boost oxygen delivery.
❖ Smilax extract to increase muscle hardness, strength, and testosterone production.
❖ Herbal supplements for muscle tone, oxygen uptake, and glandular activity, such as Crystal Star SUPERMAX™, HIGH PERFORMANCE™ or MASTER BUILDER™ capsules; or Strength Systems WILD YAM for stamina and energy.
❖ An anabolic natural steroid, such as Weider ANABOLIC PAK, or Twin Lab AMINO FUEL.
❖ Carnitine 500mg. to help muscles use stored fat for energy.
❖ Inosine or BCAAs to increase endurance, and ATP build-up.

See supplements section after this diet for additional suggestions.

Mid-morning: have an Amazake rice drink;
or carrot juice with 1 teasp. Bragg's LIQUID AMINOS;
or Sun CHLORELLA or Crystal Star ENERGY GREEN™;
or a natural food concentrated energy bar, such as Power Foods POWER BARS, Hoffman'S ENERGY BARS, Bear Valley Pemmican bars, TIGER MILK BARS, or Excel ULTRA ENERGY bars and a bottle of mineral water;
or a dried fruit or nut snack mix;
or yogurt with fresh fruit or nuts;
or Alacer HIGH K COLA mineral drink.

Lunch: whole grain or veggie pasta; hot, with veggies and a light sauce, cold, with greens or seafood and a light dressing;
or an omelet or crepes filled with veggies or seafood;
or a high energy sandwich on whole grain bread, with turkey, cheese, avocado and sprouts;
or a baked potato with 1 teasp. butter and 1 teasp. Bragg's LIQUID AMINOS, and a green salad;
or a tofu, brown rice and veggie frittata/casserole;
or some low-fat cheeses or cottage cheese with fresh fruit and whole grain muffins or bread;
or a seafood, chicken or other high protein salad and whole grain bread.

Mid-afternoon: Amazake rice drink, or yogurt with fresh fruit;
or a bean dip, kefir cheese, soy cheese or low-fat cheese with whole grain crackers, or raw veggies;
or a hard boiled egg with sesame salt dip, some whole grain crackers, and an energizing herb tea, such as Crystal Star HIGH ENERGY TEA™ or RAINFOREST ENERGY TEA™, or Siberian ginseng tea;
or fruit juice sweetened cookies or granola bars;
or a high energy sports bar.

Dinner: Whole grain or veggie pasta Italian style with a light sauce and whole grain bread;
or a hearty soup or stew with a green salad and whole grain bread;
or a brown rice or other whole grain and vegetable casserole;
or whole grain and bean Mexican meal (easy on the salsas, fats and sweeteners; no fried food);
or baked, grilled or broiled poultry or seafood with a soup and green salad;
or a vegetarian pizza with chapati or flour tortilla crust, or an egg pizza with vegetable toppings;
or a vegetable quiche with whole grain crust.
✓ Have a little red or white wine with dinner for relaxation, minerals and polyphenols.

At bedtime: 1 teasp. VEGEX yeast extract paste in a cup of hot water for relaxation and B vitamins.
For both training and off days, this is a good time to take the following supplements:
❖ High potency calcium /magnesium capsules, 1000mg.
❖ Amino acid diet capsules, such as Source Naturals SUPER AMINO NIGHT DIET caps.
❖ Stress B Complex 100 to125mg.

✓ **Don't forget** the importance of juices and bottled water during the day. Good hydration is necessary for high performance, blood circulation, cardiovascular activity and overheating. A good electrolyte re-placement such as Alacer HIGH K COLA, or Knudsen RECHARGE is great after a workout, or anytime during the day.

❧ *Supplements for the training diet*

*Nutritional supplements are almost indispensable for the serious athlete because the body is under so much stress. They can improve overall strength, endurance and power, build muscle tissue and help to maintain low body fat. They assist recuperation time between workouts and speed healing from sports-related injury. **How** you take train- ing supplements is as important as **what** you take. A training program will be much more productive if supple- ments are balanced between workout days and rest days. Muscle growth occurs on the "off" days, as the body uses the exercise and augmentation you have been giving it. Supplements are a proven adjunct to fitness and muscle growth. In general, vitamins, minerals and glandulars work best taken on "off" days. Proteins, amino acids, anabol- ics, and herbs work best taken on your "on" days, before exercise or a workout.*

✷ Training days; before you work out:

❖ Ninety percent protein, muscle builder, or body shaper drinks, such as Twin Lab AMINO FUEL or DIET FUEL, or Strength Systems 100% EGG PROTEIN.

❖ Oxygenators, such as CoQ 10 60mg. or B_{15} (DMG).

❖ Free form amino acids that act as pro-proteins during a workout to increase performance - full spec- trum pre-digested or individual, such as argenine/ornithine/lysine to reduce and metabolize useless body fats, carnitine to strengthen muscle activity, and inosine to reduce the stress of a heavy workout, metabolize sugars and provide oxygen uptake.

❖ Natural anabolic steroids, such as Natural Health 100% NATURAL STEROIDS, or Weider ANA- BOLIC 2 PAK.

❖ Gamma Oryzonal (GO) - a pituitary stimulant for maximum weight gain.

❖ Enzymatic Therapy LIQUID LIVER w/SIBERIAN GINSENG.

❖ Branched chain amino acids (BCAAs) - for ATP energy conversion.

❖ Herbal supplements, such as Crystal Star GINSENG 6 SUPER ENERGY CAPS™;
        HIGH PERFORMANCE™ - for endurance and stamina;
        IRON SOURCE CAPS™ - highly absorbable, non-constipating.
        CALCIUM SOURCE EXTRACT™ - very absorbable, for bone strength esp. for women.

❖ Smilax extract - to increase muscle hardness, and testosterone.

❖ Bee pollen - a natural amino acid source.

❖ Siberian ginseng, Crystal Star GINSENG ACTIVE ENERGY EXTRACT™ and Biosource GINSAVENA for increased glandular activity.

☛ **In between workout sessions**, take natural power bars for an energy boost, such as Power Foods POWER BARS, Hoffman ENERGY BARS, or Excel ULTRA ENERGY bars.

☛ **After you work out**, take an electrolyte replacement to bring lost minerals and energy back faster: Knudsen RECHARGE drink, Alacer's HIGH K COLA, and/or Excel ANTI-FATIGUE tablet.

✷ Rest day supplements:

❖ ALL 1 vitamin/mineral drink, or other high potency multiple, such as Energen STRESS PAK.

❖ Raw glandulars - especially pituitary, adrenal, and liver.

❖ B Complex 100 to 150mg.

❖ Ascorbate vitamin C 2000 to 3000mg. with bioflavonoids and rutin, Crystal Star DAILY BIOFLAVO- NOID SUPPORT™ DRINK, or ESTER-C with minerals and electrolytes.

❖ Bromelain 500mg., or bromelain/magnesium/potassium.

❖ Crystal Star ADRN-ALIVE™ EXTRACT, GINSENG 6 MENTAL INNER ENERGY EXTRACT, GIN- SENG 6 DEFENSE RESTORATIVE SUPER TEA™.

❖ Lipids - choline/methionine/inositol to clean the liver, or Strength Systems FAT BURNERS.

❖ Mezotrace SEA MINERAL COMPLEX, 2-4 tablets, or Crystal Star MINERAL SPECTRUM EXTRACT.

The following products are natural steroids and anabolic precursers for the serious athlete, supplying far more than the usual level of supplementation. They are super-nutrients. The doses are not for regular maintenance.

❀ **Anabolics, Megabolics, Ultrabolics, Aminobolics,** etc., 4 to 6, or 1 to 2 packs daily - the mainstay of the dedicated athlete's program. They improve power, strength and endurance, build muscle tissue and help healing of damaged muscles.

❀ **Tyrosine/arginine/tryptophane/glycine/ornithine,** needed in multigram doses for desired effect, - to stimulate GH release.

❀ **Gamma Oryzonal (G0),** 500 to 1500mg. daily - a hypothalamus and pituitary stimulator to increase testerone secretion; primarily for maximum weight gain and calorie use, with a noticeable gain in muscle mass and reduction of body fat in 3-4 weeks.

❀ **Beta Sitosterol,** 2 to 4 daily - to keep blood fats and cholesterol low, and circulation clear.

❀ **Inosine,** 500 to 1500mg. daily - to increase endurance, energy and ATP build up, take 30 minutes before working out.

❀ **Dibencozide B12** - the most active form of B12 as a steroid alternative.

❀ **Chromium Picolinate,** 250-500mcg. daily - enhances muscle growth.

❀ **CoQ 10,** 60mg. daily - for enhanced flow of oxygen to the cells.

✱ *Herbs For A Winning Body*

*Herbs offer concentrated whole nutrients for muscle building, energy and endurance. They work best when taken on training days; in the morning with a good protein drink or 30 minutes before exertion. **The following products are effective for both serious training and casual exercise:***

✤ **Smilax** 1 to 2 times daily - an extract of sarsaparilla bark and root. Coaxes the body to produce greater amounts of the anabolic hormones, testosterone, cortisone, progesterone.

✤ **Siberian Ginseng extract** daily - clinically proven to increase stamina, endurance, gland activity, and lean muscle mass, with higher tolerance for stress.

✤ **Spirulina,** 1000mg. tabs daily - natural source amino acids, proteins and chlorophyll.

✤ **Bee Pollen and Royal Jelly,** 2 teasp. or capsules daily - a perfect concentrated food, with essential amino acids, proteins, enzyme stimulants and B Vitamins.

✤ **Crystal Star** GINSENG 6 ACTIVE PHYSICAL ENERGY™ - for stamina and endurance.

✱ *Bodywork Watchwords for Training & Competition*

✚ Besides your major sport or activity, supplement and strengthen it with other fitness activities such as, bicycling, jogging/walking, swimming or aerobics. This will balance muscle use and keep heart and lungs strong.

✚ Recuperation time is essential for optimum growth and strength. Muscles do not grow during exercise. They grow during rest periods. Alternate muscle workouts and training days with rest days, or exercise different muscle sets on different days, resting each set in between.

✚ Deep breathing and lung capacity are prime training factors. Muscles and tissues must have enough oxygen for endurance and stamina. Breathe in during exertion, out as you relax for the next rep. Vigorous exhaling is as important as inhaling for the athlete, to expel all carbon dioxide and increase lung capacity for oxygen.

❋ *Sample Recipes That Work For A Training Diet*
By section and recipe number:

HEALTHY DRINKS, JUICES & WATERS - 43, 55, 60, 66, 70, 71

BREAKFAST & BRUNCH - 78, 81, 83, 85, 90, 92, 99, 100, 102, 104, 106, 107

LOW-FAT & VERY LOW-FAT RECIPES - 240, 244, 245, 247, 249, 253, 259, 268, 270, 284, 293, 294, 300

SOUPS - LIQUID SALADS - all

SANDWICHES - SALADS IN BREAD - all

STIR-FRIES - all

HIGH MINERAL FOODS - all

HIGH COMPLEX CARBOHYDRATES FOR ENERGY - all

HIGH PROTEIN COOKING WITHOUT MEAT - all

FISH & SEAFOODS - all

GREAT OUTDOOR EATING - 875, 876, 878, 884, 886, 887, 889, 891, 892, 895, 897, 899, 900, 908, 909.

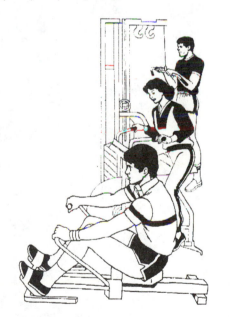

❋ *Sample Meal Planning*
Some recipe combinations that work for this diet:

A SPECIAL DINNER FOR TWO - 908, 613, 546, 758, 909, 296, 55

AN EASY RISING BREAKFAST - 70, 71, 96, 98, 85, 104

A HEARTY WINTER MEAL - 250, 745, 463, 652, 643, 661, 67

A LIGHT SUMMER MEAL - 549, 477, 299, 45

A WEEKEND PICNIC - 646, 898, 50, 621, 784

SUNDAY BRUNCH - 635, 653, 47, 662, 538

AN EASY WEEKNIGHT DINNER - 647, 782, 300, 779

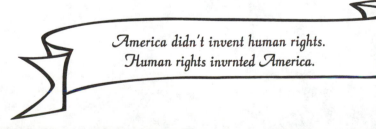

America didn't invent human rights.
Human rights invrnted America.

Dishonesty creates a failure force that manifests itself in many ways - often not apparent at the moment or to an outside observer. Cheating affects the life of the cheater far more than the person he cheats.

Sugar Imbalances; Diabetes & Hypoglycemia

The inability to properly process glucose, the body's number one energy source, affects millions of Americans today. Twenty five million of us suffer from diabetes (high blood sugar) or hypoglycemia (low blood sugar). While seeming to be opposite problems, these two conditions really stem from the same cause - an imbalance between glucose and oxygen in the system, putting the body under stress and leading to gland exhaustion. Poor nutrition is a common cause of both disorders, and both can be improved with a high mineral, high fiber diet, adequate usable protein, small frequent meals, and regular mild exercise.

✳ HYPOGLYCEMIA is one of the most widespread disorders in modern industrial nations today. It is a direct effect of our excess intake of refined sweets, low fiber foods, and other processed carbohydrates. The pancreas reacts to this overload by producing too much insulin to reduce the blood sugar, and hypoglycemia results. Typical hypoglycemic symptoms include extreme irritability, fatigue, manic/depressive states, hunger and great cravings, over-eating, restlessness and insomnia, and mental confusion. After many years of this type of diet and pancreatic reaction, the whole endocrine system, especially the adrenals, reacts to hyper-insulinism, sometimes causing hypoglycemia to become a precursor of diabetes. Many people, in fact, exhibit symptoms of both diseases during blood sugar curve tests.

✳ DIABETES is also a disease of the modern diet, in which people regularly eat too much sugar, refined carbohydrates and caffeine. When excess carbohydrates are not used correctly, blood sugar stays too high because too little balancing insulin is produced. The pancreas becomes exhausted, and glucose cannot enter the cells to provide body energy. Instead it accumulates in the blood, resulting in various symptoms from mental confusion to coma. Typical diabetic symptoms include excessive thirst and urination, failing vision, dry, itchy skin, poor circulation, lack of energy and kidney malfunction. Type 1, or juvenile onset diabetes is the more severe. Little or no insulin is produced, and insulin injections must be taken to sustain life. Type 2, or adult diabetes accounts for 90% of all cases. Pancreatic secretions which control the enzyme activity for digestion and food assimilation are inhibited, so obesity almost always results from diabetes. Enzymes relating to immune health also stem from the pancreas, so diabetics easily fall prey to other degenerative conditions as well.

☞☞ For people with these sugar imbalances there must be diet and lifestyle change for there to be a real cure. Alcohol, caffeine, refined sugars and tobacco must be avoided.

Recent clinical testing with crystalline fructose, and the herbs stevia rebaudana and gymnema sylvestre have produced some valid good news for sugar reaction disorders.

Crystalline fructose (a commercially produced sugar with the same molecular structure as that found in fruit), is low on the glycemic index, meaning that it releases glucose into the bloodstream slowly. It is metabolized by the liver and kidneys in a process that is not regulated by insulin supply; and thus produces liver glycogen rapidly making it a more   efficient energy supply than other sweeteners. It is almost twice as sweet as sugar, so that less is needed for the same sweetening power, especially in cold foods like desserts. In dental health studies, less dental plaque was reported with fructose than with sugar. It is reactive to heat, and lower cooking temperatures should be used.

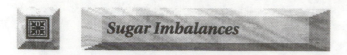
Stevia Rebaudana, also known as "sweet herb," is a South American sweetening leaf. It is totally non-caloric, and approximately 25 times sweeter than sugar when made as a concentrated infusion of 1 tsp. leaves to 1 cupful of water. Two drops equal 1 teaspoon of sugar in sweetness. In baking, 1 teaspoon of finely ground stevia powder is equal to 1 cup of sugar. Clinical studies indicate that stevia is safe to use even in cases of severe sugar imbalance.

Gymnema Sylvestre is an herb that blocks sugar assimilation into the bloodstream. Recent Japanese research indicates that gymnema can sharply reduce blood sugar levels following sugar consumption. Both gymnema and sugar are digested in the small intestine, and both have similar molecular structure, but that of gymnema is much larger, and cannot be fully absorbed. If taken before eating sugar, gymnema blocks the pathways through which sugar is normally absorbed, and fewer sugar calories are assimilated. The remaining sugar is eliminated as waste.

These substances may be seen as blood sugar balance heros, especially in the effort to control sugar intake and sugar cravings, but **they do not eliminate hypoglycemia or diabetes reactions.** Only diet improvement along with regular exercise can make a permanent difference.

The following diets for sugar balance are also effective for:
EPILEPSY HYPERACTIVITY DIABETIC RETINOPATHY MOOD and PERSONALITY SWINGS SCHIZOPHRENIA CATARACTS and GLAUCOMA DRUG or ALCOHOL ADDICTION and WITHDRAWAL ADRENAL EXHAUSTION MALE IMPOTENCE UNEXPLAINED WEIGHT GAIN GUM DISEASE and GINGIVITIS

Even though poor blood sugar metabolism is the cause of both diabetes and hypoglycemia, the different effects of each problem call for specific modifications. More rapid body response can be attained by approaching low blood sugar and high blood sugar diets separately.

Blood Sugar Balancing Diet For Diabetes Control

Diabetic proneness is often hereditary, and may be brought on by dietary habits that include too many sugary foods and refined carbohydrates. Pancreatic activity and other vital organs become damaged, the body loses the ability to produce enough insulin, and high blood sugar results. As less and less insulin is produced, these simple carbohydrates and sugars, which require a large secretion of insulin for metabolism, keep accumulating in the body and **are stored as fat.** The following diet, in addition to reducing insulin requirements and balancing sugar function in the bloodstream, has the nice "side effect" of healthy weight loss.

The key to this diet is in supplying slow-burning complex carbohydrate fuels to the body that do not need much insulin for metabolism. Meals are small, frequent, largely vegetarian, and low in fats of all kinds. Proteins come from soy foods and whole grains that are rich in lecithin and chromium. Fifty to 60% of the diet is in fresh and simply cooked vegetables for low calories and high digestibility.
All sugars, refined, fried and fatty foods are excluded.

On rising: take two lemons in a glass of water with 1 teasp. Spirulina or 2 teasp. Chlorella granules.

Breakfast: take a heaping teaspoon of Crystal Star CHOL-LO FIBER TONE' or other natural high fiber drink mix, in apple juice or water, to regulate and balance the sugar curve;
and/or make a mix of 2 TBS. **each:** brewer's yeast, wheat germ, lecithin granules and rice or oat bran. Sprinkle some daily on your choice of breakfast foods; ✦ poached egg on whole grain toast, ✦ muesli, whole grain or granola cereal with apple juice or vanilla soy milk, ✦ buckwheat or whole grain pancakes with apple juice or molasses; **or** simply mix into yogurt with fresh fruit.

Mid-morning: have a green drink such as Crystal Star ENERGY GREEN™ or Sun CHLORELLA;
and some whole grain crackers or muffins with a little soy spread or kefir cheese.
and a refreshing, sugar balancing herb tea, such as licorice, dandelion, or pau d' arco tea.

Lunch: have a green salad, with celery, sprouts, green pepper, marinated tofu, and mushroom soup;
or baked tofu or turkey with some steamed veggies and rice or cornbread;
or a baked potato with a little yogurt or kefir or soy cheese and some miso soup with sea vegetables;
or a whole grain sandwich, with avocado, low-fat or soy cheese and a low fat sandwich spread.

Mid-afternoon: have a glass of carrot juice;
and/or fruit juice sweetened cookies with a bottle of mineral water or herb tea;
or a hard boiled egg with sesame salt, or a veggie dip, and a bottle of mineral water.

Dinner: have a baked or broiled seafood dish with brown rice and peas;
or a Chinese stir-fry with rice, veggies and miso soup;
or a Spanish beans and rice dish with onions and peppers;
or a light northern Italian polenta with a hearty vegetable soup, or whole grain or veggie pasta salad;
or a mushroom quiche with whole grain crust and yogurt/wine sauce, and a small green salad.
✓A little white wine is fine at dinner for relaxation and surprisingly high chromium content.

Before bed: take another 1 TB. CHOL-LO FIBER TONE™ mix in apple juice;
and/or a VEGEX yeast broth (1 teasp. in water).

✓*Avoid caffeine and caffeine-containing foods, tobacco, hard liquor, food coloring and sodas. (Even "diet" sodas have phenylalanine in the form of Nutra-Sweet, and will affect blood sugar levels).*

✓*Avoid tobacco in any form. Nicotine increases sugar and sugary foods desire.*

✓*Sprinkle some brewer's yeast flakes on your salad, popcorn or soup for delicious, extra B vitamins.*

❋ *Supplements & Herbs for the Diabetes Control Diet:*
Never stop or reduce insulin without monitoring by your physician.

❖ To increase insulin tolerance and normalize pancreatic activity, take Alta Health CANGEST, Twin Lab LIQUID K, or Ester C 1000 to 2000mg. daily.

❖ To regulate and help utilize blood sugars and carbohydrate assimilation, take GTF chromium or chromium picolinate 200mcg., or Solaray CHROMIACIN and B Complex 100mg. daily

❖ To encourage adrenal activity, take pantothenic acid 500mg. **and** zinc 30mg. daily.

❖ To help keep arteries and circulatory system free of fats, take Omega-3 flax or fish oils 3x daily, **with** B12 sublingual or internasal gel, **and** carnitine 500mg.

❖ To help flatten sugar curve, take an Ayurvedic guggul capsule blend before meals.

❖ Take Crystal Star SUGAR STRATEGY D™ capsules as effective herbal therapy to help balance blood sugar use; and ADRN-ALIVE™ CAPS, or ADRN™ EXTRACT to stimulate exhausted adrenals.

❋ Bodywork for the Diabetes Control Diet

✚ Get regular daily exercise to increase metabolism and reduce need for insulin.

✚ Alternating hot and cold hydrotherapy will help stimulate circulation. Massage therapy has long been used to help regulate sugar use in the body.

❋ Sample Recipes for the Diabetes Control Diet
By section and recipe number:

BREAKFAST & BRUNCH - 74, 75, 76, 79, 81, 83, 86, 87, 92, 94, 96, 99, 103, 104, 106, 108

SALADS HOT & COLD - all

LOW-FAT & VERY-LOW FAT DISHES - all

SUGAR FREE SWEET TREATS - 414, 415, 416, 419, 420, 426, 428, 429, 431, 432, 433, 437, 439, 440, 441
These sugar free treats are for those who can allow some natural non-sugar sweetners in the system. If you cannot - delete these recipe numbers from your diet.

SANDWICHES - SALADS IN BREAD - 473, 482, 484, 483, 486, 489, 490, 494, 496, 498, 500

FISH & SEAFOOD - all

TOFU FOR YOU - 572, 574, 573, 578, 580, 585, 588, 589, 592, 594, 596, 575, 599, 601, 602, 606, 609, 610

HIGH COMPLEX CARBS - 743, 747, 751, 753, 756, 757, 758, 759, 761, 762, 763, 765, 766, 770, 773, 776

HIGH PROTEIN WITHOUT MEAT - 696, 697, 699, 701, 702, 704, 705, 711, 715, 716, 717, 720, 724, 729

HEALTHY FEASTING & ENTERTAINING - 826, 829, 835, 840, 844, 846, 848, 849, 850, 864, 865, 867

❋ Sample Meal Planning
Some recipe combinations that work with this diet:

AN EASY RISING BREAKFAST - 76, 74, 264, 97, 79

AN EASY WEEKNIGHT DINNER - 724, 213, 661

SUNDAY BRUNCH - 261, 242, 222, 267, 663, 699

A LIGHT SUMMER MEAL - 220, 263, 597, 300

A HEARTY WINTER MEAL - 705, 586, 742

A FAMILY MEAL - 602, 229, 294

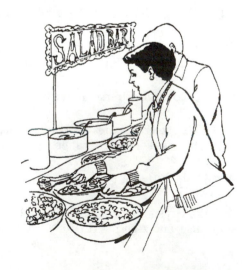

Blood Sugar Balancing Diet For Hypoglycemia:

The two key factors in hypoglycemia, low blood sugar, are stress and poor diet. Both are a result of too much sugar and refined carbohydrates. These foods quickly raise glucose levels, causing the pancreas to over-compensate and produce too much insulin, which then lowers body glucose levels too far and too fast. The following diet supplies the body with high fiber, complex carbohydrates and proteins - slow even-burning fuel, that prevents these sudden sugar elevations and drops. It consists of small frequent meals, with unrefined fresh foods to keep sugar levels more stable.

As with diabetes, sugars must be avoided. This includes natural sugars such as honey, molasses, maple syrup and hard alcohol until sugar balance is achieved. Full fat dairy foods, fried and oily foods, saturated fats, fast foods, pastries, and prepared meats should be sharply decreased. Refined foods, caffeine, preserved foods and red meats should be avoided on a permanent basis.

On rising: take a "hypoglycemia cocktail": 1 teasp. <u>each</u> in apple or orange juice to give energy and control morning sugar drop: glycine powder, powdered milk, protein powder, and brewer's yeast;
or a protein/amino drink, such as Nature's Plus SPIRUTEIN or Crystal Star SYSTEM STRENGTH DRINK™.

Breakfast: a very important meal for hypoglycemia; have some oatmeal with yogurt and fresh fruit;
or poached or baked eggs on whole grain toast with a little butter or kefir cheese;
or a whole grain cereal or granola with apple juice, soy milk or fruit yogurt and nuts;
or some whole grain pancakes with an apple or fruit sauce;
or some tofu scrambled "eggs" with bran muffins, whole grain toast and a little butter.

Mid-morning: have a green drink (page 240) or Sun CHLORELLA or Green Foods GREEN MAGMA with 1 teasp. Bragg's LIQUID AMINOS, or Crystal Star ENERGY GREEN DRINK™;
and/or a balancing herb tea, such as licorice, dandelion, or Crystal Star SUGAR STRATEGY LOW™ TEA;
and some crisp, crunchy vegetables with kefir or yogurt cheese;
or corn bread or whole grain crackers, or bran muffins with butter or kefir cheese.

Lunch: have a fresh salad, with a little cottage cheese or soy cheese, nut, noodle or seed toppings, and lemon/oil dressing;
and/or a high protein sandwich on whole grain bread, with avocados, low-fat cheese, and mayonnaise;
or a bean or lentil soup with a tofu or shrimp salad or sandwich;
or a seafood and whole grain pasta salad;
or a vegetarian pizza on a chapati crust with low-fat or soy mozarrella cheese.

Mid-afternoon: have a hard boiled egg with sesame salt, and whole grain crackers with yogurt dip;
and/or an herb tea, such as Crystal Star LICORICE MINTS, another green drink, or a small bottle of mineral water;
or yogurt with nuts and seeds.

Dinner: have some steamed veggies with tofu, or baked or broiled fish and brown rice;
or an oriental stir-fry with seafood and vegetables, and miso soup with sea vegetables;
or a whole grain or vegetable Italian pasta dish with a verde sauce and hearty soup;
or a Spanish beans and rice dish, or paella with seafood and rice;
or a veggie quiche on whole grain crust and a small mushroom and spinach salad;
or roast turkey with cornbread stuffing and a light soup.

Before bed: have a cup of VEGEX yeast paste broth;
or another cup of Crystal Star SYSTEM STRENGTH™ drink;
or papaya juice with a little yogurt.

❋ Supplements & Herbs for the Hypoglycemia Control Diet

❖ To support adrenal glands depleted by stress and hypoglycemic reactions, take vitamin C 3000 to 5000mg. daily, (or immediately during a sugar drop attack), and B complex 100mg. daily;
or Crystal Star ADRN-ALIVE™ caps or ADRN™ extract.
and/or add 2 teasp. daily of high potency royal jelly to a protein or green drink.

❖ To balance sugar use in the bloodstream, take GTF Chromiumor Chromium picolinate 200mcg. or Solaray CHROMIACIN daily, **with** DMG B15 sublingual.

❖ To improve carbohydrate digestion, take Alta Health CANGEST, guggul capsules with spirulina or bee pollen granules, morning and evening.

❖ To increase oxygen uptake and add minerals, take CoQ10 10-30 to 60mg. and Mezotrace SEA MINERAL COMPLEX daily.

❋ Bodywork for the Hypoglycemia Control Diet

✜ Get some aerobic exercise every day to work off unmetabolized acid wastes.

✜ Eat relaxed, never under stress.

✜ A massage therapy treatment once a month is especially beneficial for someone with hypoglycemia to help realign body meridians.

❋ Sample Recipes For the Hypoglycemia Control Diet
By section and recipe number:

BREAKFAST & BRUNCH - 73, 77, 81, 83, 85, 88, 89, 93, 97, 100, 102, 103, 104, 107

SALADS HOT & COLD - all

DAIRY FREE RECIPES - all

SANDWICHES - SALADS IN BREAD - all

SUGAR-FREE SPECIALS - 412, 417, 418, 423, 425, 427, 430, 434, 436, 443

HIGH MINERAL FOODS - all

HIGH PROTEIN COOKING WITHOUT MEAT - all

HIGH COMPLEX CARBOHYDRATES FOR ENERGY - all

HOLIDAY FEASTING & ENTERTAINING - 831, 832, 838, 841, 843, 846, 849, 852, 855, 865, 869, 871

✱ Sample Menu Plans
Some recipe combinations that work with this diet:

A FAMILY MEAL - 352,198, 487, 366

A HEARTY WINTER MEAL - 349, 204, 654, 374, 111

A LIGHT SUMMER MEAL - 195, 564, 712

A SPECIAL DINNER FOR TWO - 710, 323, 558, 735, 737, 372

AN EASY RISING BREAKFAST - 81, 73, 80, 96

AN EASY WEEKNIGHT DINNER - 350, 721, 568, 369

LUNCH FOR TWO - 479, 218, 373

The importance of correct diagnosis and treatment of sugar imbalances is essential. The following questionnaire is one we frequently give for self-determination in these cases, reprinted from the Enzymatic Therapy notebook. It can help you decide, in cooperation with a health care professional whether you need low blood sugar support, and whether professional help is needed. Read over the symptoms on this page, and mark them as follows if they pertain to you: (1) for mild symptoms, occuring once or twice a year; (2) for moderate symptoms, occuring several times a year; (3) for severe symptoms, occuring almost constantly.

A score of 6 from a combination of one's and two's indicates a need for support; a total of 3 or more of the threes indicates professional help is needed.

LOW BLOOD SUGAR TEST

( ) Poor concentration
( ) Digestive problems
( ) Blurred vision
( ) Forgetfulness
( ) Twitching/involuntary muscle jerks
( ) Constant worry and anxiety
( ) Lots of sighing and yawning
( ) Insomnia, the inability to return to sleep after awakening
( ) Nightmares
( ) Phobias, fears
( ) Mental confusion, spaciness
( ) Suicidal intent
( ) Nervous breakdown

( ) Frequent headaches
( ) Nervousness
( ) Heart palpitations
( ) Irritability and crying spells
( ) Craving for sweets
( ) Exhaustion
( ) Convulsions, trembling
( ) Faintness , dizziness
( ) Rapid pulse
( ) Cold sweats, shaking
( ) Antisocial behavior
( ) Weak spells
( ) Indecisiveness
( ) Unexplained depression

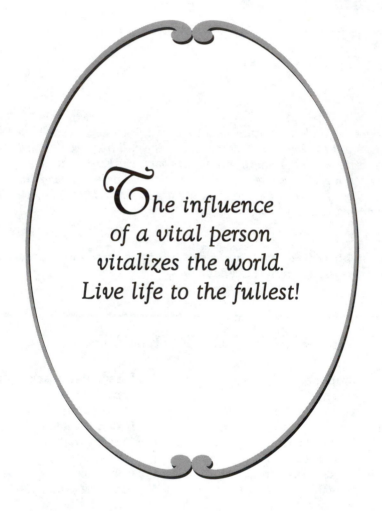

The influence
of a vital person
vitalizes the world.
Live life to the fullest!

Waste Management
Colon, Bowel & Bladder Problems

Much pain and disease that we endure extends from deficient drainage. One of the greatest factors in acquiring health is removing toxic waste from the system. It starts with back-up and fermentation in the colon, like a walking pressure cooker, and ends with the body actually re-absorbing unreleased waste material, which settles in weak cells unable to "clean house." Continuing accumulation of this acid, poisonous build-up results in disease.

The following problems are extensions of poor waste elimination and consequent weakened organs and tissue. The diets in this section can greatly improve these conditions. CHRONIC CONSTIPATION or DIARRHEA IRRITABLE BOWEL SYNDROME COLITIS and SPASTIC COLON CROHN'S DISEASE DIVERTICULITIS GAS and BLOATING FLATULENCE HEMORRHOIDS LOW ENERGY and IMMUNE RESPONSE CYSTITIS BLADDER and PROSTATE INFECTIONS VARICOSE VEINS BLADDER INCONTINENCE KIDNEY MALFUNCTION BAD BREATH and BODY ODOR INTESTINAL PARASITES

A fiber rich diet is a key to treating and preventing most of these problems. Daily vegetable fiber insures a fully active elimination system, digestive regulation, cholesterol and blood sugar balance. A gentle, gradual change from a low fiber, low residue diet will help almost immediately, and is often better than a drastic program in relieving pain and inflammation in the colon and bladder. A complete change, over several months, to unrefined whole foods with all their nutrients intact, is much better for therapeutic results than continuing with refined foods, and just adding a fiber supplement or a few fiber foods to the diet.

The protective level of fiber in your diet can be easily measured. The following GOOD PROTECTION TEST can help you monitor your support-system health on a regular basis. Essentially it is a dietary fiber check; enough soluble fiber in the diet to make the stool float is the protective level against poor waste elimination diseases.
* Bowel movements should be regular daily, and almost effortless.
* The stool should be almost oderless (signalling increased transit time in the bowel with no fermentetion) .
* There should be very little gas or flatulence.
* The stool should float rather than sink.

While improvement of waste elimination problems can be felt fairly quickly after diet improvement, it takes from 3 to 6 months to rebuild the bowel and colon to adequate tone and elasticity with good systol/diastol action. A good herbal colon health formula can help in this effort in terms of support and normalization. There is no instant, easy route, but the rewards of a regular, healthy, energetic life are worth it.

If you use over-the-counter antacids or take frequent rounds of anti-biotics, remember that they may do more harm than good. They neutralize stomach HCl needed for digestion and food assimilation, and inhibit production of friendly digestive bacteria. In addition, the continual use of laxatives to correct poor elimination can irritate bowel membranes, and in the end, almost bring normal systol/diastol activity to a halt preventing the body from working on its own. A whole foods, high vegetable fiber diet is both prevention and cure.

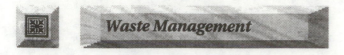

Colon & Bowel Health

It has been estimated that 95% of all disease is linked to constipation and colon toxicity. Elements causing this toxicity come from three basic areas:

1) **non-food chemicals in our food and pollutants in the environment, ranging from relatively harmless to very dangerous.** A clean, strong system can metabolize and excrete many of these, but when the body is weak or constipated, they are stored as unusable substances. As more and different chemicals enter the body they tend to interreact with those that are already there, forming mutant, second generation chemicals far more harmful than the originals. Evidence in recent years has shown that most bowel cancer is caused by environmental agents taken in through diet and air pollution.

2) **over-accumulated body wastes and metabolic by-products that are not excreted properly.** These wastes can also become a breeding ground for parasite infestation. A new nationwide survey has revealed that **one in every six people studied** had one or more parasites living somewhere in the body.

3) **slowed elimination time**, allowing waste materials to ferment, become rancid, and then recirculate through the body as toxic substances.

These and other factors, result in sluggish organ and glandular functions, poor digestion and assimilation, lowered immunity, faulty circulation, and tissue degeneration.

The body can tolerate a certain level of contamination. But when that individual level is passed, and immune defenses are low, toxic overload causes illness.

The key to avoiding bowel and bladder problems is usually nutritional. Fortunately, correcting the diseases they cause can also be brought about through diet improvement.

The following program includes a short liquid fast **with specifics for both bowel and bladder areas**, a rebuilding and tissue restoration phase, and a maintenance diet, so that problems don't return and the solution becomes long term.

Stage One; Colon & Bowel Elimination/Cleansing Diet: 3 to 5 Days

On rising: take a glass of aloe vera juice with herbs, or Sonne's LIQUID BENTONITE, with 2 teasp. acidophilus liquid added;.
or Crystal Star CHOL-LO FIBER TONE™ drink mix, 1 heaping teasp. in water or apple juice.

Breakfast: take a glass of apple, papaya, grape or prune juice;
or a potassium broth or juice, with 1 teasp. spirulina added.

Mid-morning: have a green drink (page 240), or Sun CHLORELLA, or Green Foods GREEN MAGMA, or Crystal Star ENERGY GREEN DRINK™;
and/or a cup of comfrey/mint leaf or alfalfa/mint tea.

Lunch: have a glass of fresh carrot juice.

Mid-afternoon: have a cup of peppermint, or spearmint tea, or Crystal Star LICORICE MINTS TEA.

Dinner: have another potassium broth, or Crystal Star SYSTEM STRENGTH DRINK™;
or carrot juice or apple juice.

Before bed: take another aloe vera and herbs juice;
or CHOL-LO FIBER TONE™ drink or capsules;
or papaya or apple juice.

✓ Drink plenty of bottled water throughout the day to flush released wastes.

✱ *Supplements for the Bowel/Colon Cleansing Diet*

Any supplementation taken during this cleanse should be liquid in form for better absorbancy.

❖ Take ascorbate vitamin C crystals with bioflavonoids throughout each day of the cleanse, dissolved in any juice or bottled water, 5 to 7000mg. daily.

❖ Take high omega-3 flax oil; add 1 teasp. to any juice or water, 3x daily.

❖ Take an acidophilus complex, such as Natren LIFE START II, 1/4 teasp. in water 3 or 4x daily, <u>with</u> 1 teasp. of Twin Lab LIQUID B COMPLEX added. (This suggestion is advisable if you are taking antibiotics or antacids. These substances kill the friendly bacteria in the digestive tract, and aggravate elimination problems).

✱ *Bodywork for the Colon/BowelCleansing Diet*

✚ Take a gentle catnip or chlorophyll enema at the start of this liquid diet if desired, to clear the way for better detoxification.

✚ Take a brisk walk daily to encourage free-flowing elimination.

✚ Get early morning sunlight on the body every day possible for purifying vitamin A and vitamin D.

✚ Apply warm ginger compresses to lower spine and stomach to stimulate systol/diastol activity.

Stage Two; Tissue Rebuilding Diet For The Colon; 1 to 2 months

The second part of a good program is rebuilding healthy tissue and body energy. This stage can usually begin after the cleansing diet above, and should be used for 1 - 2 months for best results. It emphasizes high fiber through fresh vegetables and fruits, cultured foods for increased assimilation and enzyme production, and alkalizing foods to prevent irritation while healing. Avoid refined foods, saturated fats or oils, fried foods, meats, caffeine or other acid or mucous forming foods,(such as pasteurized dairy products,) during this diet stage.

On rising: take a glass of aloe vera juice with herbs;
<u>or</u> Sonne's LIQUID BENTONITE, with 1 teasp. liquid acidophilus added;
<u>or</u> Crystal Star CHO-LO FIBER TONE™ capsules, or drink mix in apple or orange juice.

Breakfast: Soak a mix of dried prunes, figs and raisins the night before; take 2 to 4 TBS. with 1 TB. blackstrap molasses, <u>or</u> mix with yogurt;
<u>or</u> make a mix of oat bran, raisins, and pumpkin seeds, and mix with yogurt or apple juice, or a light vegie broth. Add 2 teasp. brewer's yeast or Lewis Labs FIBER YEAST;
<u>and</u> have some oatmeal or a whole grain cereal, granola or muesli with yogurt or apple juice;
<u>or</u> have a bowl of mixed fresh fruits with apple juice or yogurt.

Mid-morning: take a green drink (page 240), Sun CHLORELLA, Green Foods GREEN ESSENCE, or Crystal Star ENERGY GREEN DRINK™;
<u>or</u> pau d' arco or comfrey/mint tea to alkalize the system.
<u>or</u> a fresh carrot juice;

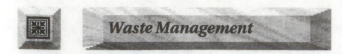

Lunch: have a fresh green salad every day with lemon/oil dressing, or yogurt cheese or kefir cheese;
or steamed veggies and a baked potato with soy or kefir cheese;
or a fresh fruit salad with a little yogurt or raw cottage cheese topping.

Mid-afternoon: have another fresh carrot juice, or Crystal Star SYSTEM STRENGTH DRINK™;
and/or mint tea or slippery elm tea, or Crystal Star LICORICE MINTS or RELAX™ TEA;
and/or some raw crunchy veggies with a vegetable or kefir cheese dip, or soy spread.

Dinner: have a large dinner salad with black bean or lentil soup;
or an oriental stir-fry and miso soup with sea vegetables snipped on top;
or a steamed or baked vegetable casserole with a yogurt or soy cheese sauce;
or a vegetable or whole grain pasta with a light lemon or yogurt sauce.

Before bed: have some apple or papaya juice;
or another glass of aloe vera juice with herbs;
or Crystal Star CHOL-LO FIBER TONE™ drink or capsules or a cup of hot ginger tea.

❋ *Supplements and Herbs for the Bowel/Colon Rebuilding Diet*

❖ Take a good food source multiple vitamin to control initial gas and stomach rumbling as the additional fiber combines with the minerals in the G.I. tract.

❖ Take vitamin C ascorbate in crystals or capsules with bioflavonoids 3 to 5000mg daily; or Crystal Star DAILY BIOFLAVONOID SUPPORT DRINK™.

❖ Take Crystal Star IBS BWL-TONE™, or Enzymatic Therapy IBS formula if there is bowel irritation.

❋ *Bodywork for the Bowel/Colon Rebuilding Diet*

✚ Be sure all food is well chewed. Eat smaller meals more frequently rather than large meals to allow the body to process easily during healing.

✚ Continue with early morning sunlight on the body, and a brisk aerobic walk every day.

❋ *Sample Recipes For The Colon & Bowel Rebuilding Diet*
By section and recipe number:

HEALTHY DRINKS, JUICES & WATERS - 47, 61, 62, 66, 69, 71

BREAKFAST & BRUNCH - 75, 76, 77, 82, 85, 93, 94, 97, 102, 104

SALADS - HOT & COLD - all

HIGH FIBER RECIPES - all

HIGH MINERAL FOODS - 612, 613, 615, 616, 623, 626, 627, 628, 641, 647, 648, 652, 656, 657

✻ *Sample Meal Planning*
Some recipe combinations that work with this diet:

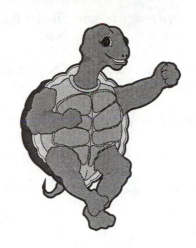

LUNCH FOR TWO - 234, 818, 824, 53

AN EASY RISING BREAKFAST - 94, 73, 76, 97, 77

AN EASY WEEKNIGHT DINNER - 809, 235, 789, 52

A LIGHT SUMMER MEAL - 238, 623, 617, 62

A HEARTY WINTER MEAL - 231, 49

A FAMILY MEAL - 228, 735, 798

Stage 1; Bladder/Kidney Elimination and Cleansing Diet; 3 to 5 days

On rising: take a glass of lemon juice and water, with 1 teasp. acidophilus liquid;
or 3 teasp. cranberry concentrate in a small glass of water with $1/4$ to $1/2$ teasp. ascorbate C crystals;
or 2 TBS. cider vinegar in a glass of water with 1teasp. honey.

Breakfast: have a glass of watermelon juice, or another glass of cranberry juice with 1/4 teasp. vitamin C crystals;
and/or a glass of organic apple juice with $1/4$ teasp. high potency acidophilus complex powder.

Mid-morning: take a cup of watermelon seed tea. (Grind seeds, steep in hot water 30 minutes, add 1 teasp. honey);
or a potassium broth or essence (page 240), with 2 teasp.Bragg's LIQUID AMINOS;
or a cup of Crystal Star BLDR-K FLUSH™ TEA.

Lunch: have a green drink (see pages 240-2), or Sun CHLORELLA, or Green Foods BARLEY GREEN MAGMA granules in water;
or a glass of carrot juice, or carrot/celery juice;
or carrot/beet/cucumber juice, every other day.

Mid-afternoon: take a cup of healing herb tea, such as parsley/oatstraw, plantain tea, or cornsilk tea;
or Crystal Star BLDR-K FLUSH™ TEA;
or another cup of watermelon seed tea.

Dinner: have another carrot juice, with some 1 teasp. liquid chlorophyll or spirulina added;
or another cranberry juice with $1/4$ teasp. ascorbate vitamin C crystals added.

Before Bed: take another glass of cider vinegar in water and honey;
and/or a glass of papaya or apple juice with $1/4$ teasp. high potency acidophilus complex powder.

✓ Be sure to drink 6 to 8 glasses of bottled water every day to flush toxins and release acid wastes.

✓ Avoid caffeine, soft drinks, salt, pasteurized dairy products, and citrus juices during this fast.

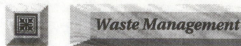

✤ *Supplements and Herbs for the Bladder/Kidney Cleansing Diet*
As with the colon cleansing fast, liquid supplementation is best during a cleanse.

❖ Take liquid chlorophyll or a liquid green supplement, such as Green Foods GREEN MAGMA, or Sun CHLORELLA.

❖ Take ¹/₄ teasp. ascorbate C crystals in juice or water 4 to 6x daily.

❖ Take a milk-free acidophilus complex, such as DDS or DOCTOR DOPHILUS, 3x daily.

❖ Take a cleansing herb tea, such as oatstraw, cornsilk, or Crystal Star BLDR-K FLUSH™ TEA.

✤ *Bodywork aids for the Bladder/Kidney Cleansing Diet*

✤ Apply hot wet compresses to the kidney area - use comfrey leaf or Epsom salts.

✤ Take alternating hot and cold sitz baths.

Stage Two; Bladder/Kidney Alkalizing/Rebuilding Diet: 2 to 3 months
This diet stage may be used for 2 to 3 months or longer for chronic problems. It emphasizes raw fresh and cultured foods to alkalize the system. It is very low in proteins, starches and carbohydrates, allowing the body to spend more energy on healing than on dealing with heavier foods. Avoid acid-forming foods, such as caffeine and caffeine-containing foods, salty, sugary and fried foods, soft drinks, alcohol, and tomatoes. Also avoid mucous-forming foods, such as pasteurized dairy products, heavy grains, starches and fats during this diet to relieve irritation and sediment formation.

✓ Drink 6 to 8 glasses of bottled water throughout the day for continued flushing of acid wastes.

On rising: take a glass of lemon juice in water with a little honey;
or 2 TBS. cranberry juice concentrate in water with ¹/₄ teasp. ascorbate vitamin C crystals added;
or take 2 TBS. apple cider vinegar in water with 1 teasp. honey.

Breakfast: have a glass of papaya or apple juice;
or a glass of fresh watermelon juice;
then some fresh tropical fruits, such as papaya, mango, or banana.

Mid-morning: have a green drink such as Sun CHLORELLA or Green Foods GREEN MAGMA, or Crystal Star ENERGY GREEN™;
or a glass of apple juice;
or dandelion or parsley tea.

Lunch: have a green salad with lots of cucumbers, spinach, watercress and celery, with lemon/oil or cottage cheese dressing;
and/or baked or marinated tofu with sesame seeds and wheat germ;
or a Chinese vegetable salad with bok choy, daikon, pea pods, bean sprouts and other Chinese greens, with a cup of miso or ramen noodle soup with sea veggies.

Mid-afternoon: have a cup of alkalizing, sediment-dissolving herb tea, such as chamomile, oatstraw or Crystal Star BLDR-K FLUSH™ tea;
or some celery and carrot sticks with kefir or yogurt cheese;
or fresh apples and pears with kefir or yogurt dip.

Dinner: have some brown rice with tofu and steamed veggies;
or steamed asparagus with miso soup and sea veggies;
or a baked potato with kefir cheese or 1 teasp. butter, and a spinach salad;
or baked or broiled salmon with millet and baked onions.
✓ A glass of white wine is fine at dinner for alkalizing and relaxation.

Before bed: have another apple or papaya/mango juice;
or miso soup with sea vegetables snipped on top;
or VEGEX yeast broth in hot water.

✓ For kidney stones, see OLIVE OIL FLUSHES under the Liver Cleansing Liquid Diet in this book.

✓ Avoid all yeast-containing foods during this diet, with no baked breads.

✱ *Supplements and Herbs for the Bladder/Kidney Rebuilding Diet*

❖ Continue with 3 to 5000mg. ascorbate vitamin C daily in juice or water (about $1/2$ teasp. every 4 hours, **and** beta carotene, or emulsified A 25,000IU 4x daily).

❖ Take alkalizing/soothing teas, such as corn silk, plantain or dandelion leaf.

❖ Take Chlorophyll liquid, or other concentrated green food supplement, such as Green Foods GREEN MAGMA, or Crystal Star ENERGY GREEN™ in water before meals.

❖ Take Enzymatic Therapy ACID-A-CAL caps to dissolve sedimentary waste, with bromelain 500mg. daily.

❖ Use Crystal Star ANTI-BIO™ CAPS or EXTRACT **with** BLDR-K™ CAPS and BLDR-K FLUSH™ TEA as needed for inflammation or irritation.

❖ Take 3 teasp. high Omega-3 flax oil in your juice or water, with Vitamin B$_6$ 250mg. 2x daily.

❖ Take DDS milk-free acidophilus powder in juice or water, as needed 2 to 3 times daily, **with** garlic oil caps 6 daily.

✱ *Bodywork for the Bladder/Kidney Rebuilding Diet*

✚ Continue with wet, hot compresses and lower back massage when there is inflammation flare up.

✚ Take hot saunas when possible to release toxins and excess fluids, and to flush acids out through the skin. A swim after a sauna is wonderful for body tone.

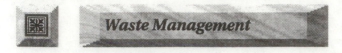

✽ *Sample Recipes for the Alkalizing/Rebuilding Diet*
By section and recipe number:

HEALTHY DRINKS, JUICES & WATERS - 46, 49, 52, 57, 62, 65

SALADS HOT & COLD - 186, 188, 189, 193, 198, 199, 201, 202, 204, 206, 209, 212, 217, 220, 233, 237

LOW-FAT & VERY LOW-FAT DISHES - all

LOW CHOLESTEROL MEALS - 302, 304, 305, 306, 307, 310, 316, 321, 322, 323, 324, 325, 326, 329, 331

DAIRY FREE COOKING - 333, 334, 336, 337, 338, 340, 342, 343, 348, 351, 352, 355, 358, 361, 329, 331

SOUPS - LIQUID SALADS - 446, 445, 447, 448, 449, 450, 451, 553, 556, 558, 564, 567

FISH & SEAFOODS - 534, 541, 542, 547, 548, 549, 550, 551, 552, 553, 556, 558, 564, 567

HIGH MINERAL FOODS - 612, 613, 617, 620, 621, 622, 624, 629, 630, 634, 640, 654, 655

HIGH FIBER RECIPES - 789, 790, 791, 794, 796, 799, 802, 807, 808, 809, 810, 812, 813, 817, 818, 819, 823

✖

Stage Three; Prevention/Maintenance Diet for Elimination Problems
*Lifelong prevention of bowel and bladder problems requires long term diet and life-style change. Modifying old patterns and habits can take a many months, and it isn't easy. But it **is** worth the trouble. A healthy elimination system can solve many other problem conditions. The good foundation established during the months of cleansing and rebuilding will lay solid building blocks for regularity, alkalinity and body energy. A comitted program for 3 to 6 months usually results in definite improvement and good waste management.*

The continuing diet should be low in salty, sugary foods, cholesterol, meats and pasteurized dairy products, and high in green foods, cultured foods and vegetable proteins. Avoid caffeine and caffeine-containing foods, fried foods, red meats, and refined carbohydrates such as white flour and sugar entirely.

On rising: take a vitamin/mineral drink, such as NutriTech ALL 1, or Nature's Plus SPIRUTEIN, in apple or orange juice.

Breakfast: have some tropical fruits (for high potassium);
and/or make a mix of dried prunes, figs and raisins, with toasted wheat germ, oat or bran flakes, and sesame or pumpkin seeds. Top this mix with a little honey, molasses, yogurt or apple juice;
or have some oatmeal with maple syrup; add some nuts and seeds or dried fruits;
or muesli or granola with yogurt or apple juice. Top either of these with 2 teasp. brewer's yeast.

Mid-morning: have a green drink such as Sun CHLORELLA or Barley Green;
or apple juice, or apple/alfalfa sprout/parsley juice;
or a tea for energy and body balance, such as Siberian ginseng, or Crystal Star FEEL GREAT™ TEA.

Lunch: have a salad with cottage cheese, a light soup and corn bread;
or a black bean or lentil soup with a high protein whole grain sandwich;
or a Mexican bean and rice meal with mild salsa and chilled gazpacho;
or an oriental stir-fry with miso soup and sea veggies;
or a baked potato with kefir or soy cheese.

Mid-afternoon: have some fresh fruits with a little cottage cheese, or kefir or yogurt cheese; **and/or** a refreshing herb tea, such as peppermint or rose hips, or Siberian ginseng tea; **or** some raw crunchy veggies with whole grain crackers and a veggie or soy spread dip.

Dinner: have a light Italian vegetable pasta meal with a spinach and mushroom sandwich; **or** baked or broiled salmon, or salmon souffle, with a yogurt/wine sauce, and brown rice and peas; **or** a light seafood dish with steamed or broiled vegetables and brown rice or millet; **or** an asparagus or artichoke quiche with a whole grain crust, and a light watercress or leek soup; **or** a vegetable-filled omelet with a light sauce and whole grain muffins .

✓ Have a little **white** wine (not red; too much high acid tannin for easy elimination) if desired for relaxation and easier digestion.

Before bed: have a glass of apple or papaya juice; **or** a relaxing herb tea, such as chamomile or mint, with lemon and honey.

✱ *Supplements and Herbs for the Prevention & Maintenance Diet*

❖ Continue with ascorbate vitamin C, or Ester C with bioflavonoids, and beta carotene at maintenance levels; about 1 to 2000mg vitamin C, and 25 to 5000IU beta carotene.

❖ Take non-dairy acidophilus or betaine HCl with meals for better digestion and food absorbancy.

❖ Take a green supplement every day, such as Sun CHLORELLA, Green Foods BARLEY GREEN MAG-MA, liquid chlorophyll, or Crystal Star ENERGY GREEN DRINK™.

❖ Take an herbal mineral supplement such as Crystal Star MEGA-MINERAL CAPS, or natural source minerals, such as Mezotrace SEA MINERAL COMPLEX.

✱ *Bodywork Aids for the Prevention & Maintenance Diet*

✚ Continue with a daily walk, and morning and evening stretching exercises to keep the system free and flowing.

✱ *Sample Recipes for the Prevention/Maintenance Diet* *By section and recipe number:*

BREAKFAST & BRUNCH - 76, 78, 81, 84, 87, 91, 92, 98, 104, 107

SANDWICHES - SALAD IN BREAD - 473, 477, 478, 481, 483, 488, 489, 491, 493, 495, 498, 500

SUGAR FREE SWEET TREATS - 413, 415, 416, 420, 423, 426, 430, 431, 433, 436, 438, 440, 439, 441, 443

FISH & SEAFOODS - 532, 537, 543, 544, 547, 552, 555, 560, 563, 569

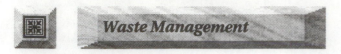
HIGH MINERAL FOODS - all

COMPLEX CARBOHYDRATES FOR ENERGY - 744, 745, 752, 756, 760, 761, 764, 767, 768, 770, 775

HIGH FIBER RECIPES - all

STIR FRIES - ORIENTAL STEAM BRAISING - all

GREAT OUTDOOR EATING - 874, 878, 879, 880, 881, 882, 883, 888, 890, 893, 894, 895, 896, 901, 908

FEASTING & ENTERTAINING - 826, 835, 838, 840, 842, 843, 844, 849, 850, 852, 853, 854, 855, 856, 865

✻ *Sample Meal Planning*
Some recipe combinations that go with the maintenance diet:

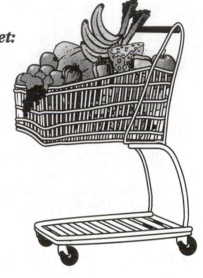

LUNCH FOR TWO - 638, 739, 663

A SPECIAL DINNER FOR TWO - 653, 630, 77, 614, 660

AN EASY RISING BREAKFAST - 81, 96, 78, 98, 74, 75

AN EASY WEEKNIGHT DINNER - 745, 755, 620, 658

A HEARTY WINTER MEAL - 800, 785, 624, 823

A LIGHT SUMMER MEAL - 788, 879, 905, 907

A WEEKEND PICNIC - 875, 893, 908, 208

SUNDAY BRUNCH - 191, 217, 808, 781, 662

HOLIDAY FEASTING - 754, 799, 806, 643, 659, 237

A FAMILY MEAL - 801, 735, 628, 652

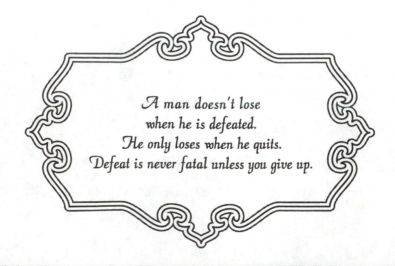

*A man doesn't lose
when he is defeated.
He only loses when he quits.
Defeat is never fatal unless you give up.*

Weight Control & Body Fat Management

Weight control today is a strategy of lifestyle. It's an attitude of eating for weight control. We used to think of a "diet" as a temporary period that we undertook until we reached a desired weight; then we reverted back to "regular" eating. But the average diet today is so nutritionally poor and so loaded with fats, sugars and refined foods that returning to these foods puts the weight right back on again.

As fried, fatty and refined foods have increased in our diets and physical labor has decreased, there has been a 500 to 800% increase in obesity in the 20th century. Most people are appearance motivated to weight loss, looking for the "miracle magic bullet" to slimness, but everyone is realizing that a good nutrition diet has to be front and center for permanent results. All signs anticipate that weight loss in the future will be a component of a sound nutritious eating plan, rather than a try at the latest fad. Many people are now also motivated for health reasons to lose weight. They are concerned about their blood pressure, cholesterol, heart problems and diabetes, and want to change their diets to insure better health.

There may be several reasons you aren't achieving your desired weight. The following conditions encourage the body to store food as fat instead of using it as fuel and energy: sluggish thyroid; lazy metabolism; glandular malfunction causing a pear-shaped figure; overeating; cellulite; habit hunger; stress eating; bloating excess fluid retention; constipation; poor liver function and circulation; hyperinsulinism; poor assimilation of foods, such as dairy or wheat products; food sensitivities and intolerances. Too much food, lack of exercise, diet composition and lifestyle are the key weight control factors.

For weight loss to be real and permanent four essential things must happen:

1) The body must be detoxified. Toxins are stored in the fat cells. Maintained weight loss depends on body cleansing and detoxification. During the first liquid diet stage in this program, the body begins heavy elimination and the breaking down of fat cells so it can remove toxic wastes and fat deposits. Wastes are discarded faster than new tissue is made, and unneeded weight is lost.

2) The craving for excess sweets and salts must be overcome. A chromium deficiency may affect the body's perceived needs for sugary, salty foods. Stress, aging and chromium-depleted soils caused by chemically-dependent agricultural practices, strip body chromium. A diet uncluding in high chromium foods, such as brewer's yeast, apples, melons, whole grains and seafoods can help overcome cravings for foods that put on weight.

3) Continual hunger must be curbed by better balance and use of nutrients. Low fat, mineral-rich complex carbohydrates are the key. You can eat two to three times more volume of these foods and still lose weight. They signal the insulin/serotonin synthesis reaction in the appestat center of the brain to communicate a feeling of fullness, even in the presence of less food intake.

4) Metabolism must be increased, so that the calories taken in are burned and used efficiently. Metabolic processes can often cause weight gain. And all metabolisms are different. Men lose weight easier on whole grains and beans for instance; women lose easier on a diet of fresh and cooked vegetables.

The importance of cutting back on fat for successful weight loss and better health cannot be over-stated. The signals of whether to eat or not are directly tied to the biochemical activity of fat cells. But fat is not all bad. It is the chief source of energy for the body, and essential for good body function in small amounts. The average overweight person often has *too high* blood sugar and *too low* fat levels. This causes constant hunger, the delicate balance between fat storage and fat utilization is upset, and the ability of the body to use fat for energy decreases. Eating too many refined carbohydrates and junk foods particularly aggravates this upset balance; the person winds up with "empty calories" and more cravings. *Fat becomes non-moving energy,* and fat cells become fat storage depots. **Saturated fats are the hardest for the liver to metabolize. Say away from them to control fat storage, and avoid cellulite deposits.**

GOOD NEWS! The newest studies show that three months of a drastically reduced fat diet can drastically reduce your body's need or craving for fat. So if you can cut out fats for 90 days, especially on salad dressings, mayonnaise, butter and dairy products you stand a good chance of staying away from them permanently.

The following health and appearance goals can be reached with this diet series:
WEIGHT LOSS CELLULITE CONTROL HIGH BLOOD PRESSURE ENERGY IMPROVE-MENT SLUGGISH THYROID and POOR METABOLISM DIABETIC OBESITY HIGH LDL CHOLESTEROL BLOATING and WATER RETENTION HEART and CIRCULATORY PROB-LEMS LIVER MALFUNCTION CONSTIPATION

Water & Weight Loss: Water is a prime factor for success.

Every effective weight loss plan should include six to eight glasses of bottled water throughout the day. No-calorie seltzers and mineral waters can also help fill this quota. When the body gets enough water, it works at its peak, fluid and salt retention decrease, glandular activity improves, the liver metabolizes more fats, and hunger is curtailed.

All of this leads to greater weight loss. Water can also carry you through the plateau experience during a weight loss program. Dieting takes away some of the foods that were providing tissue hydration, so if you don't drink enough water, fluid levels go out of balance, and the body retains more fluid in an effort to compensate. Besides fluid retention, lack of water leads to poor muscle tone, sagging skin, constipation and even weight **gain.** When calories are severely limited, water is pulled out of the tissues to metabolize stored sugars for fuel. Three to four pounds of water are lost for every pound of fuel burned. You become lighter, but you aren't losing fat. You are losing water and muscle tissue, *the very things that can give you the look and health you are dieting to accomplish.*

Exercise & Weight Loss: No diet will work without exercise; with it, almost every diet will.

Daily exercise is the key to permanent, painless weight control. Food in and energy out are the ingredients of weight loss. Even if eating habits are changed very little, you can still lose weight by expending more energy with a brisk hour's walk, or 15 minutes of aerobic exercise. A 3 mile walk will burn up about 250 calories, and a pound of fat contains 3500 calories. In about 2 weeks you will have lost a pound of real fat, not water weight. That amounts to 3 pounds a month and 30 pounds a year without changing anything in your diet. It's easy to see how cutting down even moderately on fatty, sugary foods **in combination with exercise** can quickly provide the look and body tone desired.

Exercise also promotes an *"afterburn"* **effect,** raising your metabolic rate from 1.00 to 1.05 to 1.15 per minute for 4 to 24 hours after exertion. This means that calories will be used up at an even faster rate after you stop exercising.

Exercise, especially weight training, increases lean muscle mass, replacing fat-marbled muscle tissue with lean muscle. Muscle tissue uses up calories for energy; fat burns nothing. The greater the amount of muscle tissue you have, the more calories you can burn. This is particularly important as aging decreases muscle mass. Low metabolism can be counteracted with weight training exercise.

Exercise before a meal raises blood sugar levels and thus decreases appetite, often for several hours afterward. Exercise after eating raises heart and metabolism rates so that food is used by the system instead of just "sitting there."

A Successful Two Stage Weight Loss Diet

Stage One is a moderate liquid diet, with all fresh foods and juices. Liquid fasting sounds like a "fast" way to lose weight, and sometimes it is, if you get enough nutrients from fresh fruit and vegetable juices. Unfortunately, there are three inherent problems with a fast for weight loss.

1)The body tends to form **more fat at first** when it receives no solid food at all. It feels threatened by the drastic decrease in its usual nutrients and tries to protect itself by forming fat for survival.

2) Fasting can be dangerous unless you are using organically grown foods. The pesticides and sprays on much of the commercial produce that we eat are very quickly absorbed into the blood stream when there is no food to slow them down. They can lodge in the bones and cause toxic reactions.

3) A fast means that that the body is cleansing and discarding wastes more rapidly than new tissue is being formed, (i.e. weight loss). A temporary degree of discomfort may be felt in terms of headache, bowel looseness or loss of energy. These symptoms are usually just initial detoxification signs. They are a small price to pay for getting rid of long accumulated fat cells. **Weight loss cannot occur until these cells are gone.** Drinking six to eight glasses of pure water a day will speed along this first flushing and release process. After a few days, as the toxic waste is eliminated, the symptoms will be also cease.

For permanent weight control, a biochemical change is necessary. *This can be achieved through the **Stage Two Diet**, "Eating Right & Light," and regular exercise. This diet emphasizes four keys for lasting weight loss: 1) low fats; 2) soluble dietary fiber from complex carbohydrates; 3) regular exercise; 4) plenty of water. (Thirst is often mistaken by the body for hunger, so drinking water or non-calorie liquids will save many calories throughout the day.) All red meats and full-fat dairy foods are omitted. All junk and processed foods are avoided. These can destroy the fat-metabolizing body system you have encouraged, causing poor nutrition, which in turn causes constant hunger, and the desire to eat "empty calorie" foods.*

Fad diets, crash diets, quick-loss diets and too-good-to-be-true diets usually send your weight up and down like a yo-yo. They are a very poor investment in both your health and your looks.

- ❖ When you begin eating regularly again after one of these diets, you will probably gain back the fat you lost, but not the muscle tissue - leaving you flabbier than ever.
- ❖ Taking in too few calories causes the body to rob energy from hard-to-replace muscle - including that of your heart.
- ❖ The first few pounds you lose are mostly water weight loss. They are quickly gained back.
- ❖ Eliminating certain foods or food groups may leave your body feeling constantly fatigued, and your brain mentally tired. It may also mean eliminating important vitamins and minerals.

❊ The Modified Liquid Diet for Intense Weight Loss; 7 to 10 Days

The following liquid diet is for intense weight loss periods. It is moderate, with plenty of nutrition, and is most effective when used for one to three weeks at a time, with light eating in between.

✓Take only fruits and fruit juices until noon, to use up glycogen reserves and stimulate optimal metabolic action.

On rising: take a glass of lemon juice and water with 1 teasp. honey to flush fats and clean the kidneys.

Breakfast: have some fresh fruit, **and** a glass of apple or pineapple/papaya juice with 1TB. psyllium husks, Crystal Star CHO-LO FIBER TONE™ or Sonné liquid bentonite for natural fiber and continued flushing of the bowels;
or a glass of aloe vera juice with herbs.

Mid-morning: have a glass of carrot/beet/cucumber juice to cleanse and scour the kidneys;
or a fresh carrot juice;
or a green drink such as Sun CHLORELLA or Green Foods GREEN ESSENCE in water.

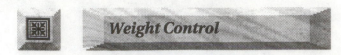
Lunch: have a meal replacement drink, such as Nature's Plus SPIRUTEIN, Crystal Star LIGHT WEIGHT™, or Lewis Labs Biochrome WEIGH DOWN;
or a meal replacement supplement, such as Rainbow Light SPIRULINA HERBAL DIET COMPLEX.

Mid-afternoon: have some crunchy raw veggies with kefir cheese, or an all vegetable puree;
and a bottle of mineral water or herb tea, such as peppermint or licorice root tea, or Crystal Star CLEANS-ING & PURIFYING TEA™ or LEAN 'N' CLEAN DIET TEA™.

Dinner: have a green leafy salad with sprouts, cucumbers, celery, carrots and a lemon/oil dressing;
and a cup of miso soup with sea vegetables snipped on top; or a cup of VEGEX yeast broth.
Before bed: have a glass of cranberry or apple juice with 1TB. liquid bentonite or psyllium:
or another glass of aloe vera juice with herbs for the night's cleanse.
✓Take a short walk before retiring, to stimulate metabolic activity during the night.

✸ *Supplements for the Modified Liquid Diet*

❖ Take 1 ESTEEM PLUS capsule daily at lunch; an effective diet aid found in health food stores.

✸ *Bodywork for the Modified Liquid Diet*

✚ Eat smaller, more frequent meals, instead of large meals.

✚ Exercise for 5 minutes before eating to raise blood sugar levels and decrease appetite.

Stage Two; Eating Right, Light, and Low-Fat for Weight Loss

*This diet should be used for at least three months to assure that your system is realigned and stabilized in your new way of eating. It gives you the diet skills to develop long term weight management - so you won't gain it back. **Keep eating plenty of raw, fresh foods. They take more time to eat so that you eat less. They don't need fattening sauces. They add more high fiber bulk than cooked foods. Their high vitamin/mineral content satifies your body's needs with less food.***
The following weight loss program is high in vegetable and whole grain fiber, full of complex carbohydrates and gland balancing foods to improve metabolism, increase the amount of excreted calories by the body, and signal a feeling of fullness to allay hunger.

See the FOREVER DIET in this book for a successful way of eating to maintain weight loss gains.

✓ Eat small meals more frequently instead of big sit-down meals. Eat only one main meal a day.

On rising: take 2 lemons squeezed in a glass of water.

Breakfast: take a cleansing/building protein drink such as Nature's Plus SPIRUTEIN, NutriTech ALL 1, or Crystal Star SYSTEM STRENGTH DRINK™ for energy and brain food without muscle wasting;
and some fresh fruits.

Mid-morning: have some yogurt with fresh fruit;
or a small bottle of mineral water;
or an herb tea, such as Crystal Star HIGH ENERGY™ or LEAN 'N' CLEAN DIET TEA™, or a mint tea; .
Lunch: have a fresh leafy green salad with lemon/oil or yogurt dressing;
with baked tofu, a baked potato or brown rice, with a low fat sauce or dressing;
or a light vegetable, black bean, lentil or miso soup, with steamed veggies and a soy/ginger sauce;
or whole grain or vegetable pasta salad, with seafood or salad veggies and a light sauce.

Mid-afternoon: have crunchy raw veggies or whole grain crackers with kefir cheese or a yogurt dip;
and a green drink such as Sun CHLORELLA or a refreshing herb tea or bottled mineral water;
and/or a hard boiled egg with a little sesame salt, and rice cakes with kefir cheese.
Dinner: have a large dinner salad with seafood and veggies, nuts and seeds, and a cup of light soup;
or a Chinese stir-fry with lots of greens, onions, mushrooms, clear soup and brown rice;
or baked or broiled fish or seafood with some steamed veggies and brown rice or millet.
or some roast turkey with light corn bread, and a salad with poppyseed dressing;
or a whole grain or veggie pasta dish with vegetables and a light sauce; and a cup of soup.
✓A little white wine with your main meal will improve digestion, and make dieting more pleasant.

T.V/Evening snack: have some un-buttered spicy popcorn. It's good for you and its airiness will fill you up and keep you from wanting heavier or "habit" foods.

Before bed: a cup of VEGEX yeast broth; **or** a glass of apple or papaya juice, or a cup of mint tea.

❧

❋ *Supplements and Herbs for Eating Right, Light and Low-Fat*

Appetite suppressants:
◆Phenylalanine 500mg., with tyrosine 500mg.
◆Rainbow Light SPIRULINA HERBAL DIET COMPLEX
◆DIET PEP and SUPER PEP CAPSULES
◆Crystal Star APPE-TIGHT DIET™ CAPS, and SCALE DOWN DIET™ EXTRACT
◆Excel SLOW RELEASE ANTI-FATIGUE formula

Fat metabolizers:
◆Carnitine 500mg. with Rainbow Light TRIM-ZYME
◆Quantum NIGHT TRIM caps with high ornithine
◆Source Naturals SUPER AMINO NIGHT caps
◆Crystal Star CEL-LEAN™ DIET SUPPORT caps, AMINO-ZYME CAPSULES and ROLL-ON GEL
◆Strength Systems FAT BURNERS capsules

Glandular imbalance:
◆Enzymatic Therapy PEAR SHAPED program, (Raw Pituitary, Mammary and Thyroid/Tyrosine)
◆Sassafras and burdock tea, bee pollen capsules or granules
◆Carnitine 250mg. with CoQ 10, 30mg, 2x daily

Metabolic increase for lazy thyroid:
◆ESTEEM DAYTIME & NIGHTIME CAPSULES
◆Crystal Star META-TABS CAPS, SUPER LEAN & CLEAN™ DIET CAPS and TEA
◆Enzymatic Therapy THYROID/TYROSINE caps with carnitine 500mg.
◆Crystal Star RAINFOREST ENERGY CAPS and THERMO-GINSENG EXTRACT with natural xanthines

Body flushing for fluid retention and bloating:
◆Crystal Star LEAN & CLEAN DIET™ CAPSULES and TEA, DIUR-CAPS™, POUNDS OFF™ BATH

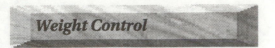

◆Laci LeBeau SUPER DIET TEAS

Controlling sugar craving and hyperinsulinism:
◆Gymnema Sylvestre caps before meals
◆SUGAR STRATEGY HIGH™ AND SUGAR STRATEGY LOW™ TEAS

Lean Muscle Mass Builders:
◆Lewis Labs WEIGH DOWN DRINK with chromium picolinate 250mcg.
◆Strength Systems CHROMAX caps, and SMILAX with chromium
◆Wakunaga PERFECT SHAPE DRINK
◆Twin Lab DIET FUEL

✦

About Caffeine and Weight Loss

Recent clinical studies have shown that the amount of caffeine in a cup of coffee increases metabolic rate by 3 to 4% for two to three hours after drinking. Calories burned with this amount of coffee increase by 8 to 11%, or 85 to 150 calories per day. Since both obesity and dieting for weight loss cause subnormal calorie burning, caffeine has received a great deal of attention as a dieting supplement. The human body uses caffeine as a short-lived, heating excitant that delivers its punch immediately to the system. In the fasting state, one to four cups of coffee cause calorie burning to increase from 5 to 15%, or 60 to 250 calories. Obviously, commonly consumed amounts of caffeine can significantly influence calorie use by the body, leading to substantial reduction in body weight over several months. Unfortunately, the hydro-carbons from heat-processed caffeine can be at the foundation of serious health problems, such as hypertension, nervousness, heart palpitations, indigestion and bladder, kidney, or prostate infections. However, if you do not have, or are not prone to a caffeine-caused health condition, and wish to try small amounts of caffeine to increase calorie burning by the body, there is clinical evidence to support its effectiveness.

About Xanthine Stimulants

Xanthines are a broad classification of stimulants that include caffeine, theine such as that found in black and green teas, guaranine as found in guarana, and maté as found in maté tea. Xanthine activity is very similar *in the laboratory,* but all authorities on xanthines make a distinction between caffeine, guaranine, maté and théine in *body* activity and effects. People who have difficulty with caffeine seldom have problems with black or green teas, guaraña or maté. Guaraña berries are particularly rich in natural oils that combine with the guaranine to block rapid absorption into the body. (This effect is very noticeable when pure, unadulterated guaraña powder is mixed with water. It does not dissolve easily, because the oils are holding it in check.) Its stimulant activity is released slowly as the oils are broken down and digested, allowing for natural time release over many hours. It is a natural, slow-release guaraña for long term stamina, stronger but softer energy. *Guaranine also potentiates lipolysis for cellulite release.*
Both guaranine and maté are cooling stimulants to the body. They re-vitalize as long range tonics, with benefits for digestion. They are naturally-occurring substances, with *chemical* similarity to caffeine, but with important subtle differences that, as in homeopathy, are uniquely understood by the human body.

❈ *Bodywork for Eating Right, Light and Low-Fat*

✚ Try to eat your last solid food before 7:00p.m. Late meals tend to settle in the waist area. If you eat later, be sure you take an after dinner walk.

✚ Chew each mouthful until finely pulverized - to ease digestion, and to satisfy hunger quicker through sublingual absorption of nutrients. Careful chewing slows down the rate of food consumption, and also causes you to pay attention to what you eat, so you don't eat out of unconscious habit.

✚ As before, exercise 5 minutes before a meal will decrease appetite, and regular daily exercise will keep fat cells lean and not used for storage.

✚ Never eat when under stress. The body converts more food to fat when it feels stress.

✚ Use dry skin brushing, an herbal body wrap, or hot and cold hydrotherapy to keep circulation stimulated and toned, especially helpful for cellulite problems.

✸ *Sample Recipes For Eating Right, Light & Low-Fat*
By section and recipe number:
Modify your favorite recipes to use less fat, avoid chemical foods, and bake instead of fry. These techniques allow lots of your favorite things without feeling guilty or deprived , and the excess weight won't come back.

LOW-FAT & VERY LOW-FAT DISHES - all

BREAKFAST & BRUNCH - 73, 74, 75, 76, 77, 78, 81, 82, 83, 84, 85, 86, 87, 92, 93, 94, 95, 97, 101, 102

SALADS HOT & COLD - 186, 187, 188, 189, 190, 193, 199, 200, 202, 210, 211, 215, 223, 229, 232, 23

SUGAR FREE SWEET TREATS - 411, 413, 414, 415, 419, 420, 426, 429, 431, 432, 434, 435, 439, 440, 443.

SOUPS - LIQUID SALADS - all

STIR-FRIES - all

FISH & SEAFOOD - all

COMPLEX CARBOHYDRATES FOR ENERGY - 743, 749, 751, 753, 757, 759, 760, 761, 763, 773, 778

GREAT OUTDOOR EATIING - 874, 875, 876, 878, 881, 883, 884, 886, 888, 890, 893, 895, 896, 901, 908

✸ *Sample Menu Plans*
Recipe combinations that work with this diet:

A SPECIAL DINNER FOR TWO - 248, 450, 195, 270, 291, 251

AN EASY RISING BREAKFAST - 74, 78, 75, 82, 264

AN EASY WEEKNIGHT DINNER - 201, 275, 263, 290

A FAMILY MEAL - 255, 300, 526, 452

AN ALL HORS D'OEUVRES PARTY - 904, 877, 299, 269, 252

SUNDAY BRUNCH - 100, 538, 258, 241, 249, 292

A LIGHT SUMMER MEAL - 451, 262, 283/287, 298, 240

A HEARTY WINTER MEAL - 445, 265, 566, 895

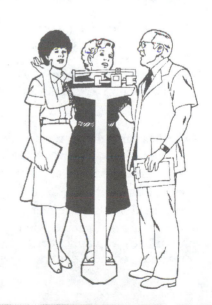

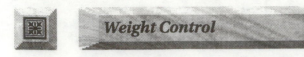

The Meal Replacement Diet

Sales of meal replacement drinks have exploded in America, and many people have turned to these low calorie powders to lose weight. Over a year of testing with numerous products has taught us three things about meal replacement diet programs: 1) Weight loss powders are not a replacement for good eating habits, and the weight lost is easily gained back. 2) They are not good as part of a fasting diet. Metabolism slows too much, and weight is harder to lose. 3) Weight loss powders work best as a temporary program to get your diet going in the right direction.

For best results, take your main meal in the middle of the day, and the meal replacement drink is taken in the morning and at night as a part of a low fat, high complex carbohydrate diet. The folowing diet has been successful both immediately and long term when used in this way.

On rising: take 2 lemons sqeezed in a glass of water.

Breakfast: take a meal replacement drink, such as Lewis Labs WEIGH DOWN with BIO-Chrome, or Crystal Star LIGHT WEIGHT™ meal replacement program;
and some fresh fruits.

Mid-morning: have some yogurt with fresh fruit;
or a small bottle of mineral water;
or a tea, such as Crystal Star RAINFOREST ENERGY™ or LEAN 'N' CLEAN DIET™ TEA, or a mint tea;.

Lunch: have a large salad with seafood and veggies, nuts and seeds, and a cup of light soup;
with baked tofu, a baked potato or brown rice, with a low fat sauce or dressing;
or a light vegetable, black bean, lentil or miso soup, with steamed veggies and a soy/ginger sauce;
or a whole grain or vegetable pasta salad, with seafood or salad veggies and a light sauce;
or a Chinese stir-fry with lots of greens, onions, mushrooms, clear soup and brown rice;
or baked or broiled fish or seafood with some steamed veggies and brown rice or millet.

Mid-afternoon: have crunchy raw veggies or whole grain crackers with kefir cheese or a yogurt dip;
and a green drink such as Sun CHLORELLA, or a refreshing herb tea such as Crystal Star CEL-LEAN RELEASE™ TEA, or bottled mineral water;
and/or a hard boiled egg with a little sesame salt, and rice cakes with kefir cheese.

Dinner: have a meal replacement drink as at breakfast;
and/or a green leafy salad with a low calorie dressing.

T.V/Evening snack: have some un-buttered, spicy savory popcorn. It's good for you and its airiness will fill you up and keep you from wanting heavier or 'habit' foods.

Before bed: have a cup of VEGEX yeast broth;
or a glass of apple or papaya juice, or a cup of mint tea.

The rules for quicker, more stable weight loss still apply:
- ☞ Fresh fruit in the morning to use up glycogen reserves, and set up good metabolic balance.
- ☞ A good meal replacement or wafers in the morning and/or evening.
- ☞ A brisk walk after dinner.
- ☞ Small meals whenever you eat.

Best results are obtained when you lose about 1% of your body weight per week. More than that results in poor body adjustment and weight **re-gain**. Shoot for an attractive body weight that you can realistically maintain without continually starving your self or exercising yourself ragged.

Weight loss is not easy in today's life style. Reaching your ideal weight is a victory. Keeping it requires vigilance, especially in light of today's processed food offerings and fast lifestyle. But living the thin life is not a lifelong deprivation sentence. Once basic metabolic processes have re-aligned and stabilized, and desired weight has been maintained for several months, you can have a few overeating days, such as when you will be eating out or with company, without losing weight control. Just balance them with undereating days, so that ideal weight can be sustained. Living thin just means knowing what it takes from you personally to maintain your weight; then it becomes automatic and intuitive.

Weight loss can be successful on a long term basis, without side effects. Don't Weight!
IT IS A REAL ACHIEVEMENT.

Weight Control for Kids ☺

Until the nineteen sixties, overweight and weight control wasn't much of a problem for kids. But ever since the fifties, over-refined and junk foods have changed parents' metabolism and cell structure. Hereditary factors from these parents of the fifties and sixties have passed the immune defense depletions, and food assimilation problems to the kids of today. And that's in addition to the wide variety of junk and chemical-laced foods, peer pressure, lack of exercise, and T.V. advertising that the kids themselves are constantly exposed to. Weight problems are mushrooming in American children. For all the current adult consciousness and attention to diet, recent statistics show that our children and teenagers are the fattest they have ever been! Obesity rates for young children jumped 54% between 1960 and 1981, and 30% for teenagers. They jumped another 50% between 1981 and 1988.

The 1985 study by the President's Council on Physical Fitness showed two very disconcerting facts: 1) 85% of the children and teenagers tested failed basic fitness tests; 2) as many as 90% of American children already have at least one risk factor for a degenerating disease.

*Poor lifestyle eating habits, with too much fat, salt, sugar and calories, and lack of exercise are at the base of this poor performance. Snacks, lunch foods and meals can be satisfying and delicious without adding significant amounts of sugar, fat or salt. In fact, young children need two or three snacks daily to have a nutritious diet, because their stomachs don't hold all they need in just three meals. Kids need mineral-rich building foods, fiber-rich energy foods, protein-rich growth foods. Changing the **type** of food eaten without restricting the amount can result in easy and spontaneous weight loss. Plenty of fresh fruit, un-buttered spicy popcorn, and sandwich fixings are good defenses against junk foods.*

*Breakfast can be a key, too. Both kids and adults who eat a high fiber breakfast don't feel as hungry at lunchtime, and eat an average of 200 **fewer calories during the day**. Your kids need you for good information, and as good diet role models to help them establish healthy eating habits. The following diet serves as an easy weight control guideline for kids. It has passed many tests on both overweight and "couch potato" kids for foods that they will eat.*

On rising: give a vitamin/mineral drink such as NutriTech EARTHSHAKE or Nature's Plus SPIRUTEIN (lots of flavors), or 1 teaspoon liquid multi-vitamin in juice (such as Floradix CHILDREN'S MULTI-VITAMIN/MINERAL).

Breakfast: have a whole grain cereal with apple juice or a little yogurt and fresh fruit;
and, if more is desired, whole grain toast or muffins, with a little butter, kefir cheese or nut butter;
add eggs, scrambled or baked or soft boiled (no fried eggs);
or have some hot oatmeal or kashi with a little maple syrup, and yogurt if desired.

Mid-morning: snacks can be whole grain crackers with kefir cheese or low-fat cheese or dip, and a sugarless juice or sparkling mineral water;
and/or some fresh fruit, such as apples with yogurt or kefir cheese;
or dried fruit, or fruit leather;
or fresh crunchy veggies, like celery, with peanut butter or a nut spread;
or a no-sugar dried fruit, nut and seed candy bar (you can easily one) or a dried fruit and nut trail mix, stirred into yogurt.

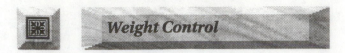
Lunch: have a fresh veggie, turkey, chicken or shrimp salad sandwich on whole grain bread, with low-fat or soy cheese and mayonnaise.

Add whole grain or corn chips with a low-fat veggie or cheese dip;

or a hearty bean soup with whole grain toast or crackers, and crunchy veggies with garbanzo spread;

or a baked potato with a butter, kefir cheese, or soy cheese, and a green salad with Italian dressing;

or a vegetarian pizza on a chapati or whole grain crust;

or whole grain spaghetti or pasta with a light sauce and parmesan cheese;

or a Mexican bean and veggie, or rice or whole wheat burrito with a light natural no-sugar salsa.

Mid-afternoon: have a sparkling juice and a dried fruit candy bar, or fruit juice-sweetened cookies;

or some fresh fruit or fruit juice, or a kefir drink with whole grain muffins and kefir cheese;

or a hard boiled egg, and some whole grain chips with a veggie or low-fat cheese dip;

or some whole grain toast and peanut butter or other nut butter.

Dinner: have a light pizza on a whole grain, chapati or egg crust, with veggies, shrimp, and soy or low-fat mozzarella cheese topping;

or whole grain or egg pasta with vegetables and a light tomato and cheese sauce;

or a baked Mexican quesadilla with soy or low-fat cheese and some steamed vegetables or a salad;

or a stir-fry with crunchy noodles, brown rice, baked egg rolls and a light soup;

or some roast turkey with corn bread dressing and a salad;

or a tuna casserole with rice, peas and water chestnuts and toasted chapatis with a little butter.

Before bed: a glass of apple juice or vanilla soy milk or flavored kefir.

✓ A snack of unbuttered, spicy, savory popcorn is good and nutritious anytime. See recipe index.

❋ *Sample Recipes For Weight Control for Kids*
By section and recipe number:

LOW-FAT & VERY LOW-FAT DISHES - all

BREAKFAST & BRUNCH - 73, 74, 77, 81, 82, 83, 84, 85, 87, 89, 90, 91, 93, 98, 99, 100, 102, 104, 106, 107

SUGAR FREE SWEET TREATS - all

SANDWICHES, SALADS IN BREAD - 473, 478, 481, 485, 486, 488, 489, 490, 491, 493, 495, 496, 500

COMPLEX CARBOHYDRATES FOR ENERGY - 743, 745, 752, 754, 758, 759, 779, 780, 781, 782, 784

HIGH PROTEIN WITHOUT MEAT - 695, 708, 712, 715, 716, 717, 718, 719, 725, 729, 730, 731, 739, 740

MINERAL-RICH FOODS - 618, 620, 628, 639, 643, 644, 646, 647, 648, 650, 651, 653, 658, 660, 662, 663

GREAT OUTDOOR EATING - 878, 879, 882, 887, 889, 891, 892, 895, 898, 900, 908, 909

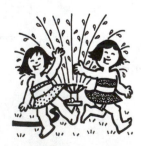

The Forever Diet
High Energy,
Abundant Nourishment,
Delicious Eating
for the Rest of your Life

The FOREVER DIET is for everyone who wants to "carry on the good work" of better nutrition for health. Altering a lifetime of poor diet and eating habits is difficult. Once they have gone through all the pain of the change, most people don't want to give up the gain that healthy eating has given them.

The "FOREVER DIET" way of eating can be the next step - one you can live with for the rest of your life. It is a natural foods program that synthesizes and synergizes the best from oriental foods, macrobiotics, and the balanced calorie/protein/complex carbohydrate diets popular in California.

The "FOREVER DIET" is high in whole grains and whole grain fiber (not yeasted breads). It is full of vegetable protein and soluble fiber, cooked, steamed and raw. It encourages fresh fruits and fruit juices for morning fiber and system flushing. It has sea foods, eggs, and low-fat cheeses for alternate proteins, and suggests the moderate use of dinner wines for flavor and digestion.
All red meats, refined sugars, full fat dairy products, fried and fatty foods of all kinds are eliminated.

The "FOREVER DIET" emphasizes fresh, natural vegetables and fruits for cleansing, regularity and body balance. It offers cooked grains, nuts, seeds and vegetables for body strength, endurance and alkalinity. It recommends baked, broiled or stir-fried seafoods, fish and vegetables for circulation and heart health.

The included recipes are simple, basic, and easy to individualize for personal taste.

❧It is easy to live with. It will fit right in with your everyday life, and family and friends.

❧It is flexible and full of variation, so you won't get bored at mealtime.

❧It is regularly cleansing, to keep the body as toxin-free as possible on a lifetime basis.

❧It has lots of solid energy for fuel foods, to keep daily strength and stamina high.

❧It includes feasting and entertaining meals, and seasonal eating, so that you can use it at Christmas or on the 4th of July.

Best of all, this way of eating is continuing support for your health.

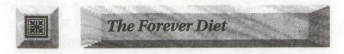

The Forever Diet

On rising: take NutriTech ALL 1 or Nature's Plus SPIRUTEIN protein drink in apple or citrus juice. Add 1 teasp. <u>each</u> brewer's yeast, wheat germ oil, and lecithin granules to either of these drinks;
<u>or</u> Crystal Star ROYAL MU TEA™ substitute.

Breakfast: always have some fresh fruits or fresh juice in the morning;
<u>then</u> choose from muesli or granola with yogurt and fruit, or apple juice or vanilla soy milk on top;
<u>or</u> whole grain toast or rice cakes with kefir cheese, butter, or 1 teasp. Bragg's LIQUID AMINOS;
<u>or</u> whole grain pancakes with maple syrup;
<u>or</u> a breakfast pilaf of whole mixed, cooked grains, such as KASHI with tamari, butter or yogurt;
<u>or</u> a poached egg on whole grain toast or English muffin.

Mid-morning: have some yogurt with fresh fruit;
<u>or</u> fresh carrot juice, potassium broth (page 240), or Crystal Star SYSTEM STRENGTH DRINK™;
<u>or</u> a cup of herb tea (see next page for suggestions);
<u>or</u> a green drink, such as Sun CHLORELLA or Green Foods BARLEY GREEN MAGMA, or Crystal Star ENERGY GREEN™ granules in water;
<u>or</u> some whole grain crackers, kefir cheese or yogurt dip, and a small bottle of mineral water.

Lunch: have a leafy green salad with miso or other clear broth and sea vegetables snipped on top;
<u>or</u> some steamed fresh veggies with Bragg's LIQUID AMINOS, light oil dressing or tamari sauce;
<u>or</u> a light veggie sandwich on whole grain toast;
<u>or</u> a baked potato with a little butter, kefir cheese, light lemon oil dressing, or tamari;
<u>or</u> a fresh fruit salad with cottage cheese or yogurt;
<u>or</u> a hot or cold a seafood or vegetable and whole grain pasta salad;
<u>or</u> a hot or cold seasonal vegetable soup with whole grain toast or muffins;
<u>or</u> marinated tofu and brown rice or other whole grain.

Mid-afternoon: have whole grain crackers or raw veggies with kefir cheese or a vegetable dip;
<u>or</u> a cup of miso soup, or ramen noodle soup;
<u>or</u> some fresh or dried fruits;
<u>or</u> rice cakes with kefir cheese or a good veggie or soy spread;
<u>or</u> fruit juice sweetened cookies or candy bar;
<u>or</u> a cup of herb tea, or bottle of mineral water.

Dinner: have a hearty vegetable salad and hot soup;
<u>or</u> baked or broiled fish or seafood (never fried) with a leafy green salad;
<u>or</u> a roast turkey salad, sandwich, or casserole;
<u>or</u> a vegetarian pizza on a whole grain or chapati crust;
<u>or</u> a whole grain or vegetable pasta dish;
<u>or</u> an oriental stir-fry with brown rice and a light broth;
<u>or</u> a tofu and whole grain casserole and salad;
<u>or</u> a baked or steamed vegetable quiche or casserole with cottage cheese, or raw cheeses.
✓ A little white wine with dinner is fine for relaxation and digestion.

At bedtime: have a cup of relaxing herb tea, (see suggestions on the next page);
<u>or</u> 1 teasp of VEGEX yeast paste in hot water for relaxation and B vitamins.

✓ Drink plenty of bottled water all through the day to keep the system hydrated, free and flowing.

✓ Eat small meals more frequently, instead of large meals.

✽ *Supplement and Herbal Suggestions for the Forever Diet*
Choose from:

❖ Ascorbate vitamin C or Ester C, 2 to 3000mg. daily with bioflavonoids.

❖ Beta carotene A 25,000IU daily.

❖ Vitamin E 400IU with selenium 200mcg. daily.

❖ Vitamin B$_{12}$, sublingual or internasal every 2 to 3 days.

❖ Bee pollen granules and/or high potency royal jelly 2 teasp. daily for prostaglandin formation.

❖ Evening primrose oil capsules, 2 to 4 daily.

❖ A green food supplement, such as Sun CHLORELLA, Green Foods GREEN MAGMA or GREEN ES-SENCE, or Wakunaga KYO-GREEN.

❖ A multimineral, such as Mezotrace SEA MINERAL COMPLEX.

❖ Suggested herbal tea choices for everyday use and benefits: (extract drops may also be put into water and drunk as a tea.)

HAWTHORN tea or extract
SIBERIAN GINSENG tea or extract
MILK THISTLE extract
PEPPERMINT tea
CHAMOMILE tea
GINGKO BILOBA tea or extract

Crystal Star herbal combinations for everyday pleasure and maintenance:
DAILY BIOFLAVONOID & C SUPPORT™ drink
ROYAL MU TEA™
SYSTEM STRENGTH DRINK™ drink
ENERGY GREEN™ drink
RELAX TEA™
LICORICE MINTS tea
FEEL GREAT™ capsules and tea
HERBAL ENZ capsules
MINERAL SPECTRUM capsules

✽ *Bodywork for the Forever Diet*

✚ Exercise every day with a brisk walk, and deep breathing and stretching exercises. An after dinner walk is an optimum choice when possible. Exercise is a nutrient in itself.

✚ Get some early morning sunlight on the body every day possible for vitamins A and D.

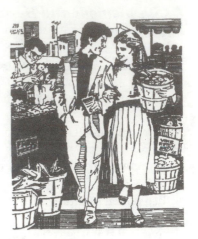

✿ *Sample Basic Recipes For The Forever Diet*

BREAKFAST & BRUNCH - all

LOW CHOLESTEROL MEALS - all

SALADS HOT AND COLD - all

SANDWICHES - SALADS IN BREAD - all

FISH & SEAFOODS - all

HIGH FIBER RECIPES - all

STIR-FRIES - all

GREAT OUTDOOR EATING - 874, 876, 878, 883, 884, 886, 890, 894, 898, 903, 904, 906, 908, 909

HOLIDAY FEASTING & ENTERTAINING - all

✿ *Sample Menus*
Some recipe combinations that work for the Forever Diet:

A WEEKEND PICNIC - 824, 905, 909, 904, 500

A SUNDAY BRUNCH - 100, 821, 495, 908, 292

AN EASY WEEK NIGHT DINNER - 453, 268, 510, 298

AN EASY RISING BREAKFAST - 73, 77, 97, 792

A SPECIAL DINNER FOR TWO - 248, 512, 552, 191, 291

A LIGHT SUMMER MEAL - 254, 876, 794, 894

A HEARTY WINTER MEAL - 558, 265, 444

A FAMILY MEAL - 519, 458, 289

LUNCH FOR TWO - 477, 300

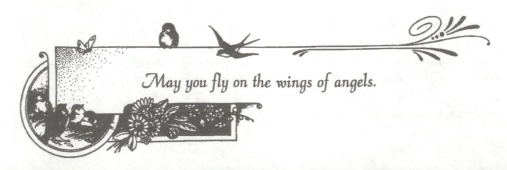

May you fly on the wings of angels.

Exercise & Spa Techniques
Bodywork for Healing
Aerobic Exercise ❧ Mineral Baths ❧ Oxygen Baths

Oxygen and minerals are the building blocks of healing, and while this book is generally about cooking, diets and nutrition for health, there are two other key elements in a successful healing program - **AEROBIC EXERCISE and THERAPEUTIC BATHING.**
Both activities exercise more than just your muscles. They effectively take nutrients into the body; often more quickly and in more concentrated form, (since the skin and lungs are large organs of ingestion), than the digestive system. Both should be included in any healthy healing program for optimal results.

Today, fitness falls somewhere between a triathlon and Zen meditation. Pushing the mind to its limits is therapeutic intelligence. Virtually everyone feels a dramatic increase in vitality and well-being when they begin an exercise program. Even with the aches, pains and strains endured by the over-zealous, exercise has one dominant effect: It makes people feel good.

We all know that exercise speeds results in weight control and heart disease recovery, but regular exercise can help any healing program. It increases metabolic rate, tissue oxygen uptake, respiratory and circulatory capacity, and muscle strength. Exercise supports whole body vitality - nerves, blood, glands, muscles, lungs, heart, brain, mind and mood. Exercise helps cleanse the body by expelling metabolic wastes through increased lung and bowel activity.

AEROBIC EXERCISE is the best for whole body tone; the key to long term weight loss, hypertension, cholesterol and stress reduction, and prevention of heart disease. It increases blood flow and supplies nutrients to muscle tissue. Lungs work harder to oxygenate more blood at a faster rate; arteries carry a greater volume of blood at higher velocity. An aerobic workout is as available as your front door if you choose to walk or jog for exercise; or more defined if you choose aerobic classes at a neraby gym. Workouts are held at convenient times every day, at very low prices, with the latest popular music and spirit-raising group energy. Comfortable workout clothes look great on everybody. They permit deep breathing, and make you feel good about your body even when you are just running around. Pick exercise activities that you like, and that work for you conveniently. Do some exercise outdoors at least once a week for healing sunlight and more oxygen. Every series of stretches and exercises that you do, tones, elasticizes, and contours the skin, muscles and body shape.

My personal favorites are walking, dancing and swimming.
❃**A daily walk**, breathing deeply, even just a mile a day, ($1/2$ mile out, $1/2$ mile back) makes a big difference in lung capacity and tissue oxygen. Vigorous exhalation releases metabolic wastes along with CO_2, and deep inhalations flood the system with fresh oxygen all at once. You can feel the difference. The circulatory system is cleansed, heart strength and muscle tone improved, and sunlight on the skin adds vitamin D for bone health - all from the simplest and easiest of exercises. Walk with a companion. The time will fly by. You won't believe it has been a mile.

❃**Dancing** is so much fun. Any kind of dancing is great. Legs get in shape fast, and the breathlessness felt afterwards is the best sign of a good aerobic workout.

❃**Swimming** tones every part of the body; very noticeable improvements come from regular swimming. 15 to 20 regular laps, three or more times a week, and a more toned, streamlined body can be yours quite rapidly.

Everyone has experienced the fact that exercise eases hunger. There is thirst after exercise, as the body calls for replacement of lost electrolytes and water, but not hunger. One of the main reasons we see such quick results in a body streamlining program when exercise is added is this phenomenon; the rise in natural glycogens that lift blood sugar levels and give a feeling of well-being. Not only do you get muscle tone, heart and lung benefits and fat loss, you also don't feel like replacing calories right away.
Even if you didn't reduce your total calorie intake, and just added exercise,
you would still lose weight and increase body tone.
Exercise becomes a nutrient in itself.
✦

If your schedule is so busy that you barely have time to breathe, let alone exercise, but still want the benefits of bodywork, there is a simple, double-quick, total body exercise. It has gotten resounding enthusiasm and excellent success rates for aerobic activity, muscle work and oxygen increase - **all in 1 minute.** It sounds very easy, but is actually very difficult, and that's why it works so well. You will be breathless and aerobically energized very quickly. Simply lie flat on your back on a rug or carpet. Rise to a full standing position any way you can, and lie back down on your back again. That's the whole thing; stand and lie down, stand and lie down, for 60 seconds.
The usual reps for most people with average body tone are 6 to 10 in one minute. Be very easy on yourself. Repeat only as many times as you feel comfortable, and work up to more. (Record time for a person in top competitive condition would only be 20 to 25 times a minute.) Try it, because it works every muscle, lung capacity and the circulatory system so well, but don't over-do it.

Whatever exercise program you choose, make rest a part of it. Spread exercise sessions throughout the week. Exercise more on one day, go easy the next; or exercise for several days and take 2 off. This is better for body balance, and will actually increase energy levels when you exercise the next time. After a regular program is begun, exercising 4 days a week will increase fitness levels. Exercise 3 days a week will maintain fitness levels. If you are doing aerobic conditioning, you should be able to continue your individual level of exercising for twenty minutes in order to improve and maintain your cardio-respiratory training. Exercise 2 or less days a week will not maintain a high level of fitness, but is better than no exercise at all.

☞ Stretch out before and after workouts to keep cramping down and muscles loose.

☞ Get some early morning sunlight on the body every day possible for best absorption of vitamins and minerals, especially healing vitamin D.

The body is an amazing, intelligent entity. It can be streamlined, toned and maintained, no matter what age or shape you are in, with just a little effort. The secret is to stick with it.
✦

THERAPEUTIC BATHS are another beneficial body activity for nutritional healing. Clinics and spas all over the world are famous for their mineral, seaweed and enzyme baths. They work, and the bath or spa in your own home can easily be used as a way of giving your body mineral, oxygen and enzyme nutrients. The skin is such a large organ of ingestion that results are almost immediately noticeable. Therapeutic baths are a pleasant, stress-free way to increase health.

❦**Mineral baths,** such as Batherapy or Abracadabra brand salts and packets, are available in most health food stores. Spa stores also carry those that can be used in a home spa. Mineral baths increase enzyme action, and therefore better food digestion and assimilation. They rapidly relax, stabilize and replenish a stressed-out system.

🌿**Seaweed baths** are Nature's perfect body/psyche balancer. Remember how good you feel after a walk in the ocean? Seaweeds purify ocean pollutants, and they can do the same for your body. Rejuvenating effects occur when toxins are released from the body. A hot seaweed bath is like a wet-steam sauna, only better, because the kelps and sea greens balance body chemistry instead of dehydrate it. The electrolytic magnetic action of the seaweed releases excess body fluids from congested cells, and dissolves fatty wastes through the skin, replacing them with depleted minerals, particularly potassium and iodine.

Iodine boosts thyroid activity, taming the appetite and increasing metabolism so that food fuels are used before they can turn into fatty deposits. Eating sea veggies regularly also has this effect. Vitamin K is another key nutrient in seaweeds. This precurser vitamin helps regulate adrenal function, meaning that a seaweed bath can also help maintain hormone balance for a more youthful body.

🌿**How to take a seaweed bath:**

If you live near the ocean, gather kelp and seaweeds from the water, (not the shoreline) in clean buckets or trash cans, and carry them home to your tub. If you don't live near the ocean, the dried kelp, sea greens or whole dulse leaves available in most herb sections of health food stores can be a good alternative. Dried sea greens granules are also available from spa and natural body care firms, such as La Costa and Zia Cosmetics.

Whichever form you choose, run very hot water over the seaweed in a tub, filling it to the point that you will be covered when you recline The leaves will turn a beautiful bright green if they are fresh. The water will turn a rich brown as the plants release their minerals. Add an herbal bath oil, if desired, to help hold the heat in, and pleasantly scent the water. Let the bath cool enough to get in. As you soak, the smooth gel from the seaweed will transfer onto your skin. This coating will increase perspiration to release toxins from your system, and replace them by osmosis with minerals. Rub the skin with the seaweed leaves during the bath to stimulate circulation, smooth the body, and remove wastes coming out on the skin surface. When the sea greens have done their therapeutic work, the gel coating will dissolve and float off the skin, and the leaves will shrivel - a sign that the bath is over. Each bath varies with the individual, the seaweeds used, and water temperature, but the gel coating release is a natural timekeeper for the bath's benefits. Forty five minutes to an hour is usually long enough to balance the acid/alkaline system, and encourage liver activity and fat metabolism. Skin tone and color, and circulatory strength are almost immediatly noticable from the iodine and potassium absorption. After the bath, take a capsule of cayenne and ginger powder to put these minerals quickly through the system.

🌿**Oxygen baths** are valuable detoxifying agents, and can noticeably increase body energy and tissue oxygen uptake. Vital Health brand **food grade** 35% hydrogen peroxide is a popular, effective product. About 1 cup per bath or spa produces significant effect for 3 to 7 days. Oxygen baths are stimulating rather than relaxing. An energy increase is usually noticed right away. Other therapeutic benefits include body balance and detoxification, reduction of skin cancers and tumors, clearing of asthma and lung congestion, arthritis and rheumatism relief, and other conditions where increased body oxygen can prevent and control disease.

Certain herbs used in the bath can also supply oxygen through the skin. Rosemary is one of the best, and most popular because of its aroma; peppermint and mullein are also effective. Just pack a small muslin bath or tea bag with the herb, drop it into the tub or spa, and soak for 15 to 20 minutes. Use the bag as a skin scrub during the bath for smoothing and tone.

🌿**Herbal baths** are wonderful therapies to improve body chemistry and replace depleted minerals quickly. Herbs can relax both mind and body, soothe aching muscles, hydrate and soften skin, provide nutritive elements through the pores, draw out toxic wastes, and neutralize acids. Herbs combined with the hot water also provides an aromatherapy treatment for the mood and spirit.

Some of the most restorative and beneficial body conditioning herbal treatments may be used in your own home. Herbal wraps, baths, oils, gels, creams and drinks can tighten, tone, alkalize and release

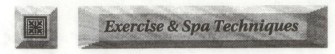

wastes from the body very quickly at a fraction of European or California spa costs.
Zia Cosmetics, Crystal Star Herbal Nutrition and Breh Sea Bath Creations among other herb and holistic companies have a wide variety of healing spa products.

❦How To Take An Herbal Therapeutic Bath:

The procedure for taking an effective infusion bath is almost as important as your choice of herbs. In essence, you are soaking in an herbal tea, allowing the large organ of your skin to take in the nutrients and healing properties instead of the mouth and digestive system.

There are two good ways to take an herbal bath:

1) Draw very hot bath water. Put the bath herbs in an extra large tea ball or small muslin bath bag, (sold in most health food stores), and steep until water cools slightly and is aromatic.

or

2) Make a strong tea infusion, strain and add to bath water. Soak for 20 to 30 minutes to give the body time to absorb the herbal properties. Brush with a dry skin brush before the bath, and rub the body with the solids in the muslin bag, during the bath for best results.

❧A baking soda alkalizing bath is a simple but remarkable therapeutic treatment for detoxification. It is especially helpful when you are suffering from the repercussions of too little sleep, too much stress, excessive alcohol, caffeine or nicotine, a "hanging on" cold or flu, or the side effects of medication. Baking soda balances an over-acid system leaving you refreshed and invigorated, with extra soft skin.

❦How to take a baking soda bath:

Fill the bath with enough pleasantly hot water to cover you when you recline. Add 8-oz. baking soda and swirl to dissolve. Soak for 20 to 30 minutes. When you get out of the bath, wrap up in a big thick towel or a blanket and lie down for 15 minutes. This will help to overcome any feelings of weakness or dizziness that might occur from the heat and rapid toxin release. Zia of Zia Cosmetics recommends this rest time for a face mask, since the hot water will have opened up the pores for maximum benefits.

❧Hot & cold hydrotherapy opens and stimulates the body's vital energies. Alternating hot and cold showers, or even alternating hot and cold compresses, are very effective in putting the body on a positive track toward healing. Hydrotherapy stimulates sluggish circulation, relieves muscle aches and cramping, alleviates bowel and bladder congestion, tones muscles, and balances system energy for relaxation and stability.

❦How to use hot and cold hydrotherapy in the home:

Begin with a comfortably hot water shower for three minutes. Follow with a sudden change to cold water for two minutes. Repeat this cycle three times ending with cold. Rub the skin briskly with a rough towel for one minute to bring up circulation. Follow with mild exercise to stretches for best results.

You don't have to change the world, just take better care of it.

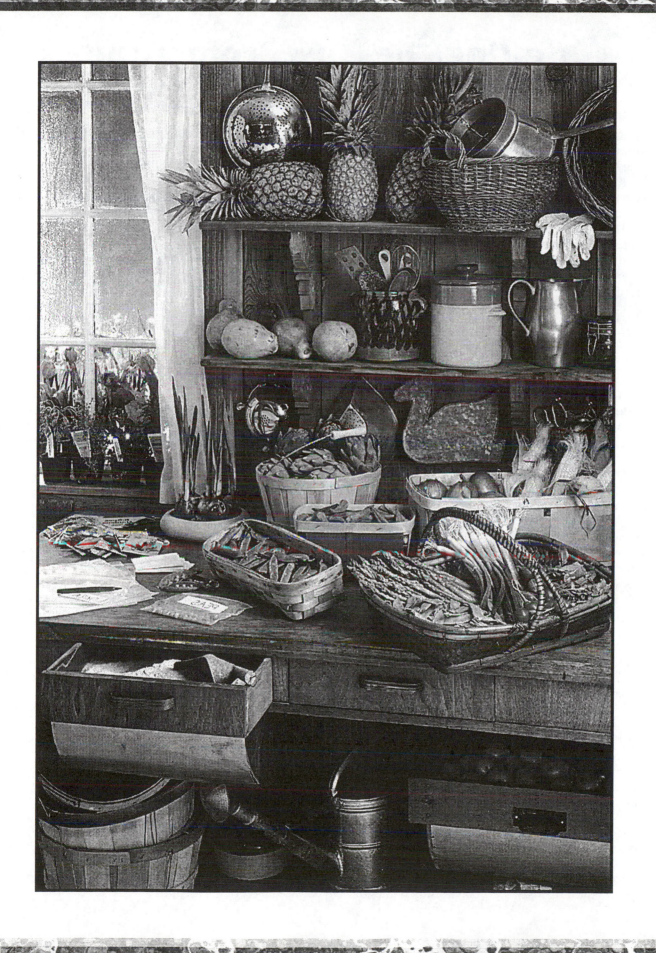

Getting The Most From Your Natural Food Pharmacy

Enjoy the changes of nature and the seasons, and flow with them for body harmony. Eat fruits in the summer for cooling, and root vegetables in the winter for building. Eating fruits and vegetables as they are harvested in your own area is a wonderful way to keep a closer touch with nature.

A personal working kitchen garden can do wonders for harmony of mind and body; even if you can't have a garden, eating the foods from your own region is a step toward being in harmony where you are. It helps keep the balance around us right, reminding us that we are all part of the natural chain.

The sun is the main energy source of the earth, and plants constitute the most direct method of conserving the energy we receive from the sun. Fruits, vegetables and grains do their best to attract us, to reach out to us, to make themselves beautiful and nourishing. There is no fear in them of being eaten as there is in animals. Their energy simply transforms into ours, and their life transmutes into the higher life form of man.

About Red Meats

Animals are closer to us on the bio-scale of life. They experience fear when killed. They don't want to be eaten. Unlike eating plants, there is no uplifting transmutation of energy. Instead our bodies become denser, with more internal fermentation and body odor. So, eating red meats tends to put us a step away from environmental harmony. Human digestive systems are not naturally or easily carnivorous, so the body has to struggle to transmute red meat energy. Meat eating is a lot like extracting oil out of the ground. It may cost more to get the oil than it is worth on the market. Thus the protein content of meat, which the body can use, is often cancelled out by the energy it takes to digest it, and the lethargic after-dinner feeling we get when a disproportionate amount of that energy goes to the task of digestion. Frequent intake of highly concentrated red meat protein can create toxic by-products of unused nitrogens that are hard for the elimination system to cope with or excrete.

In addition to humanitarian reasons, people are developing a new awareness about what meat-eating does to the body. Crop animals today are shot through with hormones and slow-release anti-biotics; their meat is preserved with nitrates and nitrites. These substances are passed into your body at the dinner table. Recent scientific studies show that human hormone activity is severely disrupted by excess exposure to the hormones and anti-biotics used on red meat animals. In addition, stockyard animals are often sick and overmedicated, and their meat is tainted, chemicalized and adulterated. Red meat is the biggest contributor to excess protein and saturated fat in the modern diet. No one argues that less fat in the diet is healthier, or that saturated fats are the most harmful. Eliminating red meat quickly reduces the saturated fat in our diets. Cooked red meats are acid-forming in the body; when cooked to well-done, the meat may create chemical compounds capable of causing many diseases.

Finally, meat eating promotes more aggressive behavior - a lack of gentleness in personality, and arrogance. From a spiritual point of view, red meats keep us tied to the material things in life, expansion of territory, and the self-righteous intolerance that makes adversaries. People who do not eat red meats have a well documented history of lower risk for heart disease, obesity, diabetes, osteoporosis and several types of cancer. These people also play an active role in conserving precious water, topsoil and energy resources that are wasted by an animal-based diet. Avoiding red meats has become one of the most important things you can do for your own health and that of the planet.

The following statistics are reprinted from Diet for a New America, by John Robbins. These incredible facts are gathered yearly by EarthSave, a non-profit organization in Felton, Ca. Environmental damage to the Earth's climate, land, water, and atmosphere tops the list of challenges for the 1990s. Many persons who are concerned about their personal health are equally concerned about the health of the planet. The information from the EarthSave study relates directly to the subject of meat-eating.

REALITIES 1990

"The diet of North Americans has changed significantly since 1900. Then, most meals were based on whole grain products, potatoes, fresh seasonal vegetables, and fruits - with meats consumed only occasionally. In recent years we have replaced this way of eating, rich in complex carbohydrates and fiber, low in fats and cholesterol, with a high-fat, low-fiber diet - largely based on meats and pasteurized dairy foods. By 1980, consumption of grains and potatoes had fallen to half of their 1900 levels, while the amount of fats has more than doubled. Such drastic dietary changes cannot occur without very significant consequences - for public health, the economy, and the environment."

☞ Human population of the United States: **260,000,000.**

☞ Human beings who could be fed by the grain and soybeans eaten by U.S. livestock: **over 1,300,000,000.**

☞ Amount of corn grown in U.S. eaten by human beings: **20%.**

☞ Amount of corn grown in the U.S. eaten by livestock: **80%.**

☞ Amount of oats grown in the U.S. eaten by livestock: **95%.**

☞ Amount of protein wasted by cycling grain through livestock: **90%.**

☞ Amount of carbohydrate wasted by cycling grain through livestock: **99%.**

☞ Amount of dietary fiber wasted by cycling grain through livestock: **100%.**

☞ How frequently a child in the world dies of starvation: **every 2.3 seconds.**

☞ Potatoes that can be grown on 1 acre of prime land: **20,000 pounds.**

☞ Beef that can be grown on 1 acre of prime land: **165 pounds.**

☞ Amount of U.S. agricultural land used to produce beef: **56%.**

☞ Grain and soybeans needed to produce 1 pound of edible flesh from feedlot beef: **16 pounds.**

☞ Protein fed to chickens to produce 1 pound of protein as chicken meat: **5 pounds.**

☞ Protein fed to hogs to produce 1 pound of protein from pork: **7.5 pounds.**

☞ Vegetarians who can be fed on the land needed to feed 1 person consuming a meat-based diet: **20.**

☞ Number of people who will die from malnutrition this year: **20,000,000.**

☞ Number of people who could be adequately fed from the land, water and energy freed from growing grains to feed U.S. livestock if Americans reduced their intake of meat by only 10%: **60,000,000.**

☞ User of more than **one half** of all water used for all purposes in the U.S.: **livestock production.**

☞ Water needed to produce 1 pound of wheat: **25 gallons.**

☞ Water needed to produce 1 pound of red meat: **2,500 gallons.**

☞ Quantity of water used in the production of the average cow sufficient to: **float a destroyer.**

♣

☞ Historic cause of downfall of many great civilations: **Topsoil depletion.**

☞ Amount of original U.S. topsoil lost to date: **75%.**

☞ Amount of U.S. cropland lost to soil erosion each year: **4,000,000 acres (the size of Connecticut)**

☞ Amount of U.S. topsoil loss directly associated with raising of livestock: **85%.**

☞ Number of acres of U.S. forest lands which have been clear cut to create cropland to produce a meat-centered diet: **260,000,000.**

☞ How often an acre of U.S. trees disappears: **Every 5 seconds.**

☞ Amount of trees spared per year by each person who switches to a vegetarian diet: **1 acre.**

♣

☞ Driving force behind the destruction of the world's tropical rain forests: **American meat diet.**

☞ Amount of meat imported annually by the U.S. from central and South America: **300,000,000 lbs.**

☞ Rate of species extinction due to destruction of tropical rain forests and related habitats: **1,000 per year.**

☞ Principle reason for U.S. military intervention in the Persian Gulf: **Dependence on foreign oil.**

☞ Length of time world's oil reserves would last if all human beings ate meat based diets: **13 years.**

☞ Length of time world's oil reserves would last if all human beings ate a vegetarian diets: **260 years.**

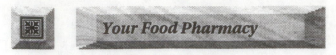

☞ Calories of fossil fuel expended to get 1 calorie of protein from beef: **78.**

☞ Calories of fossil fuel expended to get 1 calorie of protein from soybeans: **2** .

☞ Amount of all raw materials consumed by the U.S.that are devoted to livestock production: **33%.**

☞ Amount of all raw materials consumed in the U.S. needed to produce a vegetarian diet: **2%.**

✣

☞ Production of excrement by total U.S. population: **12,000 pounds per second.**

☞ Production of excrement by U.S. livestock: **250,000 pounds per second.**

☞ Sewage systems in U.S. cities: **Common.**

☞ Sewage systems in U.S. feedlots: **None.**

☞ Annual waste produced by U.S. livestock in feedlot operations which is not recycled: **1 billion tons.**

☞ Concentration of feedlot wastes compared to raw household sewage: **Ten to several hundred times more concentrated.**

☞ Where feedlot wastes often end up: **streams, rivers and ground water.**

✣

☞ Number of U.S. medical schools: **125.**

☞ Number of U.S. medical schools with required course in nutrition: **30.**

☞ Nutrition training received during 4 years of medical school by average U.S. physician: **2.5 hours.**

☞ Most common cause of death in the U.S.: **Heart attack.**

☞ How frequently a heart attack strikes in the U.S.: **Every 25 seconds.**

☞ How frequently a heart attack kills in the U.S. : **Every 45 seconds.**

☞ Risk of death by heart attack of average American man: **50%.**

☞ Risk of death by heart attack by the average U.S. vegetarian man: **15%.**

☞ Risk reduction for heart attack by reducing consumption of meat and dairy products by 10%: **9%.**

☞ Risk reduction for heart attack by reducing consumption of meat and dairy products by 50%: **45%.**

☞ Average cholesterol level of people eating a meat-centered diet: **210mg/dl.**

☞ Chance of dying from heart disease for a male with blood cholesterol of 210mg/dl: **Greater than 50%.**

☞ Chance of dying from heart disease if you do not eat cholesterol loaded red meats: **4%.**

☞ Leading sources of saturated fat and cholesterol in the American diet: **Red meat and dairy products.**

☞ Risk of breast cancer in women who eat meat daily compared to less than once a week: **4 times higher.**

☞ Risk of ovarian and breast cancer for women who eat butter and cheese 2 to 4 times a week compared to once a week: **3.2 times higher.**

☞ Risk of prostate cancer for men who eat red meat and dairy products daily as compared to sparingly: **3.6 times higher.**

♣

☞ Diseases linked to excess animal protein consumption: **Osteoporosis and kidney failure.**

☞ Number of cases of osteoporosis and kidney failure in the U.S.: **Tens of millions.**

☞ Average measurable bone loss of female meat-eaters at age 65: **35%.**

☞ Average measurable bone loss of female vegetarians at age 65: **18%.**

☞ Meat Board advertisements claim: **Today's meats are low in fat.**

☞ The Meat Board shows us: **A serving of beef they claim has 200 calories.**

☞ Reality: **The servings of beef they show us are only 3 oz. (half the size of an average serving of beef); and they have been surgically defatted with a scalpel.**

☞ The Dairy Industry claims: **Whole milk is only 3.5% fat.**

☞ Reality: **The 3.5% figure is based on weight and most of the weight in milk is water. The amount of** *fat* **calories in whole milk is 50%.**

☞ Dairy Industry advertising claims that: **Milk is nature's most perfect food.**

☞ Reality: **Milk is nature's most perfect food for a calf, who has four stomachs, will double its weight in 47 days, and can weigh up to 1000 pounds within a year.**

☞ Dairy Industry advertising claims: **To grow up big and strong, drink lots of milk.**

☞ Reality: **The enzyme for digestion of milk is lactase. 20% of Caucasians, and almost 90% of blacks and Asians have no lactase tolerance. They get cramps, bloating and diarrhea from drinking milk.**

❦

☞ The meat and dairy industries claim: **Animal products constitute 2 of the 4 basic food groups.**

☞ Reality: There were originally **12 official food groups before these industries applied enormous pressure on behalf of their products.**

☞ The meat and dairy industries claim: **We are well-fed with animal products.**

☞ Reality: **Listed below are the diseases which can be commonly prevented, consistently improved, and sometimes cured by a low-fat diet free of saturated-fat animal products include:**

❦Stroke and Heart Disease ❦Kidney and Gall Stones ❦Prostate Cancer ❦Cervical and Ovarian Cancer ❦Diabetes ❦Ulcers ❦Hiatal Hernia ❦Asthma ❦Irritable Bowel Syndrome ❦High Blood Pressure ❦Diverticulitis ❦Colon Cancer ❦Pancreatic Cancer ❦Endometrial Cancer ❦Stomach Cancer ❦Trichinosis ❦Hypoglycemia ❦Hemorrhoids ❦Constipation ❦Obesity ❦Osteoporosis ❦Breast Cancer

⚜

☞ Pesticide residues in the U.S. diet from meat: **55%.**

☞ Pesticide residues in the U.S. diet supplied by dairy products: **23%.**

☞ Pesticide residues in the U.S. diet supplied by vegetables: **6%.**

☞ Pesticide residues in the U.S. diet supplied by grains: **1%.**

☞ Pesticide residues in the U.S. diet supplied by fruits: **4%.**

☞ Amount of pesticide residues in breast milk of meat-eating U.S. mothers: **99%.**

☞ Amount of pesticide residues in breast milk of vegetarian mothers: **8%.**

☞ Percentage of male college students sterile in 1950: **0.5%.**

☞ Percentage of college students sterile in 1980: **27%.**

☞ Sperm count of average American male compared to 30 years ago: **Down 30%.**

☞ Principle reason for sterility and low sperm counts in U.S. males: **Chlorinated hydrocarbon pesticides.**

☞ Meat industry advertises that pesticides in our beef are not a concern because: **Quantities are so small.**

☞ Reality: **One ounce of dioxin can kill 1 million people.**

☞ Common belief: **The USDA protects our health through meat inspection.**

☞ Reality: **Less than 1 out of every quarter million slaughtered animals are tested for toxic residues.**

☞ Number of animals killed for meat in U.S.: **500,000 per hour.**

☞ Cost to render an animal unconscious prior to slaughter humanely with captive bolt bullet: **1 penny.**

☞ Reason given by meat industry for not using captive bolt pistol: **Too expensive.**

☞ Percentage of antibiotics routinely fed to U.S. livestock: **55%**

☞ Staphylococcus infections resistant to penicillin in 1960: **13%.**

☞ Staphylococcus infections resistant to penicillin in 1988: **91%.**

☞ Effectiveness of all antibiotics to staph infections: **Declining rapidly.**

☞ Major contributing cause: **The breeding of antibiotic resistant bacteria in factory farms due to routine feeding of antibiotics to livestock.**

☞ Response of entire European Economic Community to routine feeding of antibiotics to livestock: **Ban**

☞ Response of American pharmaceutical industry to routine feeding of antibiotics to livetock: **Full and complete support.**

☞ Health status of vegetarians from many world populations according to the Food & Nutrition Board of the National Academy of Sciences: **Excellent.**

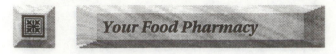

✳ *About Water*

Water is second only to oxygen in importance for health. It makes up 65 to 75% of the body, and every cell requires water to perform its essential functions. Water maintains system equilibrium, lubricates, flushes wastes and toxins, hydrates the skin, regulates body temperature, acts as a shock absorber for joints, bones and muscles, adds needed minerals, and transports nutrients, minerals, vitamins, proteins and sugars for assimilation. Water cleanses the body inside and out.

When the body gets enough water, it works at its peak. Fluid and sodium retention decrease, gland and hormone functions improve, the liver breaks down and releases more fat, and hunger is curtailed. To maintain this wonderful internal environment, you must drink plenty of water every day, at least six to eight glasses to replace lost electrolytes and metabolic waste fluid.

Thirst is not a reliable signal that your body needs water. Thirst is an evolutionary development designed to indicate **severe dehydration.** You can easily lose a quart or more of water during activities such as skiing or running before thirst is even recognized. The thirst signal also shuts off before you have had enough for well-being. You must pay conscious attention to getting enough water every day.

Plain or carbonated cool water is the best way to replace lost body fluid. Second best are unsweetened fruit juices diluted with water or seltzer, and vegetable juices. Alcohol and caffeine-containing drinks are counter-productive in replacing water loss because of their diuretic properties. Drinks loaded with dissolved sugars or milk **increase** the body's water needs, instead of satisfying them.

Unfortunately, most of our tap water today is chlorinated, fluoridated, and treated to the point where it can be an irritating disagreeable fluid instead of a delicious elixir. Some city tap water may contain as many as 500 different disease-causing bacteria, viruses and parasites. Toxic chemicals and heavy metals used by industry and agriculture have found their way into ground water, adding more pollutants. Some tap water is now so bad, that without the enormous effort our bodies use to dispose of these chemicals, we would ingest enough of them to turn us to stone by the time we were thirty! Concern about this lack of purity is leading more and more people to bottled water.

For a healing program, several types of water are worth consideration.

❦**Mineral water** - usually comes from natural springs with varying mineral content and widely varying taste. The naturally occurring minerals are beneficial to digestion and regularity, and in Europe this form of bottled water has become a fine art. Only government regulated for purity in California and Florida.

❦**Distilled water** - either from a spring or tap source, is "de-mineralized" so that only oxygen and hydrogen remain. This is accomplished by reverse osmosis, filtering or boiling, then conversion to steam and recondensing. It is the purest water available, and ideal for a healing program.

❦**Sparkling water** - from natural carbonation in underground springs. Most are also artificially infused with CO_2 to maintain a standard fizz. An aid to digestion, and excellent in cooking to tenderize and give lightness to a recipe.

❦**Artesian well water** - the cadillac of natural waters, it always comes from a deep pure source, has a slight fizz from bubbling up under rock pressure, and is tapped by a drilled well. It never comes in contact with ground contaminants.

Note: Beyond buying bottled water, you can also take steps as an individual to conserve water and diminish pollution: ♣Use biodegradable soaps and detergents. ♣Don't use water fresheners in your toilets. ♣Avoid pouring hazardous wastes such as paint, solvents, or petroleum-based oils into drains or sewers. ♣Use natural fertilizers such as manure and compost in your garden. ♣Avoid using non-biodegradable plastics and polystyrene. ♣Conserve water with conscious attention to what you really need for a shower, bath, laundry or cooking.

※ *About Caffeine*

Like most of mankind's other pleasures, there is good news and bad news about caffeine. Moderate use of caffeine has been hailed for centuries for its therapeutic benefits. Every major society uses xanthine-containing plants stimulants like caffeine in some food form to overcome fatigue, handle pain, open breathing, control weight and jump-start circulation. Caffeine is a part of both foods and medications today; coffee, black and green tea, colas, sodas, analgesics such as Excedrin, over-the-counter stimulants, such as Vivarin, chocolate and cocoa to name a few.

There is solid evidence for the positive effects of caffeine on mental performance, clearer thinking, shortened reaction time, and increased capacity for attention-requiring tasks. It can increase alertness through the release of adrenaline into the bloodstream. It mobilizes fatty acids into the circulatory system, facilitating greater energy production, endurance and work output. Its benefits toward weight loss have long been known since caffeine promotes enhanced metabolism and the burning of fat. It has a direct potentiating effect on muscle contraction for both long and short-term sports and workout activity.

Some of the health problems it can cause are also well known - headaches and migraines, irritability, stomach and digestive problems, and chronic fatigue. As an addictive stimulant it works as a drug, causing jumpiness and nerves, heart disease, heart palpitations.

Caffeine can produce oxalic acid in the system, causing a host of problems waiting to become diseases. It leaches B vitamins out of the body, particularly thiamine (which controls stress). It can lodge in the liver restricting its proper function, and constrict arterial blood flow. Over-use of caffeine affects the glands, particularly the adrenals, to exhaustion, causing hormonal imbalances to the point of becoming a major factor in the growth of breast and uterine fibroids in women, and prostate trouble in men. It is definitely indicated in PMS symptoms, bladder infections, hypoglycemic and diabetic sugar reactions.

Specific areas of health and the effects of caffeine include:

♣**Caffeine and Pregnancy** - caffeine should be avoided during pregnancy. Like alcohol, it can cross the placenta and affect the fetus' brain, central nervous system and circulation.

♣**Caffeine and Breast Disease** - there is official uncertainty about the link between caffeine and breast fibroids, **but our own experience shows improvement when caffeine intake is decreased or avoided.**

♣**Caffeine and Heart Disease** - heavy coffee drinking has been directly implicated in heart disease.

♣**Caffeine and Sleep Quality** - caffeine consumed late in the day or at night jeopardizes the quality of sleep by disrupting brain wave patterns. It also means you will take longer to get to sleep.

♣**Caffeine and Ulcers** - caffeine stimulates gastic secretions, sometimes leading to a nervous stomach, but it has not been linked to either gastric or duodenal ulcers.

♣**Caffeine and Headaches** - caffeine definitely causes headaches in some people - and causes withdrawal headaches when avoided after regular use.

♣**Caffeine and PMS** - caffeine causes congestion through a cellular overproduction of fibrous tissue and cyst fluids. Reducing or abstaining from caffeine affords PMS relief.

Caffeine is just as difficult as any other addiction to overcome, but if you have any of the above-mentioned problems, it is worth going through the temporary withdrawal symptoms. Improvement in the problem condition is often noticed right away.

However the carcinogenic effects often blamed on caffeine are now thought to be caused by the roasting process used in making coffee, tea and chocolate. Since even decaffeinated coffee has been implicated in some forms of organ cancer, conclusions are being drawn that caffeine is not the culprit - the roasted hydro-carbons are.

There are lots of good foods to help break the caffeine habit: herbs teas, delicious coffee substitutes such as Roma, carob treats instead of chocolate, plain aspirin in place of Excedrin, and energy supportive herbal pick-me-ups with no harmful stimulants of any kind.

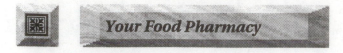

✖ *About a Low Salt Diet*

In the past generation, Americans have consumed more salt than ever before; too much restaurant food, too many processed and refined foods, too many animal foods. Most people are aware that excessive salt causes heart disease, hypertension, and blood pressure problems. Circulation is constricted, kidneys malfunction, fluid is retained, and migraines occur frequently. Too much salt can produce hyperactivity, aggressive behavior, and poor glandular health.

A salt free diet is obviously desirable for someone who eats too much salt. However, once the body's salinity normalizes, some salt should be brought back into the diet quickly. Adequate salinity is needed for good intestinal tone, strong blood, tissue transportation of nutrients, healthy organs and glands. Too little, or no salt can lead to lack of vitality, stagnated blood and loss of clear thinking.

Regular table salt is almost totally devoid of nutritional value, but there are many other ways to get the good salts that the body needs. Tamari, soy sauce, shoyu, misos, umeboshi plums, sea plants and washed, sun-dried sea salt, herb salts and seasonings, sesame salt, and naturally fermented foods such as pickles, relishes and olives all have enzymes and alkalizing properties that make salts usable and absorbable. **LOW SALT, NOT NO SALT, is best for a permanent way of eating.**

✖ *About Fats & Oils*

We all know that there is a direct relationship between the quantity of fat we consume and the quality of health we can expect. During this century, Americans have increased their intake of fat calories by over 33%. The link between high salt and fat intake has also become clear. Excess salt inhibits the body's capacity to clear fat from the bloodstream. Warnings and discussions about fat have filled the media in America for a decade. But much of the information is contradictory and inaccurate. This section should simplify the confusion, especially as it relates to choices made for a healing diet.

Saturated & Unsaturated Fats:

All foods contain saturated and unsaturated fats in various proportions, the difference is in molecular structure, with animal foods higher in saturated fat, and except for tropical palm and coconut oils, vegetable foods higher in unsaturated fat. Saturated fats are solid at room temperature, as in butter or meat fat. They are the culprits that clog our arteries, and lead to heart and degenerative disease. Unsaturated fat. (mono-or-poly-unsaturated) is liquid at room temperature, as in vegetable or nut oils. Although research supports unsaturates as helping to reduce serum cholesterol, just switching to unsaturated fats without increasing dietary fiber will not bring about improvement. In fact, consuming moderate amounts of both kinds of fats, should be coupled with a high fiber diet to benefit most people.

Hydrogenated fats:

Hydrogenation is the process of taking a poly-unsaturated oil and bubbling hydrogen through it to cause reconstruction of the chemical bonds to delay rancidity. It makes unsaturated fats such as corn oil into saturated fats such as margarine. Much testing has shown that these altered fats are comparable to animal fats in terms of saturation and lack of usability by the body. A good alternative to margarine or shortening, much lower in saturated fat, is a combination of equal amounts of warm butter with vegetable oil.

Omega-3 & Omega-6 Fatty Acids:

◆**Omega-3 oils** are a family of fatty acids high in EPA (eicosapentaenoic acid), DHA (dihomogammalinolenic acid), and gamma linolenic acid. They include cold water fish oils, walnut oil, canola oil, wheat germ oil, evening primrose oil and flax oil. Research has indicated that treatments for P.M.S, high blood pressure and rheumatoid arthritis benefit from the use of these fatty acids. Omega-3 oils are also a specific for the 30% of the population trying to keep serum cholesterol levels low.

*Omega-6 oils** are the group of fatty acids high in linoleic and arachadonic acids, and include sesame, sunflower, safflower and corn oil. Both Omega-3 and Omega-6 fatty acids stimulate the formation of prostaglandins.

*Prostaglandins** are produced by every cell in the body, and control such things as reproduction and fertility, inflammation, immunity and communication between cells. They also inhibit the over-production of thromboxane, a substance in the body that promotes clotting. Because blood clots in narrowed arteries, (the major cause of heart attacks), they are essential to health.

Lipids: Cholesterol & Triglycerides:

*Lipid** is an inclusive term for a group of fats and fat-like substances essential to human health. Lipids are found in every cell, and are integral to membrane, blood and tissue structure, hormone/ prostaglandin production, and nervous system functions.

*Triglycerides** are dietary fats and oils, used as fuel by the body, and as an energy source for metabolism.

*Phospholipids** are fats such as lecithin, and **cholesterol,** vital to cell membranes, nerve fibers and bile salts, and a precursor for sex hormones.

HDLs & LDLs (High and Low Density Lipo-proteins):

*Lipoproteins**, water-soluble, protein covered bundles, transport cholesterol through the bloodstream, and are synthesized in the liver and intestinal tract. LDLs, (low-density lipo-proteins, or "bad cholesterol,") carry cholesterol through the bloodstream for cell-building needs, but leave behind the excess on artery walls and tissues. HDLs, (high density lipo-proteins, or "good cholesterol,") help prevent narrowing of the artery walls by removing the excess cholesterol and transporting it to the liver for excretion as bile.

Mono-&-Poly-unsaturated fats:

*Olive oil** is a mono-unsaturated fat that reduces the amount of LDL in the bloodstream. Research shows that it is even more effective in this process than a low-fat diet. Another oil high in mono-unsaturated fats is canola or rapeseed oil.

*Poly-unsaturated vegetable oils** are the chief source of the "essential fatty acids" (linoleic, linolenic and arachidonic) so necessary to cell membrane function, prostaglandin production and many other metabolic processes. Good poly-unsaturates include sunflower, safflower, sesame oil, and flax oil, one of the greatest sources of essential fatty acids.

Vegetable oils:

All vegetable oils are free of cholesterol, but some contain synthetic preservatives and are heavily refined, bleached and deodorized with chemical solvents. Others are simply mechanically pressed, filtered and bottled. The highest quality fresh vegetable oils are rich in Omega fatty acids and essential to health in their ability to stimulate prostaglandin levels.

*Unrefined oils** that are expeller or mechanically pressed go through the least processing and are the most natural. (**Cold pressing** applies only to olive oil.) They are dark with some sediment, and a taste and odor of the raw material used.

*Solvent extracted oil** is a second pressing from the first pressing residue. Hexane is generally used to enable the most efficient extraction, and is then burned off at about 300∞ to evaporate the hexane. Even though small amounts of this petroleum chemical remain, it is still considered an unrefined oil.

*Refined oils** go through several other processing stages, such as de-gumming, which keep the oil from going rancid quickly, but also removes many nutrients, including vitamin E. It is de-pigmented through charcoal or clay, clarified through deodorizing under very high temperatures, and preservatives are added. At this final stage , the oil is clear, odorless, and almost totally devoid of nutrients.

See the WHOLE FOODS GLOSSARY on page 228 for a complete listing and description of oils.
Note: Natural oils are fragile and become rancid quickly. They should be stored in a dark cupboard or in the refrigerator. Purchase small bottles if you don't use much oil in your cooking.

※ *About Sea Vegetables & Iodine Therapy*

Sea vegetables and iodine-rich herbs have superior nutritional content. They transmit the energies of the sea and earth as rich sources of vitamins, minerals, proteins, and complex carbohydrates. **Ounce for ounce they are higher in vitamins and minerals than any other food group,** and are rich in Omega-3 oils. They convert inorganic minerals into organic mineral salts that combine with amino acids. Our bodies use this combination as an ideal way to get effective nutrients for structural building blocks. In fact, sea vegetables combined with some specific herbs contain all the necessary trace elements for life, many of which are depleted in the earth's soil.

Sea vegetables and herbs are almost the only non-animal sources of Vitamin B12, which is necessary for cell growth and nerve function. They also provide effective carotene, chlorophyll, enzymes and fiber. The mineral balance of sea plants is a natural chelated combination of potassium, sodium, calcium, phosphorus, magnesium, iron, and trace minerals. It is a natural tranquilizer for building sound nerve structure, and good metabolism. These plants alkalize the body, lower cholesterol, reduce excess stores of fluid and fat, and work to neutralize toxic metals in the system (including radiation), into harmless salts that the body can eliminate. They purify the blood from acidic effects of the modern diet, allowing for better absorption of nutrients. They strengthen the body against disease.

In this era of processed foods and iodine-poor soils, **sea vegetables, sea foods and certain iodine containing herbs** stand almost alone as potent sources of natural Iodine. Iodine is essential to life, since the thyroid gland cannot regulate metabolism without it. Iodine is an important element of alert, rapid brain activity, and a prime deterrent to arterial plaque. Iodine is also a key factor in the control and prevention of many gland deficiency conditions that are prevalent today; breast and uterine fibroids, tumors, prostate inflammation, adrenal exhaustion, and toxic liver and kidney states. Pregnant women who have inadequate iodine are more prone to giving birth to cretin babies, a form of retardation.

Preventive nutritional measures may be taken against these problems by adding 2 tablespoons of snipped or crushed dried sea vegetables and/or iodine-rich herbs to your daily diet.

In addressing the concern about harvests coming from polluted waters, two inherent properties and one fact about sea vegetables should be noted:

1) The alginic acids in sea vegetables bind with the ions of heavy metals which are then converted to harmless salts that are not soluble in the intestine, and are naturally excreted.

2) Sea vegetables **actually chelate radioactive matter already in the body**, and bind it for elimination via the large intestine.

3) Macrobiotic quality sea vegetables are gathered from waters noted for their cleanliness.

※ *About Green Superfoods*

Green foods are a rich source of essential nutrients. We are all adding more salads and green vegetables to our diets for better health. However, because of the great concern for the nutritional quality of produce grown on mineral depleted soils, supplemental green superfoods, such as chlorella, spirulina, barley green, wheat grass and alfalfa have become popular. Nutritionally more potent than regular foods, they are carefully grown and harvested to maximize vitamin, mineral and amino acid concentrations.

Green, and blue-green algae have been called perfect superfoods because of their abundant, easily assimilable amounts of high quality protein, fiber, chlorophyll, vitamins, minerals and enzymes. They are therapeutically successful with the power to stimulate immune response, improve digestion, detoxify body systems, accelerate healing with healthy tissue growth and repair, protect against radiation toxins, help prevent degenerative disease and promote longer life.

The green grasses contain all the known mineral and trace mineral elements, a balanced range of vitamins, and hundreds of enzymes for digestion and absorption. The small molecular proteins in these plants can be absorbed directly into the blood for cell metabolism. They are highly therapeutic from the chlorophyll activity absorbed directly through the cell membranes.

Chlorella contains a higher concentration of chlorophyll than any other known plant. It is a complete protein food, including the B vitamins, vitamin C and E and many minerals in amounts high enough to be considered supplementary. The cell wall material of chlorella has a particular effect on intestinal and bowel health, detoxifying the colon, stimulating peristaltic activity, and promoting the growth of beneficial bacteria. Chlorella is effective in eliminating heavy metals, such as lead, mercury, copper and cadmium. Anti-tumor research has shown that it is an important source of beta carotene. It strengthens the liver, the body's major detoxifying organ, so that it can rid the system of pathogenic infective agents that destroy immune defenses. It helps arthritis stiffness, lowers blood pressure, relieves gastritis and ulcers. Its rich nutritional content has made it effective in weight loss programs, both for cleansing ability, and in maintaining muscle tone during reduced food intake. But its most importent benefits come from a combination of molecules that biochemists call the *Controlled Growth Factor*, a unique composition that provides a a noticeable increase in sustained energy and immune health when eaten on a regular basis.

Spirulina is the original high nutrient superfood, an easily produced algae with the ability to grow in both ocean and alkaine waters. It is ecologically sound because it can be cultivated without prime land or fresh water, in extreme environments which are useless for conventional agriculture. It can be grown on small scale community farms, in such a variety of climates and growing conditions that it can significantly improve the nutrition of local populations currently on the brink of starvation. Research has shown that spirulina alone could double the protein available to human beings on a just a fraction of the earth's land, while helping to restore a balanced environment to the planet. It is a complete protein, providing all 21 amino acids, and the entire B complex of vitamins, including B12. It is rich in beta carotene, in minerals, trace minerals, and essential fatty acids. As with chlorella, digestibility is high, stimulating immediate, long range energy.

Barley Grass contains a broad spectrum of concentrated vitamins, minerals, enzymes, proteins and chlorophyllins. It has eleven times the calcium of cow's milk, five times the iron of spinach, and seven times the amount of vitamin C and bioflavonoids as orange juice. One of its most important contributions is to a vegetarian diet where it is difficult to get B_{12}, because it has 80mcg of vitamin B_{12} per hundred grams of powdered juice. Much research has been done on barley grass with encouraging results for DNA damage repair and anti-aging activity.

Wheat Grass has great curative powers when taken as a fresh liquid for many degenerative, "incurable" diseases. Fifteen pounds of fresh wheat grass are equal in nutritional value to 350 pounds of the most choice vegetables. In tablet or powder form it provides highly concentrated food for both people and animals who need more dietary greens and roughage.

Alfalfa is one of the world's richest mineral foods, pulling up earth resources from root depths as great as 130 feet! It is the basis for liquid chlorophyll, with a balance of chemical and mineral constitutuents almost identical to human hemoglobin.

In essence, eating any of these green superfoods is like giving yourself a little transfusion to help treat illness, enhance immunity and sustain well-being. They have a synergistic and beneficial effect when added to a normal diet. The green superfoods are valuable in almost every healing diet. Over the years we have found the incredible claims about their valuable benefits to have substance and truth.

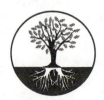

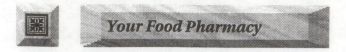

❋ *About Natural Wines*

Naturally fermented wine is more than an alcoholic beverage. It is a complex biological fluid possessing definite physiological values. Wine is still a living food, and can combine with, and aid the body like yogurt or other fermented foods. Many small, family owned wineries make chemical and additive-free wines that retain the inherent nutrients from the grapes, including absorbable B vitamins, and minerals and trace minerals such as potassium, magnesium, organic sodium, iron, calcium and phosphorus.

Wine is a highly useful drink for digestion, and in moderation, as a calmative for the heart, arteries and blood pressure. In fact, tests have shown that a glass or two of white wine with dinner can cut heart disease risk by 50%.

Recent studies at U.C. Berkeley have shown that red wine contains the extremely potent anti-carcinogen quercetin, a chemical that can reverse tumor development.

Because of its high density lipoproteins, wine can free the circulation, relieve pain and reduce acid production in the body. It is superior to tranquilizers or drugs for relief of nervous stress and tension.

Wine's importance should not be overlooked in a weight loss or fitness program, because a little wine relaxes. When you are relaxed, you tend to eat less.

ALWAYS USE IN MODERATION.

Note: Liquor other than wines is not recommended, even for cooking, when you are involved in a healing program. Although most people can stand a little hard spirits without undue effect, and alcohol burns off in cooking, the concentrated sugar residues won't help a recovering body.

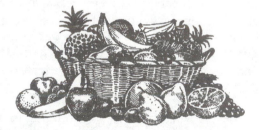

❋ *About Fruits*   **Fresh fruits are nature's way of smiling.**

Fruits are wonderful for a quick, internal system wash and cleanse. Their high natural water and sugar content speeds up metabolism to release wastes rapidly. Fresh fruit has an alkalizing effect in the body, and is high in vitamins and nutrition. The easily convertible natural sugars transform into quick non-fattening energy that speeds up the calorie burning process.

But these advantages are only true of **fresh** fruits. With fruit, the way that you eat it is as important as what you eat. Cooking fruits changes their alkalizing properties to acid-forming in the body. This is also true of sulphured dried fruit, and the combination of fruit with vegetables or grains. Eating fruits in these fashions causes digestion to slow down, and usually causes gas, as the high fruit sugars stay too long in the stomach allowing rapid fermentation instead of assimilation.

Fruits have their best healing and nutritional effects when eaten alone or with other fruits, as in a fruit salad, separately from grains and vegetables. With a few exceptions, both fruits and fruit juices should be taken before noon for best energy conversion and cleansing benefits.

Eat organically grown fruits whenever possible. The quick metabolism of fruits allows pesticides, sprays to enter the body very rapidly.

❈ *About Medicinal Herbs*

Herbs as natural medicines have a unique healing spirit, with wide ranging properties, and far reaching possibilities for therapeutic activity. We are just beginning to scratch the surface of their forgotten magnitude and acclaim. The history of herbal healing is long and rich from the beginning of man's rise on earth, yet it is also perfectly adaptable to today's requirements, with the same focused strength and reliability. Herbs are more than a scientific, or even a natural healing system. Universal truths show through herbs; we can see them as an art, as tools of metaphysical Nature as well as of Science. Herbs react integrally with each individual person. They can help with almost every aspect of human need, and like all great realities of Nature, there is so much more than we shall ever know.

Many men and women today realize the value of herbs as alternative therapy that they themselves can use safely and easily. Hundreds of herbs are regularly available in several usable forms and at all quality levels. Worldwide communications and improved storage allow us to simultaneously obtain and use herbs from different countries and different harvests, an advantage ages past did not enjoy. Even standardized active ingredients from herbs are widely available in extractions if desired.

How Herbal Formulas Work

Herbs are concentrated foods, whole essences, with the ability to address both symptoms and causes of a problem. As nourishment, herbs can offer the body nutrients it does not always receive, either from poor diet, or environmental deficiencies in the soil and air. As medicine, herbs are essentially body balancers, that work with the body functions, so that it can heal and regulate itself.

Herbs pave the way for the body to do its own work, by breaking up toxins, cleansng, lubricating, toning and supporting. Herbal combinations are not addictive or habit-forming, even in extract form, and very small doses can be used over a period of time to help build a healthy base for restoring body balance. When correctly used, herbs promote the elimination of waste matter and toxins from the system by simple natural means. They support nature in the fight against disease. Like Nature, and all natural processes, there are no instant panaceas. But herbs are powerful agents that are cumulative in the body and should be used with care.

While herbs certainly have medicinal qualities, they are not drugs. Do not expect the activity or response that form the basis for chemical anti-biotics or tranquilizers. These agents only treat the symptoms of a problem. Herbal healing works differently than drug-based medicine. Results will seem to take much longer. But this fact only shows how herbs actually work, at a deeper level of the body processes, acting as support in controlling and reversing the cause of the problem, a much more permanent effect. Even so, some improvement from herbal treatment can usually be felt in three to six days. Chronic and long standing degenertion will, of course take longer. A good rule of thumb is generally one month of healing for every year of the problem.

As in other forms of natural therapeutics, there is sometimes a "healing crisis" in an herbal healing program. This is traditionally known as the "Law of Cure," and simply means that sometimes you will seem to get worse before you get better. The body frequently begins to eliminate toxic wastes quite heavily during the first stages of a system cleansing therapy. This is particularly true in the traditional three to four day fast that many people use to begin a serious healing program. Herbal therapy without a fast works more slowly and gently. Still, there is usually discomfort and weakness felt as disease poisons are released into the bloodstream to be flushed away. Strength and relief shortly return when this process is over. We have found that watching for this phenomenon allows you to observe your body processes at work toward healing, - a very interesting experience indeed.

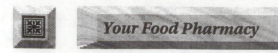
Tips on taking herbal combinations:

1) A 24 hour juice fast before starting an herbal formula will often produce greater effectiveness.

2) Take capsules with a warm drink for faster results. (Do not take with citrus juice if the formula contains a Ginseng.)

3) Abstain from alcohol, red meat, caffeine and tobacco if possible during use to give the herbs a cleaner environment in which to work.

4) Herbs work best with a natural foods diet. Everyone can benefit from herbal mixtures, but the more you are eating naturally, the more you can expect to receive their advantages.

5) Herbs are concentrated foods, and are identified by the body as such. They are quickly assimilated by digestive enzyme action. With a few exceptions, they should be taken before or with meals.

6) Herbs work better in combination than they do singly. Most combinations should be taken no more than 6 days in a row, with a rest on the seventh day before resuming, to allow the body to regularly restore its own balance.

Therapeutic herbs work best when combined with a natural foods diet. Everyone can benefit from an herbal formula, but results increase dramatically when fresh foods and whole grains form the basis of the diet. Subtle healing properties are more effective when they don't have to labor through excess waste material, mucous, or junk food accumulation. (Most of us carry around 10-15 pounds of excess density.)

Interestingly enough, herbs themselves can help counter the problems of "civilization foods." Herbs are high in minerals and trace minerals, the basic elements missing or diminished in today's "quick-grow," over-sprayed, over-fertilized farming. In addition to their other attributes, minerals and trace minerals are the bonding agents between you and your food, and a basic element in food assimilation. Mineral-rich herbs provide not only the healing essences to support the body in overcoming disease, but also the foundation that allows it to take them in!

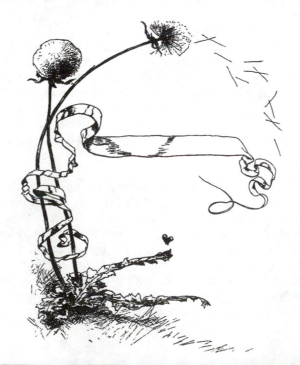

Balancing Your System Type

Over the years, we have seen and heard from literally thousands of people with individual nutritionally related health problems. We have gradually noticed that people with the same food preferences and much the same eating habits, fall prey to the same type of disease conditions.

❦Congestive diseases, like arthritis, constipation, eczema, bursitis, respiratory problems, gallbladder and kidney stones, blood pressure and heart problems, arterioscleriosis, hemorrhoids, overweight, candida and vaginal yeasts, diverticular disease, varicose veins, and hypoglycemia, seem to afflict people who like soft, creamy foods. Ice cream and other creamy desserts, potatoes and squashes, chocolate, pastas with creamy sauces, macaroni and cheese, dairy products, especially milk and cheeses, soft breads and sandwiches, cakes and pastries, Italian foods, and creamy fruits are good examples of these kinds of foods.

❦Corrosive diseases, like staph and strep infections, virus infections like Epstein Barr virus and chronic fatigue syndrome, liver problems, mononucleosis; degenerative diseases like cancer, leukemia, multiple sclerosis and muscular dystrophy; digestive problems, colitis and spastic colon, hiatal hernia, herpes, hepatitis, toxic shock, ulcers, and skin cancers, seem to affect people who eat lots of hard, brittle, crunchy foods. Crackers, sodas, cookies, celery, carrots and broccoli, Chinese and Mexican foods, spicy and condiment seasoning foods, hard candies, coffee, crunchy fruits, etc. are good examples of these kinds of foods.

We have noticed this so many times, it is worth consideration as part of identifying an individual imbalance for yourself. Consider using it to provide more balancing foods to achieve better body equilibrium and harmony.

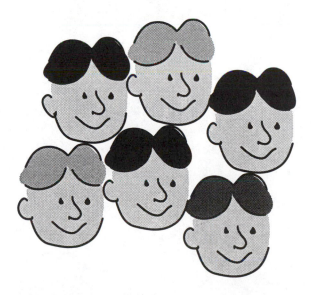

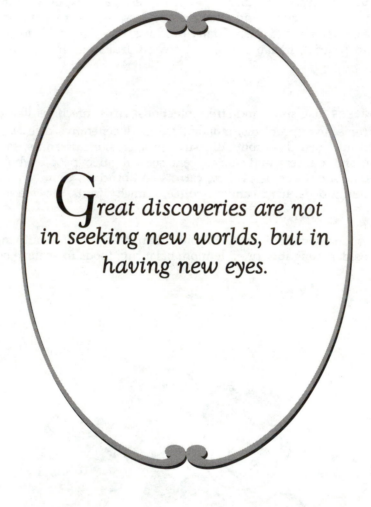

Great discoveries are not in seeking new worlds, but in having new eyes.

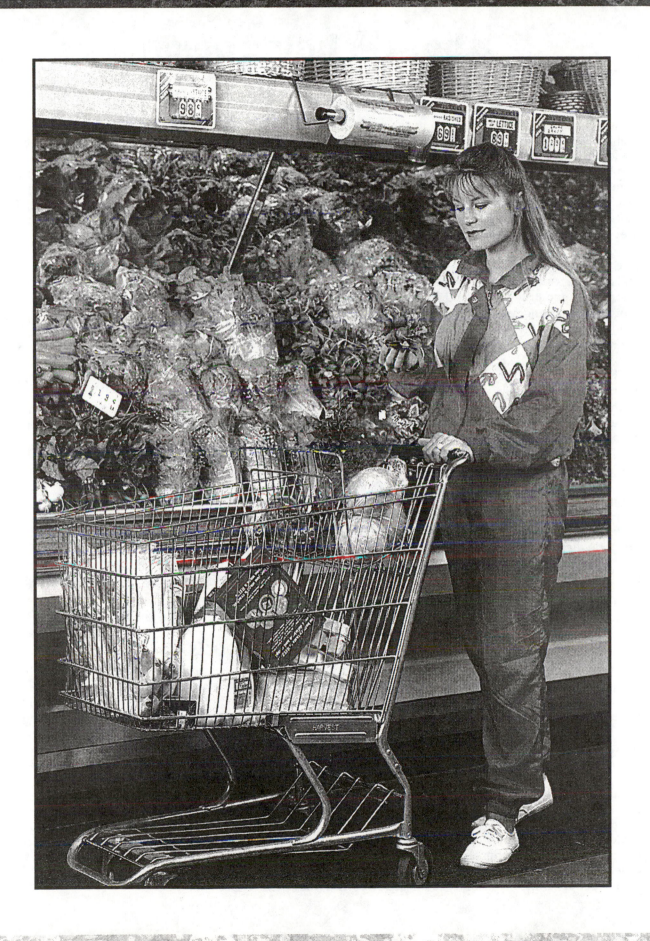

About Whole Foods

✴ *Whole Foods and the Senses*

Sometimes we get so caught up in the nutritional values of our foods, or the separate components as fuel and healing factors (the amount of fat, the number of calories, the concentration of proteins, etc.) that we lose the enjoyment of eating, and the oneness we share with the living growing things that nourish us. Food affects the way we feel more than just through assimilation and digestion. Cooking creates health. It is an end as well as a means; a source of relaxation and pleasure. It is something we are involved with and react to every day. Appreciation of the way foods influence our senses can make meal planning much more interesting, and add other dimensions to a healing diet. The beauty and anticipation of a carefully prepared meal are well known, but the ingredients themselves in the fresh state are also beautiful.

The natural colors of foods for instance, can generate many subtle feelings. Fresh foods are "solar grown and cooked," and contain the inherent solar vibrations from their growing, visible to us by a predominate color. Light and brightly colored foods, such as fruits, make us feel lighter, and expansive. Darker colored root vegetables and grains make us feel more solid and earthbound. Traditionally, red-toned foods seem to increase vigor and elimination, blue and violet foods relax, green foods give strength and balance to life, yellow and orange foods increase circulation and brain activity.

The touch of fresh foods, their shape and feel, communicate to us even before we eat them, providing a certain anticipation about texture and temperature in the mouth.

The aroma and smell of foods, increases the appetite and starts the digestive process when the "mouth waters." As the diet becomes fresher and more natural, this sense sharpens, and even familar scents become enhanced. Could the smell of a fresh lemon drive you wild?

Food sounds can be pure enjoyment; the crunch of a tart apple, the snap of a carrot or celery, the tender crisp sizzle of a fresh stir-fry, the slow bubble of a soup pot. Sound can tell you when just the right amount of cooking has been done.

But the taste is the test. Taste buds originally served the function of telling us what was good and what was harmful to the body. For most of us, years of eating refined, over-processed and non-food foods have dulled this sensibility. Taste buds can be fooled by tobacco, chemical foods and drugs. The optimal nutrition diets and recipes in this book can greatly improve the sense of taste.

A healing diet can be pleasant, and an important part of the rest of your life. People are always amazed at how really good food tastes when the body begins to rebuild and rebalance with diet improvement.

⚜

✴ *Avoiding Refined and Processed Foods*

Much has been said about the health problems from eating refined, preserved, pasteurized, waxed, hydrogenated, canned, smoked, cured, irradiated, colored, additive-laden, adulterated foods. Some of it bears discussion here. Refining and processing removes many needed minerals, trace minerals and vitamins from foods, and these can't be chemically "added back" later in their original state to make the food wholesome again. Not only are additives and chemicals incapable of supporting life themselves, when combined with whole foods, the food itself is chemically changed, and the life-sustaining ability diminished. In addition, microorganisms and bacteria can develop resistance to ion radiation and other preservatives, so that food can still appear edible when it is seriously contaminated.

All refining processes lower nutrient and life-support value. Even when food values are given on a package, they are derived from standard testing results done on the food in its fresh unsprayed state, not its processed state. All of us have washed heads of lettuce, or greens, and seen the water turn soapy, or peeled cucumbers, apples or eggplant to remove the wax. Many grocery markets brag that their produce is in the store the day after it is picked; surely freshness-retaining chemicals are not needed for so short a time. Most processing is needed for economic, not nutritive, reasons; for longer shelf life, unnatural perfection of appearance, the ability to offer strawberries from Chile in December, etc.

Below are some startling new facts released by Omni Magazine and The Fact Book on Food Additives about the effect of food additives and preservatives.

☞Over **10,000 chemicals** are used as food additives in one way or another in pre-prepared foods before they reach our tables.

☞More than 1000 of these chemicals **have never been tested** for the potential to cause cancer, genetic damage or birth defects. Modern processing methods compound the problem by removing many nutrients that could naturally protect the body from harmful effects.

☞More than 80% of all food purchased in grocery stores today is processed or refined. The typical fast food meal of a hamburger, shake and french fries, **contains 22 chemical additives**, 12 of which even in fairly small amounts are known to be toxic.

☞The average American consumes over **nine pounds of additives** annually.

☞According to the AMA, autopsies of American soldiers between the ages of 18 and 22 killed in World War II showed no signs of atherosclerosis. In autopsies of American youths killed in Viet Nam, **almost all had atherosclerosis at some stage.**

☞Rejection of Armed Forces volunteers for physical and mental deficiencies is well over **40%.**

☞In tests of 10,000 business executives, doctors found only **1 in 10** to be in general good health.

☞In the last 10 year period, the number of patients admitted to hospitals for serious degenerative diseases has increased **5 times faster** than the growth of the population as a whole.

☞In "The Impact of Nutrition on the Health of Americans," Dr. Joseph Beasley states that some conditions and symptoms of degenerative disease now afflict upward of **100,000,000 Americans.** Dr Beasley calls this phenomenon the Malnutrition-Poisoning Syndrome.

What can you do? Buy seasonal produce, locally and organically grown whenever possible. Fix it yourself for the best results on a healing diet. It can make a big difference to the success of your program. **Remind yourself that only whole foods are wholesome.**

⚜

✿ *Cooking Essentials & Techniques with Whole Foods*

A healthy healing diet can change your way of cooking because it incorporates new, different ingredients. This may be a bit daunting and frustrating to handle all at once - especially when you have a family, and want to keep everybody happy by fixing their favorite meals.

*This section can help. We've "done it all" over the last twenty years; changing over to whole foods and ingredients, substituting other high protein foods for meats, making recipes rich without dairy products, lightening heavy dishes - and lowering fat in everything. The recipes in this book are essentially a synthesis of these changes and techniques. A good starting point is deciding **what to avoid**. None of the following things are in this book:*

☛**Red meats of any kind:** both for ecological and health reasons. (See About Red Meats, page 206).

☛**Table salt:** the recipes in this book use sesame salt, herbal blends, natual sea salt, and low salt tamari instead of table salt; and only low sodium relishes, olives and condiments. (See page 642, Making Your Own Salts & Seasonings.)

☛**Fried and deep fried foods:** all become saturated with fat, hard to digest, and hard on the arteries. (See page 344, Low-Fat & Very Low-Fat section.)

☛**White flour, or refined flours of any kind:** flour in most of the recipes in this book is a mix of whole flours, easy to buy and make.

☛**Pasteurized dairy products:** they are too mucous-forming, allergy-aggravating, and clogging for a cleansing or healing diet. Happily, they are not necessary for richness or good taste. There are many other healthy choices; raw milk and cheeses, yogurt and yogurt cheese, soy milk and soy cheeses, kefir and kefir cheese, and almond milk. (See page 391, Dairy Free Cooking.)

☛**Too much caffeine:** coffee, black tea, chocolate, cocoa, soft drinks, or caffeine-containing analgesics such as Excedrin, or other oxalic acid-producing foods, (See page 211, About Caffeine.)

☛**Hard Liquor or Beer:** we cook frequently but lightly with dry wines, to "keep the pipes clean," relax the body, ease digestion, and lend a delicious rich taste to foods that are low in fats and calories. But we use no other alcoholic products in this book. Beer is too high in calories. Hard liquor and liqueurs are too high in sugars. (See page 216, About Natural Wines.)

☛**Pre-prepared, processed, or convenience foods:** they usually have too much salt, and other, "hidden" ingredients that won't help a healing diet. Optimal nutrition needs fresh, untreated foods.

✤

▒ *The Art of Substituting*

When you move away from a meat-based, saturated fat, sugary foods diet, it is important to know that you can still enjoy most of your favorite dishes simply by making substitutions. If you have food allergies, sensitivities or intolerances, substitutions become necessary to be able to enjoy eating without the foods that are causing the problems. The healing diets and recipes in this book successfully substitute healthy foods for many traditional popular dishes. The following section includes easy, delicious, healthier exchange foods for meats, dairy products, wheat, salt, and sugar, so that you can substitute in your own favorite recipes.

❦ *Substitutes for Meats:*

❀Tofu - may be used as a one-for-one substitute for ground meat in recipes. Use tofu fresh, or frozen, thawed, squeezed out, and sliced or crumbled. It may be baked or sautéed. You can prepare tofu in almost every way you would use meat.

❀Tempeh - plain or frozen and thawed, as a one-for-one substitute for red meats.

❀Dried beans and legumes - soaked and cooked; then used as a one-for-one substitute for red meats.

❀Falafel or grain burger mixes - mix with water as directed, and substitute for any ground meat.

❦ *Substitutes for Dairy Products:* (See also DAIRY-FREE COOKING in this book.)

Milk & Cream Substitutes:

❀Soymilk - plain, or vanilla; substitute equal amounts for milk or cream.

❀Yogurt and water mixed to the consistency of milk; use in equal amounts for milk or buttermilk. Yogurt can also be homemade with soy milk or nut milk.

❀Kefir - plain flavor may be substituted in equal amounts for milk, buttermilk or half-and-half.

❀Almond milk, or other nut milks - an excellent substitute in gravies, soups and sauces. (See recipe on page 391 .) Use cup for cup in place of milk in recipes.

❀Tahini milk - made by adding 1 TB. sesame tahini to 8-oz. water with a little honey; use equally as milk in recipes.

❀Amazake rice drink - blend 1/2 cup with 2 cups of water to use equally as milk in recipes.

❀Fruit juice -use to taste to replace milk in recipes, or on dry cereals.

❀Water - use to replace milk in hot cereals, and in baked recipes for a dry, crunchy taste, instead of smooth, moist texture.

❦Chickpea miso - mix with stock and seasonings and use in equal amounts for milk, especially in macrobiotic diets.

❦Lecithin granules - mix into sauces or gravies to emulsify and thicken without using milk or cream.

Ice Cream Substitutes:

❦Rice Dream, or soy-based ice cream desserts.

❦Bananas - peeled and frozen, then cut into chunks, blended with fruits or juices and re-frozen.

❦Lecithin granules - mix one to two tablespoons into frozen desserts to emulsify without cream.

Cheese Substitutes:

❦Tofu -sliced, marinated, and used in cold or hot sandwiches.

❦Yogurt cheese - see how to make on page 392. Use as a substitute for cream or cottage cheese.

❦Kefir cheese - use in equal amounts as a substitute for sour cream, cream cheese or cottage cheese.

❦Soy cheese - comes in many different consistencies and flavors. Use in equal amounts as a substitute for mozzarella, cheddar, jack or cream cheese.

❦Low-fat or non-fat cottage cheese - a healthy substitute for cream cheese, mozzarella, ricotta and full fat cottage cheese. Use one-for-one as a replacement value.

❦Mochi - grate and substitute for cheese toppings for melted cheese texture.

Sour Cream Substitutes:

❦Tofu -see recipe in the DAIRY-FREE COOKING section.

❦Yogurt - substitute equal amounts for sour cream.

❦A half and half mix of yogurt and mayonnaise - use as an equal amount substitute for sour cream.

Butter Substitutes:

❦Vegetable oil - use in equal amounts for butter in sauces, dressings, gravies, baking, and sautéing.

❦Vegetable or onion broth - substitute for butter in sautées, braising, sauces and gravies.

❦Clarified butter - for less saturated fat, simply melt butter and skim off top foam. Use the clear butter in recipes as a substitute for full fat butter.

Egg Substitutes:

❦Egg Replacers - use as directed for leavening and binding in recipes.

❦Dry yeast or sourdough - use as a leavening agent in place of eggs.

❦Starchy vegetables, applesauce, flaxseed and water mix, or almond butter - use as a substitute binding agent in place of eggs.

❦Tofu - fresh and crumbled in place of scrambled eggs, and in some recipes. Experiment to your taste.

✶Substitutes for Wheat, Gluten, Yeast: (See also Wheat-Free Baking in this book.)

❦Yeasted bread substitutes - Rye breads, rice cakes, mochi, corn tortillas, chapatis, Essene bread, flat bread, quick breads, and pancakes made with baking powder.

❦Corn, vegetable pasta, 100% buckwheat soba, frozen/thawed tofu -use as substitute for wheat pasta.

❦Crackers - made with 100% rye or rice flour are available everywhere.

❦Cooked grains - substitute barley, millet, buckwheat.

❦Cereals - including cream of rice, puffed rice, rice crispies and rice flakes; cream of rye and rye flakes; corn flakes, puffed corn and corn germ; puffed millet, cream of buckwheat, oat bran and oatmeal, wheat free granola.

❦Starchy vegetables - puree and substitute in recipes for bread, grains or pasta.

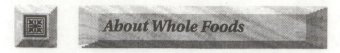

☙ *Substitutes for Salt:*

● Mineral salts and seasonings - robust kelp, sea vegetables and herbs mixes. Use to taste.

● Herbal seasonings - these have no or very low sodium. Use to taste.

● Miso - use to taste in casseroles, gravies, soups and sauces; a little goes a long way.

● Shoyu or tamari - use to taste in any dish needing more salt.

● Spices and citrus zests - use singly or mixed to taste in place of salt in sweet or savory recipes.

☙ *Substitutes for Sugar:*

● Honey - Use $1/2$ cup to replace 1 cup of sugar; reduce recipe liquid by $1/4$ cup.

● Maple syrup - use $1/2$ to $2/3$ cup to replace 1 cup of sugar; reduce recipe liquid by $1/4$ cup.

● Molasses -use $1/2$ cup to replace 1 cup of sugar; reduce recipe liquid by $1/4$ cup.

● Malt syrup - use 1 to 1 1/4 cups to replace 1 cup of sugar; reduce recipe liquid by $1/4$ cup.

● Apple juice or other fruit juice - use 1 cup to replace 1 cup of sugar; reduce recipe liquid by $1/4$ cup.

● Fructose - use $1/3$ to $2/3$ cup to replace 1 cup of sugar.

● Date sugar - use one-for-one to replace 1 cup of sugar.

● Sucanat - use one-for-one to replace 1 cup of sugar.

● Stevia ribaudana (sweet herb) - make into a strong liquid infusion; store tightly covered in the refrigerator, and use sparingly in beverages and recipes (25 times sweeter than sugar).

● Vanilla, cinnamon, cardamom - use to replace sugar toppings and in sweet dessert sauces.

☙ *Substitutes for Citrus:*

● Apple Cider vinegar - substitute one-for-one in recipes.

⚜

▨ *Healthy Cooking Techniques with Whole Foods*

*Sometimes it isn't just **what** you eat, its the **way** you cook it that means success for a healing diet. The following section includes the best methods for getting the optimum nutrition and healing benefits from food.*

☙ *Healthy Techniques with Vegetables :*

● When steaming vegetables, always have water boiling first. Add a few liquid smoke drops to the water for an outside grill taste if desired, then add the veggies.

● Parboil vegetables in seasoned water or light broth for crunchiness, color and flavor. Boil liquid first, add veggies, and just simmer until color changes. (Save the cooking liquid for use in the recipe.) Drain immediately, run under cold water to set color, then chill for a salad, or toss in a hot pan with a little butter, broth or tamari to heat through. Squeeze a little lemon juice over for tang.

● Concentrate flavors of zucchini, tomatoes and eggplant by sprinkling with sesame or herb salt. Let sit in a colander over the sink for 10 to 15 minutes, then press out moisture. It really makes a difference.

● Dry salad greens thoroughly after washing by rolling them in paper towels, or by using a salad spinner. The greens will be crisper, and need less dressing for taste.

● Invest in a Salad Shooter. It makes your salad look and taste professional. Keep it out on your work area. It's small, easy to clean, and will encourage you to have a salad every day.

● When stir-fry/steaming, heat the wok first; then add oil, and heat to very hot. Then add veggies and stir-fry fast to seal in nutrients. Turn down heat to low, add sauce, cover, and steam til sauce bubbles.

● If you are using a juicer in your healing diet, use the carrot and apple pulp from juicing in place of grated apples or carrots in recipes, such as in muffins or quick breads, or other baked dishes.

● Lightly steaming carrots releases bio-available carotenoids, (cancer preventing substances) better.

❦ *Healthy Techniques with Poultry:*

- Have poultry at room temperature before cooking. Pat meat dry.
- Freeze bones and trimmings in plastic bags to use for making stock. Oven roast bones and carcasses before making stock to add even richer flavor.
- When baking stuffings or cornbread separately for a roast turkey or chicken dinner, use a cast iron skillet for increased flavor and texture.

❦ *Healthy Techniques for Eggs:*

- When beating eggs to "stiff but not dry," always add a pinch of cream of tartar to maintain lightness and puff. Another secret for lightness in soufflés, dumplings, crepes, and omelets is simply gentleness. Work with a light hand when you work with eggs - no vigorous stirring or beating.
- Poach eggs in a light broth or bouillon instead of water for better flavor and to maintain shape.

❦ *Healthy Techniques with Pasta:*

Mushy, or tough pasta can ruin a meal. Attention is the key. Stay with it all the way once the cooking has started.

- Be sure you use a very large pot. Probably the largest one you have will be perfect.
- Use a lot of water, so pasta can easily swim and separate when cooking. The more water, the less gummy the pasta. Add 1 TB. oil to the water so it won't boil over and pasta strands will separate.
- Bring the water to a swift rolling boil. Add 1 teasp. salt to lift the flavor.
- **Be sure your sauce is ready by this point.**
- Add pasta to the water slowly, in batches so the water won't stop boiling. Stir after each batch to keep pasta separated. Keep the water at a fast boil, even covering it briefly to insure continuous boiling.
- Fresh pasta cooks very fast, in 2 to 6 minutes. Watch it every second, and start testing for doneness in 2 or 3 minutes. Dry pasta cooks in about 8 to 20 minutes, depending on its size and shape. Start testing for doneness at about 6 to 7 minutes. Remove a strand or piece with a fork and bite into it. If it isn't still hard, and it isn't mushy, it's al dente (to the tooth) and it's done.
- Drain immediately, adding a little cold water to the pot first to stop the cooking. Draining into a colander is the easiest way. Do not rinse unless pasta is to be used for a cold salad.
- Add sauce right away and serve. If sauce can't be added right away, toss with a little oil. (To re-heat pasta before saucing, put it in a bowl of hot water, and stir to let pieces gently separate.)

❦ *The Healthy Way to Use Oils*

- Use only vegetable, nut or seed oils, mechanically, expeller, or cold-pressed.
- Use oils for quick sautées, in salad dressings, and as a replacement for butter in baking and sauces. **Never deep-fat fry when you are on a healing program**.
- Don't re-use cooking oils that have been heated.
- Store all cooking oils in the refrigerator after they have been opened.

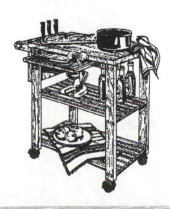

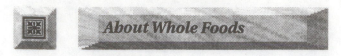
❧ *Healthy Crusts, Toppings, and Coatings:*

Crusts, toppings, sprinkles and coatings are an important part of a recipe. The foundation should be as healthy as the filling. A quiche, pie, or casserole is a layered dish, to be built from the bottom up. (Also see the index for individual crust and topping recipes).

Low-fat, thin crusts for pizzas, quiches, and vegetable tarts:

- Use crushed, whole grain cracker crumbs, either plain, or sprinkled with a little low oil dressing or tamari. Bake until crispy; about 10 minutes at 375°; then fill.
- Split chapatis or pita bread halves **horizontally**, or use whole wheat or corn tortillas. Toast briefly for crispiness; lay on the bottom of your baking dish and top with filling.
- Thin slice tofu blocks horizontally. Bake with a little oil at 350° for firmness before filling.
- Spread crispy Chinese noodles on the bottom of the baking dish. Toast in the oven; then add filling.
- Sprinkle toasted nuts and seeds to cover bottom of the baking dish. Add seasoning salt, and fill.
- Spread cooked brown rice to cover the bottom and sides of a lecithin-sprayed baking dish. Toast at 375° to crisp and dry slightly; then fill.
- For the ultimate easy crust, use **any cooked whole grain or vegetable leftovers,** and whirl in the blender to a paste. Press into a lecithin-sprayed baking dish, crisp in a 400° oven for 10 minutes, and voila! you have an original, easy crust for a new quiche, casserole, or savory pie.

Low-fat crusts for dessert pies, tarts and custards:

- Toast wheat germ in the oven. Mix with a little date sugar or honey to sweeten, and spread on bottom and sides of baking dish. Toast again briefly and fill.
- Use toasted nuts and seeds, ground and sweetened with a little date sugar or honey. Spread on the bottom and sides of baking dish. Toast again briefly for crunch, and fill.
- Use juice-sweetened sugarless cookie crumbs. Press onto bottom and sides of baking dish. Toast briefly and fill.
- Sprinkle date sugar (ground up dates), or maple syrup granules, or maple sugar on bottom of a custard or dessert dish. Broil briefly to caramelize; then fill and bake as usual. Yum.

See page 647 for a gourmet flour mix if you wish to make a healthy conventional crust. Whole grains produce a lighter, slightly nutty pastry.

Casserole foundations -a unique cooking art;

Avoid the calories and density of a crust a casserole foundation. Quiches and casseroles become new dishes, but still give a favorite filling something good to rest on. Cover the bottom of the baking dish with any of the following:

- Hard boiled eggs;
- Left over cooked brown rice or other whole grain;
- Spaghetti squash, cooked and briefly toasted;
- Zucchini or tomato rounds.

For both bottoms and toppings:

- Chinese-noodles, toasted;
- Whole grain granola, toasted;
- Whole grain chips, crushed slightly and toasted.

Healthy low-fat, low salt coatings for seafood, poultry and veggies:

Mix any of the following with yogurt, or mixed egg and water; coat food and chill briefly before baking.

- Toasted wheat germ;
- Crushed whole grain chips;
- Falafel or tofu burger mix.

※ *About Culinary Herbs*

*Cooking with fresh herbs is an easy, healthy way to season food. One of the nicest things you can do for your kitchen is to plant an herb garden. It can be any size, from raised beds to a window box. Whatever you can manage is worth it for taste and health. Pick fresh only the amount you need each time. Dry the rest on screens or an herb drying rack when the season for an is over. **Basil, chervil, chives and parsley** are mild and compatible with almost all other herbs. They are best fresh-chopped right before use. **Bay, marjoram, oregano, savory and thyme** are congenial with other herbs, stand up well in cooking, and may be used fresh or dried. **Coriander, dill, mints, rosemary, sage and tarragon** add distinct flavors, and should be used with a light hand, since their strong tastes do not work with everything. To substitute fresh herbs for dried in recipes, use three times as much as is called for.*

♣**Basils** have a peppery, clove/anise taste. Add them freshly chopped to vegetable sautées, omelettes and sauces, or toss onto salads. They are especially compatible with all squashes, tomatoes, eggs and vinaigrette dressings, and are the basis for traditional pestos. Store by drying the leaves on screens, pureeing in olive oil and freezing; or mincing, blending into butter and freezing.

♣**Bay leaves** have a complex, spicy, scent. They are not meant to be eaten, but are excellent in marinades for fish or seafood, and for simmering in soups, stews or tomato sauces. Preserve by hanging sprigs upside down to dry, and store in airtight containers.

♣**Chervil** looks and tastes like parsley with a hint of anise. Add freshly chopped at the last minute, to eggs, peas, mushrooms, soups and fish. To store, add minced to butter and freeze.

♣**Chives** have a mild, sweet, oniony flavor. Add them freshly chopped at the last minute to vegetables, soups, mayonnaise, dressings and sauces. To store, add chopped to butter and freeze.

♣**Coriander (cilantro)** may be used like parsley, but has a very different taste - citrusy, cool and minty. The seeds have an orangy flavor, excellent in teas and baking. Add freshly chopped at the last minute to seafood, vegetables, guacamole or curries. Coriander is a specific for Indian, Asian and southwestern cooking. To preserve, puree in olive oil and freeze.

♣**Dill weed** has a caraway taste. It is best used fresh, but is a good dry substitute for flavoring yogurt dips and dressings, soups, sauces and vegetables. To store, steep sprigs in vinegar, or hang them upside down to dry, then keep in an airtight container.

♣**Marjoram** has a mild, earthy taste similar to oregano. It is good in egg and cheese recipes, and with avocados, mushrooms, tomatoes and potatoes. To dry, hang upside down, and store air tight.

♣**Mints** have light to very potent flavor. They are good fresh in salads, for savory sauces, for sweet dishes such as custards, and as flavoring for drinks, or in tea. They are specifics in Middle Eastern and Asian cooking. Hang upside down to dry.

♣**Oregano** has a bittersweet, spicy taste. Use in marinades for seafoods, or in dressings for salads. It is compatible with cheeses, salsas, yogurt, beans and rice and South-of-the-Border cooking. Hang upside down to dry on the stem. Store airtight.

♣**Parsley** is mild, fresh-tasting and full of chlorophyll. Add it just before serving. Chop and steep it in olive oil as a base for sautées or soup. It is so available and easy to grow, that there is no need to store it.

♣**Rosemary** has a strong, piny taste. Use fresh or dry in marinades, simmered soups and sauces. It is excellent with pizza or potatoes. A little goes a long way. Dry upside down, or steep in olive oil.

♣**Sage** has a warm, potent musky taste. A specific for poultry and stuffing seasoning, sage is also compatible with tomato, egg and cheese dishes. Cook fresh leaves in butter until crisp to lightly top pasta. Hang upside down to dry, and store air tight.

♣**Savory** has a lemony taste. Use with fish and sea foods, beans, tomato sauce and dressings. Hang sprigs upside down to dry, and store airtight.

♣**Tarragon** has a sweet, spicy, licorice taste. Add chopped to tomato-based soups, mushrooms, beets, salads, eggs amd poultry. Steep in vinegar to store; then drain and chop leaves as needed.

♣**Thyme** has a balmy, pungent taste. It is an essential for stocks, soups, sauces and marinades. Thyme is excellent with roast poultry, egg dishes, seafood and fish. Hang bunches upside down to dry, then freeze or store airtight.

The Inside Story
Special ingredients that make your diet more healthy

We use many ingredients of exceptional quality and kind in the healing diets. The following pages are a glossary of the properties and benefits of each, to offer you more understanding about what these high nutrition foods can do for your health. An added advantage about many of these unusual foods is that they are also a part of gourmet cooking. While you are improving your health, you can also improve your palate!

ADUKI BEANS - Japanese beans which are very low-fat and easily digested.

AGAR-AGAR - a good vegetarian substitute for gelatin; derived from several species of sea algae. Buy it in flakes, and use it like gelatin - 1 TB. of flakes to gel 1 cup of liquid. Let it slowly soften in cold water, and then slowly simmer to dissolve. Agar-Agar has almost no taste, no calories, and is mostly fiber.

ALOE VERA - long in use for burns and skin care in gel form, aloe juice is now becoming widely known for its digestive and soothing laxative properties.

AMARANTH - an ancient Aztec grain, now being rediscovered in America, amaranth contains very high quality protein, as well as a high concentration of the amino acid lysine. This grain has been found compatible with a diet to control candida albicans yeast overgrowth.

AMAZAKE - a thick, rich pudding-like mixture made from fermented sweet brown rice. It can be eaten like pudding, used as a base for desserts, or as a high protein, satisfying beverage.

ARROWROOT - powdered cassava plant, used as a thickener when a shiny sauce is desired. It can be used as a less processed substitute for cornstarch, without the digestive problems cornstarch can cause.

BAKING POWDER - aluminum free, such as Rumford's.

BARLEY - a low gluten flour with a slightly sweet malty taste. We use it as part of a four and whole grain mix to lend a nice chewy texture to cookies and muffins.

BARLEY GRASS - see GREEN SUPERFOODS SECTION.

BARLEY MALT SYRUP - a mild natural sweetener made from barley sprouts and water, and cooked to a syrup. It has a pleasant flavor that is delicious in cookies, muffins and quick breads, and is only 40% as sweet as sugar.

BASMATI RICE - a uniquely delicious aromatic whole grain rice, originally from India, but now also being grown as a hybrid in Texas. In our opinion, this is the Cadillac of rice; better for you than white rice, lighter, easier to digest than brown rice.

BEE POLLEN - collected by bees from male seed flowers, mixed with secretion from the bee, and formed into granules. Bee pollen is a highly concentrated, perfectly balanced food, notable for possessing all the essential amino acids. It is often used as an antidote during allergy season. 2 teasp. daily is the usual dose.

BEE PROPOLIS - a product collected by bees from the resin under the bark of certain trees. It is an antibacterial and antibiotic substance that stimulates the thymus gland and thus boosts immunity, and resistance to infection.

BLACK BEANS - a Mexican staple with rice. Black beans are an excellent source of absorbable protein; and particularly good as an alkalizing soup.

BRAN - often called miller's bran, the outside shell of the grain, well known these days for its fiber content. Use it as part of a flour mix for texture. A dose of 1 to 2 tablespoons a day with liquid is plenty for regularity and digestion.

BREWER' S YEAST - an excellent source of protein, B vitamins, and some amino acids and minerals. Easy to take, 1 to 2 teaspoons in a protein drink offer an excellent daily lift. Brewer's yeast is not the same as candida albicans yeast. It is one of the best-immune-enhancing supplements available in food form.

BUCKWHEAT - when this grain is roasted, it is known as kasha, a nutty seed popular in casseroles and pilafs. Use the flour as part of a baking mix for milder taste.

CANOLA OIL - from the rapeseed plant; high in mono-unsaturated fats, with 10% omega-3 fatty acids, and half the amount of saturated fat found in other vegetable oils.

CAPERS - the flower buds of a Mediterranean shrub, pickled in salt water and vinegar, and used as a condiment.

CAROB POWDER - a sweet powder with 45% natural sugars, made from the seed pods of a Mediterranean tree. It has a flavor similar to chocolate, but contains less fat and no caffeine. It may be used raw or roasted as a substitute for cocoa in recipes.

CHAPATIS - Indian flat bread; use as a whole grain pizza crust or sandwich "wrap."

CHEESE - (see page 223, and 391-392 on essentials of low-fat, raw, and non-dairy cheeses). Rennet free cheeses use a bacteria culture, instead of calves enzymes to separate curds and whey. Goat cheese (chevre) and sheep's milk cheese (feta) are both lower in fat than cow's milk cheeses, and are more easily digested. Authentic mozzarella cheese is made from buffalo milk, and is now becoming available on the west coast and in New York - absolutely delicious! Low sodium cheeses are now made in almost every type of cheese, and are an obviously better choice for a healing program. You'll never miss the high salt taste.

CHILI PEPPERS - the immature pods of various peppers, such as anaheim, ancho, cayenne, jalapeno, etc., used to add heat and color to Mexican dishes. Fresh chilies can burn both eyes and skin. Be careful. Handle them with gloves. Broil them until blistered, then allow them to steam in a paper bag. Run under cold water, slip off skin, and remove seeds and veins before using.

CHLORELLA - a tiny one-celled algae plant, known and grown as a superfood; full of proteins, high chlorophyllins, fiber, beta-carotene and many other high quality nutrients. The list of chlorella benefits is long and almost miraculous, from detoxification to energy enhancement, to immune system restoration. (See GREEN SUPERFOODS SECTION, pages 214 and 215.)

CHUTNEY - a sweet, spicy relish condiment of Indian cooking. Natural food stores carry fruit and honey-sweetened varieties.

CILANTRO - fresh coriander leaves, used in Mexican, Chinese and Spanish cooking. The dried herb has almost no flavor. Use cilantro fresh, or substitute parsley.

COUSCOUS - precooked semolina, very light, low calorie; easy and quick to fix.

CRACKERS, WHOLE GRAIN - much more flavorful than those made with white flour; an excellent choice for complex carbohydrates without the density of breads. There are many varieties and flavors to choose from, with no lard preservatives or colors, and lower salt content.

CREAM OF TARTAR - tartaric acid, commonly used as a leavening in baking, and to help incorporate into egg whites. Substitute $1/2$ teasp. cream of tartar and $1/2$ teasp. baking soda for 1 teasp. double acting baking powder.

DAIKON RADISH - a mild, almost sweet radish used in macrobiotic and Japanese cooking; it may be eaten shredded fresh or stir-fried, and has the therapeutic benefit of gentle diuretic action.

DASHI - a basic healing soup stock and broth used in macrociotic and Japanese cooking. Make it by simmering a 6" peice of Kombu sea weed with 1 or 2 chopped shiitake mushrooms and 2 teasp. tamari in water.

DATE SUGAR - ground up dates. When used in baking, mix with water and then add to recipe to prevent burning. Sprinkle on as a sweet topping **after** removing your dish from the oven or stove.

DULSE - the most often eaten sea vegetable, with excellent taste and good alkalizing properties. Crumble over vegetables, soups and salads, use in seasonings and savory dishes, or as an effective dieting tea.

EGG REPLACER - a combination of starches and leavening agents used to replace those qualities of eggs in baking. It is a vegetarian product, cholesterol free.

ENOKI MUSHROOMS - very tender tiny mushrooms with long slender stems, they are delicious barely heated or eaten raw in a salad for exotic taste.

ESSENE BREAD - a sprouted bread of wheat or rye, with no flour, oil , sweetener, salt or leavening. Perfect for those on a restricted, initial diet for allergies, food intolerances or candida albicans.

FENNEL/ANISE - a wonderful licorice flavored vegetable that is mild enough to use fresh in salads, and good in stuffing mixes. Very exotic; a little goes a long way.

FLAX SEED OIL - a high omega-3 oil that has medicinal and cooking uses. An excellent source of unsaturated fatty acids. (See ABOUT OILS, page 225, and 212.)

FRUCTOSE - a highly refined sweetener that is twice as sweet as white sugar. It is, however, absorbed more slowly into the bloodstream than sugar and does not require insulin for assimilation. Use only half the amount as regular sugar in cooking. However, if you are hypoglycemic or diabetic, fructose is still sugar and should be used very carefully.

GARBANZO BEANS - meaty, high protein beans. They take a long time to ccok, but are excellent in dips and authentic falafels.

GINGER - a flavorful, aromatic, spicy herb, both fresh and dried ginger have therapeutic properties for digestive and other problems. Use pickled ginger in oriental dishes, and fresh ginger in many recipes to lend a different flavor to old favorites. There is an easy way to have fresh ginger on hand without spoilage. Peel fresh roots, chop in the blender, put in a plastic bag, and freeze. Ginger thaws almost immediately. In about 10 minutes, it' s ready for use.

GOMASHIO - a mixture of sesame seeds and sea salt. Originally only used in oriental cooking, it is a delicious lower sodium alternative to table salt, and an excellent cooking and baking salt.

GRANOLA - for healing purposes, granola can be good high fiber nutrition; but check ingredients carefully, so the kind you eat isn't high in fat or sweeteners.

KASHI - a delicious 7 grain pilaf mix, available puffed for a cold cereal, & cooked as a grain base for almost any rice or pasta type dish. It has a chewy, nutty texture, and a taste unlike any single grain. Kashi is an excellent source of protein, complex carbohydrates and fiber. Ground into a flour, it is healthy and delicious for all baked goods.

KEFIR - a fermented milk product, it comes plain or fruit-flavored, and may be taken as a liquid or used like yogurt or sour cream. Kefir provides friendly intestinal flora.

KUZU - a Japanese and macrobiotic diet powdered thickening root. Kuzu is superior for imparting a shine and sparkle to stir-fried foods and clear sauces.

LECITHIN - a soy derived granular product, used as a stabilizer and emulsifier to improve smoothness and may be substituted for one-third of the oil in recipes for a healing diet. It is also a therapeutic food, and 2 teasp. daily may be added to almost any food for its superior phosphatides, choline, inositol, potassium and linoleic acid.

LEMON JUICE POWDER - dehydrated lemon juice, lemon solids and lemon oil; much easier to keep on hand than fresh lemons, it may be substituted for fresh lemon juice in dressings, beverages, or baking.

MILLET - a quick-cooking, balanced amino acid grain, acceptable for those with wheat allergies and candida albicans yeast.

MISO - is a fermented soybean paste that is a basic medicinal food. It is very alkalizing to the system, lowers cholesterol, represses carcinogens, helps neutralize allergens, pollutants, and the effects of smoking on the body, and provides an immune-enhancing environment. Unpasteurized miso is preferred for a healing diet, since beneficial bacteria and other enzymes, as well as flavor is still intact. Miso is also a tasty base for soups, sauces, dressings, dips, spreads and cooking stock, and is a healthy substitute for salt or soy sauce. There are many kinds, strengths and flavors of miso, from chickpea (light and mild) to hatcho (dark, and strong). **Natto miso** is the sweetest, a chunky mix of soybeans, barley and barley malt, kombu, ginger and sea salt. Delicious as a relish, sandwich spread, chutney with grains and many other uses. **Miso is very concentrated; use no more than $1/2$ to 1 teasp. of dark misos, or 1 to 2 teasp. of light misos per person.** Dissolve in a small amount of water to activate the beneficial enzymes before adding to a recipe. Omit salt from the recipe if you are using miso.

MOCHI - is a chewy rice "bread" made from sweet brown rice. It is baked very hot, at 450∞ and puffs up to a crisp biscuit that can be filled, used as big croutons in soup, or as a delicious casserole topping.

MOLASSES - blackstrap, unsulphured - although a by-product of the sugar refining process, molasses has very high mineral content, particularly iron and potassium. It can be taken plain as a supplement for hair regrowth and color, or used in baking and cooking for distinctive flavor.

MUSHROOMS, WILD -
  Cepe (King Boletus) - a rich, meaty mushroom particularly good in soups, stews and stuffings.
  Chanterelle - golden, trumpet-shaped mushrooms with a light delicate flavor. They are most often used in French and gourmet sauces, or as a special vegetable delicacy.
  Enoki - long stemmed, tiny-capped mushrooms with a delicate flavor, most often used as a garnish.
  Morel - brown, spongy mushrooms with a deep, rich flavor. They go particularly well with eggs and omelettes, and broiled tofu or tempeh.
  Oyster - fan-shaped pale mushrooms, with a taste somewhat like oysters; a delicate flavor often used in Japanese and French sautées.
  Porcini - Italian mushrooms with large caps, fat stems and deep, rich flavor. Use in soups and stews.
  Shiitake - often called oyster mushrooms when fresh, these usually are sold dry. To use, just soak in water until soft then remove the woody stem and slice for use in dressings, soups and salads. Shiitake mushrooms have been linked to cures for cancers and tumors, because of their ability to stimulate inter-

feron in the body; we use them frequently as a preventive medicine food. Their distinctive taste creates a whole new dish when substituted for regular button mushrooms. Use just a few each time; a little goes a long way.

NUTRASWEET - combines the amino acids phenylalanine and aspartic acid. It is 200 times sweeter than sugar, and has been linked to several problems involving sugar use in the body, such as PKU seizures, high blood pressure, headaches, insomnia and mood swings. Nutrasweet has taken the place of saccharin in pre-prepared foods, and that means we get a lot of it. Read the labels if you have sugar sensitivities.

OATS & OAT BRAN - an excellent fiber grain source, to help lower cholesterol and promote regularity. An excellent addition to any grain or flour mix.

OILS, NATURAL VEGETABLE - these should be unrefined, either cold or expeller pressed, and stored in the refrigerator after opening. Natural oils provide vitamins A, E, lecithin and essential fatty acids. Use olive oil in salads, Italian and Middle Eastern cooking for its superior flavor and poly-and mono-unsaturated composition. For other uses, we make or buy a blend of pressed oils - usually a mixture of safflower, peanut, corn and soy, with a little sesame seed for flavor.

   Olive Oils -
- Extra Virgin - from the first pressing, with no additives; highest quality; best flavor and aroma.
- Fine Virgin - good flavor, no additives, but with higher acid content.
- Plain Virgin - slightly off flavor and the highest acidity.
- Pure - from the second pressing with additives to mellow bitter taste; includes pulp, pit and skin.

   Avocado Oil - a rich, sweet oil used mainly in salad dressings and for grilled greens.
   Corn Oil - a rich, buttery-flavored oil for baking, sautéing and salad dressings.
   Peanut Oil - ideal for stir-frying at high temperatures to seal in juices and nutrients.
   Safflower Oil - light and mild; excellent for sautéing and baking.
   Sesame Oil - made from toasted sesame seeds, and used as a flavoring agent for both Chinese and Middle Eastern stir-frying.
   Soy Oil - a mild, light oil used in dressings and for vegetables or sautéing greens.
   Sunflower Oil - a delicate poly-unsaturated oil, good for stir-frys, salads, dressings and light cooking.
   Coconut Oil - highly saturated; not recommended for cooking; useful for massage, dry skin and hair.
   Palm Kernal Oil - highly saturated, with few essential fatty acids. We recommend avoiding this oil.
   Walnut Oil - a robust oil with a distinctive flavor; used most often blended with lighter oils in baking.

OMEGA-3 OILS - see index for more on the health benefits of these oils. For cooking purposes, flax oil and olive oil have the best LDL reducing properties.

PASTA - versatile, whole grain, vegetable, low-fat, low calorie - quick and easy to make, compatible with Oriental, Italian, modified macrobiotic, and healthy diets. It's hard to have problems with pasta. We use Japanese noodles made from buckwheat (Soba), whole wheat (Udon and Somen), rice (Rice Sticks and Saifun), and combination grain ramens. High complex carbohydrate Italian pastas include sesame, spinach, artichoke, and soy, in all sorts of shapes and sizes.

PINE NUTS - from Mediterranean pine cones, they have a sweet, delicate flavor used in appetizers, pestos and stuffing dishes.

PITA BREAD - a low calorie, low-fat, whole wheat flat bread that can be opened and filled, for a healthy salad in bread.

QUINOA - an ancient Inca supergrain, containing complete protein from amino acids, and good complex carbohydrates. It is light and flavorful, and can be used like rice or millet as a diet staple.

RICE - There is a taste for everybody in brown rice - all healthy, all good. Use a mix of rices for a more complex and individual flavor. Try your own blend. Long grain is dry and fluffy; short grain is soft and sticky (good for molds and shaping). Sweet brown can be used for desserts, wehani for its nutty light texture, basmati for aroma, and wild rice for its distinctive chewiness.

RICE SYRUP - a subtle sweetener, this syrup and malt syrup come in many different consistencies and flavors, easily digestible, with slow, steady energy-producing complex carbohydrates.

ROYAL JELLY - the milk-like secretion from the head glands of the queen bee's nurse-workers. It is a powerhouse of vitamins, minerals, enzyme precursers and amino acids. It is a natural anti-biotic, a stimulant to the immune system, and has been found effective for many health problems.

RYE FLOUR - a low gluten grain, rye flour products are usually moist and dense. But the delicious solid flavor is excellent as part of a grain or flour mix.

SEA VEGETABLES - these foods have superior nutritional content; a rich source of proteins, carbohydrates, minerals and vitamins. They are good alkalizers for the body, and can add an exotic taste to almost any recipe. Most of us are familiar with nori, used to wrap sushi ingredients, but we also like several other sea veggies that have different tastes; we have made up a **SEA VEGGIE COMBO** (see page 294) that we sprinkle on lots of dishes in place of salt or other seasonings.

    Arame - a mild Japanese sea vegetable with high natural sugars, often used to flavor sauces and soups.

    Bladderwrack - a specific for iodine therapy, it is also used in therapeutic baths and herbal compounds.

    Dulse - a popular, delicious sea vegetable; soft and chewy, delicious in soups, stews, salads and sandwiches, or sautéed into chips.

    Hijiki - a popular oriental sea vegetable, with a nutty taste and crisp texture. It is protein-and calcium-rich, with absorbable B Complex vitamins.

    Kelp - a good salt substitute and high mineral sea vegetable.

    Kombu - a delicious iodine-rich sea vegetable, with sweet taste. Just boil until tender and use in soups, snip over salads, or wrap vegetable or rice hors d'oeuvres.

    Nori - also known as laver, this thin dried sea vegetable is used for sushi wrapping, snipped in soup, or dry roasted for a sweet, nutty taste. Nori is very high in beta carotene and usable proteins.

    Wakame - best when sun-dried, wakame has a delicate, mild taste, excellent with tofu, miso soup or fish. It is also delicious roasted and tossed with a little sesame oil and sesame seeds.

SEMOLINA - the authentic taste of Italian pasta comes from this flour. It is soft wheat with the bran removed.

SEEDS - many seeds are good sources of protein and minerals. Our favorites are sesame, sunflower and pumpkin seeds. All can be used for healthy benefits in cereal mixes, salads, dips, spreads, grain mixes for pilaf and veggie burgers, and as toppings.

SHOYU - a deep, rich soy sauce containing soy, wheat, koji and salt.

SOY MILK - SOY CHEESE - see pages 391, 392, and 222 .

SPIRULINA - another of the high protein algae-source superfoods; spirulina is also rich in B vitamins and beta-carotene. The high chlorophyll content enhances enzyme production and digestion.

SPROUTS - are delicious, highly nutritious, inexpensive food. Sprouts are a wonderful source of protein in the form of amino acids, chlorophyll, enzymes and plant hormones. They are good sources of vitamins A, C, B, and E, with balanced minerals and trace minerals. Sprouts are easy to grow in a sprouting jar or trays at home. Mix and match different kinds for your own personal taste. Sprouts can enhance almost any vegetarian recipe, from salads, sandwiches and tacos to soup toppings, from omelettes and stir-fries to rice pilafs. Use quality organic seeds for best nutritional results.

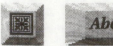

Alfalfa sprouts - use alone as an excellent fresh protein source, or in a sprout mix in salads, with radish, clover and sunflower sprouts, for more crunch and tang.

Red Clover Sprouts - these sprouts are like light, sweet alfalfa sprouts. They have therapeutic properties, and are delicious as part of a sprout mix in sandwiches and salads.

Mung Bean Sprouts - mild, crunchy sprouts especially good in salads and stir-fries. Steam slightly first when using raw to enhance the flavor and tenderness.

Radish Seeds - tangy, spicy taste with therapeutic properties.

Sunflower Sprouts - excellent in stir-fries, with a longer freshness life than mung bean sprouts.

SUCANAT - the trade name for a natural sweetener made from dried granulated cane juice. Use 1 to 1 in place of sugar. Nothing is added, only the water removed; all sucanat is from organically grown cane. It is still a concentrated sweetener, however. Use carefully if you have sugar balance problems.

TAHINI - ground sesame butter, that can be used in healthy candies and cookies, and on toast in place of peanut butter, or as a dairy replacement in soups and dressings or sauces without the cholesterol and all the protein.

TAMARI - a wheat free soy sauce, lower in sodium and richer in flavor than soy sauce. Bragg's Liquid Aminos, a wonderful energizing protein broth, is also of the tamari family, but unfermented, lower in sodium, and with 8 essential amino acids.

TAPIOCA - this sweet sun-dried starch is made by crushing cassava roots with water. The starch is separated, dried, crumbled through a sieve, and tumbled in barrels to form little round, gelatin pearls. It can be used as a thickener in cooking, or as a sweet mild dessert that is a great favorite with children.

TEAS, BLACK & GREEN - All black, green and Oolong teas come from *thea sinensis* an evergreen shrub that ranges from the Mediterranean to the tropics, and from sea level to 8000 feet. It can be harvested every 6 to 14 days depending on the area and climate, and yields tea leaves for 25-50 years. The kind of tea produced is differentiated by the manner in which the leaves are processed. For green tea, the first tender leaves of spring are picked, then partially dried, rolled, steamed and dried with hot air. Oolong tea leaves have been allowed to semi-ferment for an hour. Black teas are partially dried, rolled on tile, glass or concrete, and fermented for 3 hours to strengthen aroma and flavor, and reduce bitterness. Black teas are often scented during fermentation with fresh flower blossoms or spices.

Tea nomenclature can be confusing. As stated above, names like oolong, black or jasmine teas refer to how the tea was processed. Names such as Assam, Darjeeling or Ceylon, etc. refer to the country or region where the tea was grown. Names such as pekoe, orange pekoe, etc. refer to the leaf size.

Bancha Leaf - the tender spring leaves of the Japanese tea plant, containing much less caffeine or tannins than other teas, with a mild taste.

Kukicha Twig - a therapeutic, smooth, roasted Japanese tea, made from the twigs and stems rather than the leaves of the tea plant. Containing less caffeine and acidic oils than the leaves, this tea is a favorite in macrobiotic diets for its blood cleansing qualities, high calcium content, and mellow flavor.

Darjeeling - the finest, most delicately flavored of the black Indian teas.

Earl Grey - a popular hearty, aromatic black tea that has been sprayed with bergamot oil.

English Breakfast - a connoisseur's rich, mellow, fragrant black tea with Chinese flavor. It is a combination of Assam flowery orange pekoe and Ceylon broken orange pekoe.

Ceylon - a tea grown in Sri Lanka with a intense, flowery aroma and flavor.

Irish Breakfast - a famous combination of Assam flowery orange pekoe and Ceylon orange pekoe.

Jasmine - a black tea scented with white jasmine flowers during firing.

Oolong - a delicate, light tea with a complex flavor, semi-fermented and fired in baskets over hot coals.

TEMPEH - a meaty Indonesian fermented soy food, containing complete protein and all essential amino acids. It has a robust texture and mushroom-like aroma. Tempeh is also a pre-digested product due to the enzyme action in the culture process, making its nutrients highly absorbable.

TOFU - bean curd; a delicious soy food. See page 502 for a complete chapter of tasty, healthy recipes.

TORTILLAS - both whole wheat and corn make good light nutritious pizza crusts, nachos, and wrappers for Mexican-style sandwiches.

TRITICALE - a hybrid flour of wheat and rye berries, containing the best properties of both and higher in protein than either.

TURBINADO SUGAR - refined sugar without all the molasses removed.

UDON NOODLES - long, thick, flatwheat noodles, like linguine; used primarily in Oriental dishes.

UMEBOSHI PLUMS - pickled Japanese apricots with alkalizing, bacteria-killing properties; part of a good macrobiotic diet.

VINEGARS - Vinegars have been used for 5000 years as healthful flavor enhancers and food preservers. As part of condiments, relishes or dressings, they help digest heavy foods and high protein meals. The most nutritious vinegars for health are not overly filtered, and still contain the "mother" mixture of beneficial bacteria and enzymes in the bottle. They look slightly cloudy.
   Brown Rice - a mild sweet vinegar made from fermented brown rice. It is used extensively in Oriental and macrobiotic dishes.
   Balsamic - barrel aged, aromatic, sweet and sour vinegar, excellent in marinades and vinaigrettes.
   Apple Cider - a therapeutic vinegar for cleansing and alkalizing, and everyday vinegar for salads.
   Herbal - these use various herbs steeped in a wine vinegar, and are best with light salads.
   Raspberry - a light, fresh flavor delicious with both vegetables and fruits, and in fish sauces.
   Ume Plum - the liquid drawn off from pickled Japanese umeboshi plums and shiso leaves. It is a good salt and lemon substitute in tart oriental dishes.

WASABI - Japanese powdered horseradish. Mix a little with a small amount of water to make a paste. Very hot.

WATERS - for healing purposes, use distilled, mineral, artesian and sparkling waters. (Page 210.)

WHEAT GERM & WHEAT GERM OIL - the embryo of the wheat berry; very high in B vitamins, proteins, vitamin E, and iron. It goes rancid quickly. Buy only in nitrogen-flushed packaging. Wheat germ oil is a good vitamin E source and body oxygenator. One tablespoon provides the antioxidant equivalent of an oxygen tent for 30 minutes.

WHEAT & WHEAT FLOUR - the ubiquitous whole grain.
   Bulgur - cracked, toasted wheat berries, quick and easy to cook, nutty and tasty.
   Whole wheat pastry flour - from a soft, low gluten wheat variety. Use it for pastries and unleavened baking.
   Unbleached white flour - ground wheat berries with the bran and germ removed, but aged naturally with no chemical bleaching or treating agents.
   High gluten flour - wheat with the starch removed to concentrate the gluten; yielding 80% protein.
   Graham flour - ground whole hard wheat, coarse in texture with a chewy, nutty taste.

WILD RICE - nutty, brown seeds of a special grass; used in rice and grain mixes for stronger flavor.

ZEST - the outermost rind of a citrus fruit, used as a flavoring or garnish.

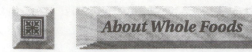

◈ About Microwaving

Since their introduction, microwave ovens have posed many safety questions. Owners were told to stand at least four feet away during use, and not to watch the food while it was cooking. New research is showing that microwaveable *packaging* is also questionable for health. Microwave"cookware" can leach chemicals into the food during microwave heating. Many of the packages for the microwave contain a "heat susceptor," a piece of metallized plastic that gets hot and fries the surface of the food to crisp or brown it.

Original testing for migration of chemicals into food was only done up to 300°F. Since microwave temperatures reach up to 500°F, newer FDA testing has been instituted. Packaging chemicals and adhesives at this temperature leach into food within 3 minutes of cooking. Many of them, such as benzene, toluene and xylene are suspected carcinogens. Plastic wraps and regular plastic containers have never been tested for the microwave. Even microwave-safe or "approved" materials are showing chemical instability at high temperatures.

➤Transfer foods that come in microwave packages into covered glass or ceramic dishes before heating.

➤If you use plastic wrap, make sure it does not come in contact with the food.

➤Use plastic containers to store foods only, not to heal them.

Recent testing in Japan has confirmed that certain foods lose 10 or more percent of vitamins E and A after only six minutes in a microwave, and 40% after twelve minutes. More testing is being done on a wider range of foods and temperatures, but if you are on a healing diet, or have great sensitivity to chemically altered foods, it might be a good idea to use a conventional oven.

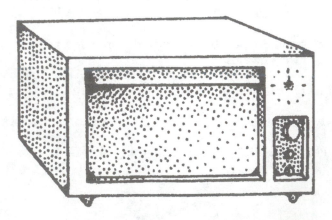

ABOUT THE RECIPES

All of the healing recipes in this book are simple, quick and easy, to keep as much food value as possible. All have taste, balance and high nutrition. Many are followed by a detailed nutritional analysis to identify specific nutrients or properties that are pertinent to a healing diet. All are very adaptable and variable to your individual taste. The best dishes for you, after all, are your own creations. Sometimes personality input is the difference between good and great. But knowing the basics, the elements, the seeds of cooking for health make it easier. The experiments and changes you make as you see your own improvement will help your program progress more rapidly, and your diet taste better.

Since this is a healing cookbook, the recipe sections are loosely ordered to reflect the stages of a healing program. The first chapters are concerned with cleansing, liquid, raw and macrobiotic foods. The middle sections pinpoint the specifics of both a rebuilding diet and those concerning a particular illness. The later sections are more general for building and maintaining continued health, with the final recipes about healthy feasting and entertaining. In an informal way, as you progress through the recipe subjects, the more you find your interests tending toward the back of the book, the better you must be getting.

While you are on a healing diet, cook from scratch whenever possible, so that you are controlling the quality of your foods. Canned and processed foods are not only less nutritious, they never taste as good once your palate and body tune in to fresh foods prepared with your own individuality.

Food can be an expression of love in many ways - a show of caring by the person who prepares it, and absorbed by those who eat it. Care is an important ingredient - flavor your food with an abundant portion. Preparing good food for a healing diet allows you to work with the most basic elements of health, and gives you an opportunity to express caring within yourself and for others. The foods and utensils you use can work together to create a feeling of well- being for yourself, family and friends.
A loving feeling creates an atmosphere of warmth in the kitchen, and adds a flavor to the dishes that can't be duplicated or equalled.

So get ready for a treat from these recipes - lots of treats. Even though you may be on a "healing diet," there is lots of variety. Whole foods are good for you. They combine easily and naturally. It's really hard to make a bad meal when you are eating naturally. As your threshhold lowers for having to overstuff the body with lots of "empty" calorie foods, your appetite will become keen for lean, whole foods. You will find yourself eating things that you like and that agree with you, eating only when you are hungry, and then a little less than possible. We hope you'll make the recipes a part of your continuing diet menu even after your health problems are solved.

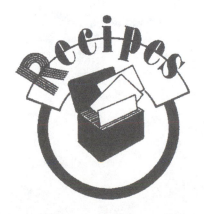

*W*hat is behind your eyes
is more important
than what is in front of them.

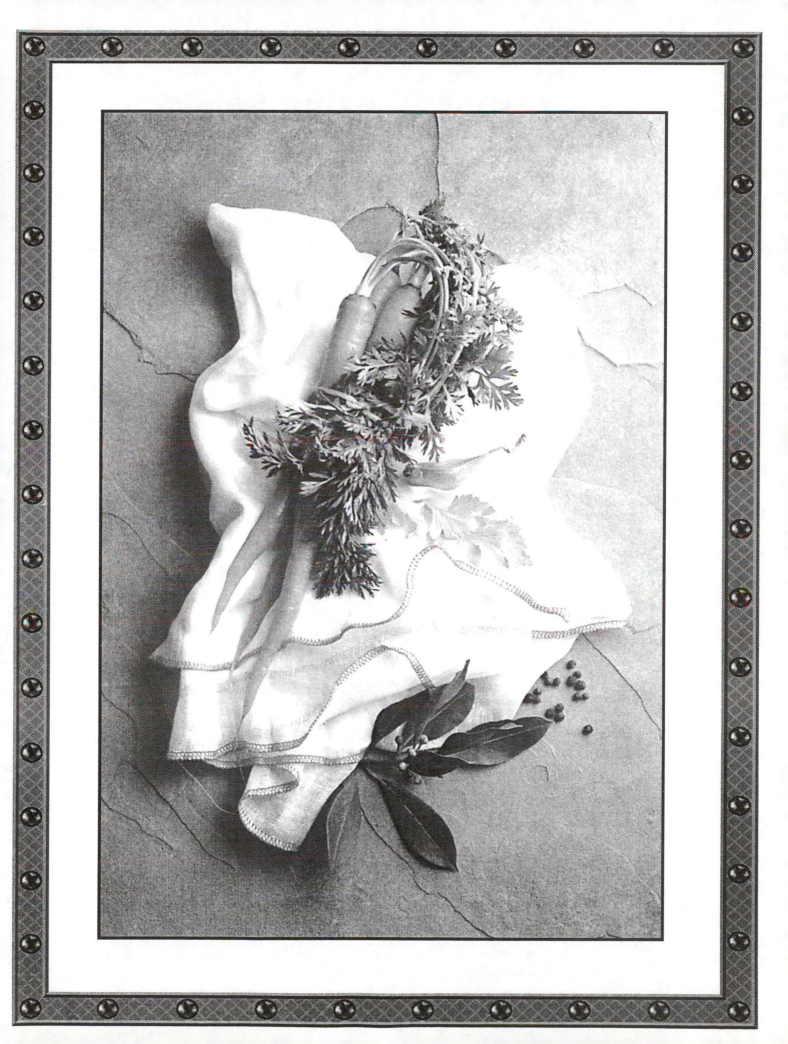

Cleansing & Fasting Foods

The recipes in this section emphasize foods with effective detoxification ability. Many are high in Vitamin C, B complex and minerals to neutralize the effects of pesticides, environmental pollutants and heavy metals, as well as toxins from the overuse of drugs, caffeine and nicotine.

Fasting and cleansing foods should be fresh, organically grown, and eaten raw for best results. Raw foods and juices retain the full complement of food nutrients, and help to stabilize and maintain the acid/alkaline balance of the body. Fruits and fruit juices eliminate wastes quickly and help reduce cravings for sweets. Fresh vegetable juices carry off excess body acids, and are rich in vitamins, minerals and enzymes that satisfy the body's nutrient requirements with less food. Chlorophyll-rich foods, such as spirulina, chlorella, and barley grass also have anti-infective properties. Since chlorophyll has a molecular structure close to our own plasma, drinking them is like giving yourself a mini transfusion. They help clear the skin, cleanse the kidneys, and clean and build the blood. Herb teas and mineral drink mixes during a cleansing diet provide energy and cleansing at the same time, without having to take in solid proteins or carbohydrates for fuel.

❋ *Tips for a successful cleansing fast:*

☞Optimize a cleansing fast with green salads, fresh fruits, and plenty of pure water the day before you begin, so that body chemistry changes will not be uncomfortable. A gentle herbal laxative taken the night before can be beneficial.

☞Avoid all dairy products and cooked foods during a cleansing fast.

☞Conserve outward activity during a fast. Allow your energy to concentrate on inner vitality. Centering the mind on internal cleansing is important, enhancing the oneness of body, mind and spirit.

☞Bathe two or more times daily while cleansing, to remove toxins coming out through the skin. Dry brush the skin with a natural bristle brush for five minutes before a bath or shower, until the skin is pink and glowing. Use a body scrub or natural "salt glow" treatment for increased results.

☞Drink 6 to 8 glasses of <u>bottled</u> water daily during a fast. Public water today is chlorinated, fluoridated, and chemically treated. It can be an irritating disagreeable fluid with caustic action.

☞Take at least one enema during the cleanse if your condition is serious, to remove old, encrusted waste from the colon, and to allow the juices and raw foods to do their best work. (See page 244 - How To Take An Enema if you need directions.)

☞Take daily fresh air walks with deep breathing to enhance aerobic activity. Sunbathe early in the morning every day possible for increased purification and fortifying vitamin D.

Mother Nature is drastically cleaning house during a liquid fast. You may eliminate accumulated poisons and wastes quite rapidly, causing headaches, slight nausea and weakness as the body purges. These reactions are usually only temporary, and disappear along with the waste and toxins. Rebuilding of healthy tissue starts right away when the detoxification foods and juices are taken in. Your body is designed to be a self-healing organism. Healing is *allowed* to occur through fasting. Hormone secretions stimulate the immune system during a cleanse to set up a disease defense environment.

This section includes the following categories:
❧CLEANSING FRUIT DRINKS ❧VEGETABLE JUICES and GREEN DRINKS ❧HERB TEAS FOR CLEANSING and FASTING SUPPORT ❧HERBAL BODYWORK TECHNIQUES FOR CLEANSING ❧THERAPEUTIC BROTHS ❧MONO DIETS ❧CLEANSING SALADS and DRESSINGS ❧

Cleansing Fruit Drinks

These are blender mixed drinks; add everything to the blender, blend it up, and drink it down. Use organically grown fruits whenever possible.

1 GOOD DIGESTION PUNCH

Natural sources of papain and bromelain for soothing and cleansing the stomach.

1 PAPAYA, peeled and seeded; or 1 CUP PAPAYA JUICE
1 PINEAPPLE, skinned and cored; or $1^1/_2$ CUPS PINEAPPLE JUICE
1 to 2 ORANGES, peeled; or $^1/_4$ to $^1/_2$ CUP ORANGE JUICE

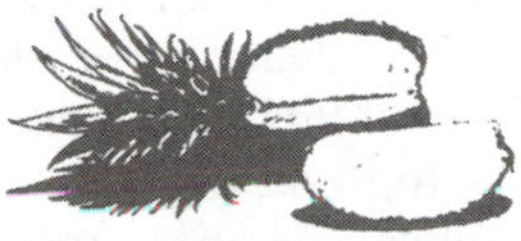

2 ENZYME COOLER

An intesinal balancer to help lower cholesterol, cleanse intestinal tract, and allow better assimilation of foods.

1 APPLE, cored and sliced; or $^1/_2$ CUP APPLE JUICE
1 PINEAPPLE, skinned and cored; or $1^1/_2$ CUPS PINEAPPLE JUICE
2 LEMONS, peeled; or $^1/_4$ CUP LEMON JUICE

3 BLOOD BUILDER

A blood purifying drink with iron enrichment.

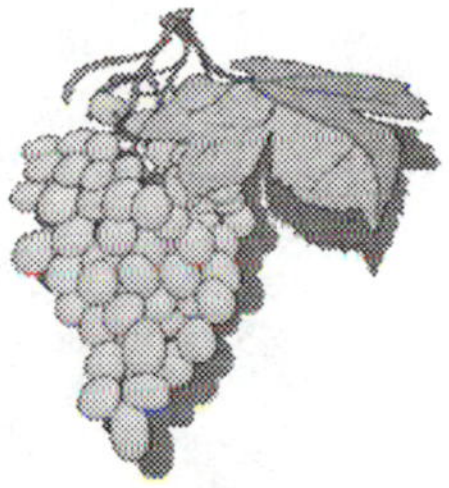

2 BUNCHES of GRAPES; or 2 CUPS GRAPE JUICE
6 ORANGES, peeled; or 2 CUPS ORANGE JUICE
8 LEMONS peeled; or 1 CUP LEMON JUICE
♣Stir in: 2 CUPS WATER and $^1/_4$ CUP OF HONEY

4 STOMACH CLEANSER & BREATH REFRESHER

A body chemistry improving drink.

1 BUNCH of GRAPES; or 1 CUP GRAPE JUICE
3 APPLES cored; or 1 CUP APPLE JUICE
1 BASKET STRAWBERRIES
4 SPRIGS OF FRESH MINT

5 PINEAPPLE CARROT COCKTAIL

Natural sources of bromelain, beta carotene and vitamin A.

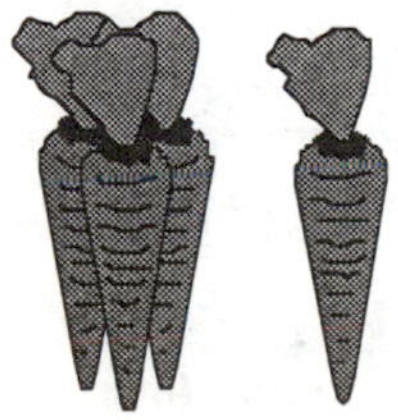

1 PINEAPPLE, skinned and cored; or $1^1/_2$ CUPS PINEAPPLE JUICE
4 CARROTS
$^1/_2$ CUP FRESH CHOPPED PARSLEY

Other good fasting fruit juices: black cherry juice for gout conditions; cranberry juice for bladder and kidney infections; grape and citrus juices for high blood pressure; watermelon juice for bladder and kidney malfunction, and apple juice to overcome fatigue.

Vegetable Juices & Green Drinks

Green drinks are potent fuel in maintaining human energy and good health. They are a wonderful nutrient source of life, rich in chlorophyll, vitamins, minerals, proteins and enzymes. Green drinks contain large amounts of vitamin C, B1, B2, B3, pantothenic acid, folic acid, carotene and choline. They are high in minerals, particularly potassium, calcium, magnesium, iron, copper, phosphorus and manganese. They are rich in chlorophyllins, and because the composition of chlorophyll is so close to that of human hemoglobin, these drinks can act as "mini-transfusions" for the blood, and tonics for the brain and immune system. They are excellent for mucous cleansing and alkalizing the body. They are full of enzymes for digestion and assimilation, some containing over 1000 of the known enzymes necessary for human cell response and growth. Many green drinks have almost twice as much protein as wheat germ, with five times the amount of minerals, and they don't come burdened by the fats that accompany animal products. The drinks included here have been used with a great deal of therapeutic success for many years. You can have every confidence in their nutritional healing and regenerative ability.

Note: A high quality juicer is the best way to get all the nutrients from vegetable juices. A blender or food processor gives only moderate results, but is definitely better than nothing at all. **Use organically grown produce whenever possible.**

6 POTASSIUM JUICE

The single most effective juice for cleansing, neutralizing acids, and rebuilding the body. It is a blood and body tonic to provide rapid energy and system balance.
For one 12-oz. glass:

♣Juice in the juicer

3 CARROTS   1/2 BUNCH PARSLEY
1/2 BUNCH SPINACH   3 STALKS CELERY
opt. 1 to 2 teasp. Bragg's LIQUID AMINOS

Nutritional analysis: per serving; 69 calories; 3gm. protein; 15gm. carbohydrate; 6gm. fiber; trace fats; 0 cholesterol; 100mg. calcium; 2mg. iron; 52mg. magnesium; 788mg. potassium; 144mg. sodium; 1mg. zinc.

7 POTASSIUM ESSENCE BROTH

If you do not have a juicer, make a potassium broth in a soup pot. While not as concentrated or pure, it is still an excellent source of energy, minerals and electrolytes.
For a 2 day supply:

♣Cover with water in a soup pot

3 to 4 CARROTS   1/2 BUNCH PARSLEY
2 POTATOES with skins   1/2 HEAD CABBAGE
1 ONION   1/2 BUNCH BROCCOLI
3 STALKS CELERY

♣Simmer covered 30 minutes. Strain and discard solids.

♣Add 2 teasp. Bragg's LIQUID AMINOS, or 1 teasp. miso. Store in the fridge, covered.

Nutritional analysis: per serving; 100 calories; 6gm. protein; 22gm. carbohydrate; 9gm. fiber; trace fats; 0 cholesterol; 141mg. calcium; 4mg. iron; 60mg. magnesium; 147mg. sodium; 1mg. zinc; 944 mg. potassium.

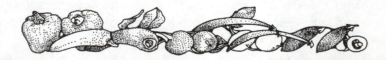

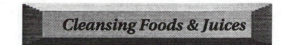

8   KIDNEY FLUSH

A purifying kidney cleanser and diuretic drink, with balancing potassium and other minerals.
For four 8-oz. glasses:

4 CARROTS
4 BEETS with tops
4 CELERY STALKS with leaves

1 CUCUMBER with skin
8 to 10 SPINACH LEAVES, washed
♣opt. 1 teasp. Bragg's LIQUID AMINOS

Nutritional analysis: per serving; 69 calories; 3gm. protein; 15gm. carbohydrates; 5gm. fiber; trace fats; 0 cholesterol; 81mg. calcium; 2mg. iron; 62mg. magnesium; 760mg. potassium; 143mg. sodium; 1mg. zinc.

9   PERSONAL BEST V-8

A delicious high vitamin/mineral drink for body balance. A good daily blend even when you're not cleansing.
For 6 glasses:

6 to 8 TOMATOES; or 4 CUPS TOMATO JUICE
1/2 GREEN PEPPER
2 STALKS CELERY with leaves
1/2 BUNCH PARSLEY
3 to 4 GREEN ONIONS with tops
2 CARROTS
1/2 SMALL BUNCH SPINACH, washed, or 1/2 HEAD ROMAINE LETTUCE
2 LEMONS peeled; or 4 TBS. LEMON JUICE
opt. 2 teasp. Bragg's LIQUID AMINOS and 1/2 teasp. ground celery seed

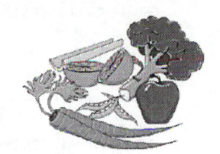

Nutritional analysis: per serving; 57 calories; 2 gm. protein; 13gm. carbohydrate; 4gm. fiber; trace fats; 0 cholesterol; 43mg. calcium; 36mg. magnesium; 2mg. iron; 606mg. potassium; 63mg. sodium; 1mg. zinc.

10   STOMACH/DIGESTIVE CLEANSER

For one 8-oz. glass:

♣Juice 1/2 CUCUMBER with skin, 2 TBS. APPLE CIDER VINEGAR and a PINCH of GROUND GINGER.
♣Add enough cool water to make 8-oz.

11   SPROUT COCKTAIL
This high protein juice is particularly good for ending a cleansing fast.
For 2 drinks:

♣Juice 3 APPLES with skin, cored, 1 TUB, (4 OZ.) ALFALFA SPROUTS and 3 to 4 SPRIGS FRESH MINT.

Nutritional analysis: per serving; 138 calories; 3gm. protein; 34gm. carbohydrate; 7gm. fiber; 1gm fats; 0 cholesterol; 37mg. calcium; 1mg. iron; 26mg. magnesium; 303mg. potassium; 6mg. sodium; trace zinc.

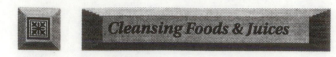

12   CARROT JUICE PLUS

For 2 large drinks:

4 CARROTS $1/_2$ CUCUMBER with skin
1 TB. CHOPPED DRY DULSE   2 STALKS CELERY with leaves

Nutritional analysis: per serving; 84 calories; 2gm. protein; 20gm. carbohydrate; 6gm. fiber; trace fats; 0 cholesterol; 88mg. calcium; 1mg. iron; 52mg. magnesium; 706mg. potassium; 119mg. sodium; 1mg. zinc.

13   SKIN TONIC
Deep greens to nourish, cleanse and tone skin tissue from the inside.
For 1 drink:

1 CUCUMBER with skin $1/_2$ BUNCH PARSLEY
1 TUB (4-OZ.) ALFALFA SPROUTS   3 to 4 SPRIGS FRESH MINT

14   EVER GREEN
A personal favorite for taste, mucous release and enzymatic action.

1 APPLE with skin   1 teasp. SPIRULINA or
1 TUB (4-OZ.) ALFALFA SPROUTS   CHLORELLA GRANULES
$1/_2$ FRESH PINEAPPLE skinned/cored   3 to 4 SPRIGS FRESH MINT

15   HEALTHY MARY COCKTAIL
A virgin mary is really a healthy green drink when you make it fresh.
For 4 drinks:

3 CUPS WATER   1 SLICE GREEN PEPPER
2 TOMATOES   1 STALK CELERY
1 GREEN ONION with tops   12 SPRIGS PARSLEY
1 TB. CHOPPED DRY SEA VEGETABLES,
    such as WAKAME or DULSE, or 1 teasp. KELP POWDER

16   GOLDEN ENZYME DRINK
A drink specifically for healing enzyme properties.
For 2 drinks:

$1^1/_2$ to 2 CUPS PINEAPPLE JUICE
4 CARROTS
1 teasp. HONEY

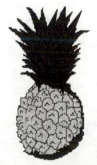

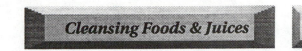

Herb Teas For Cleansing Support

Herbal teas are the most time-honored of all natural healing mediums. Essentially body balancers, teas have mild cleansing and flushing properties, and are easily absorbed by the system. Herbs and the important volatile oils in them, are released by the hot brewing water, and when taken in small sips throughout the cleansing process, they flood the tissues with concentrated nutritional support to accelerate regeneration, and the release of toxic waste.

In general, herbs are more effective in combination than when used singly, providing a broader range of activity when taken together in a blend. I have listed several favorites in each area - blood cleansing, mucous cleansing, and bowel cleansing - that may be combined for your own particular needs.

✸ How to Take Medicinal Teas for Therapeutic Results:

1) Pack a small tea ball packed with herbs.
2) Bring 3 cups of cold water to a boil. Remove from heat. Add herbs, and steep covered; 10 to 15 minutes for a leaf and flower tea, 20 to 25 minutes for a root and bark tea.
3) Use a glass, ceramic or earthenware pot. Stainless steel is acceptable, but aluminum negates the herbal effects, and the metal often washes into the tea and gets into the body.
4) Keep lid tightly closed during steeping and storage. Volatile herbal oils are the most valuable part of the drink, and will escape if left uncovered.
5) Drink teas in small sips over a long period of time rather than all at once, to allow the tissues to absorb as much of the medicinal value as possible.
6) Take two to three cups of tea daily for best medicinal effects.

✦ EFFECTIVE HERBS FOR BLOOD CLEANSING

Echinacea (Angustifolia and Purpurea), Red Clover, Chaparral, Pau d' Arco, Licorice, Burdock Root, Oregon Grape Root, Dandelion, Garlic.

A sample tea combination for blood cleansing might include: Red Clover, Hawthorn, Pau d' Arco, Nettles, Sage, Alfalfa, Milk Thistle Seed, Echinacea, Hoesetail, Gotu Kola, and Lemon Grass.

✦ EFFECTIVE HERBS FOR MUCOUS CLEANSING

Garlic, Chlorella, Mullein, Elecampane, Ephedra, Comfrey Root, Pleurisy Root, Fenugreek Seed, Ginger, Cayenne, Hawthorn, Licorice.

A sample tea combination for mucous cleansing might include: Mullein, Comfrey, Ephedra, Marshmallow, Pleurisy Root, Rosehips, Calendula, Boneset, Ginger, Peppermint, and Fennel Seed.

✦ EFFECTIVE HERBS FOR COLON BOWEL CLEANSING

Psyllium Seeds, Flax Seed, Butternut Bark, Cascara Sagrada, Rhubarb, Fennel Seed, Acidophilus, Senna Leaf and Pod, Peppermint.

A sample tea combination for cleansing the bowel and digestive system might include: Senna Leaf, Papaya Leaf, Fennel Seed, Peppermint, Lemon Balm, Parsley Leaf, Calendula, Hibiscus, and Ginger Root.

Effective Herbal Bodywork For Cleansing

❧**Herbs are effective in enema and compress solutions for use during a cleanse.** An enema can greatly aid the release of old, encrusted colon waste, making the whole body cleansing process easier and more thorough. The addition of herbs in the enema water serves to immediately alkalize the bowel area, help control irritation and inflammation, and provide local healing activity where there is ulceration or distended tissue.

We recommend three herbs regularly for enemas; catnip and pau d'arco, (use 2 cups of very strong brewed tea to 1-quart of water), and liquid chlorophyll, (use 3 TBS. to 1-quart water) or spirulina, (2 TBS. powder to 1-quart water). Catnip is effective for stomach and digestive conditions, and for childhood diseases. Pau d' Arco is used to balance the acid/alkaline system, as in chronic yeast and fungal infections. Chlorophyll-source herbs are successful for blood and bowel toxicity.

During a liver or serious blood cleanse where degenerative disease is present, coffee enemas have become almost standard as a natural healing technique. Caffeine used in this way stimulates the liver and gallbladder to remove toxins, opens bile ducts, and produces enzymatic activity for healthy red blood formation and oxygen uptake. Use 1 cup of strong brewed cool coffee to 1-quart of water.

❧**How to take an enema:** place solution in an enema bag and hang or hold about 18 inches higher than the body. Attach colon tube. Lubricate tube with vaseline or K-Y jelly. Lie on the left side and slowly insert about 18 inches into the colon. Rotate the tube gently for ease of insertion, making sure there are no kinks so liquid flows freely. When all the solution has entered the colon, slowly remove the tube, and remain on the left side for about 5 minutes. Roll on the back for another 5 minutes, then onto the right side for 5 minutes, so that each portion of the colon is reached. Get up and quickly expel fluid into the toilet.

❧**Compresses** are used during a cleanse to draw out waste residues such as cysts, growths and abscesses through the skin. Use hot and cold alternating compresses for best results - applying the herbs to the hot compress, and leaving the cold compress plain. Cayenne, ginger and lobelia are all effective as compress herbs. Simply make a solution of 1 teasp. of powdered herb in a bowl of very hot water. Soak a washcloth and apply to the affected area until the cloth cools. Then apply a cloth dipped in ice water until it reaches body temperature. Repeat several times daily during a cleanse.

Green clay compresses are also effective toxin-drawing agents for growths, and may be applied to gauze, placed on the area, covered, and left for 24 hours at a time. Simply change as you would any dressing when you bathe.

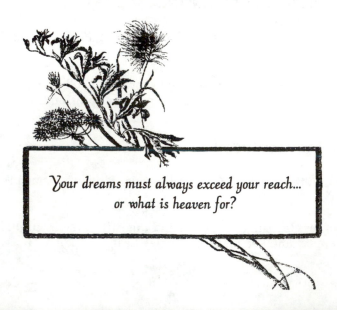

Your dreams must always exceed your reach... or what is heaven for?

Therapeutic Alkalizing Broths

Clear soups and broths are a satisfying form of nutrition during a cleansing fast. They are simple, easy, inexpensive, can be taken hot or cold any time, and provide an uncomplicated means of "eating" and being with others at mealtime without going off your liquid program. This is more important than it might appear, since any solid food taken after the body has released all of its solid waste, but before the cleanse is over, will drastically reduce the diet's success. Broths are also alkalizing, and contribute toward balancing body pH.

17 PURIFYING DAIKON & SCALLION BROTH

Daikon, a cleansing diuretic food, and scallions, a sulphur-rich digestive vegetable are synergistic together.
For one bowl.

♣Heat gently together for 5 minutes
4 CUPS VEGETABLE BROTH
ONE 6" PIECE DAIKON RADISH, peeled and cut into matchstick pieces
2 SCALLIONS, with tops
1 TB. TAMARI, or 1 TB. BRAGG'S LIQUID AMINOS
1 TB. FRESH CHOPPED CILANTRO
PINCH of PEPPER

Nutritional analysis: per serving; 25 calories; 1 gm. protein; 2gm. fiber; 0 fat; 1 gm. carbo.; 0 cholesterol; 31mg. calcium; trace iron; 15mg. magnesium; 172mg. potassium; 194mg. sodium; trace zinc.

18 ONION & MISO SOUP

A therapeutic broth with anti-biotic and immune-enhancing properties.
For 6 small bowls of broth:

♣Sauté 1 CHOPPED ONION in 1/2 teasp. SESAME OIL for 5 minutes.
♣Add 1 STALK CELERY WITH LEAVES, and sauté for 2 minutes.
♣Add 1 QUART WATER or VEGETABLE STOCK. Cover and simmer 10 minutes.
♣Add 3 to 4 TBS. LIGHT MISO. Remove from heat.
♣Add 2 GREEN ONIONS with tops, and whirl in the blender.

Nutritional analysis: per serving; 42 calories; 7gm carbohydrate; 1gm. fat; 2gm. protein; 2mg. iron; 0 cholesterol; 27mg. calcium; trace iron; 12mg. magnesium; 121mg. potassium; 410mg. sodium; trace zinc.

19 ONION/GARLIC BROTH

A therapeutic broth with anti-biotic properties to reduce and relieve mucous congestion.
For 1 bowl:

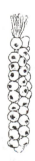

♣Saute 1 ONION and 4 CLOVES GARLIC in 1/2 teasp. SESAME OIL until very soft.
♣Whirl in the blender. Eat in small sips.

Nutritional analysis: per serving; 103 calories; 3gm. protein; 18gm. carbohydrate; 3gm. fiber; 3gm. fats; 0 cholesterol; 56mg. calcium; 1mg. iron; 20mg. magnesium; 315mg. potassium; 7mg. sodium; trace zinc.

20 COLD DEFENSE CLEANSER

Make this broth the minute you feel a cold coming on.
Heat for 2 drinks:

1½ CUPS WATER
1 teasp. GARLIC POWDER
1 teasp. GROUND GINGER
1 TB. LEMON JUICE

1 TB. HONEY
½ teasp. CAYENNE
3 TBS. BRANDY

♣Simmer gently 5 minutes. Drink in small sips for best results.

Nutritional analysis: per serving; 95 calories; trace protein; 19gm. carbohydrate; trace fiber; trace fats; 10mg. calcium; trace iron; 6mg. magnesium; 53mg. potassium; 7mg. sodium; trace zinc.

21 COLDS & FLU TONIC

This drink really opens up nasal and sinus passages fast. We tried a version of this in Morocco several years ago. It was something not easily forgotten.
For 2 drinks:

♣Toast in a dry pan until aromatic
4 CLOVES MINCED GARLIC or 2 teasp. GARLIC/LEMON SEASONING (page 644)
¼ teasp. CUMIN POWDER
¼ teasp. BLACK PEPPER
½ teasp. HOT MUSTARD POWDER
♣Add 1 TB. OIL and stir in. Toast a little more to blend.

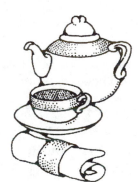

♣Add
1 CUP WATER
1 teasp. TURMERIC
½ teasp. SESAME SALT.
½ teasp. GROUND CORIANDER or 1 TB. FRESH CILANTRO
1 CUP COOKED SPLIT PEAS or 1 CUP FRESH FROZEN
♣Simmer gently for 5 minutes, and whirl in blender. Very potent.

22 MUCOUS CLEANSING BROTH

Your and grandmother were right. Hot chicken broth really does clear out chest congestion faster.
For 4 bowls:

♣Use 1-QT. <u>HOMEMADE</u> CHICKEN STOCK (boil down bones, skin and trimmings from 1 fryer in 2-qts. water, and skim off fat).

♣In a large pot, saute 3 CLOVES MINCED GARLIC, 1 teasp. HORSERADISH, and a PINCH of CAYENNE until aromatic for 5 minutes.

♣Add chicken stock and simmer for 7-10 minutes.
♣Top with NUTMEG and SNIPPED PARSLEY.

23 CHINESE MAMA'S CHICKEN SOUP

All over the world, people have found that chicken really works. This is a clear, healing oriental version.
For 2 large bowls of broth:

♣Combine and bring to a simmer
3 to 4 CUPS OF STRAINED HOMEMADE CHICKEN BROTH
1/2 CUP BEAN SPROUTS

♣Add and simmer for 10 minutes
1 CUP SHREDDED CHICKEN   2 THIN SLICES GINGER
2 TBS. TAMARI   1/2 CUP CARROTS, in thin matchsticks

♣Add 1/2 CUP FRESH TRIMMED PEA PODS and 1/2 CUP SHREDDED CHINESE CABBAGE and heat
for 3 minutes.
♣Serve with more dashes of tamari or Bragg's LIQUID AMINOS BROTH.

Nutritional analysis: per serving; 98 calories; 13gm. protein; 7gm. carbohydrate; 2gm. fiber; 2gm. fats; 29mg. cholesterol; 36mg. calcium; 1mg. iron; 31mg. magnesium; 275mg. potassium; 251mg. sodium; 1mg. zinc.

24 HERB & VEGETABLE HEALING BROTH

For 4 cups of broth:

♣Heat 3 CUPS OF HOMEMADE VEGETABLE STOCK (see page 652) in a soup pot.

♣Add and heat gently
1 to 2 TBS. MISO dissolved in 1 CUP WATER   1 TB. BREWER'S YEAST FLAKES
1 TB. CHOPPED GREEN ONIONS   1/2 CUP TOMATO JUICE
1/2 teasp. <u>each</u>: DRY BASIL, THYME, SAVORY, and MARJORAM

25 ALKALIZING APPLE BROTH

This drink alkalizes, gives a nice spicy energy lift and helps lower serum cholesterol.
For 4 drinks:

♣Sauté 1/2 CHOPPED RED ONION and 2 CLOVES MINCED GARLIC in 1 teasp. OIL until soft.

♣While sautéing, blend in the blender
1 SMALL RED BELL PEPPER
2 TART APPLES cored and quartered
1 LEMON partially peeled, with some peel on
2 TBS. FRESH PARSLEY
2 CUPS KNUDSEN'S VERY VEGGIE-SPICY (or any good spicy tomato juice)

♣Add onion mix to blender and puree. Heat gently and drink hot.

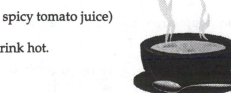

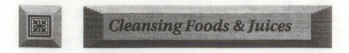
26   MINERAL RICH ENZYME BROTH

For 6 cups of broth:

♣Put in a large soup pot

3 SLICED CARROTS

1 CUP CHOPPED FRESH PARSLEY

1 LARGE ONION, chopped

2 POTATOES, diced

2 STALKS CELERY with tops

♣Add 1½ QTS. WATER, and bring to a boil. Reduce heat and simmer for 30 minutes. Strain and serve with 1 TB. Bragg's LIQUID AMINOS.

Nutritional analysis: per serving; 40 calories; 1gm. protein; 3gm. carbohydrate; trace fiber; trace fats; 0 cholesterol; 21mg. calcium; 2mg. iron; 18mg. magnesium; 146mg. potassium; 21mg. sodium; trace zinc.

27   GOURMET GAZPACHO

A classic gourmet favorite with healing properties. Whirl all in the blender and chill.
For 6 servings:

4 TOMATOES

4 GREEN ONIONS with tops

½ GREEN PEPPER

½ CUCUMBER

4 SPRIGS PARSLEY

2 TBS. LEMON JUICE

1 teasp. BRAGG'S LIQUID AMINOS

1 CUP WATER

1 teasp. CRUMBLED WAKAME or DULSE

2 CLOVES GARLIC

Nutritional analysis: per serving; 46 calories; 2gm. protein; 10gm. carbohydrate; 3gm. fiber; trace fats; 0 cholesterol; 39mg. calcium; 1mg. iron; 28mg. magnesium; 443mg. potassium; 48mg. sodium; trace zinc.

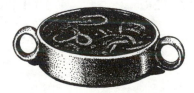

Mono Diets For Specific Problems

Mono diets are sometimes effective for particular problems where specific body areas need alkalizing/balancing.
Use them for 1 or 2 days, at the end of an all-liquid fast, and before other solid foods are taken.

♣**Carrots/Carrot Juice:** for stomach and digestive balance; very beneficial when incorporated into a diet for arthritis and colon inflammation.

♣**Grapefruit/Citrus Fruit:** to stimulate an exhausted liver for better metabolism, and for heavy mucous elimination from the lungs.

♣**Apples/Apple Juice:** for digestive and colon problems; beneficial in lowering blood pressure and cholesterol, and balancing body pH.

♣**Grapes/Grape Juice:** may be used for an entire fast as a primary blood cleanser, heart tonic and source of energy.

Simple Raw Salads & Dressings For Cleansing

A simple fruit or vegetable salad is the best way to begin and end a liquid fasting diet.
A small salad the night before prepares the body gently for light food, and starts the cleansing process.
A salad on the last night of a fast begins the enzymatic and systol/diastol activity of digestion again.
The following salads are light combinations that may be used any time you want to put less strain on your system.

28   LETTUCE POTPOURRI

For one salad:

♣ Make a mix of your favorite lettuce greens.
♣ Then mix together

2 TBS. FRESH LEMON JUICE	1 TB. OLIVE OIL
1 TB. FRESH LIME JUICE	1 teasp. ITALIAN HERBS
1 teasp. HONEY	A PINCH OF GROUND PEPPER

♣ Toss with the lettuces until they glisten.

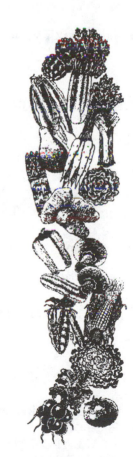

29   SWEET & SOUR CUCUMBERS

For one salad:

♣ Slice 1 CUCUMBER and $1/4$ CUP RED ONION.
♣ Mix together
2 teasp. OLIVE OIL,
2 teasp. HONEY
3 teasp. CIDER VINEGAR.
♣ Chill, and top with 1 tablespoon of plain yogurt

30   NO OIL SWEET & SOUR SALAD

For one salad:

♣ Slice very thin
1 CUCUMBER
$1/2$ GREEN or RED BELL PEPPER
♣ Heat together until aromatic
1 teasp. HONEY
$1/4$ CUP TARRAGON VINEGAR.
3 THIN SLICES RED ONION
♣ Toss with veggies. Chill and serve on lettuce with 1 teasp. fresh DAIKON RADISH chopped on top.

Nutritional analysis: per serving; 91 calories; 3gm. protein; 23gm. carbohydrate; 5gm. fiber; trace fats; 0 cholesterol; 61mg. calcium; 1mg. iron; 42mg. magnesium; 665mg. potassium; 9mg. sodium; 1mg. zinc.

31   SPROUTS PLUS

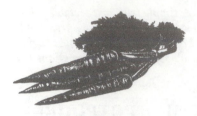

For 2 salads:

♣Toss together
1 TUB ALFALFA SPROUTS
2 CUPS GRATED CARROTS
1 CUP MINCED CELERY

♣Stir together to make a dressing
6 TBS. OLIVE OIL   4 TBS. LIME JUICE
4 TBS. TOMATO JUICE   1 teasp. SESAME SALT

♣Toss with veggies. Delicious!

Nutritional analysis: per serving; 332 calories; 4gm. protein; 19gm. carbohydrate; 7gm. fiber; 28gm. fats; 0 cholesterol; 83mg. calcium; 2mg. iron; 47mg. magnesium; 680mg. potassium; 449mg. sodium; 1mg. zinc.

32   CARROT & LEMON SALAD

For 2 salads:

♣Grate 2 CUPS CARROTS

♣Mix together
$1^1/_2$ TBS. LEMON JUICE   2 teasp. FRESH CHOPPED PARSLEY
$1^1/_2$ TBS. LIGHT OIL   1 teasp. MAPLE SYRUP
$1/_4$ teasp. 5 SPICE POWDER   2 TBS. RAISINS
2 teasp. FRESH CHOPPED MINT

♣Toss dressing with carrots and chill.

33   CARROT & CABBAGE SLAW

For 2 salads:

♣Whirl $1/_2$ HEAD CHINESE CABBAGE and 1 CARROT in a food processor.

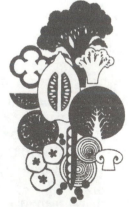

♣Mix together for dressing
2 teasp. HONEY
3 TBS. TARRAGON VINEGAR,
$1/_2$ teasp. FRESH MINCED GINGER,
$1/_4$ teasp. SESAME SALT
1 GREEN ONION minced with tops.
♣Toss with veggies. Cover and chill for an hour to marinate flavors.

34   SUNNY SPROUTS & CARROTS

For 2 salads:

♣Grate 2 to 3 CARROTS into a bowl.
♣Add 1 LARGE HANDFUL OF SUNFLOWER SPROUTS or a SPROUT MIX.
♣Add 2 or 3 MINCED SCALLIONS with tops.

♣Mix together for a dressing
2 TBS. OLIVE OIL   1 teasp. DIJON MUSTARD
1 TB. CIDER VINEGAR   1 teasp. DRIED DILL
1 teasp. HONEY   PINCH PEPPER
♣Toss with veggies and chill.

Nutritional analysis: per serving; 198 calories; 3gm. protein; 18gm. carbohydrate; 5gm. fiber; 14gm. fats; 0 cholesterol; 62mg. calcium; 2mg. iron; 34mg. magnesium; 464mg. potassium; 76mg. sodium; 1mg. zinc.

35   FRESH FRUITS & YOGURT

For 4 salads:

♣Slice or chop together in a bowl   ♣Add and mix through
1 BANANA   2 TBS. RAISINS
1 PEACH OR PEAR   2 TBS. TOASTED SUNFLOWER SEEDS
1 APPLE   1/2 CUP LEMON/LIME YOGURT
1/4 FRESH PINEAPPLE
1 MANDARIN ORANGE
♣Toss together and serve in lettuce cups. Top with 2 TBS. COCONUT/ALMOND GRANOLA.

Nutritional analysis: per serving; 177 calories; 4gm. protein; 35gm. carbohydrate; 5gm. fiber; 4gm. fats; 1mg. cholesterol; 74mg. calcium; 1mg. iron; 35mg. magnesium; 431mg. potassium; 13mg. sodium; 1mg. zinc.

36   SPINACH & BEAN SPROUT SALAD
An excellent protein and greens salad to end a fasting diet.
For 2 salads:

♣Wash, drain, and toss together
1 SMALL BUNCH FRESH SPINACH
8-OZ. FRESH BEAN SPROUTS
2 CAKES OF FIRM DICED TOFU or 4-OZ. FRESH SLICED MUSHROOMS

♣Toss with 2 TBS. SESAME OIL, 2 TBS. BROWN RICE VINEGAR, 2 teasp. TAMARI, 1 teasp. chopped fresh GINGER (or 1/4 teasp. GINGER POWDER) and 1 teasp. SESAME SALT. Chill before serving.

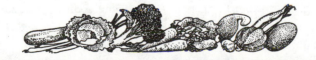

Light Dressings For Cleansing Salads

37   NO OIL TAMARI LEMON

For 1 salad:

Mix

2 TBS. LEMON JUICE

1 TB. TAMARI

1 TB. HONEY

1 teasp. SESAME SEEDS

1/4 teasp. GINGER ROOT

Nutritional analysis: per serving; 101 calories; 2gm. protein; 22gm. carbohydrate; trace fiber; 2gm. fats; 0 cholesterol; 11mg. calcium; 1mg. iron; 21mg. magnesium; 105mg. potassium; 178mg. sodium; trace zinc.

38   LOW FAT NORTHERN ITALIAN

For 1 salad:

Blender blend

1 TB. FRESH CHOPPED PARSLEY

A PINCH GARLIC/LEMON SEASONING

2 teasp. OLIVE OIL

2 teasp. WINE VINEGAR

2 teasp. LEMON JUICE

1 TB. WATER or WHITE WINE

Nutritional analysis: per serving; 86 calories; 2gm. protein; 2gm. carbohydrate; trace fiber; 9gm. fats; 0 cholesterol; 8mg. calcium; trace iron; 3mg. magnesium; 44mg. potassium; 72mg. sodium; trace zinc.

39   HERBS & LEMON DRESSING

For 1 salad:

Mix

1 teasp. CIDER VINEGAR

1 teasp. LEMON JUICE

2 teasp. OLIVE OIL

1/4 teasp. LEMON HERB SEASONING

1/4 teasp. DIJON MUSTARD

1 teasp. FRESH MINCED BASIL

1/4 teasp. DRY TARRAGON

1/4 teasp. DRY OREGANO

1 TB. FRESH CHOPPED PARSLEY

1/4 teasp. HONEY

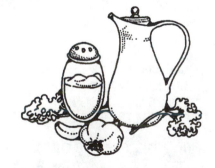

Nutritional analysis: per serving; 96 calories; trace protein; 3gm. carbohydrate; trace fiber; 9gm. fats; 0 cholesterol; 35mg. calcium; 1mg. iron; 10mg. magnesium; 81mg. potassium; 195mg. sodium; trace zinc.

40   SESAME VINAIGRETTE

For 3 salads:

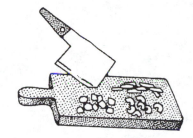

♣Mix together
1/4 CUP TAMARI
3 TBS. RICE VINEGAR
1 TB. WHITE WINE or SPARKLING WATER
2 teasp. HONEY
1 teasp. SESAME SEEDS
1 TB. SESAME OIL
PINCH SESAME SALT

Nutritional analysis: per serving; 78 calories; 2gm. protein; 7gm. carbohydrate; trace fiber; 5gm. fats; 0 cholesterol; 7mg. calcium; 1mg. iron; 13mg. magnesium; 68mg. potassium; 258mg. sodium; trace zinc.

41   ORIGINAL HONEY FRENCH

For 6 salads:

♣Mix together

1 CUP BALSAMIC VINEGAR	PINCH SESAME SALT
2 TBS. HONEY	PINCH DRY MUSTARD
4 TBS. OLIVE OIL	PINCH PEPPER

Nutritional analysis: per serving; 106 calories; trace protein; 8gm. carbohydrate; trace fiber; 9gm. fats; 0 cholesterol; 3mg. calcium; trace iron; 1mg. magnesium; 45mg. potassium; 13mg. sodium; trace zinc.

42   GINGER LEMON/LIME DRESSING

For 4 salads:

♣Blend in the blender
1 CUP LEMON OR PLAIN YOGURT, OR YOGURT CHEESE (see page 392)
1 TB. LIME JUICE
1 TB. LEMON JUICE
1/2 teasp. GINGER POWDER
1/4 teasp. TAMARI

Nutritional analysis: per serving; 36 calories; 3 gm. protein; 5gm. carbohydrate; trace fiber; trace fats; 3mg. cholesterol; 105mg. calcium; trace iron; 11mg. magnesium; 145mg. potassium; 23mg. sodium; trace zinc.

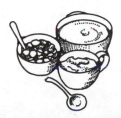

If you can imagine it, you can achieve it. If you can dream it, you can become it...but almost never in the way you imagined it.

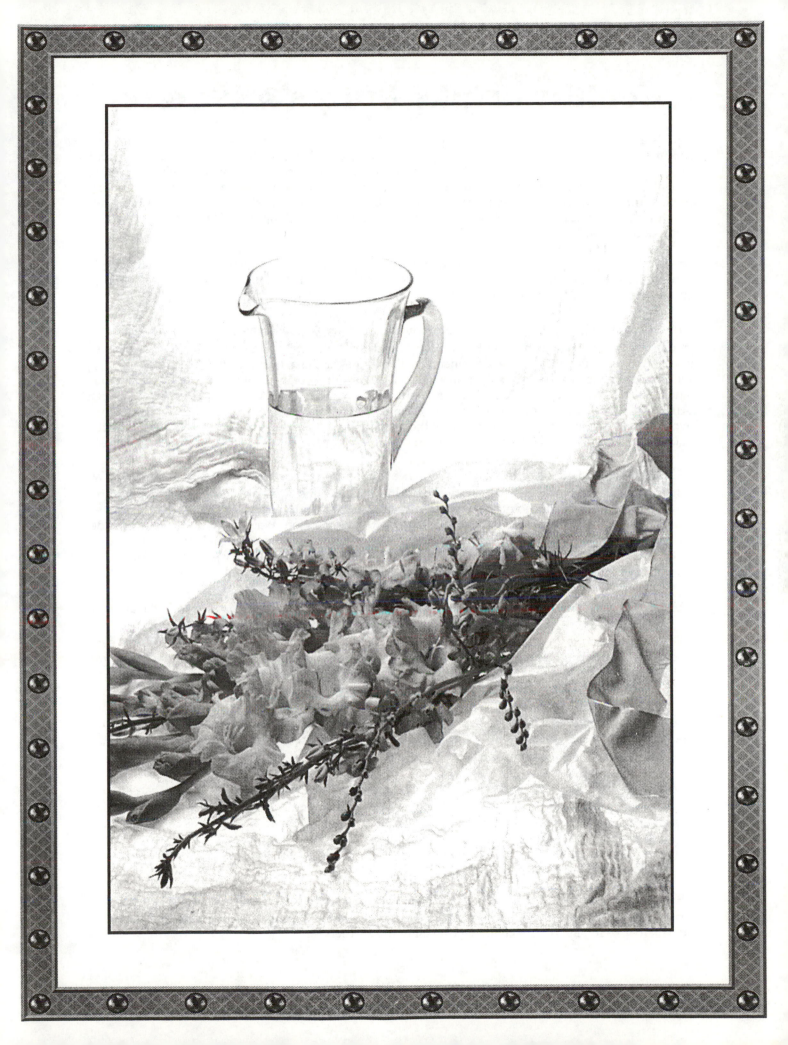

Healthy Drinks, Juices & Waters

Liquids are a fast, easy way to take absorbable, usable nutrients into the system. They are the least concentrated form of nutrition, but have the great advantage of easy assimilation; they break down and flush out toxins quickly, and provide lubrication to the system. Tissues are flooded with therapeutic nutrients in a gentle and often delicious way. In fact, since many natural liquids are rich in minerals, proteins and chlorophyll (nutrients often deficient in our bodies), the drinks in this section, even though rich in medicinal qualities sometimes taste better than anything else. The body often craves what it needs most.

Several types of beneficial drinks are included in this chapter for a variety of tastes and healing activity. ❧FRUIT SMOOTHIES ❧FROSTS and SLUSHES ❧COFFEE SUBSTITUTES ❧HERB TEAS FOR PLEASURE and THERAPY ❧COOLERS ❧HOT TONICS ❧NUTRITIVE MEAL REPLACEMENTS ❧

❋ *About Milk -* Almost no milk is used in healing recipes, because of its clogging and mucous-forming properties. Pasteurized milk is a pretty dead food for rebuilding body nutrition. Even raw milk is often difficult to assimilate for someone with allergies, asthma, or respiratory problems.
 But there are delicious, healthy substitutes that can be used in cooking: soy milk, almond milk, plain yogurt mixed with water or white wine, tofu, kefir, tahini, etc. See THE ART OF SUBSTITUTING and DAIRY FREE COOKING in this book for specific methods and ratios. We find these foods to be more flavorful than milk in almost every case, with the advantages of richness without fat, digestibility without clogging, and taste without excess mucous formation.

❋ *About Water -* I can't say enough good things about drinking plenty of pure water every day. Water lubricates the body, flushes out waste and toxins, hydrates the skin, regulates body temperature, acts as a shock absorber for joints, bones and muscles, supplies natural earth minerals, and dissolves organic minerals, vitamins, proteins and sugars for body assimilation. Water cleanses the body inside and out. Concern about the lack of purity in our water supply is leading many people to bottled water. See **About Water** (Page 210) in the GETTING THE MOST FROM YOUR NATURAL FOOD PHARMACY section for a complete discussion about available waters, their properties and qualities.

❋ *About Black Teas -* Black teas contain caffeine and tannins, but differ from coffee in the amount and kind of caffeine they have. **Black teas**, do not raise blood cholesterol, or lower vitamin C levels, and can be useful in counteracting depression. In addition, cold wet black tea bags placed over the eyelids are proven eye brighteners, and help clear red, tired eyes. **Green teas**, whose leaves are dried without fermentation, do not interfere with iron or calcium absorption, and have some of the same spirit lifting qualities as black teas. **Bancha green tea** is an especially good blood cleansing tea.

❋ *About Coffee Substitutes -* These are grain or chicory based drinks, roasted and ground, often with a little molasses or herbs added for flavor. They are caffeine-free, and some of the newest ones such as ROMA are delicious.

❋ *About Herb Teas -* The herb teas in this secton are there more as pleasureable drinks than for medicinal qualities. They are caffeine-free, and can be enjoyed on a regular basis. Favorite single herb teas are peppermint, spearmint, licorice, rose hips, hibiscus, and lemon grass. Spices such as cinnamon, nutmeg, cloves, lemon peel and star anise are wonderful brewed as teas, and can be drunk alone or mixed with other spices and herbs for exotic tastes. Herbs and spices are also delicious mixed with fruit juices for tangy taste, and are at their best as sun-brewed, iced drinks.

☞**How to make sun tea:** For 1 gallon. Use 10 to 12 tea bags or 8 to 10 TBS. loose tea to a gallon jar. Place in the sun or a sunny window, and let steep 5 or 6 hours until tea is twice as dark and strong as you usually like it. Fill with ice cubes, let chill a minute and serve.

Fruit Smoothies

There is nothing like a fresh fruit smoothie for rich refreshment. Smoothies have remained popular ever since their beginnings in the juice bars of the California sixties. They taste decadently sinful, but are a wonderful way to get your fresh fruits for the day while satisfying sweet and sugar cravings. The key to perfect taste as well as convenience is keeping a couple of bunches of peeled bananas (and other fruits) in the freezer - so you can just pop them in the blender any time. (You can also add 4 or 5 ice cubes while blending, instead of freezing the bananas, but it won't taste quite as rich). All of these drinks are blender blended.

43   APRICOT ORANGE CREAM

For 1 drink:

4 FRESH APRICOTS, halved
1 PEELED ORANGE sectioned
1 FROZEN BANANA chunked

1 TB. CHOPPED PECANS
1 TB. SHREDDED COCONUT
enough APPLE JUICE to blend

44   BERRY-NECTARINE SHAKE

For 2 drinks:

2 NECTARINES, chopped
1 FROZEN BANANA chunked
1 PINT BOX of BERRIES

1 HANDFUL PITTED DATES
1 teasp. CINNAMON
enough APPLE JUICE to blend

45   PEACHY SWEET

For 2 drinks:

2 CUPS FRESH PEACHES, chunked
2 FROZEN BANANAS, chunked

1 CUP APPLE JUICE

Frosts & Slushes

*These partially frozen blender drinks are a delicious dessert-y way to get your daily fruits.
Just freeze the fruit first, or add ice cubes to the blender while you blend.*

46   PINEAPPLE BERRY FROST

For 1 drink:

1/2 CUP PINEAPPLE CHUNKS
1/2 CUP STRAWBERRIES

1/2 CUP CRUSHED ICE

47   FRESH FRUIT SLUSH

For 2 drinks:

1 FROZEN BANANA
1 PEAR sliced
1 PEACH sliced

1 ORANGE peeled and sectioned
1 teasp. NUTMEG
2 CUPS CRUSHED ICE

48   CITRUS SLUSH

For 2 drinks:

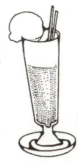

1 CUP CUBED PINEAPPLE
1 MANDARIN ORANGE, peeled, sectioned
1/2 CUP ORANGE JUICE

1 TB. LEMON JUICE
1 TB. LIME JUICE
2 CUPS CRUSHED ICE

Coolers

Healthy coolers are wonderful on a hot day or after exertion to keep the body hydrated and energized. Each of the following recipes makes a big pitcher to keep in the fridge.

49   STRAWBERRY APPLE LEMONADE

This is a unique, delicious cooler we have been making for years to compliments.

1 1/2 QUARTS ORGANIC APPLE JUICE
1 1/2 CUPS LEMON JUICE
1 CUP SLICED STRAWBERRIES

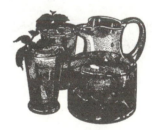

50   EASY HAWAIIAN PUNCH

1 CUP PAPAYA JUICE
1 1/2 CUPS PINEAPPLE/COCONUT JUICE

1/4 CUP ORANGE JUICE
JUICE OF 1 LIME

51   SUMMER LIME COOLER

1 CUP FRESH LIME JUICE
2 QUARTS ICE WATER

1/4 CUP HONEY
1 LIME SLICED IN RINGS

52   CARDAMOM ICED TEA

♣Add 18 DARJEELING TEA BAGS and 18 CARDAMOM PODS to 6 CUPS LUKEWARM WATER in a pitcher. Let sit for 12 hours.
♣Strain, and add 6 TBS. HONEY, or 3 TBS. FRUCTOSE, and 6 TBS. LEMON JUICE. Pour into glasses of crushed ice. Top with 6 SPRIGS FRESH MINT.

53   HIBISCUS ICED TEA

24 BAGS (1 BOX) HIBISCUS TEA
♣Add tea bags to 8 CUPS WATER and let sit for 5-6 hours in a sunny spot until quite dark red.
♣Strain. Add 8 TBS. HONEY or 4 TBS. FRUCTOSE, 1/4 CUP LIME JUICE and 1 LIME sliced in circles.
♣Serve over ice.

🌿*Herbs and wines make beautiful music together! For a different gourmet drink try your next wine cooler with herbs and spices instead of fruit juice. Here are two of our favorites:*

54   LEMON MINT SANGRIA

For 1 big pitcher:

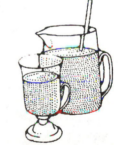

1 BOTTLE DRY WHITE WINE
1/2 CUP WHITE GRAPE JUICE
1 10-OZ. BOTTLE SPARKLING MINERAL WATER (OR KIWI FRUIT SODA)
3 TBS. DRY SHERRY
4 SPRIGS FRESH MINT or 3 SPEARMINT TEA BAGS
2 TBS. LEMON PEEL
2 TBS. LEMON GRASS
♣Combine all together. Float 1 KIWI in slices on top. Let steep several hours. Remove lemon peel, lemon grass or mint sprigs and tea bags before serving.

55   HIBISCUS WINE COOLER

For 1 pitcher:

1 BOTTLE WHITE or BLUSH WINE   1/2 QUART APPLE JUICE
10 to 12 HIBISCUS TEA BAGS   1 1/2 to 2 CUPS WATER
1 SMALL BOTTLE SPARKLING GRAPE JUICE
♣Place tea bags in bottom of large pitcher. Bring water to boil, and pour over bags. Let steep 5 minutes.
♣Remove bags and let cool. Add rest. Pour over ice cubes. Garnish with grape halves or lemon slices.

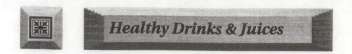

Making Your Own Herbal Teas

Blending your own herb teas can be a rewarding experience for both individual pleasure and health.
This section includes some basic complementary herbs to get you started, and examples of traditional blends
that are valuable for a healing diet. (See CLEANSING & PURIFYING CHAPTER for brewing instructions.)

♣Mints are on everybody's favorite list: **Peppermint, Spearmint and Lemon Balm** are delicious by themselves and make any herb blend palatable. They also aid digestion and help purify the system.

♣Lemon or citrus favorites include **Lemon Grass, Lemon Peel and Orange Peel.** They also blend well with most other herbs for taste, vitamin C, and liver cleansing/stimulating properties.

♣Berries such as **Hawthorn Berries, Juniper Berries and Rose Hips** are tangy, pleasant-tasting herbs for vitamin C and circulation stimulation.

♣Blossoms and flowers such as **Red Clover, Calendula Flowers (Marigold), Yarrow and Chamomile** often taste as good as they look, and have mild blood purifying activity.

♣Roots and barks, such as **Cinnamon, Licorice Rt., Wild Cherry Bark, and Ginger Rt.** add spiciness and substance to a tea, as well as detoxification and alkalizing qualities for the body.

Simple Medicinal Blends for Healing Diets

Use one small packed tea ball for 2 to 3 cups of tea.

56   A RELAXING TEA FOR STRESS, TENSION AND HEADACHE

2 PARTS ROSEMARY
2 PARTS SPEARMINT OR PEPPERMINT
1 PART CATNIP
1 PART CHAMOMILE

57   A DIURETIC TEA FOR GENTLE BLADDER FLUSHING

2 PARTS UVA URSI
2 PARTS JUNIPER BERRIES
1 PART GINGER
1 PART PARSLEY LEAF

58   A DECONGESTANT TEA FOR CLOGGED CHEST & SINUSES

2 PARTS MARSHMALLOW ROOT
2 PARTS MULLEIN LEAF
2 PARTS ROSE HIPS
2 PARTS FENUGREEK SEED

59   A WARMING TEA FOR COLDS & CHILLS

2 PARTS WILD CHERRY BARK
2 PARTS LICORICE ROOT
1 PART ROSE HIPS
1 PART CINNAMON CHIPS

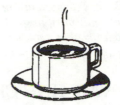

60   AN ENERGIZING TEA FOR FATIGUE

2 PARTS GOTU KOLA
2 PARTS PEPPERMINT
2 PARTS RED CLOVER
1 PART CLOVES

61   A DIGESTIVE TEA FOR GOOD ASSIMILATION

2 PARTS PEPPERMINT
2 PARTS HIBISCUS
1 PART PAPAYA LEAF
1 PART ROSEMARY

62   HOMEMADE GINGER ALE

This is a delicious sparkling tea for both children and adults to settle the stomach, and help elimination during a cold, flu or fever. Drink this tea freely as part of your increased liquid intake during illness.
For 1 quart:

♣Bring to a boil and simmer for 5 minutes
3 CUPS WATER
1 teasp. FRESH GRATED GINGER ROOT, or $1/2$ teasp. POWDERED GINGER
1 teasp. DRY RED RASPBERRY LEAVES
1 teasp. DRY SASSAFRAS ROOT CHOPPED

♣Remove from heat and let steep for 10 to 15 minutes. Strain and add just before serving
1 CUP SPARKLING WATER, such as Evian or Calistoga
2 FRESH LEMON SLICES

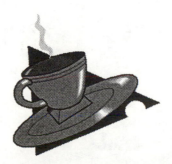

Hot Tonics

The drinks in this section are neither soups nor broths nor teas, but unique hot combinations of vegetables, fruits and spices with purifying, cleansing or energizing activity. The ingredients provide noticeable synergistic action when taken together - with more medicinal benefits than the specific foods alone. Try them - we know you'll agree. Morning and evening seem to be the best times to take these drinks.

63 WARMING CIRCULATION TONIC

Immediate body heat against aches, shakes and chills.
For 4 drinks:

1 CUP CRANBERRY JUICE
1 CUP ORANGE JUICE
2 TBS. HONEY
4 to 6 WHOLE CLOVES
4 to 6 CARDAMOM PODS

1 CINNAMON STICK
4 TBS. RAISINS
4 TBS. ALMONDS chopped
1 teasp. VANILLA

♣Heat all gently for 15 minutes. Remove cloves, cardamom and cinnamon stick. Serve hot.

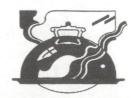

64 MEDITATION TONIC

To clear the head and stimulate the brain.
For 4 drinks:

1 teasp. BUTTER
2 WHOLE CLOVES
1 CINNAMON STICK
PINCH CUMIN POWDER
PINCH CAYENNE

PINCH DRY MUSTARD
1 teasp. FRESH GRATED GINGER
1 CARDAMOM POD
2 CUPS ORANGE JUICE

♣Heat all together for 15 minutes. Remove solid spices and serve in small cups. Very potent.

65 PURIFYING CLEAR BROTH

Very high in potassium and minerals.
For 6 cups:

♣Saute in 2 TBS. OIL until tender crisp
1/4 CUP CHOPPED CELERY
1/4 CUP DAIKON RADISH

1/2 CUP BROCCOLI chopped
1/4 CUP CHOPPED LEEKS
1/4 CUP GRATED CARROTS

♣Add
6 CUPS RICH VEGETABLE STOCK (page 652)
2 TBS. FRESH SNIPPED LEMON PEEL

2 teasp. BRAGG'S LIQUID AMINOS
1/4 CUP SNIPPED PARSLEY

♣Heat for 1 minute, then serve hot.

66 RICE PURIFYING SOUP

For 6 cups:

♣Toast in a large pan until aromatic for 5 minutes
²/₃ CUP LENTILS
²/₃ CUP SPLIT PEAS
²/₃ CUP GOURMET GRAIN BLEND (page 647) or BROWN RICE

♣Add rest and cook over low heat for 1 hr. stirring occasionally

2 CLOVES MINCED GARLIC
1 ONION CHOPPED
1 STALK CELERY, chopped
1 CARROT CHOPPED

3 CUPS WATER
3 CUPS ONION OR VEGGIE BROTH
1 teasp. CAYENNE
¹/₂ teasp. PEPPER
¹/₂ teasp. GINGER POWDER

67 HOT JULEPS

For 2 drinks:

3 PEPPERMINT TEA BAGS, or 2 CUPS STRONG PEPPERMINT TEA
JUICE OF 2 ORANGES   2 teasp. HONEY
2 CUPS HOT WATER   2 MINT SPRIGS
♣Heat all together for 10 minutes. Do not boil. Pour into cups.

68 REVITALIZING TONIC

This is the one from the movies...minus the valet and the raw egg. You know, where smoke comes out of your ears after one sip. Very good for a "morning after hangover." Effective hot or cold. Works every time.
Enough for 8 drinks:

♣Mix in the blender.
ONE 48-OZ. CAN TOMATO JUICE or KNUDSEN'S SPICY VERY VEGGIE JUICE
1 CUP MIXED CHOPPED GREEN, YELLOW, and RED ONIONS
2 STALKS CHOPPED CELERY
1 BUNCH OF PARSLEY, chopped
2 TBS. CHOPPED FRESH BASIL, or 2 teasp. dried
2 teasp. HOT PEPPER SAUCE
1 teasp. ROSEMARY LEAVES
¹/₂ teasp. FENNEL SEEDS
1¹/₂ CUPS WATER
♣1 teasp. BRAGG'S LIQUID AMINOS
♣Pour into a large pot. Bring to a boil and simmer for 30 minutes.

Representative nutritional analysis for hot tonics: per serving: 42 calories; 2gm. protein; 10gm. carbohydrate; 2gm. fiber; trace fat; 41mg. calcium; 2mg. iron; 26mg. magnesium; 487mg. potassium; 637mg. sodium.

Nutritive Meal Replacement Drinks

Meal replacement drinks have become a popular, convenient mainstay for dieters and sports enthusiasts. They are essentially high quality, nutrient dense protein powders, with large amounts of added vitamins, minerals and electrolytes. For weight loss, meal replacement drinks are effective in lowering calorie and food quantity intake while keeping nutrition balanced and adequate. They are best used to replace either the morning or midday meal. For athletes, especially those on training diets including three or more meals a day, these drinks can increase calorie, protein and amino acid intake without the usual accompanying fats.

Making your own meal replacement drinks is a good way to address individual needs easily and conveniently. Think about what foods and food supplements can offer you the nutritive elements you want, put them in the blender or a soup pot, and custom-make a quick, liquid, low-fat meal. We have included four examples here to use for inspiration.

69   MORNING MEAL REPLACEMENT

Effective non-dairy protein. Blender all until mixed.
For 2 drinks:

1 CUP STRAWBERRIES, sliced
1 BANANA, sliced
1 CUP PAPAYA, chunked
8 OZ. SOFT TOFU
or 1 CUP AMAZAKE RICE DRINK

2 TBS. SWEET CLOUD SYRUP
 or BARLEY MALT
1 CUP PINEAPPLE/COCONUT JUICE
$1^1/_2$ teasp. VANILLA
1 TB. TOASTED WHEAT GERM

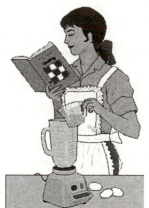

70   HEAVY DUTY PROTEIN DRINK

Blender blend all. A training drink for optimal athletic performance.
For 2 drinks:

1 CUP WATER
6 TBS. DRY NONFAT MILK
1 BANANA, sliced
1 EGG
2 TBS. PEANUT BUTTER
1 TB. CAROB POWDER

1 CUP YOGURT (ANY FLAVOR)
2 TBS. BREWER'S YEAST
1 TB. TOASTED WHEAT GERM
1 teasp. SPIRULINA POWDER
2 teasp. BEE POLLEN GRANULES

Nutritional analysis: per serving; 241 calories; 17gm. protein; 28gm. carbohydrate; 5gm. fiber; 10gm. fats; 283mg. calcium; 2mg. iron; 78mg. magnesium; 774mg. potassium; 156mg. sodium.

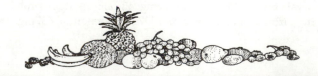

71   MINERAL-RICH AMINOS DRINK

This is an easy, short version of the Crystal Star Herbal Therapy SYSTEM STRENGTH™ drink. It is a complete, balanced food-source vitamin/mineral supplement that is rich in greens, amino acids and enzyme precursers.

♣Make up a dry batch in the blender, then mix about 2 TBS. powder into 2 cups of hot water. Let flavors bloom for 5 minutes before drinking. Add 1 teasp. BRAGG'S LIQUID AMINOS to each drink if desired.
♣Sip over a half hour period for best assimilation.
♣Enough for 8 drinks:

4 to 6 PACKETS MISO CUP SOUP POWDER (Edwards & Son Co. makes a good one.)
1/2 CUP SOY PROTEIN POWDER
1 TB. BREWER'S YEAST FLAKES
2 TBS. BEE POLLEN GRANULES
1 TB. CRUMBLED DRY SEA VEGETABLES (Kombu, Wakame, or Sea Palm)
1 teasp. ACIDOPHILUS POWDER
1 PACKET INSTANT GINSENG TEA GRANULES
1 teasp. or 1 PACKET SPIRULINA OR CHLORELLA GRANULES
1 teasp. DRY CRUMBLED PARSLEY LEAF
♣Add 1 teasp. BRAGG'S LIQUID AMINOS for more flavor.

Nutritional analysis: per serving; 85 calories; 9gm. protein; 10gm. carbohydrate; 2gm. fiber; 2.5gm. fats; 24% calories from fat; 0 cholesterol; 21mg. calcium; 1mg. iron; 8mg. magnesium; 179mg. potassium; 383mg. sodium.

72   DIETER'S MID-DAY MEAL REPLACEMENT DRINK

This drink is good-tasting, filling and satisfying. It is full of foods that help to raise metabolism, cleanse and flush out wastes, balance body pH, and stimulate enzyme production.

♣Blend a dry batch in the blender. Use 1 TB. per glass.
♣Drink slowly.
♣Makes enough for 12 drinks.:

6 TBS. RICE PROTEIN POWDER
4 TBS. OAT BRAN
2 TBS. FLAX SEED
2 TBS. BEE POLLEN GRANULES
2 teasp. SPIRULINA POWDER
1 teasp. ACIDOPHILUS POWDER
1 teasp. LEMON JUICE POWDER
2 teasp. FRUCTOSE (or to taste)
1/2 teasp. GINGER POWDER

Nutritional analysis: per serving; 45 calories; 4gm. protein; 7gm. carbohydrate; 2gm. fiber; 2gm. fats; 29% calories from fat; 21mg. calcium; 1mg. iron; 17mg. magnesium; 124mg. potassium; 23mg. sodium, trace cholesterol.

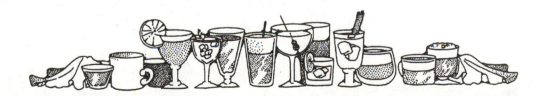

$\mathcal{L}$ife is a splendid torch.
Hold it high.
Make it burn bright.
Nothing is too good to be true.
Everything is possible.

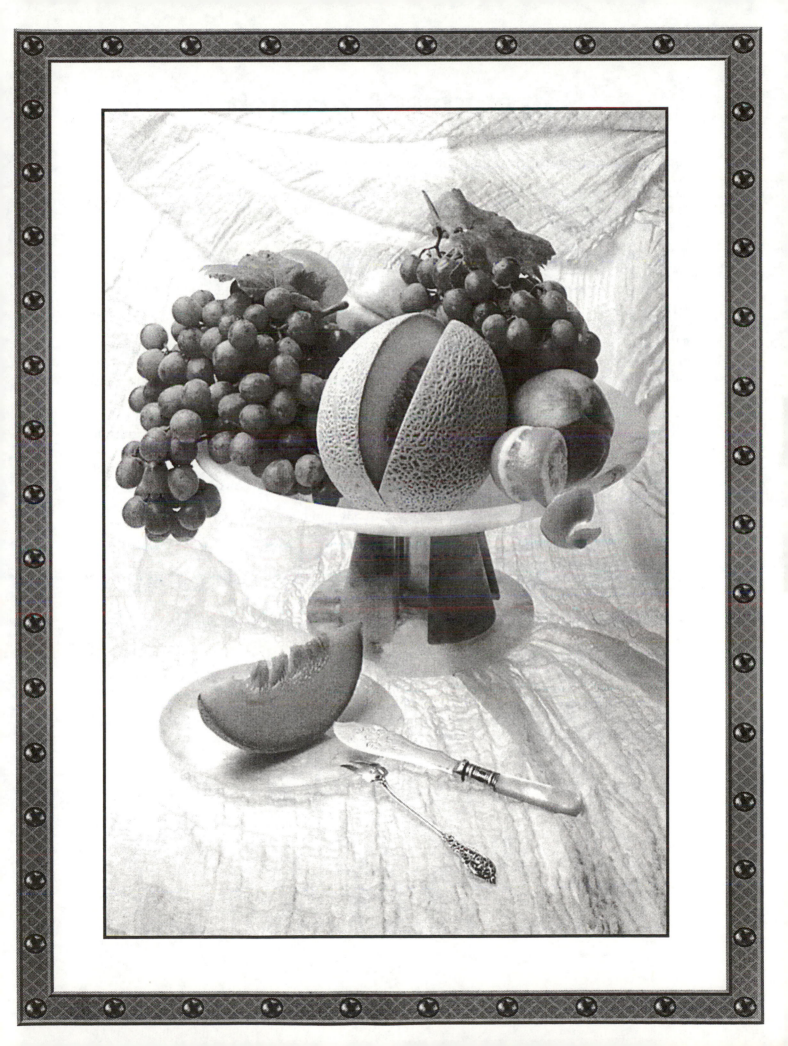

Breakfast & Brunch

Today, people are increasingly realizing the importance of breakfast for health. Morning nutrients are more than just early fuel. They are a key factor in a healing diet. The foods taken on rising, at breakfast and mid-morning, lay the foundation for daily improvement in body chemistry balance. Healing progress can be noticeably accelerated through conscious attention to the nutritional content of the foods you eat before noon.

♣Cleansing, detoxification, and blood purification can be established and stimulated for the next 24 hour period.

♣Liver function can be encouraged to better metabolize fats and to form healthy red blood cells.

♣The body's glycogen supply can be maximized in the morning hours for better sugar tolerance and energy use.

♣Broad spectrum enzyme production can be established through the pancreas for increased assimilation of nutrients and better tolerance of food sensitivities.

♣Brain and memory functions make maximum use of food fuel in the morning, especially after a restful night. Consider a good breakfast for the the health of your head.

♣If you have hypoglycemia, a good solid breakfast is almost a must.

♣Breakfast is also the day's best opportunity to get high fiber foods like whole grains and fruits, for regularity and body balance.

♣Metabolism is at its highest in the morning to burn up excess calories. Low-fat, high energy breakfast foods can help keep you away from junk foods and unconscious nibbling all day.

The recipes in this chapter can help accelerate the above body improvement objectives for healing. They include sections on:

❧MORNING DRINKS ❧FRESH and DRIED FRUITS ❧BREAKFAST GRAINS and CEREALS ❧ BREADS, MUFFINS and PANCAKES ❧EGGS and OMELETS ❧VEGETARIAN BREAKFAST SOY FOODS ❧HEALTHY BREAKFAST BARS ❧

Morning foods are linked with our earliest health awareness nutrition; whole grain granolas, fresh or dried fruits, nut butters, yogurt and protein drinks. As the value of these foods has become better realized, breakfast has come to include other healthy food categories, such as whole grain sandwiches, pitas, muffins and pancakes, brown rice with dried fruits, nuts or vegetables, tofu, tempe, tahini and low-fat spreads such as hummus, or cottage cheese.

Ideally, the body needs to get about one third of its daily nutrients in the morning. Enjoy a quick, nourishing morning meal. What you put in your stomach at the start of the day affects how your whole day goes.

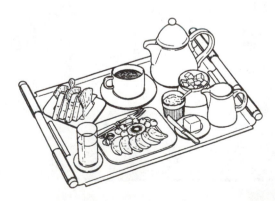

Morning Drinks

73   NON-DAIRY MORNING PROTEIN DRINK

You must have protein to heal. The new breed of protein drinks are a wonderful way to get protein without meat, bulk or excess fat. This drink obtains protein from several food sources so that a balance with carbohydrates and minerals is achieved, and a real energy boost felt. Blender blend all until mixed.
For 2 drinks:

1 CUP STRAWBERRIES or KIWI, sliced
1 BANANA, sliced
1 CUP PAPAYA or PINEAPPLE, chunked
8-OZ. SOFT TOFU
or 1 CUP AMAZAKE RICE DRINK

2 TBS. MAPLE SYRUP
1 CUP ORGANIC APPLE JUICE
1 teasp. VANILLA
1 TB. TOASTED WHEAT GERM
1/2 teasp. GINGER POWDER

Nutritional analysis: per serving; 156 calories; 6gm. protein; 28gm. carbohydrate; 3gm. fiber; 3gm. fats 18% calories from fat; 0 cholesterol; 90mg. calcium; 4mg. iron; 85mg. magnesium; 12mg. sodium; 417mg. potassium.

74   MORNING ORANGE SHAKE

For 2 drinks:

2 ORANGES peeled and sectioned
1 FROZEN BANANA chunked
1/4 CUP ORANGE JUICE

2 TBS. YOGURT
1 teasp. VANILLA

Nutritional analysis: per serving; 135 calories; 3gm. protein; 33gm. carbohydrate; 4gm. fiber; 1gm. fat 4% calories from fat; trace cholesterol; 84mg. calcium; trace iron; 10mg. sodium; 35mg. magnesium; 558mg. potassium.

75   MOCHA MOCHA COFFEE SUBSTITUTE

Use 1 to 2 teasp. per cup of this caffeine-free mix. Steep and strain just like a tea.

♣Mix 2 parts <u>each</u>:
CAROB CHIPS
BARLEY MALT POWDER
ROAST CHICORY GRANULES

♣Add 1/2 part <u>each</u>:
CLOVES
CARDAMOM PODS

♣Add 1 part <u>each</u>:
CINNAMON CHIPS
ALLSPICE BERRIES
LICORICE ROOT CHIPS

♣Add flavoring drops of:
VANILLA EXTRACT

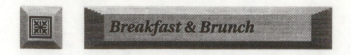

76   MORNING & EVENING FIBER DRINK

This is an excellent health drink mix for daily regularity. It may be used as needed with confidence in its efficiency, without concern about dependency. Take 1 heaping teaspoon in water or juice in the morning and at bedtime.

♣Mix in the blender
3 PARTS OAT or RICE BRAN 1/2 PART ACIDOPHILUS LIQUID
2 PARTS FLAX SEED 1/4 PART FENNEL SEED
1 PART PSYLLIUM HUSK POWDER

Nutritional analysis: per serving; 20 caloties; 1gm. protein; 3gm. carbohydrate; 1gm. fiber; 1gm. fats; 37% calories from fat; 23mg. 0 cholesterol; calcium; trace iron; 11mg. magnesium; 8mg. sodium; 51mg. potassium.

✳

♣Note: Black, green or herbal teas in the morning can also satisfy that need for a little lift at the beginning of the day. Our favorite black teas are Darjeeling, English Breakfast and Earl Grey, all of which may be bought caffeine-free. (See **About Black Teas** in the HEALTHY DRINKS, JUICES & WATERS section of this book.)
Green teas, such as Bancha leaf, are "bitters" teas, proven body cleansers. They stimulate the production of bile for better digestion, food assimilation and liver health.
Good herbal morning teas include red raspberry for body balance, gotu kola for mental energy, and ginseng teas for rejuvenation.

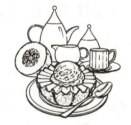

Fresh & Dried Fruits

77   HIGH PROTEIN FRUIT BREAKFAST MIX

There are two delicious variations for this morning fruit mix. The first is especially good for skin health and tone. The second is effective for regularity and extra minerals. Each makes enough for two.

♣Mix together <u>either</u> FRESH CHOPPED PEACHES, PAPAYA, and STRAWBERRIES with
1/4 CUP TOASTED SLICED ALMONDS
1/4 CUP TOASTED SESAME SEEDS
1/4 CUP CHOPPED DRIED PRUNES
1/4 CUP CHOPPED DRIED PAPAYA
1/4 CUP PLAIN YOGURT

<u>or</u> FRESH SLICED GRAPES, PEARS, BANANAS and PINEAPPLE with
1/4 CUP TOASTED WALNUTS or CASHEWS
1/4 CUP TOASTED SUNFLOWER SEEDS
1/4 CUP CHOPPED DRIED PRUNES
1/4 CUP RAISINS
1/4 CUP PLAIN YOGURT

♣Mix together the topping in a small bowl and pour over either fruit mix
2 TBS. TOASTED WHEAT GERM   2 teasp. HONEY
1 teasp. LECITHIN GRANULES   2 teasp. LEMON JUICE
2 teasp. BREWER'S YEAST FLAKES

✳

78   SMOOTH PRUNES
A delicious, creamy way to keep regular.
For 4 bowls:

♣Soak 2 CUPS PITTED PRUNES IN WATER in the fridge until soft, or overnight.

♣Blender blend with 1 PINT of PLAIN YOGURT, 1 TB. HONEY, and 1 teasp. VANILLA.
♣Whirl until smooth, and mound in small open bowls. Sprinkle with NUTMEG.

Nutritional analysis: per serving; 292 calories; 8gm. protein; 66gm. carbohydrate; 8gm. fiber; 2gm. fat; 7mg. cholesterol; 6% calories from fat; 252mg. calcium; 2mg. iron; 59mg. magnesium; 83mg. sodium; 903mg. potassium.

79   GINGER GRAPEFRUIT WITH MERINGUE TOPPING
A gourmet, Sunday morning treat.
Topping for 4 grapefruit halves:

♣Whip 2 EGG WHITES to soft peaks. Add $1/4$ CUP THIN HONEY and $1/4$ teasp. POWDERED GINGER and whip to meringue consistency.

♣Spread meringue on grapefruit halves, and bake at 300° for 15 to 20 minutes.

Nutritional analysis: per serving; 110 calories; 3gm. protein; 27gm. carbohydrate; 1gm. fiber; trace fat; 0 cholesterol; 15mg. calcium; trace iron; 13mg. magnesium; 194mg. potassium; 28mg. sodium.

80   MORNING LUNG TONIC PEARS
A good choice during high risk, respiratory problem seasons.
For 2 Servings:

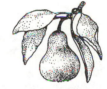

♣Core and slice 2 HARD WINTER PEARS.
♣Drizzle with 2 teasp. honey, and sprinkle with $1/2$ teasp. ground cardamom per pear. Bake or broil until brown and caramelized.

YOGURT CHEESE TOPPING FOR FRESH FRUIT OR GRANOLA

♣Mix together and spoon onto fresh fruits, granola or hot cereal.
$1/2$ CUP YOGURT CHEESE (See How To Make on page 392.)
1 TB. LIGHT HONEY

1 TB. LEMON JUICE
GRATED ZEST of 1 LEMON

Nutritional analysis: per serving; 146 calories; 6gm. protein; 28gm. carbohydrate; trace fiber; 1gm. fat; 10% calories from fat; 7mg. cholesterol; 226mg. calcium; trace iron; 23mg. mag.; 80mg. sodium; 315mg. potass.

Morning Cereals & Grains

Whole grains and cereals in the morning are becoming an increasingly preferred way to start daily nutrition. Hot or cold, they offer full, satisfying calories with low-fat, sustaining energy, and lots of taste.

81   HOT OR COLD BREAKFAST GRAINS

You can use the grain mix recommended here, or any single grain or blend you like. You can't go wrong.
For 4 servings:

♣Bring 1 CUP APPLE JUICE, or PINEAPPLE JUICE to a boil
♣Add 1 CUP GOURMET GRAIN MIX. (page 647) and 1 CUP WATER.

♣Reduce heat to medium and cook until liquid is absorbed, about 25 minutes.

♣Serve hot with a handful of TOASTED SLICED ALMONDS and SUNFLOWER SEEDS, DASHES of CINNAMON and a HANDFUL OF RAISINS.
♣Serve cold with 1 or 2 teasp. HONEY and FRUIT YOGURT to taste.

Nutritional analysis: per serving; 213 calories; 5gm. protein; 43gm. carbohydrate; 5gm. fiber; 2gm. fat; 0mg. cholesterol; 10% calories from fat; 24mg. calcium; 1mg. iron; 74mg. magnesium; 271mg. potassium; 11mg. sodium.

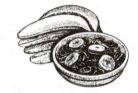

82   ISLAND MUESLI

For 6 servings:

♣Toast in the oven until coconut is golden brown
1/4 CUP SHREDDED COCONUT
1/4 CUP CHOPPED PECANS
1/4 CUP SUNFLOWER SEEDS
1/4 CUP SLICED ALMONDS
1/4 CUP ROLLED OATS

♣Chop in chunks
1 MANGO or 1 PEACH
1/4 FRESH PINEAPPLE
1 PAPAYA
2 BANANAS

♣Mix all together lightly with grains and seeds.
♣Pour over 1/2 CUP PINEAPPLE or ORANGE JUICE.
♣Top with 1/2 CUP RAISINS.

MAKE YOUR OWN GRANOLA

♣Granola is a hearty blend of whole grains, nuts, seeds and dried fruits, lightly coated with honey, maple syrup or molasses and an unsaturated oil, and oven-roasted. It is as robust, nutritious and delicious as it has been from the beginning of the healthy food consciousness days of the sixties. Unfortunately most mass-market granolas now have coconut, or partially hydrogenated oils instead of high quality oils, brown sugar or corn syrup instead of the natural sweeteners, sulfur dried fruits and all kinds of sugary bits added. These two recipes bring you back to the basics with the original, wholesome, high-density energy foods. They both make enough for a week of breakfasts for 2 people.
♣Store air-tight to maintain crispness.

83   REAL GRANOLA

Enough for 20 servings: Preheat oven to 150°.

♣Mix together in a large bowl
8 CUPS ROLLED OATS OR BARLEY
2 CUPS WHEAT GERM
1 CUP SHREDDED COCONUT
1/2 CUP BUCKWHEAT OR GRAPENUTS
2 CUPS CHOPPED ALMONDS
1 CUP SUNFLOWER SEEDS

♣Blender blend next 4 ingredients, and pour over first mixture
1/2 CUP LIGHT VEGETABLE OIL
1/2 CUP MAPLE SYRUP
1/3 CUP APPLE OR PEAR JUICE
2 teasp. VANILLA or ALMOND EXTRACT
♣Spread on baking sheets. Bake in low oven for 1 hour until crunchy and golden. Stir every 10 minutes.
♣Add 1 CUP CHOPPED DATES or RAISINS.

84   FRUIT & NUT GRANOLA

Enough for 18 to 20 servings: Preheat oven to 350°.

♣Mix together in an extra large bowl
6 CUPS ROLLED OATS
2 1/2 CUPS SUNFLOWER SEEDS
1 CUP SESAME SEEDS
2 CUPS WHEAT BRAN
1 CUP OAT BRAN
1 CUP WALNUT PIECES
2 CUPS SLICED or SLIVERED ALMONDS

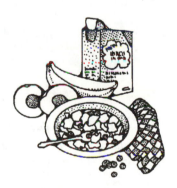

♣Warm in a small saucepan
1/2 CUP LIGHT VEGETABLE OIL
1 1/2 CUPS HONEY
♣Pour over and toss with granola.
♣Spread on two 11 x 17 jelly roll pans, and bake for 15 minutes. Remove and stir.
♣Reduce oven temperature to 325°, and bake for 30 minutes. Stir every 10 minutes or so, and switch pans so browning will be even.
♣Return to the large bowl and add 4 CUPS MIXED DRIED CHOPPED FRUITS, such as RAISINS, CUR-RANTS, APRICOTS, DATES AND PITTED PRUNES. Toss to blend and let cool before storing.

Nutritional analysis: per serving; 669 calories; 18gm. protein; 85gm. carbohydrate; 12gm. fiber; 35gm. fat; 0 cholesterol; 43% calories from fat; 121mg. calcium; 257mg. magnesium; 6mg. iron; 805mg. potass.; 11mg. sodium.

Breads, Muffins & Pancakes

85   ORIGINAL BRAN MUFFINS

We made these almost every day in the Rainbow Kitchen. This is the original popular recipe, and it is obviously for a crowd. But it is easily cut down to a one muffin tin batch. Tasty and high in cereal fiber.
For 6 dozen muffins: Preheat oven to 350°.

♣Pour 2 CUPS BOILING WATER over 2 CUPS GRAPENUTS and set aside to work.

♣Cream together in a large bowl

3/4 CUP BUTTER	1/2 CUP FRUCTOSE
1/4 CUP OIL	1/2 CUP DATE SUGAR
1 CUP HONEY	

♣Add 4 EGGS and 4 CUPS BUTTERMILK or PLAIN YOGURT mixed with WATER to milk consistency. Mix in well.

♣Mix together in another bowl

5 CUPS WHOLE WHEAT PASTRY FLOUR	4 teasp. BAKING POWDER
4 CUPS BRAN FLAKES CEREAL	5 teasp. BAKING SODA

♣Combine the two mixtures together gently to moisten, and mix in 1¹/2 CUPS CHOPPED DATES or WALNUTS or RAISINS.
♣Spoon into paper-lined or lecithin sprayed muffin cups and bake for 20 minutes until a toothpick inserted in the center of a muffin comes out clean.
♣This batter stores very well in the fridge for a short while, or in the freezer for quite a while. You can make up the whole amount and use it as needed.

Nutritional analysis: per serving; 121 calories; 3gm. protein; 23gm. carbohydrate; 3gm. fiber; 3gm. fat; 17mg. cholesterol; 23% calories from fat; 41mg. calcium; 2mg. iron; 37mg. magnesium; 209mg. potass.; 140mg. sodium.

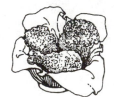

86   TOASTED WHEAT GERM MUFFINS

These are a delicious way to enjoy the health advantages of wheat germ.
For 12 muffins: Preheat oven to 375°.

♣Combine 1 CUP TOASTED WHEAT GERM (you can use raw wheat germ, but the flavor is much better, and the health advantages only minimally impaired if you toast it briefly in the oven before using), and 1/2 CUP PLAIN YOGURT mixed with 1/2 CUP WATER. Let stand for 1 hour.

♣Add 1 BEATEN EGG and 2 TBS. OIL.
♣Add 1 CUP WHOLE WHEAT FLOUR or FLOUR BLEND (see page 647), 4 teasp. BAKING POWDER, and 1/2 teasp. SEA SALT to liquid ingredients.
♣Mix all ingredients together lightly, and fill lecithin-sprayed or paper-lined muffin tins 2/3 full.
♣Bake for 15 to 20 minutes until a toothpick inserted in the center comes out clean.

87   RAISIN OAT BRAN MUFFINS

♣For 6 big deli-style Sunday breakfast muffins, use 4 greased pyrex custard cups, and bake at 375°.

♣For 8 regular size muffin, put batter in a 6-cup greased muffin tin and bake at 400° until a toothpick inserted in the center comes out clean.

♣Mix the dry ingredients
1 CUP UNBLEACHED FLOUR
1/2 CUP WHOLE WHEAT PASTRY FLOUR
1 CUP GRAPENUTS or a favorite BRAN CEREAL
1 CUP ROLLED OATS
1 1/2 teasp. BAKING SODA

♣Form a well in the center, and pour in
1 CUP PLAIN YOGURT
1/2 CUP HONEY
1 EGG
1/4 CUP OIL
1/2 CUP RAISINS

♣Stir all together until lumpy, and bake as above.

Nutritional analysis: per serving for large muffins; 352 calories; 8gm. protein; 62gm carbo.; 4m. fiber; 9gm. fat; 28mg. choles.; 22% calories from fat; 76mg. calcium; 5mg. iron; 51mg. magn.; 289mg. potass. 270mg. sodium.

88   WHOLE GRAIN BISCUITS

For 6 biscuits: Preheat oven to 400∞.

♣Cut in and stir everything together to make the dough
1 CUP GOURMET BAKING MIX or UNBLEACHED FLOUR
1/2 teasp. BAKING POWDER
1/2 teasp. BAKING SODA
PINCH SEA SALT
1/3 CUP TOASTED WHEAT GERM

3 TBS. OIL
1 EGG
1/3 CUP LOW-FAT YOGURT

♣Using a spoon, drop dough into lecithin-sprayed muffin cups, or pat out onto a floured board, cut or shape 6 biscuits, and put on a lecithin-sprayed baking sheet. Bake about 20 minutes til golden.

89   HONEY NUT SWEET BREAD

Much better than a Danish in the morning.
For 12 servings: Preheat oven to 375∞.

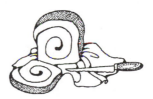

Mix all together just to moisten. Batter will be very light.
1/4 CUP OIL
1/2 teasp. SEA SALT
1 CUP HONEY
2 TBS. MAPLE SYRUP
1/2 CUP PLAIN LOW-FAT YOGURT

2 EGGS
1 1/2 CUPS WHOLE GRAIN FLOUR MIX
1 1/2 teasp. BAKING SODA
1 teasp. ALMOND EXTRACT
3/4 CUPS CHOPPED WALNUTS

♣Pour batter into a lecithin-sprayed round baking pan.

♣Top with 1/4 CUP CHOPPED NUTS, and bake for 35 minutes until springy when touched on top.

♣Cut in wedges to serve.

Nutritional analysis: per serving; 253 calories; 4gm. protein; 38gm. carbohydrate; 2gm. fiber; 10gm. fat; 36mg. cholest. 35% calories from fat; 39mg. calcium; 1mg. iron; 37mg. magnesium; 151mg. potass.; 211mg. sodium.

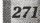

90   FOUR GRAIN FLAPJACKS

These hearty pancakes lay a solid foundation for a day's hard work.
For 18 pancakes: Preheat griddle or cast iron skillet until a drop of water skitters on the surface.

♣Combine in a bowl and let stand for 10 minutes
3/4 CUP ROLLED OATS
1/2 CUP COTTAGE CHEESE
1/2 CUP WATER

♣Put 1 CUP COLD WATER into a small saucepan. Whisk in 1/2 CUP CORNMEAL.
♣Bring to a boil over high heat, stirring constantly until thickened. Reduce heat and cook 2 to 3 minutes more, until mixture is quite thick. Scrape into a bowl, and let cool slightly.
♣Whisk in
1/2 CUP BUTTERMILK or YOGURT
   and WATER mixed   1/4 CUP MOLASSES
1/4 CUP OIL   2 EGGS

♣Stir in OATS and COTTAGE CHEESE MIXTURE and set aside.

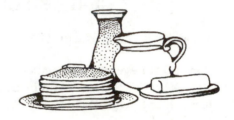

♣Mix together
1 CUP WHOLE WHEAT PASTRY FLOUR
1/2 CUP BUCKWHEAT FLOUR
2 teasp. RUMFORD'S BAKING POWDER
1/2 teasp. BAKING SODA
1/2 teasp. SEA SALT

♣Stir wet and dry mixtures together until just blended. Let stand 10 minutes to work, for lightness.
♣When skillet is ready brush on some oil lightly, and ladle in 2 to 3 pancakes at a time. Cook until bubbles burst on the surface. Flip and cook until golden. Oil cooking surface between each batch.
♣Serve with maple syrup or honey.

✷

91   OAT BRAN BANANA PANCAKES

High in fiber, and a treat for kids of all ages.
For 18 pancakes: Preheat griddle or cast iron skillet until a drop of water skitters on the surface.

♣Toss together   ♣Add
1 CUP OAT BRAN   1 VERY RIPE BANANA, mashed
1 CUP BAKING SODA   2 teasp. VANILLA
2 teasp. FRUCTOSE   1 1/2 CUPS PLAIN YOGURT

♣Beat 4 EGG WHITES to soft peaks. Fold into batter, and stir in 2 TBS. melted butter.
♣Ladle 2 to 3 pancakes onto griddle or skillet, and spread into circles. Cook until bubbles appear on the surface, about 1 minute. Flip and cook until bottoms are brown, about 1 minute more.
♣Serve hot with maple syrup or honey.

✷

92   HEALTHY HASH BROWNS

This traditional hearty favorite is perfect for an active weekend, I'm-really-hungry breakfast.
For 8 servings:

♣Boil 5 RED or WHITE ROSE POTATOES in water over high heat for 5 minutes. Drain and set aside.

♣Dry roast 2 TBS. SOY BACON BITS in a large skillet until aromatic, about 5 minutes.
♣Add 2 TBS. OIL and 2 LARGE SLICED ONIONS and sauté for 25 minutes, covered until softened and <u>brown</u>. Remove and set aside.

♣Grate the potatoes in a salad shooter or food processor and season with $1/2$ teasp. SALT, $1/2$ teasp. FRUCTOSE, and $1/4$ teasp. PEPPER.
♣Add 2 TBS. OIL and THE POTATOES to the skillet. Press against bottom and sides to form a crust.
♣Cook for 15 minutes over medium heat until nice and brown on the bottom.

♣Drizzle on 1 TB. OLIVE OIL, $1/2$ teasp. GARLIC/LEMON SEASONING and 1 teasp. ROSEMARY.
♣Mix in onions, and run under the broiler for 1 minute to brown and crisp. Serve hot.

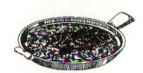

Breakfast Soy Foods

Soy foods offer an excellent vegetarian source of protein for morning fuel.

93   BREAKFAST, NO DAIRY PANCAKE PIZZA

This is a very unusual recipe; but try it - you'll like it.
For 10 to 12 pieces: Preheat oven to 425°.

♣Heat a round pizza pan or baking sheet in the oven until the batter is ready.

♣Mix the batter briefly in the blender.
2 EGGS
$1^3/4$ CUPS PLAIN or VANILLA SOY MILK
2 TBS. OIL
2 CUPS BUCKWHEAT PANCAKE MIX
♣Spray the hot pizza pan with lecithin spray, and pour on the batter.

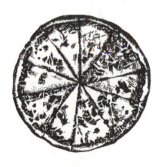

♣Sprinkle with
$3/4$ CUP GRANOLA (page 273)
$3/4$ CUP CHOPPED PECANS
A HANDFUL OF RAISINS
♣Bake 12 to 15 minutes until brown at the edges. Cut in wedges or squares. Serve with maple syrup.

Nutritional analysis: per serving; 218 calories; 6gm. protein; 21gm. carbohydrate; 3gm. fiber; 12gm. fat; 47mg. cholesterol; 47% calories from fat; 115mg. calcium; 1mg. iron; 45mg. magnesium; 248mg. potass. 150mg. sod.

94   HIGH PROTEIN TOFU PANCAKES

For 18 easy pancakes: Preheat a griddle or cast iron skillet until a drop of water skitters on the surface.

♣Make it all in the blender

1 CUP PLAIN YOGURT	1 teasp. BAKING POWDER
1/2 CUP WATER	PINCH SEA SALT
3 EGGS	1 CUP GOURMET FLOUR MIX (p. 647)
1 TB. OIL	1 LB. VERY FRESH TOFU, mashed
2 TBS. MAPLE SYRUP	11/2 teasp. VANILLA

♣Whirl until smooth, and pour onto the hot griddle in 1/3 to 1/2 cup circles. Flip when bubbles appear, and stack on a serving platter. Serve with more maple syrup.

Nutritional analysis: per serving; 112 calories; 9gm. protein; 12gm. carbohydrate; 2gm. fiber; 5gm. fat; 54mg. cholesterol; 36% calories from fat; 105mg. calcium; 3mg. iron; 58mg. magnes. 226mg. potass. 76mg. sodium.

95   PUFFY TOFU POPOVERS

These are very light. The secret is to heat the Pyrex custard cups or the popover pan in a hot oven <u>first</u>. Remove them only when batter is ready, fill and immediately return to the hot oven. They will puff beautifully.

For 6 big popovers: Preheat oven to 400°.
♣Put 1 TB. BUTTER in each of 6 custard or popover cups. Put the cups on a baking sheet and heat in the oven while you make the batter. They must be *very* hot.

♣Make the batter in the blender

3 EGGS	1 teasp. SESAME SALT
4 CAKES TOFU crumbled	3/4 CUP UNBLEACHED FLOUR

♣Pour the batter slowly over the butter in the cups. <u>Do not stir</u> together. Bake for 20 minutes. Reduce heat to 350°.and bake for 15 more minutes.

96   TAHINI TOFU BREAKFAST SLICES

For 8 slices: Preheat oven to 400°.

♣Slice 1 LB. TOFU IN 8 SLABS (cut each cake in half <u>lengthwise</u>)

♣Combine in a bowl and spread some sauce on each slab
1/4 CUP SESAME TAHINI or ALMOND BUTTER
1/4 CUP WHITE MISO PASTE
1 TB. SOY BACON BITS

♣Sprinkle with TOASTED WHEAT GERM, and place on oiled sheets in the oven, or under a broiler for 1 minute, until crusty. Turn slabs and spread on rest of sauce. Sprinkle with more wheat germ.
♣Bake or broil until crusty.

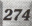

Breakfast Eggs & Omelet Art

Eggs are finally getting the "break" they deserve as researchers learn how to consider the whole food and not just its parts in their findings. Recent studies show what the health food world has long known; that an egg's cholesterol content is balanced by its lecithin and phosphatides. Eggs are still one of nature's premier foods.

97 BOUILLON POACHED EGGS

Simple gourmet eggs the way the pros do it. A most healthful way to enjoy eggs.
For 2 breakfast servings:

♣Heat 1 quart of WATER and 1 TB. VINEGAR in a heavy skillet to boiling. Add 2 BOUILLON CUBES, or 2 teasp. VEGETABLE or CHICKEN BROTH POWDER.
♣Crack an egg into a teacup, and lower the cup into the broth - let the egg slide out. Repeat three times.
♣Cook to medium firm, **for 3 minutes**. Lift eggs out gently with a slotted spoon. Serve immediately.

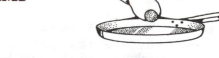

98 SCRAMBLED EGGS SPECIAL

For 4 servings: Preheat a griddle or skillet until a drop of water skitters on the surface.

♣Sauté 1/4 CUP MINCED ONION in 2 TBS. OIL, or braise in 2 TBS. ONION or VEGETABLE BROTH until brown and aromatic.
♣Meanwhile, whirl in the blender

6 EGGS
1/2 teasp. SESAME SALT
1/4 teasp. PEPPER

2 teasp. PARSLEY FLAKES
1/3 CUP COTTAGE CHEESE
1 teasp. YELLOW MUSTARD

♣Add to hot onion sauté and cook slowly, stirring frequently but gently until eggs are set.

Nutritional analysis: per serving; 162 calories; 12gm. protein; 3gm. carbohydrate; trace fiber; 11gm. fat; 300mg. cholesterol; 60% calories from fat; 57mg. calcium; 1mg. iron; 11mg. magnesium; 135mg. potasssium; 378mg. sod.

99 SCRAMBLED EGGS WITH BABY SHRIMP

A better way to have a little meat protein at breakfast.
For 4 servings:

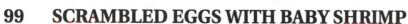

♣Mix briefly in a bowl
6 EGGS
2 GREEN ONIONS, chopped
1/2 teasp. SALT
2 PINCHES OF PEPPER
♣Add 5 to 6-oz. COOKED BABY SHRIMP.
♣Stir and cook until set. Serve hot.

♣Heat over medium hot heat
2 TBS. OIL

♣When hot, add ONION/EGG MIX and
stir until half cooked.

Nutritional analysis: per serving; 213 calories; 17gm. protein; 2gm. arbohydrate; trace fiber; 14gm. fat; 380mg. cholesterol; 60% calories from fat; 64mg. calcium; 2mg. iron; 195mg. potassium; 23mg. mag.; 440mg. sodium.

100   HUEVOS RANCHEROS CUSTARD FRITTATA
This is very rich. Great for small brunch portions.
For 8 to 10 brunch portions: Preheat oven to 350°.

♣Arrange a 7-OZ. CAN WHOLE GREEN CHILIS face open in a single layer on the bottom of a 3-qt. baking dish. Sprinkle with 1 CUP LOW-FAT CHEDDAR CHEESE, 1 CUP LOW-FAT JACK CHEESE, and 2 teasp. CAPERS or 1 TB. GREEN CHOPPED OLIVES.
♣*Repeat layers of cheeses and olives.*

♣Beat 3 EGGS, 1 CUP PLAIN YOGURT and 1 DICED TOMATO together in a bowl. Pour over cheeses, and bake for 30 minutes until edges are just beginning to brown.
♣Garnish with MORE CHOPPED TOMATO and DRIZZLES of MILD SALSA (page 100).

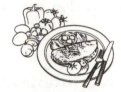

101   EASY VEGETABLE HERB FRITTATA
This is a breakfast, brunch, and simple supper favorite.
For 8 wedge portions: Preheat oven to 350°.

♣Sauté 1/4 CUP CHOPPED RED ONION in 2 TBS. OIL, or 2 TBS. ONION or VEGETABLE BROTH.
♣Add 1 CUP CHOPPED FRESH TOMATOES and turn off heat.
♣Whirl 8 EGGS, 1/4 CUP PLAIN LOW-FAT YOGURT and 1 teasp. ITALIAN HERBS in the blender.
♣Pour over tomatoes in the skillet. Sprinkle with 1/2 CUP CHOPPED GREEN PEPPER, 1/4 CUP MINCED OLIVES, and 1 CUP GRATED PART SKIM MOZARRELLA CHEESE.
♣Bake for 15 to 20 minutes until eggs are set. Garnish with SNIPPED PARSLEY and cut in wedges.

Nutritional analysis: per serving; 159 calories; 10gm. protein; 3gm. carbohydrate; 1gm. fiber; 12gm. fat; 223mg. cholesterol; 63% calories from fat; 131mg. calcium; 17mg. mag. 1mg. iron; 169mg. potassium; 260mg. sodium.

102   BREAKFAST POLENTA
This hearty Italian whole grain is great for breakfast/brunch, too.
For 4 servings: Preheat oven to 350°.

♣Bring 1 CUP ONION or CHICKEN STOCK to a boil in a heavy pot. Add 1/2 CUP POLENTA and stir until it masses together and pulls away from the sides of the pan, about 10 minutes.
♣Add 1 TB. BUTTER or OIL, 1/4 CUP GRATED PARMESAN or ROMANO CHEESE, and 2 PINCHES BLACK PEPPER.
♣Spoon 1/2 cup of mixture into each of four individual ramekins or custard cups. Make an indentation in the middle and crack 1 EGG into each. Cover with more polenta to enclose. Sprinkle each ramekin with 1 TB. LOW-FAT WHITE CHEDDAR.
♣Place the ramekins on baking sheets; bake until cheese melts and browns, about 10 minutes. Serve hot.

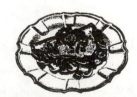

103 ZUCCHINI OPEN FACE OMELET

Nice and spicy. Serve with a dollop of homemade tomato sauce.
For 4 to 5 wedge portions: Preheat oven to 350°. Use a cast iron or oven-approved skillet.

♣Sauté 1/2 CHOPPED GREEN PEPPER and 2 CHOPPED MEDIUM ZUCCHINIS over medium high heat in 2 TBS. OIL or 2 TBS. ONION or VEGETABLE BROTH for 5 minutes.

♣Whirl in the blender
1 TB. PLAIN YOGURT   6 EGGS
1 teasp. SESAME or HERB SALT   1 TB. OIL
2 PINCHES PEPPER

♣Add to skillet and cook for 2 minutes, until eggs are just set on the bottom.

♣Put skillet in the oven and bake for 4 minutes until eggs set on the top. Cut in wedges, and top with an AVOCADO SALSA (pg. 456), or TOMATO SAUCE. (pg. 462).

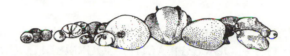

Healthy Breakfast Bars & Munches

104 TRIPLE FIBER COOKIES

For 36 cookies: Preheat oven to 375°.

♣Mix the wet ingredients until fluffy   ♣Mix the dry ingredients
1 STICK BUTTER   1 CUP OAT BRAN
1/4 CUP OIL   1/2 CUP WHOLE WHEAT FLOUR
4 TBS. BROWN SUGAR   1/2 teasp. BAKING SODA
1/2 CUP HONEY   3 CUPS ROLLED OATS
2 TBS. MAPLE SYRUP   1 CUP CHOPPED PITTED PRUNES
1 EGG   1/2 CUP CHOPPED WALNUTS
1 teasp. VANILLA

♣Mix all ingredients together until just blended. Form 1" balls. Flatten to discs, and place 1" apart on greased baking sheets. Bake for 12 to 15 minutes until golden. Cool on racks.

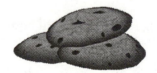

105 FIG AND HONEY BARS

For 24 bars:

♣Toast 3 to 4 TBS. SESAME SEEDS in the oven. Sprinkle over the bottom of an 8 x 8" baking pan.
♣Cook and stir 1/2 CUP HONEY, 1/2 CUP ALMOND BUTTER and 4 TBS. UNSALTED BUTTER over low heat until smooth and melted, about 5 minutes.
♣Remove from heat and mix in 2 1/2 CUPS GRANOLA and 1/2 CUP CHOPPED DRIED FIGS.
♣Press into prepared pan and cool 1 hour before cutting.

106   BREAKFAST FRUIT NACHOS

For 18 wedges: Preheat oven to 375°.

♣Split 3 pita breads horizontally and cut each in 6 wedges. Toast on baking sheets briefly to crisp.
♣Spread half with RASPBERRY or BLUEBERRY PRESERVES, and the other half with ORANGE MAR-MALADE. Top with granola sprinkles and a pineapple wedge. Sprinkle on GRATED CHEDDAR. Broil 2 to 3 minutes until cheddar melts.

✻

107   THICK & CHEWY ORANGE GRANOLA BARS

For 36 bars: Preheat oven to 350°.

♣Combine crust ingredients, and press into the bottom of a 9 x 13" baking pan.
1 CUP WHOLE WHEAT PASTRY FLOUR or HEALTHY GOURMET FLOUR MIX (pg. 647)
$1/_4$ CUP FRUCTOSE
$1/_4$ CUP DATE SUGAR
$1/_3$ CUP UNSALTED BUTTER
♣Bake for 10 minutes until just pale gold in color. Remove and set aside for filling.

♣Combine filling ingredients, and spread on top of crust.

$1/_2$ CUP HONEY	2 CUPS GRANOLA
$1/_2$ CUP DATE SUGAR or 1 CUP CHOPPED DATES	2 EGGS
1 CUP UNSALTED BUTTER	1 teasp. SEA SALT
1 CUP SHREDDED COCONUT	1 teasp BAKING SODA
$1/_2$ CUP CHOPPED PECANS	$1 1/_2$ teasp. VANILLA
1 TB. GRATED ORANGE RIND	

♣Bake for 35 minutes until done, but still chewy.

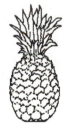

108   PINEAPPLE DATE BARS

Fruit juice sweetened bars. Especially good for those with sugar regulation problems.
For 24 bars: Preheat oven to 350°. Spray a square baking pan with lecithin spray.

♣Cook filling ingredients until liquid is absorbed: 1 CUP PACKED, CHOPPED DATES, 3/4 CUP PINE-APPLE JUICE, and $1/_2$ CUP CRUSHED DRAINED PINEAPPLE.

♣Mix the bar layer ingredients: $1 1/_2$ CUPS OATS, $1 1/_2$ CUPS OAT FLOUR, 2 teasp. BAKING POWDER, 2 teasp APPLE PIE SPICE, $1 1/_2$ teasp. VANILLA, 1 EGG, 1 TB. HONEY or APPLE JUICE, and $1/_4$ CUP BUTTER.
♣Pat half of the bar layer mix in to the prepared pan. Top with all of the filling mix. Sprinkle on rest of the oat mix. Pat down. Bake for 30 minutes. Let stand for 1 hour after removing from the oven to get a moister, sweeter bar.

✻

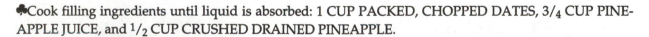

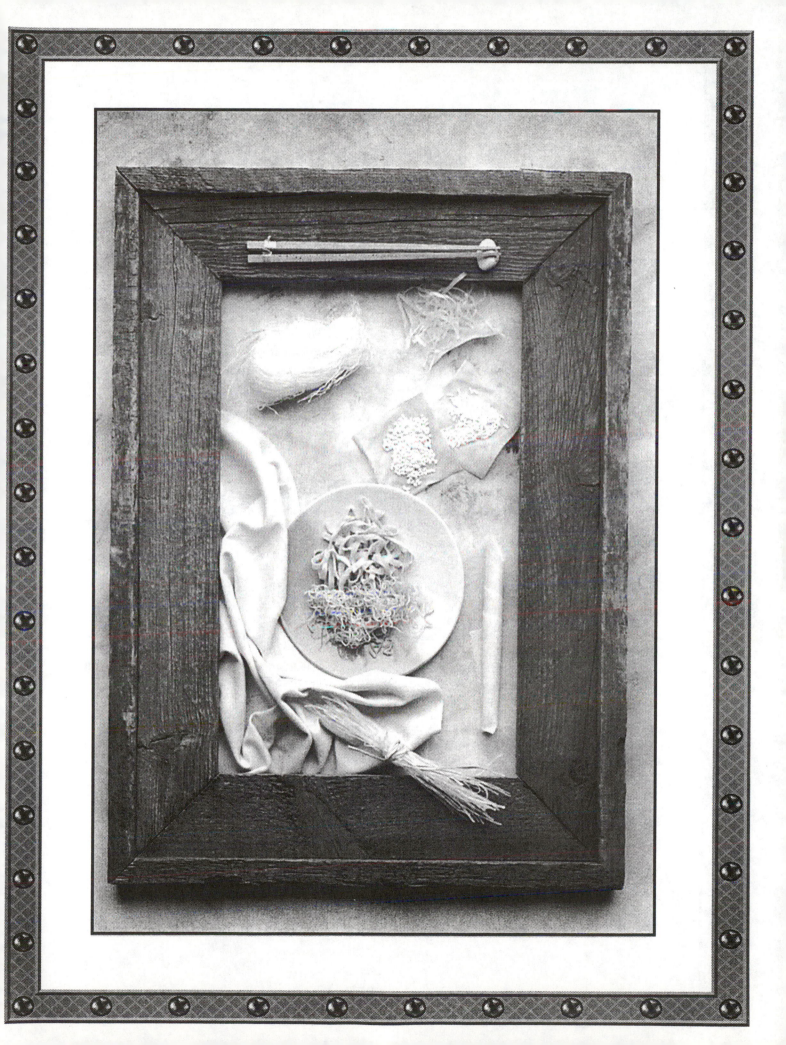

Oriental & Light Macrobiotic Eating

The recipes in this section arise not only from the Oriental, particularly Japanese, way of eating, but also from the Eastern philosophy of life. Macro (long) - biotics (life) considers the seasons, climate, activity level, farming methods, traditional customs, and an individual's condition, in determining the way to eat. Other aspects of the macrobiotic way of life have also been adopted by those using this diet; daily exercise, avoiding synthetic clothing, aluminum, Teflon, and microwave ovens, expressing gratitude and appreciation, "early to bed and early to rise," and living life positively. Proper orientation to these considerations, according to this philosophy, leads to happiness, health, freedom, and appreciation for all of life - its bounties and its boundaries.

The macrobiotic diet is designed in the orient to prevent illness and degenerative disease. In America, it has rightly become popular as a therapeutic diet, encouraging harmony and balance in the body. Thousands of people suffering from cancer, heart disease, diabetes, arthritis and other illnesses are using the macrobiotic system as part of an approach to healing. It is non-mucous forming, low in fat, high in vegetable proteins and fiber, and very alkalizing. Refined foods, and those with flavor or coloring additives are avoided. Brown rice and other whole grains, and fresh in-season foods are the mainstays.

A macrobiotic diet is not a set pattern, but instead flexible for a person's individual needs. In general, this way of eating consists of about 45 to 55% whole grains and beans for good plant proteins, 25 to 30% vegetables, 10% soy foods, such as tofu, tempeh, miso and tamari, about 5% fruit, 5% sea vegetables, nuts and seeds, and 5% cultured foods, such as kefir, kefir cheese and yogurt, with occasional fish and eggs. Condiments and seasonings are an important part of macrobiotic cooking, not only to enhance flavor, but to promote good enzyme and digestive activity.
Favorite macrobiotic seasonings include gomashio (sesame salt), kuzu starch, sea salt, daikon radish, ginger pickles, umeboshi plums, tamari sauce, tekka, brown rice vinegar, wasabi horseradish, toasted sesame and corn oils, and occasional maple syrup, rice syrup or barley malt for sweetening.

A macrobiotic diet is stimulating to the heart and circulatory systems by keeping the body alkaline and balanced in iodine and potassium. Its emphasis on foods such as miso, bancha (kukicha) tea, sea vegetables, shiitake mushrooms, tofu, other soy foods, and umeboshi plums, make it a diet resistant to disease. In strict form, macrobiotics is a way of eating that is cleansing and balancing at the same time. In a modified, lighter form, it is a way of eating you can live with in health on a lifetime basis.

Recipes are included here for both strict and light diets, and include the following chapters:
❧SNACKS and APPETIZERS ❧TREATS ❧SANDWICHES ❧ORIENTAL and MACROBIOTIC SOUPS ❧MACROBIOTIC SEA VEGETABLES ❧ORIENTAL SEAFOOD DISHES ❧ORIENTAL SALADS ❧MACROBIOTIC SALADS ❧MACROBIOTIC GRAINS and PASTAS ❧HEALTHY GRAIN ONE DISH MEALS ❧

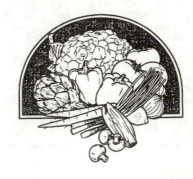

Snacks & Appetizers

109   CHINESE STUFFED MUSHROOMS

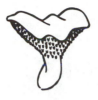

For 20 large stuffing mushrooms: Preheat oven to 350°.

♣Stem MUSHROOMS and wipe clean. Chop stems.

♣Mix filling in a bowl
1 TB. TAMARI
1 TB. MIRIN SEASONING (or SHERRY)
1 CUP MIXED MINCED CHINESE GREENS (SCALLIONS, BOK CHOY, BEAN SPROUTS, etc.)
4 to 6 CHOPPED WATER CHESTNUTS

1 teasp. ARROWROOT
$1/2$ teasp. FRUCTOSE

♣Sprinkle a little ARROWROOT POWDER on the open side of each mushroom cap. Fill. Press a cilantro leaf on top. Coat a round baking pan with oil and arrange mushrooms in 1 layer.
♣Mix $1/4$ CUP ONION STOCK with 2 TBS. OYSTER SAUCE and pour around mushrooms
♣Cover with foil and bake 15-20 minutes. Remove foil. Baste and heat again briefly. Remove with slotted spoon to serving plate.

110   MACROBIOTIC MUSHROOM PATÉ

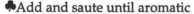

For 16 appetizer servings: Preheat oven to 400°.

♣Sauté briefly in a hot skillet
$2/3$ CUP CHOPPED LEEKS OR SCALLIONS
1 CHOPPED CELERY STALK
1 TB. OIL
♣Remove from heat.

♣Add and saute until aromatic
5 CUPS SLICED MUSHROOMS (about 1 $1/4$ LBS.)
$1/2$ teasp. DRY BASIL (or 1 TB. FRESH)
$1/4$ teasp. DRY THYME
$1/2$ teasp. TARRAGON
$1/4$ teasp. ROSEMARY
PINCH CAYENNE (or PAPRIKA)

♣Add and toss all together to coat
1 CUP WHOLE GRAIN BREAD CMBS.
1 CUP CHOPPED WALNUTS
1 CAKE CUBED TOFU

♣Mix together for sauce and add to paté
$1/4$ CUP SESAME TAHINI
1 TB. MIRIN or SHERRY
2 TBS. TAMARI
BLACK PEPPER to taste

♣Oil a loaf pan, and line it with <u>oiled</u> waxed paper. Spoon in paté, and fold extra waxed paper over top. Bake about 1 $1/4$ hrs. until a toothpick comes out clean.
♣Cool in pan. Invert on a plate, peel off paper and surround with greens. Serve with rice crackers.

Nutritional analysis: per serving; 114 calories; 4gm. protein; 7.6gm. carbohydrate; 2.2gm fiber; 8.4gm. fat; 0 cholesterol; 175mg. sodium; 32mg. calcium; 1.6mg. iron; 45mg. magnesium;230mg. potassium; 1mg. zinc.

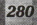

111 BROCCOLI PUREE

This delicious mix is wonderful for dipping up with toasted pita or chapati pieces. Serve hot.
For 12 servings:

♣Sauté in a hot skillet until aromatic
2 TBS. OIL
2 CUPS CHOPPED ONIONS
1/2 teasp. SESAME OR HERB SALT
1/4 teasp. BLACK OR GREEN PEPPER
1/2 teasp. DRY BASIL (or 1 TB. FRESH)
1 CLOVE GARLIC (or 1/2 teasp. LEMON/GARLIC SEASON)

♣Add
11/2 to 2 CUPS DICED BROCCOLI
1 CUP CHOPPED ZUCCHINI
1 BELL PEPPER CHOPPED, any color
2 TBS. WINE or WINE VINEGAR
1/4 teasp. DRY THYME

♣Steam and braise covered for about 5 minutes. Let cool in pan.
♣Puree in the blender. Put into a shallow serving bowl and top with TOASTED SESAME SEEDS and/or TOASTED SUNFLOWER SEEDS, CHOPPED BLACK OLIVES and BLACK PEPPER.

Nutritional analysis: per serving; 50 calories; 1gm. protein; 4gm. carbohydrate; 1gm. fiber; 3.4gm. fat; 0 cholesterol; 20mg. calcium; trace iron; 11mg. magnesium; 2mg. potassium; 75mg. sodium; trace zinc.

112 CAULIFLOWER & RED PEPPER PUREE

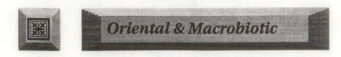

For about 2 1/2 to 3 cups: Preheat oven to 400°.

♣Roast in the oven until soft - about 45 minutes
4 PEELED SHALLOTS Steam
1 TB. OLIVE OIL
1 RED BELL PEPPER

1 LARGE CAULIFLOWER HEAD
    cut in florets until tender

♣Puree all in blender with 11/2 TB. OIL, 1 teasp. TAMARI, and 1/2 teasp. PEPPER.

♣Serve warm, sprinkled with chopped green onions or chives.

113 ROAST POTATO & SWEET POTATO STICKS

Try either of the above purees with these delicious appetizer sticks.
Makes enough for 4 people: Preheat oven to 500°.

♣Oil a baking sheet.

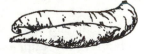

♣Cut 2 YAMS and 2 BAKING POTATOES in 1/2" x 1/4" MATCHSTICKS.
♣Toss with 1 to 2 TBS. OIL.
♣Place side by side, *not touching* on baking sheet.
♣Bake for 10 minutes til brown and crusty.
♣Season with SEA SALT and PEPPER, or SPIKE or GREAT 28 SEASONING MIX (pg. 645).

114   DOUG'S "DA KINE" GUACAMOLE

This mix is from Hawaii where Doug lived and surfed away the seventies. (We should all be so lucky!) He also got into natural foods during those years and developed this delicious recipe.
For about 1¹/₂ to 2 cups:

♣Amounts may vary depending on the size of the avocado. Taste as you add seasonings.
♣Mash together and mix

1 LARGE AVOCADO   ¹/₂ CUP PLAIN LOW-FAT YOGURT
1 to 2 TBS. CHUNKY SALSA or PICANTE SAUCE   1 to 2 teasp. LEMON JUICE
2 to 3 teasp BRAGG'S LIQUID AMINOS or TAMARI
2 DASHES SPIKE or other natural seasoning salt

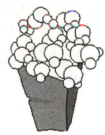

115   GREEN & RED GUACAMOLE

This is a definite favorite.
For about 2 cups:

♣Mix and mash together
2 to 3 AVOCADOS seeded   1 SMALL TOMATO chopped
¹/₂ SMALL RED ONION finely diced   JUICE of 1 LIME
1 to 2 GREEN CHILIS chopped   ¹/₂ teasp. LEMON PEPPER

116   DOUG'S POPCORN

Doug makes a great popcorn mix, too.

♣Make up a batch of hot air popcorn, then mix this blend and pour over it.

2 TBS. OIL   1 teasp GROUND CUMIN
2 TBS. BRAGG'S LIQUID AMINOS   1 teasp. CHILI POWDER
♣Sprinkle on BREWER'S YEAST FLAKES to taste.
♣Top with a little SPIKE if desired.

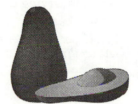

117   TOMATO BASIL SWIRL

This is especially good for cold cucumber or yellow squash sticks.

♣Heat in a pan
1 CUP TOMATO SAUCE (or CANNED UNDILUTED SOUP)
1 CUP PASTA SAUCE WITH MUSHROOMS, or 2 CUPS PASTA, PIZZA or TOMATO SAUCE
1 BAY LEAF (Remove when ready to serve.)
2 TBS. CHOPPED FRESH BASIL (or 1 teasp. DRY)
♣Put into serving dish. Scissor snip fresh mint leaves on top.

118   DESERT DIP

Another good 'scoop' for toasted chapati or pita pieces. It is equally good with eggplant or zucchini.
For 12 servings: Preheat oven to 400°.

♣Pierce and roast 2 LBS. of EGGPLANT until crinkly and soft; **or** steam or parboil 2 LBS. SLICED ZUC-CHINI in vegetable broth until just tender. Scoop out eggplant meat into blender.

♣Add to eggplant meat or zucchini in blender and puree until smooth with

6 TBS. FRESH LEMON JUICE	2 TBS. CHOPPED PARSLEY
4 TBS. SESAME TAHINI	1/4 teasp. CUMIN POWDER
2 TBS. CHOPPED GREEN ONION	1/2 teasp. LEMON PEPPER

♣Turn into a shallow serving dish and top with CHOPPED TOMATOES.

Nutritional analysis: per appetizer serving; 54 calories; 2gm. protein; 7gm. carbohydrate; 3gm. fiber; 3gm. fats; 0 cholesterol; 37mg. alcium; 1mg. iron; 28mg. magnesium; 216mg. potassium; 5mg. sodium; 1mg. zinc.

119   LINDA RAE'S FAMOUS SOY BEAN SPREAD

This mix is justifiably popular with almost everybody. Use it for raw veggies, crackers, chips, or rolled up in romaine or Boston lettuce leaves.
Enough for 12 people:

♣Cook 1 LB. SOY BEANS (2 1/2 CUPS DRY) very well.
♣Mix together

1/2 CUP OLIVE OIL	3/8 teasp. ONION POWDER
3/8 CUP TAMARI	2 TBS. MINCED FRESH PARSLEY
3/8 CUP LEMON JUICE	3/8 teasp. PAPRIKA
3/8 teasp. GARLIC POWDER	1/4 teasp. CUMIN POWDER

♣Combine and mash sauce with beans and chill until flavors bloom.

Nutritional analysis: per 2-oz. serving; 248 calories; 14gm. portein; 13gm. carbohydrate; 2gm. fiber; 16gm. fats; 0 cholesterol; 111mg. calcium; 6mg. iron; 113mg. magnesium; 729mg. potassium; 516mg. sodium; 2mg. zinc.

120   DOUG'S TAHINI DIP & SPREAD

Another specialty from our resident macrobiotic expert.
For about 1 cup:

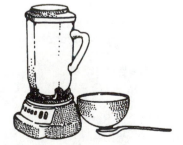

♣Mix together
1/4 CUP TAHINI
1/2 CUP PLAIN YOGURT
1/4 CUP BREWER'S YEAST FLAKES
2 TBS. SESAME OIL
2 or 3 TBS. TAMARI or Bragg's LIQUID AMINOS
♣Cover and chill to let flavors bloom before serving.

121   SWEET HOT ORIENTAL MUSHROOMS

Just mound these on a plate, surround them with chopped greens, and offer a cup of toothpicks.
Enough for 4 people:

♣Sauté in 10 DROPS of SAMBAL OELEK HOT SAUCE or SZECHUAN CHILI OIL and 3 to 4 CUPS WHOLE BUTTON MUSHROOMS in 2 TBS. OIL in a hot skillet for 5 minutes.

♣Add and toss until hot
1 teasp. FRESH MINCED GINGER   4 TBS. TAMARI
1 TB. FRUCTOSE (or 1 TB. HONEY)   1 CLOVE MINCED GARLIC
1 teasp. MIRIN (or 1 teasp. SHERRY)
♣Add a few more drops HOT CHILI SAUCE or SAMBAL OELEK HOT SAUCE. Serve hot.

Nutritional analysis: per person; 61 calories; 3gm. protein; 10gm. carbohydrate; 2gm. fat; 0 cholesterol; 8mg. calcium; 1mg. iron; 14mg. magnesium; 302mg. potassium; 1032mg. sodium; 1mg. zinc.

122   AUTHENTIC TABOULI

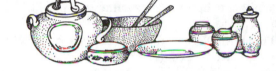

Enough for 6 appetizer servings:

♣Combine 1 CUP RAW BULGUR and 1½ CUPS HOT WATER in a bowl and allow to sit til soft, about 30 minutes to 1 hour. Drain off excess water, and combine with rest of ingredients

1 CUP FINELY CHOPPED GREEN ONIONS   ¼ CUP OLIVE OIL
1 CUP CHOPPED FRESH PARSLEY   2 CHOPPED TOMATOES
1 teasp. LEMON/GARLIC SEASONING   1 teasp. DRIED MINT
♣Toss well and chill 1 hour. Top liberally with FRESHLY GROUND PEPPER at serving.

Nutritional analysis: per appetizer serving; 178 calories; 4gm. protein; 22gm. carbohydrate; 7gm. fiber; 10gm. fats; 0 cholesterol; 38mg. calcium; 2mg. iron; 52mg. magnesium; 417mg. potassium; 107mg. sodium; 1mg. zinc.

123   BULGUR APPETIZER RELISH

Serve this zesty mix like a tabouli with chapatis or roll in romaine leaves.
Enough for 6 appetizer servings:

♣Sauté 2 SHREDDED CARROTS, 2 SHREDDED ZUCCHINI and 1 RED or GREEN BELL PEPPER, seeded and slivered in 1 TB. OIL or VEGETABLE BROTH for 5 minutes until aromatic.
♣Add ⅓ CUP RAW BULGUR, 1 CUP VEGETABLE or ONION BROTH, and 2 TBS. TAMARI and sauté for 5 more minutes. Bring to a boil, cover and remove from heat. Let stand until liquid is absorbed and bulgur is tender - about 20 minutes.
♣Chill overnight if serving as an appetizer. Or use as a side dish for broiled fish.

Nutritional analysis: per ¼ cup serving; 59 calories; 2gm. protein; 13gm. fats; 11gm. carbohydrate; 0 cholesterol; 20mg. calcium; trace iron; 27mg. magnesium; 456mg. potassium; 538mg. sodium; trace zinc.

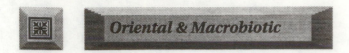

124   GINGER SHRIMP MUSHROOMS
You will need a steamer for these stuffed mushrooms. We use a simple round rack placed above boiling water in a wok, but bamboo and stainless steel steamers also work fine.
For 24 appetizers:

♣Soak 24 LARGE SHIITAKE MUSHROOMS in enough water to cover until soft. Save soaking water.

♣Blend the shrimp paté in the blender

1/2 LB. COOKED SHRIMP PIECES
1 TB. SHERRY or SAKÉ
1 teasp. GARLIC/LEMON SEASONING)
1/2 teasp. SESAME SALT (GOMASHIO)
1/2 teasp. CHILI OIL or TOASTED SESAME OIL

1 TB. SHREDDED FRESH GINGER
2 EGG WHITES
1 teasp. FRUCTOSE
1/4 teasp. PAPRIKA

♣Stuff mushrooms with the paté, and place filled side up on the steamer rack. Press frozen peas into the tops. Chill briefly to set. Steam over simmering water until paté feels firm when pressed.

♣While mushrooms are steaming, mix a little dipping sauce
2 TBS. TAMARI
1 TB. SHREDDED GINGER (or 1 teasp. GINGER POWDER)
1 teasp. FRUCTOSE (or 2 teasp. HONEY)
1 teasp. HOT CHILI OIL
1 MINCED GREEN ONION
♣Place mushrooms on crisp greens. Put a small dish of dipping sauce in the center and serve.

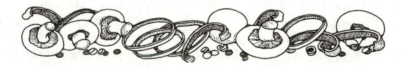

Treats For A Macrobiotic Diet
We made these snacks almost every week during the Rainbow Kitchen restaurant years.
They fit in with macrobiotic diet needs while providing tasty energizing treats.

125   CHINESE 5 SPICE NOODLES
A very unusual sweet munch.
Enough for 4 people: Preheat oven to 350°.

♣Bring 1 CUP HONEY and 1 CUP WATER to a boil and simmer til slightly thickened.
♣Toast 2 to 3 CUPS CRISP CHINESE CHOW MEIN NOODLES in 2 TBS. OIL in a skillet.

♣Pour honey syrup over noodles. Bring to a boil. Simmer for 8 to 10 minutes, stirring.
♣Spread the sweet noodles on a baking sheet and sprinkle with 1/2 teasp. CHINESE 5 SPICE POWDER.
♣Bake for 10 minutes until all liquid is absorbed and noodles are crisp and brown.
♣Serve warm if possible.

126   NUT BUTTER HONEY BALLS

For about 8 balls:

♣Blender blend all.

3 TBS. TOASTED SUNFLOWER SEEDS   3 TBS. SESAME TAHINI
3 TBS. TOASTED SESAME SEEDS   3 TBS. HONEY
1/2 CUP TOASTED CHOPPED ALMONDS   1 TB. PEANUT BUTTER

♣Toast 1/2 CUP SHREDDED COCONUT in the oven until golden, and roll balls in it. Chill.

❈

127   CASHEW DELIGHT

For one 8 x 8" square pan:
For 12 servings:

♣Blend and mix all to candy consistency. Press into pan. Cut and chill.

2 CUPS TOASTED CASHEW PIECES   2 to 3 TBS. HONEY
1/2 CUP TOASTED SUNFLOWER SEEDS   1/4 CUP DATE PIECES
1/2 CUP TOASTED CHOPPED ALMONDS   1 teasp. VANILLA EXTRACT
1/2 CUP TOASTED COCONUT SHREDS

Representative nutritional analysis: per serving; 245 calories; 6gm. protein; 18mg. carbo; 4gm. fiber; 18gm. fats; 0 cholesterol; 33mg. calcium; 2mg. iron; 89mg. magnesium; 271mg. potassium; 6mg. sodium; 2mg. zinc.

❈

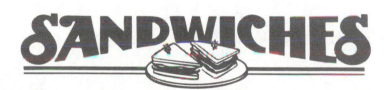

*Sometimes we think of sandwiches as the essence of "fast" or even "junk" food,
but they can be healthy convenience meals with a little time and attention.
The four here are favorites from The Rainbow Kitchen restaurant, and fit well with a macrobiotic diet.*

128   HOT CLOUD

For 2 sandwiches:

♣Split an extra large PITA BREAD *horizontally*. Lay each circle flat, and spread with HUMMUS (cooked garbanzo and tahini spread), or TABOULI, or SOY SPREAD (page 283) or SPICED MAYONNAISE.
♣Top each circle with <u>2 TBS. each:</u>
CHOPPED GREEN ONION, SLICED BLACK OLIVES, SLICED CUCUMBERS, SLICED MUSHROOMS or TOFU CUBES, SLICED TOMATOES and PARMESAN CHEESE.
♣Toast or broil to bubble slightly and top with ALFALFA SPROUTS.

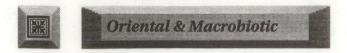
129   THE WEDGE

For 2 sandwiches:

♣ Cut 1 PITA BREAD in half. Open each pocket and line with ALFALFA SPROUTS.
♣ Stuff each side with <u>1 TB. each:</u>
SHREDDED CARROT, SLICED CUCUMBER, CHOPPED BLACK OLIVES, CHOPPED TOMATO, TOASTED SUN SEEDS, and A SLICE OF RED ONION.
♣ Top with a GRATED SOY PARMESAN CHEESE or SPICED LIGHT MAYONNAISE. Eat hot or cold.

130   HOT ZUCCHINI POCKET PIZZAS

For 2 sandwiches:

♣ Sauté 2 SMALL ZUCCHINI cut in rounds in 2 TBS. OIL or VEGETABLE BROTH until color changes.

♣ Add and heat
1 TOMATO chopped
1 TB. TAMARI
A PINCH <u>EACH</u>: SAVORY and OREGANO

♣ Grate a little LOW-FAT CHEESE or SOY CHEESE on top. Cover pan, and remove from heat. Leave a few minutes to heat. Stuff into hot pita pockets.

131   TERIYAKI MUSHROOM MELT

For 1 big sandwich:

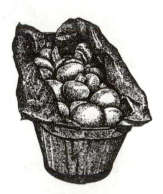

♣ Sauté in 1 TB. oil until aromatic
1 CUP SLICED MUSHROOMS
1/4 teasp. GARLIC POWDER or GARLIC LEMON SEASONING
1/4 teasp. GINGER POWDER

♣ Add
2 teasp. TAMARI
1 teasp. SNIPPED SEA VEGGIES such as WAKAME or DULSE
1 teasp. HONEY
♣ Reduce heat to low and simmer for 2 minutes.

♣ Pile onto a piece of WHOLE GRAIN TOAST. Sprinkle with 1 CHOPPED GREEN ONION, and some GRATED PARMESAN or SOY CHEESE. Run briefly under broiler to melt. Serve hot.

Representative nutritional analysis: per serving; 178 calories; 5gm. protein; 22gm. carbo; 4gm. fiber; 10gm. fats; 0 cholesterol; 66mg. calcium; 3mg. iron; 45mg. magnesium; 162mg. potassium; 348mg. sodium; 1.3mg. zinc.

Oriental Soups

Oriental soups are an expression of the "essence" of the Eastern culture. Light, clear, uncluttered, with depth and unfailing good taste - like many other Oriental arts. They are high in nutrition, and may be any part of a meal - as a first course, main dish, or as a light broth to clear the palate after a strong dish.

We use so many of these in connection with healing diets that it is hard to present just a few. All are dairy free, low in fat, and alkalizing to the system. Many may even be used as part of a liquid cleansing diet.

132 MUSHROOM HEAVEN SOUP

For 4 to 6 servings:

♣Soak 1-oz. DRY SHIITAKE BLACK MUSHROOMS in a bowl of hot water until soft. Reserve water, and slice mushrooms thin. Discard woody stems.

♣Chop lower woody stems from 1 bunch or bag of FRESH ENOKI MUSHROOMS (canned enokis from a Japanese market also work well. Just rinse them.)

♣Separate green and white from a BUNCH of SCALLIONS. Chop into separate piles and set aside.

♣Sauté white parts with 1¹/₂ teasp. fresh GRATED GINGER and 1 TB. PEANUT OIL.

♣Add and sauté til fragrant

8 OZ. SLICED BUTTON MUSHROOMS	2 TBS. TAMARI
THE SLICED SHIITAKE MUSHROOMS	¹/₄ CUP MIRIN
	¹/₂ teasp. BLACK PEPPER

♣Mix 1 TB. KUZU or ARROWROOT into reserved mushroom soaking water. Add to mushrooms and stir to coat. Add 1 CUP LIGHT STOCK, 1 teasp. HONEY, and 1 TB. BROWN RICE VINEGAR.

♣Add ONE SMALL CAN SLICED WATER CHESTNUTS and the ENOKI MUSHROOMS. Cover and simmer 10 minutes.

♣Ladle into serving bowls. Top with GREEN ONION TOPS and drops of TOASTED SESAME OIL.

Nutritional analysis: per serving; 110 calories; 3gm. protein; 17gm. carbohydrate; 4gm. fiber; 3gm. fats; 0 cholesterol; 24 mg. calcium; 2mg. iron; 24mg. magnesium; 400mg. potassium; 490mg. sodium; 1mg. zinc.

133 ONION GINGER BROTH

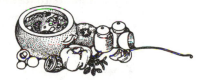

A healing broth with a French/Vietnamese touch.
For 4 to 6 servings:

♣Sauté in 3 TBS. ONION BROTH or OIL til soft but not browned, about 2 to 3 minutes

¹/₂ CUP CHOPPED SCALLIONS	2 TBS. CHOPPED FRESH GINGER
¹/₂ CUP MINCED SHALLOTS	1 teasp. TOASTED SESAME OIL

♣Add and bring to a boil	♣Remove from heat, and stir in
2 teasp. GROUND CORIANDER	¹/₂ CUP PLAIN LOW-FAT YOGURT
1 TB. HONEY	¹/₂ CUP FRESH CHOPPED CILANTRO
4 CUPS ONION BROTH	¹/₄ CUP MINCED CHIVES
PINCHES of SEA SALT and PEPPER	

♣Puree in the blender. Return to heat briefly just to warm. Garnish with fresh cilantro leaves.

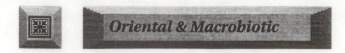

134   HOT & SOUR SOUP

For 6 servings:

♣Soak 5 or 6 SHIITAKE BLACK MUSHROOMS in water. Reserve soaking water. Slice softened mushrooms into thin strips and discard woody stems.

♣Make a LIGHT MISO SOUP. Bring 4 CUPS WATER to a boil. Add 1 TB. MISO PASTE for each cup water. Use mushroom soaking water for part of the soup liquid.
♣Add

2 CLOVES MINCED GARLIC	1 teasp. HONEY
2 teasp. WORCESTERSHIRE SAUCE	1 TB. TAMARI
2 TBS. BROWN RICE VINEGAR	1/2 teasp. SESAME SALT
1 teasp. TOASTED SESAME OIL	1/2 teasp. PEPPER

♣Reduce heat and add 2 CAKES CUBED TOFU, the SHIITAKE MUSHROOM SLICES, and 1 teasp. KUZU OR ARROWROOT dissolved in 1 TB. WATER. Simmer gently about 5 minutes.
♣Add 3 GREEN ONIONS CHOPPED. Remove from heat, and serve.

Nutritional analysis: per serving; 82 calories; 5gm. protein; 10gm. carbohydrate; 2gm. fiber; 3gm. fats; 0 cholesterol; 59mg. calcium; 3mg. iron; 54mg. magnesium; 22mg. potassium; 721mg. sodium; 1mg. zinc.

135   FAMOUS SOUP

We call this soup "famous" because it is requested so much.
For 6 cups:

♣Toast 1/2 CUP SLICED ALMONDS and 1 TB. SESAME SEEDS in a 350° oven until golden.

♣Bring 4 CUPS CHICKEN BROTH or LIGHT MISO SOUP to a boil.

♣Add 1 CUP DICED MIXED VEGGIES such as RED ONION, CELERY, CARROT or JICAMA to soup.
♣Simmer gently for a *few minutes* til just tender crisp.

♣Add
2 TBS. SHERRY or MIRIN or SAKE
ONE 3-OZ. PKG. RAMEN NOODLES

♣Mix

1 TB. BROWN RICE VINEGAR	4 OZ. BUTTON MUSHROOMS, or
1 teasp. FRUCTOSE	1-OZ. DRIED BLACK MUSHROOMS
4-OZ. DICED TOFU CUBES or DICED SHRIMP	soaked and sliced
1 TB. TAMARI	

♣Add to soup and stir in. Bubble briefly for about 2 minutes. Remove from heat.
♣Top immediately with 1 CUP SHAVED HEAD LETTUCE SHREDS and the toasted nuts and seeds.

Nutritional analysis: per serving; 198 calories; 8gm. protein; 21gm. carbohydrates; 4gm fiber; 10gm. fats; 0 cholesterol; 65mg. calcium; 3mg. iron; 64mg. magnesium; 272mg. potassium; 668mg. sodium; 1mg. zinc.

136   TRADITIONAL SHABU - SHABU

This is a delicious whole meal Japanese stew, with many different tastes and ingredients for very little calorie or fat cost. It may be made with either seafoods or chicken.
For 8 servings:

♣Press a 1 LB. BLOCK of TOFU between 2 plates with a weight on top. Let stand for 30 minutes to press out excess fluid. Slice in $1/4$" strips and set aside.

♣Have ready 1 RINSED CAN of SHIRATAKE (YAM THREADS), **or** soak about the same amount of dried BEAN THREADS in water til soft.

♣Slice 1 LB. CHICKEN BREASTS **or** 1 LB. mixed PRAWNS and SCALLOPS into bite size slices.

♣Slice 1 LARGE ONION in half rings. Shred $1/2$ HEAD CHINESE NAPPA CABBAGE. Soak 8 BLACK SHIITAKE MUSHROOMS. Slice thin when soft. Save soaking water, discarding woody stems. Chop $1/2$ to 1 BUNCH of *washed* SPINACH, and mix with about 4-OZ. BEAN SPROUTS.

♣Assemble the stew. Bring 4 CUPS LIGHT MISO SOUP to a boil. Add mushroom soaking water and 2 TBS. MIRIN. Add tofu strips and chicken or seafood, and let boil until meat is white and firm. Remove with a slotted spoon and put in individual shallow soup bowls. Add vegetables, cabbage, onion and mushrooms, and simmer until just tender. Remove and ladle into soup bowls. Add sprouts and spinach for about 30 seconds just to wilt. Remove to soup bowls. Add yam or bean threads and stir until soft and heated through. Divide the liquid between each bowl and serve with dipping sauces.

DIPPING SAUCES: *Each of these is different and delicious. Make up some of each and put in small individual bowls near each person's plate. Serve with chopsticks so pieces of the stew can be easily picked up and dipped into the sauces.*

✽**ORANGE TAMARI:** Squeeze 1 ORANGE into a measuring cup. Add an equal amount of TAMARI and 1 teasp.GROUND GINGER.

✽**TOASTED SESAME:** Toast $1/2$ CUP SESAME SEEDS until brown. Crush slightly and add 2 TBS. BROWN RICE VINEGAR, 3 TBS. TAMARI, 2 TBS. MIRIN or SHERRY, and 1 teasp. HONEY.

Nutritional analysis: per serving; 249 calories; 24gm. protein; 5gm. fiber; 18gm. carbohydrate; 38mg. cholesterol; 633mg. sodium; 9gm. fats; 119mg. calcium; 139mg. magnesium; 5mg. iron; 536mg. potassium; 3mg. zinc.

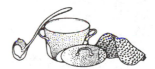

137   TOFU DUMPLINGS for Oriental Soups

These are a tasty addition to any of the soups in this section. They add protein and make the soup a full meal.
For 4 to 6 dumplings:

♣Mix and mash all together and form into balls

1 TB. LIGHT MISO

$1/2$ teasp. TOASTED SESAME OIL

1 teasp. ARROWROOT or KUZU dissolved in 1 teasp. WATER or BROTH

1 LB. FRESH TOFU

1 TB. WHOLE WHEAT FLOUR

♣Drop balls into any simmering soup, and let bubble for 10 to 15 minutes.

Nutritional analysis: per serving; 72 calories; 7gm. protein; 3gm. carbohydrate; 1 gm. fiber; 4 gm. fats; 0 cholesterol; 81 mg. calcium; 4 mg. iron; 80 mg. magnesium; 101mg. potassium; 110 mg. sodium; trace zinc.

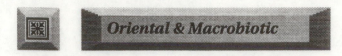

138   LEMON SHRIMP SOUP

We love Thai cooking. This is a favorite based on a recipe from The Rice Table resataurant in San Rafael, Ca.
For 8 servings:

♣Combine in a soup pot
8 CUPS CHICKEN or FISH STOCK
3 to 5 DRIED WHOLE CHILI PEPPERS
2 TBS. DRIED LEMON GRASS (or 3 LEMON GRASS TEABAGS).
♣Simmer covered about 15 minutes until you can smell the lemon spiciness.

♣Add 1 LB. SHELLED SHRIMP and 1/3 CUP LEMON JUICE.
♣Remove from heat and add 3 CHOPPED GREEN ONIONS and 2 TBS. CHOPPED FRESH CILANTRO.
♣Serve hot and fragrant.

Nutritional analysis: per serving; 60 calories; 10gm. protein; 3gm. carbohydrate; trace fiber; 1gm. fats; 69mg. cholesterol; 35mg. calcium; 1mg. iron; 24mg. magnesium; 157mg. potassium; 297mg. sodium; trace zinc.

139   GREEN GINGER SOUP

It takes a little more time to make this delicate broth from scratch, but it makes all the difference, and the soup is so delicious.
For 10 bowls:

♣Make the GINGER BROTH. Combine in a large pot and bring to a boil
1 LARGE CHOPPED ONION
6 CLOVES GARLIC, minced
4 to 6 SLICES FRESH PEELED GINGER
7 CUPS WATER
1 teasp. SESAME SALT (Gomashio)
♣Partially cover and simmer about 45 minutes until aromatic. Strain and discard solids. Return to pot.

♣Add, bring to a boil, partially cover and simmer for 5 minutes.
10 to 12 FRESH SLICED MUSHROOMS
1 SMALL CAN WATER CHESTNUTS, sliced
2 CAKES TOFU in small cubes
2 TBS. TAMARI
4 to 6 <u>STALKS</u> BOK CHOY STEMS (reserve leaves)

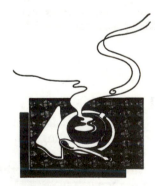

♣Add
3 to 4 CHOPPED SCALLIONS
4 OZ. FRESH STRUNG SNOW PEAS
1 CUP FROZEN PEAS
THE RESERVED BOK CHOY <u>LEAVES</u> chopped
♣Simmer briefly until everything is hot, tender and aromatic. Put in individual soup bowls.
♣Drizzle a little rice vinegar and toasted sesame oil over top, and snip on some green onion tops.

Nutritional analysis: per serving; 62 calories; 4gm. protein; 9gm. carbohydrates; 3gm. fiber; 1gm. fats; 0 cholesterol; 36mg. calcium; 2mg. iron; 45mg. magnesium; 269mg. potassium; 1mg. zinc.

Light Macrobiotic Soups

These soups retain their high quality vegetable protein, complex carbohydrate, low-fat character through the use of whole grains and legumes. They are satisfying without being dense, filling without being heavy.

140 LENTILSTRONE

For 8 servings:

♣ Bring 8 CUPS WATER or VEGETABLE or ONION STOCK to a boil in a large soup pot. Add 1 CUP WASHED LENTILS. Cook for 30 minutes.
♣ Add

3 DICED CARROTS	2 DICED ZUCCHINI
2 STALKS DICED CELERY with leaves	2 TBS. LIGHT CHICKPEA MISO
4 CHOPPED GREEN ONIONS	1 CUP FROZEN PEAS
12 MINCED CLOVES GARLIC	2 teasp. DILL WEED
1 LARGE CHOPPED RED ONION	1/2 teasp. THYME
3 CUPS CHOPPED BOK CHOY or SWISS CHARD	1/2 teasp. CUMIN
2 CUPS CHOPPED CABBAGE	1/2 teasp. PEPPER
1 CUP FROZEN or FRESH CORN	1 teasp. GREAT 28 MIX (pg. 645)
1/3 CUP FRESH CHOPPED BASIL (or 3 teasp. dry)	

♣ Cover and simmer for 15 minutes. Turn off heat and add 2 TBS. CHOPPED PARSLEY and 1 CHOPPED TOMATO. Serve hot.

Nutritional analysis: per serving; 121 calories; 8gm. protein; 23gm. carbohydrate; 5gm. fiber; trace fats; 0 cholesterol; 68mg. calcium; 3mg. iron; 53mg. magnesium; 506mg. potassium; 252mg. sodium; 1mg. zinc.

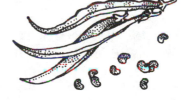

141 MIXED BEAN & VEGETABLE SOUP

For 4 to 6 servings:

♣ Soak 1 CUP MIXED DRIED BEANS, such as split peas, small white beans, black turtle beans, pinto beans and garbanzos. Soak overnight, or in the morning for the evening meal. It's a pain to remember this, but worth it in terms of taste and digestibility.
♣ Drain off soaking liquid. Add fresh water to beans, and cover by 1/2" to 1". Bring to a quick boil and cook, covered at a simmer for one hour. Drain into a cup measure and <u>reserve cooking water</u>. Add fresh water to make 3 CUPS LIQUID.
♣ Put into a big pot with 1 CUP RESERVED LIQUID

1 ONION CHOPPED	1 CARROT, DICED
1 BUNCH BROCCOLI chopped small	2 STALKS CELERY w/ LEAVES, sliced
1 ZUCCHINI, DICED	1 teasp. DRY OREGANO

♣ Bring to a boil. Reduce heat. Cover and cook 10 minutes.
♣ Add beans and rest of the reserved water. Bring to a boil again. Stir in 2 TBS. LEMON JUICE, 1 TB. MOLASSES, 1/4 teasp. CAYENNE. Add more water if desired, adjust seasoning. Stir in 1/2 CUP MINCED PARSLEY. Serve hot.

Nutritional analysis: per serving; 162 calories; 11gm. protein; 27gm. carbohydrate; 6gm. fiber; 3gm. fat; 0 cholesterol; 131mg. calcium; 5mg. iron; 98mg. magnesium; 947mg. potassium; 39mg. sodium; 1mg. zinc.

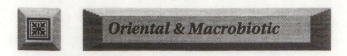

142   CARROT & LEMON SOUP

A cleansing soup with plenty of vitamin A.
For 6 to 8 servings:

♣ Sauté 1 CHOPPED ONION and 1 CLOVE MINCED GARLIC until translucent in 4 TBS. OIL or ONION BROTH.

♣ Add 2 TBS. MORE OIL or BROTH and stir in

1½ LBS. CARROTS, sliced	3 TOMATOES, sliced
¼ CUP FRESH MINCED BASIL (or 1 TB. dry)	1½ teasp. SALT
1 POTATO, peeled and sliced thin	½ teasp. PEPPER
4 CUPS VEGETABLE STOCK	

♣ Bring to a boil, reduce heat and simmer for 45 minutes. Remove vegetables with a slotted spoon and puree in the blender.

♣ Add back to the pot with 1 CUP PLAIN YOGURT, or ¾ CUP YOGURT and ¼ CUP LIGHT MAYONNAISE and ¼ teasp. LIQUID HOT SAUCE.

♣ Heat 15 minutes and ladle in ¼ CUP LEMON JUICE. Top with snipped cilantro leaves. Serve hot.

✳

143   MILLET & LENTIL SOUP

For 8 servings:

♣ Sauté 4 CLOVES CHOPPED GARLIC, 2 YELLOW ONIONS, and 1 teasp. HOT PEPPER FLAKES in 2 TBS. OLIVE OIL for about 10 minutes until aromatic and soft.

♣ Add 2 TBS. FRESH CHOPPED CILANTRO LEAVES and ½ CUP LENTILS.

♣ Sauté briefly until coated and add
1 teasp. SESAME SALT
1 teasp. LEMON PEPPER
½ teasp. CUMIN POWDER
½ teasp. GROUND CORIANDER
¼ teasp. LEMON PEEL POWDER
7 CUPS WATER and 1 CUP WHITE WINE (or 8 cups water)
♣ Cover and simmer for 20 minutes.

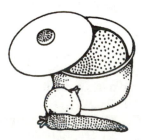

♣ Add
½ CUP MILLET GRAINS
1 ZUCCHINI SLICED
♣ Cover and cook 30 minutes until tender. Top each serving with more chopped cilantro

Nutritional analysis: per serving; 167 calories; 6gm. protein; 22gm. carbohydrate; 4gm. fat; 0 cholesterol; 1 gm. fiber; 144 mg. sodium; 32mg. calcium; 2mg. iron; 47mg. magnesium; 279mg. potassium; 1mg. zinc.

✳

Sea Vegetables
CORNERSTONES OF A HEALING DIET

Sea vegetables are a veritable medicine chest of proteins, complex carbohydrates, minerals, (especially iron, calcium, potassium, and iodine) all forty-four trace minerals, and vitamins A, C, E, and B Complex. They are the only vegetarian source of measureable B_{12}. **Ounce for ounce sea weeds are higher in vitamins and minerals than any other food group.** *They are one of nature's richest sources of carotene, chlorophyll, enzymes and soluble fiber. Just two tablespoons of chopped dried sea vegetables go a long way toward fulfilling the healing requirements for many nutrient deficiencies.*

Sea vegetables build strong teeth, bones, nails and hair. They strengthen nerves synapses, and digestive, circulatory and nervous system functions. They help reduce cholesterol and regulate blood sugar levels. **See page 214 for more about Iodine Therapy in regard to other healing benefits.**

Since most sea vegetables are hand-gathered and dried by small companies of individuals, the question regarding ocean pollution is valid. Our research with Ocean Harvest Company and Maine Coast Sea Vegetables indicates that the alginic acids in sea vegetables perform a dual miracle. "First, they bind with the ions of toxic heavy metals which are then converted to harmless salts. These salts are insoluble in the intestine, and are excreted. Second, they actually chelate radioactive matter <u>already present</u> in the human body and bind it for elimination via the large intestine." Sun-dried and packaged sea vegetables retain almost all of the health advantages, and are the perfect medium for an easy -to- use addition to your soups, salads, steamed veggies, or grain dishes.

144   SEA VEGGIES SUPREME

This blend is both flavor enhancer, and a nutritional part of your recipe. Crumble into a bowl, and then just barely blend in the blender, so that there are still sizeable chunks of the different vegetables. They will expand in any recipe with liquid, and when heated, return to the beautiful fresh green color they had in the ocean. Use freely as a seasoning salt on salads, soups and rice.

$3/4$ CUP CHOPPED DRIED DULSE
$1/4$ CUP CHOPPED DRIED WAKAME
$1/4$ CUP CHOPPED DRIED KOMBU
$1/4$ CUP DRIED CHOPPED NORI OR SEA PALM
$1/2$ CUP TOASTED SESAME SEEDS

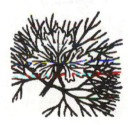

145   DOUG'S MISO SPECIAL

Doug has been fixing foods 'macrobiotically' long before most of us even knew about this way of eating. This is one of his favorites. Now that he has become a brother-in-law, I hope we will see more.

For about 4 bowls:

♣Bring 3 to 4 CUPS OF WATER to a boil. Reduce to a simmer. Add 3 to 4 TBS. WHITE or RED MISO.

♣Add 2 CHOPPED GREEN ONIONS, $1/2$ LB. TOFU in small cubes, and $1/4$ to $1/3$ CUP DRIED WAKAME snipped into small bits.

♣Simmer for 2 minutes. Remove from heat and add $1/2$ CUP SOY CHEESE or MOZZARELLA CHEESE in small cubes. Sprinkle on 3 teasp. BREWER'S YEAST FLAKES. Let cheese melt 30 seconds and serve.

Nutritional analysis: per serving; 128 calories; 11gm. protein; 9gm. carbohydrate; 3gm. fiber; 6gm. fats; 9mg. cholesterol; 188mg. calcium; 4mg. iron; 87mg. magnesium; 200mg. potassium; 645mg. sodium; 2mg. zinc.

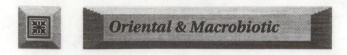

146   SESAME NORI NO-OIL SALAD DRESSING

This recipe is an easy way to introduce sea vegetables - as a condiment for a low-fat diet.
For about 2 cups:

♣Combine in a jar and shake vigorously to blend

1 CUP TOASTED, CRUMBLED NORI SHEETS
3 TBS. PAN ROASTED SESAME SEEDS
1/2 teasp. TAMARI or BRAGG'S LIQUID AMINOS

4 TBS. BROWN RICE VINEGAR
1 CUP WATER or ONION BROTH

♣Serve over vegetable salads, ramen noodles, or rice salads.

Nutritional analysis: per serving; 25 calories; 2gm. protein; 1gm. carbohydrate; 1gm. fiber; 2gm. fat; 0 cholesterol; 7mg. calcium; 1mg. iron; 15mg. magnesium; 40mg. potassium; 37mg. sodium; trace zinc.

�֎

147   SEA PALM & TOFU CASSEROLE

Sea Palm is a rare vegetable that attaches to the rocks off the California coast and lives in the pounding surf of the shoreline. It has become very popular in macrobiotic diets for its sweet taste and versatility.
For 6 servings:

♣Soak 1 OUNCE DRIED SEA PALM FRONDS in water. Drain and cut in 2-inch lengths. Place in a pan with a little water, cover and simmer for 20 minutes until tender, adding more water if necessary.
♣Mash 1 LB. TOFU with the tender sea vegetables and toss with 1 teasp. DRY BASIL and 1 teasp. DRY OREGANO, **or** 2 teasp ITALIAN SEASONING.

♣Make the sauce. Dice 1 LARGE ONION and 1 1/2 LBS. CARROTS. Sauté in 2 TB. OIL or ONION BROTH for 10 minutes. Remove from heat, and puree in the blender with 3 TBS. UMEBOSHI PASTE **or** 3 TBS. SWEET AND SOUR SAUCE. Toss with tofu and palm fronds in a skillet to heat.

♣Meanwhile make the topping. Puree 1/3 CUP TOASTED SESAME SEEDS in the blender with 1 teasp. TAMARI, some FRESH CHOPPED PARSLEY and enough water to make a thick sauce.
♣Cover tofu mixture in the skillet, and cook for 5 more minutes to heat. Serve hot.

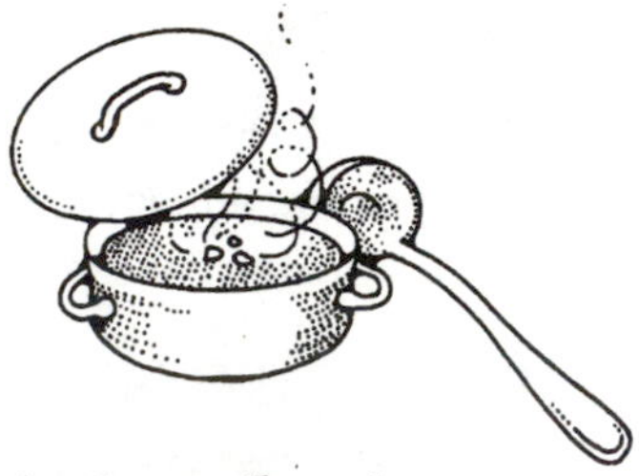

✖

148   QUICK & EASY WAKAME SUCCOTASH

For 4 servings:

♣Soak 1-OZ. DRIED WAKAME in water for 30 minutes. Drain and steam for 10 minutes until tender.
♣Snip into 1 inch pieces, removing the tough stems.
♣Cook ONE 10-OZ. PKG. FROZEN SUCCOTASH VEGETABLES and 1 CUBE CRUMBLED TOFU in a pan according to package directions.

♣Sauté 1 THIN-SLICED RED ONION in 2 teasp. OIL until fragrant. Toss with vegetables and wakame.
♣Toss with 2 TBS. MINCED CHIVES and 2 TBS. UMEBOSHI or BROWN RICE VINEGAR, and let marinate for 3 to 4 hours before serving.

✖

149 SHRIMP & SEA VEGETABLES WITH VINEGAR SAUCE

This seafood salad comes from a booming health food store in Kauai, Hawaii, where sea veggies are a staple.
For 4 salads:

♣Cut 1/2 package of WAKAME or KOMBU into 1-inch lengths. Soak for 1 hour in water, or vinegar or lemon juice. (Acidity tenderizes the sea vegetables). Rinse, drain and set aside.

♣Peel and halve 1/2 to 1 EUROPEAN-TYPE CUCUMBER and cut into half circles or julienne. Sprinkle with 1/2 to 1 teasp. SEA SALT and put in a colander over a pan to drain for 15 to 30 minutes.
♣Squeeze out any remaining excess water and set aside.

♣Rinse 8-OZ. TINY COOKED SHRIMP (or cooked crabmeat) and set aside.

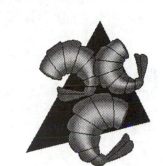

♣Make the VINEGAR SAUCE. Mix together
1 TB. BROWN RICE VINEGAR
1 teasp. CHILI POWDER or DROPS of HOT SAUCE
1 CLOVE CRUSHED GARLIC
1 TB. FRUCTOSE or HONEY
1 TB. PAN ROASTED SESAME SEEDS
1/2 BUNCH GREEN ONIONS with tops, finely chopped.
♣Toss with cucumber, shrimp and sea vegetables. Serve on tiny appetizer plates.

Nutritional analysis: per serving; 89 calories; 8gm. protein; 11gm. carbohydrate; 3gm. fiber; 2gm. fats; 43mg. cholesterol; 84mg. calcium; 2mg. iron; 69mg. magnesium; 237mg. potassium; 400mg. sodium; 1mg. zinc.

150 FRIED RICE WITH SEA VEGETABLES

Sea vegetables go especially well with brown rice for protein complementarity.
For 3 to 4 servings:

♣Sauté 1 CUP DICED RED ONIONS and 1 TB. SHREDDED FRESH GINGER in 2 teasp. TOASTED SESAME OIL or 1 TB. ONION BROTH until soft and fragrant.

♣Add 1/2 CUP CARROTS, julienned, and 1 CUP TOASTED CRUMBLED NORI or SNIPPED DRIED WAKAME and stir-fry for 5 minutes.

♣Add and stir fry for 3 minutes
1/2 CUP DICED CELERY
1/2 CUP DICED BOK CHOY STALKS
2 TBS. TAMARI
1 TB. TAMARI

♣Add and stir-fry for 2 to 3 minutes
2 CUPS COOKED BROWN RICE
1 TB. MIRIN or SAKE
3 TBS. WATER

♣Top with 2 TBS. TOASTED, SLIVERED ALMONDS.
♣Heat to hot and serve.

Nutritional analysis: per serving; 188 calories; 6gm. protein; 33gm. carbohydrate; 5gm. fiber; 4gm. fats; 0 cholesterol; 91mg. calcium; 2mg. iron; 97mg. magnesium; 310mg. potassium; 1047mg. sodium; 1mg. zinc.

Sea vegetables are also good for snacks and munches, especially for a very strict healing diet. Here are a few simple, quick ways to fix sea plant treats.

151 KOMBU OR DULSE CHIPS

♣Snip dry KOMBU or DULSE into bite size pieces. Then either sauté in an oiled pan until leaves turn dark and crisp, **or** roast for 3 to 5 minutes in a 325° oven until vegetables bubble on the surface. Cook a moment more to get very crispy, but watch closely. Sea vegetables scorch easily. Serve with dips.

152 KELP OR KOMBU HONEY BITS

♣Soak dried Kelp or Kombu pieces in water until soft. Drain and snip into bite size pieces to fill 1/2 cup. Bring 1/4 CUP HONEY and 1/2 CUP WATER to a boil. Reduce heat, add sea vegetables and simmer until liquid is evaporated, about 1 to 1 1/2 hours. Spread 1 CUP TOASTED SESAME SEEDS, or 1 CUP GROUND ALMONDS on a baking sheet, and arrange sea vegetables on top, turning to coat with tongs or chopsticks. Bake in a 300∞ oven for 25 to 30 minutes. Turn halfway through baking.

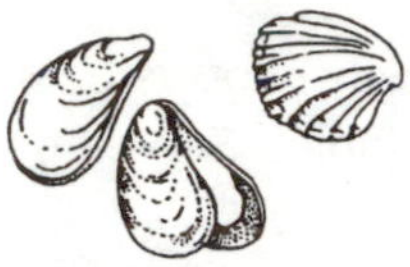

Oriental Seafood Dishes

FOOD FOR THE HEART

Light, low in fat, high in Omega-3 oils and always tasty, the oriental technique in fixing foods from the sea is a delicious way to get these benefits.

153 WHITE FISH TERIYAKI

For 4 servings:

♣Make a fresh teriyaki sauce. Mix all in a pan and simmer til aromatic, about 5 minutes.

1 TB. HOT ORIENTAL MUSTARD
1/4 CUP TAMARI
1/4 CUP MIRIN OR SHERRY
1/2 CUP FISH STOCK (See Page 652)
1 TB. FRUCTOSE or HONEY

♣Add 2 teasp. KUZU or ARROWROOT mixed in 1 TB. WATER and stir over low heat until mixture thickens to a clear glaze. Pour into a dish and set aside.

♣Coat a broiler rack with oil. Rinse four 8-OZ. THICK WHITE FISH FILETS and place skin side down on the rack. (RED SNAPPER , HALIBUT and SHARK are all good.)

♣Brush with the TERIYAKI GLAZE, and broil 4" from heat about 5 to 6 minutes. Baste often. Check for doneness and opaque firmness often so the fish will be at the peak of tenderness when you eat it. Fish is tricky. See page 484 for more information about cooking it to perfection.

♣Garnish with cilantro or parsley and serve immediately.

Nutritional analysis: per serving; 291 calories; 43gm. protein; 9gm. carbohydrate; trace fiber; 6gm. fats; 109mg. cholesterol; 50mg. calcium; 1mg. iron; 80mg. magnesium; 877mg. potassium; 586mg. sodium; 1mg. zinc.

154   YOSENABE - JAPANESE BOUILLABAISSE

This is very good with Japanese soba noodles.
For 8 servings:

♣In a heated wok, sauté until aromatic

3 TBS. PEANUT OIL

2 TBS. FRESH CHOPPED GINGER

3 CLOVES MINCED GARLIC

1 teasp. TOASTED SESAME OIL

♣Add and bring to a boil

1 CUP BOTTLED CLAM JUICE

2 LOBSTER TAILS SPLIT and CHUNKED, or 2 LARGE KING CRAB LEGS IN BIG CHUNKS.

1 LB. CALAMARI IN BITE SIZE CHUNKS

1 DOZEN FRESH or CANNED CLAMS

1 DOZEN LARGE SHELLED PRAWNS

1/2 LB. THICK WHITE FISH FILLET in bite size chunks.

2 TBS. CILANTRO chopped

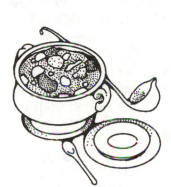

♣Let bubble a minute while you make the sauce. Mix together

1 MORE CUP CLAM JUICE

2 TBS. MIRIN or SAKE

2 TBS. OYSTER SAUCE

1 TB. KUZU CHUNKS or ARROWROOT POWDER

2 teasp. grated LEMON PEEL

1 teasp. DUCK SAUCE, HONEY or FRUCTOSE

♣Add to YOSENABE and stir in until thickened and glossy.

Nutritional analysis: per serving; 247 calories; 41gm. protein; 6gm. carbohydrate; 1gm. fiber; 5gm. fats; 80mg. calcium; 6mg. iron; 86mg. magnesium; 727mg. potassium; 486mg. sodium; 4mg. zinc.

155   BABY LOBSTER TAILS SHANG-HAI STYLE

For 2 main dishes:

♣Cook 1 LB. SMALL LOBSTER TAILS in boiling salted water 1 1/2 minutes and remove with slotted spoon. Cut away shell with kitchen shears, and slice meat in big chunks.
♣Heat wok. Add 1 1/2 TBS. PEANUT OIL and stir-fry 3 SLICES FRESH PEELED GINGER and 3 CRUSHED GARLIC CLOVES for 30 seconds until aromatic. Discard Ginger and garlic pieces.
♣Add LOBSTER PIECES and stir-fry for 1 minute until just opaque and tender. Remove and drain.

♣Add 1 TB. OIL to wok and stir-fry for 2 minutes

1 CUP LEEKS chopped

1 teasp. HONEY or FRUCTOSE

1 TB. MIRIN or SHERRY

1 teasp. SESAME SALT

1/4 CUP CHICKEN STOCK

1 teasp. RED WINE VINEGAR

2 teasp. TOASTED SESAME OIL

♣Return lobster and toss until coated. Serve hot with spicy rice.

Nutritional analysis: per serving; 286 calories; 30gm. protein; 13gm. carbohydrate; 1gm. fiber; 12gm. fat; 142mg. cholesterol; 83mg. calcium; 2mg. iron; 54mg. magnesium; 521mg. potassium; 759mg. sodium; 5mg. zinc.

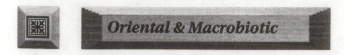

156   RICE PAPER SHRIMP

Traditionally served as a first course or side dish, these were a favorite with Americans in Viet Nam. Buy the rice papers in oriental markets. They are inexpensive, are made of rice and water only, and keep forever.
For 8 rolls:

♣Make these rolls about an hour ahead of serving time so rice paper won't crack or fall apart.

♣Make filling. Mix and let chill in the fridge

1 LB. COOKED TINY SHRIMP	$1/2$ teasp. FRUCTOSE or HONEY
$1/2$ CUP BROWN RICE VINEGAR	1 TB. LIME JUICE
$1/2$ CUP CHOPPED GREEN ONION	3 TBS. CHOPPED FRESH MINT
$1/2$ teasp. HOT PEPPER SAUCE, or SAMBAL OELEK (or 2 teasp. dry mint)	
3 TBS. FRESH CHOPPED CILANTRO	

♣Lay dry wrappers on a flat surface or cutting board. Brush with water. Let sit 2 minutes to soften.
♣Only work with one or two at a time. Put $1/8$ of the filling on the bottom half of each wrapper. Fold bottom up and over. Fold in sides, and roll up into a tight cylinder. Put on a baking sheet, cover with plastic wrap, and let chill while you make the **DIPPING SAUCE.**

♣Mix

1 teasp. CRUSHED RED PEPPER	1 SMALL MINCED CARROT
1 TB. BROWN RICE VINEGAR	$1/2$ teasp GARLIC POWDER
$1/2$ CUP FISH STOCK (page 704)	$1/3$ CUP HONEY
1 $1/2$ CUP WATER	

♣Heat and boil down to about 2 cups.
♣Cool and serve on the side for dipping rolls

Nutritional analysis: per serving; 127 calories; 13gm. protein; 18gm. carbohydrate; 1gm. fiber; 1.5gm. fats; 111mg. cholesterol; 38mg. calcium; 3mg. iron; 60mg. magnesium; 220mg. potassium; 133mg. sodium; 1mg. zinc.

157   GRILLED PRAWNS WITH VEGGIES & SESAME SAUCE

For 4 servings:

♣Make a mix of $1/2$ CUP MIRIN or SAKE, 2 TBS. TAMARI, and 1 TB. SESAME OIL. Use half to marinate 1 LB. PRAWNS, and the other half to marinate the vegetables.

8 GREEN ONIONS SLICED
4 SMALL ZUCCHINI SLICED
8 LARGE MUSHROOMS or BLACK SHIITAKE MUSHROOMS
♣Chill both ingredient mixes.

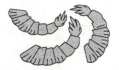

♣Grill prawns on a griddle, or outside grill or in the broiler until just opaque and tender. Grill vegetables until light browned and tender. Baste twice. Remove from heat immediately when done. Keep warm.

♣Make a **SESAME SAUCE.** (See next page.)

♣Sauté or toast in the oven 1/2 CUP SESAME SEEDS until golden. Whirl in the blender with

3 TBS. OIL

1/4 CUP WATER or WHITE WINE

2 TBS. LEMON JUICE

2 TBS. FRESH MINCED GINGER

1 TB. FRUCTOSE OR HONEY

PINCH of GARLIC POWDER

PINCH OF PAPRIKA

♣Blend until smooth and serve over the prawns and veggies.

158   MISO MARINADE FOR FISH

Enough for 2 lbs. of fish or seafood:

♣Mix the marinade together. Pour over fish; cover and let marinate overnight.

1/2 CUP MISO BROTH

1/2 CUP SHERRY

1/3 CUP TAMARI 1

1 TB. GRATED FRESH GINGER

1 tsp. GARLIC/LEMON SEASONING

1/2 TB. HONEY or FRUCTOSE

♣Broil or grill fish about 3 minutes each side, basting several times during cooking.

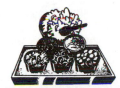

Oriental Salads

Fresh vegetables and greens are a mainstay of oriental meals, and as salads they offer unique combinations.
But the main delight of these dishes are the distinctive spicy dressings that appeal to western tastes.

159   SUSHI SALAD
California maki in a bowl - much easier to make, but with the same great taste of sushi rolls.
For 4 salads:

♣Use 1 CUP BROWN RICE, or KASHI, or WILD and BROWN RICE mixed. Toast until aromatic in a dry pan, or in a little oil until grains are coated.

♣Add 2 CUPS WATER or LIGHT STOCK. Bring to a boil, cover and simmer about 30 minutes until all liquid is absorbed. Remove from heat.

♣Add the following. Mix and toss

A PINCH OF WASABI POWDER

2 TBS. BROWN RICE VINEGAR

1 AVOCADO chopped

3 SCALLIONS minced

1/2 CUP KING CRAB PIECES

♣Crumble a toasted SUSHI NORI SHEET or snip several WAKAME PIECES over the top.

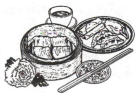

♣Serve with a dab of **HOT MUSTARD DRESSING:**

For 1 cup, mix

4 teasp. CHINESE HOT MUSTARD

ONE PINCH WASABI POWDER (optional)

1/4 CUP LEMON JUICE

2 teasp. TAMARI

6 TBS. OIL

1/2 teasp. GROUND PEPPER

160   EASY GINGER SHRIMP SALAD

For 6 salads:

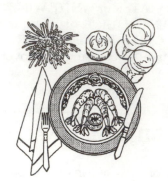

♣Mix and toss together
1¹/₄ LB. COOKED SHRIMP, rinsed and drained
3 TBS. BROWN RICE VINEGAR
2 TBS. SLIVERED PICKLED RED GINGER
1 TB. OIL
¹/₂ teasp. TOASTED SESAME OIL
♣Pile onto rinsed, crisped greens

♣Blend to a paste
2 TBS. WASABI POWDER
1 TB. WATER
♣Put a dollop on each salad plate and pinch into a little cone. Dip shrimp in cones.

Nutritional analysis: per serving; 148 calories; 24gm. protein; 3gm. carbohydrate; trace fiber; 4gm. fats; 221mg. cholesterol; 69mg. calcium; 4mg. iron; 45mg. magnesium; 330mg. potassium; 264mg. sodium; 2mg. zinc.

161   SWEET & SOUR SEAFOOD SALAD

We have made this recipe more times than we can count. It is a perfect opening to any meal.
4 to 6 servings:

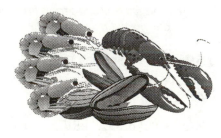

♣Sauté in 2 TBS. LIGHT OIL until golden brown
¹/₂ CUP SLICED or SLIVERED ALMONDS
2 TBS. SESAME SEEDS
4-OZ. CRISPY CHINESE NOODLES
♣Remove and drain on paper towels.

♣Add to pan and sauté briefly until just opaque and firm.
2 CUPS SHELLED and SPLIT SHRIMP, PRAWNS or CRAB MEAT

♣Shred into a large salad bowl
4 CUPS GREEN CABBAGE or 4 CUPS CHINESE CABBAGE
♣Toss in ¹/₂ CUP CHOPPED GREEN ONIONS with tops

♣Add seafood, nuts, seeds and noodles, and toss everything with the following mixed dressing:
5 TBS. LIGHT OIL
6 TBS. BROWN RICE VINEGAR
4 teasp. FRUCTOSE or 4 teasp. HONEY
¹/₂ teasp. BLACK PEPPER
♣Serve right away so nuts and noodles will be crispy.

Nutritional analysis: per serving; 402 calories; 20gm. protein; 22gm. carbohydrate; 4gm. fiber; 27gm. fats; 133gm. cholesterol; 96mg. calcium; 4mg. iron; 86mg. magnesium; 399mg. potassium; 247mg. sodium; 2mg. zinc.

162   SPICY THAI SALAD WITH PEANUT SAUCE

For 4 salads:

♣Sauté 4 to 6-OZ. SHRIMP in 1 TB. OIL or BROTH til opaque and firm. Remove and set aside.

♣Add A LITTLE WATER or LIGHT STOCK to the pan, and add
2 CUPS SHREDDED GREEN CABBAGE or CHINESE CABBAGE
1 PACKAGE (10-oz.) FROZEN PEAS
♣Braise and toss briefly til shiny and green.
♣Remove from heat, mix with shrimp and toss with the following PEANUT SAUCE:

♣Mix together
3 TBS. PEANUT BUTTER
2 TBS. OIL
2 TBS. TAMARI
1 TB. HONEY or 2 teasp. FRUCTOSE

1 TB. BROWN RICE VINEGAR
1/2 teasp. TOASTED SESAME OIL
1/4 teasp. BLACK PEPPER

♣Pan roast 1/2 CUP WALNUTS in the oven while you make the dressing.
♣Toss the dressing with the salad to coat. Snip over 2 GREEN ONIONS and top with the WALNUTS.

Nutritional analysis for this salad; per serving; 357 calories; 17gm. protein; 22gm. carbohydrate; 6gm. fiber; 24gm. fats; 69mg. cholesterol; 93mg. calcium; 3mg. iron; 86mg. magnesium; 464mg. potassium; 340mg. sodium; 2mg. zinc.

163   CHICKEN TERIYAKI SALAD
This recipe came from a favorite restaurant in Atlanta, Ga., now closed, but the good dish lives on.
For 6 salads:

♣Poach 3 BONELESS CHICKEN BREASTS, skinned and cut in 1/4" wide strips in 1/2 inch VEGETABLE BROTH until white and firm. Remove and place in a bowl.

♣Julienne 1 SWEET RED BELL PEPPER and 4 GREEN ONIONS and add to bowl with chicken.

♣Add 50 to 60 SNOW PEAS, strung and blanched to bright green in hot water.

♣Add 1 CUP CHOPPED CASHEWS, toasted to golden in the oven.

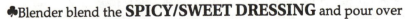

♣Blender blend the **SPICY/SWEET DRESSING** and pour over
2 TBS. SNIPPED PARSLEY
2 CLOVES GARLIC, minced fine
1/2 CUP TAMARI
1/4 CUP SESAME TAHINI
1/4 CUP LIGHT OIL
DASHES HOT PEPPER or HOISIN SAUCE

3 TBS. BROWN RICE VINEGAR
2 TBS. SHERRY or MIRIN
2 teasp. FRUCTOSE or 1 TB. HONEY
2 teasp. CHINESE 5 SPICE POWDER
2 teasp. TOASTED SESAME OIL

♣Mix and toss with all salad ingredients. Top with more TOASTED SESAME SEEDS. Chill.

 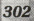

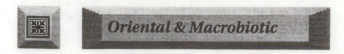

164 QUICK NAPPA & NOODLE SALAD

For 8 salads:

♣Put the noodles from one 3-OZ. PACKAGE RAMEN in boiling water to cover for <u>1 minute only.</u> Drain and combine with
4 CUPS SHREDDED CHINESE NAPPA CABBAGE and 1 SMALL FINE CHOPPED CUCUMBER.

♣Sauté in 2 teasp. OIL or BROTH for 3 minutes. Remove from heat and set aside 2 TBS. SESAME SEEDS and 1/3 CUP MINCED GREEN ONIONS.

♣Blend the salad sauce in a bowl and pour over cabbage mix
THE SEASONING PACKET FROM THE RAMEN NOODLES
3 TBS. BROWN RICE VINEGAR
1 1/2 TBS. HONEY or 1 TB. FRUCTOSE
2 TBS. OIL
1 teasp. TOASTED SESAME OIL
1/4 teasp. SESAME SALT (GOMASHIO)
♣Top with GREEN ONIONS and SESAME SEEDS and serve chilled.

Nutritional analysis: per serving; 99 calories; 2gm. protein; 10gm. carbohydrate; 2gm. fiber; 6gm. fat; 0 cholesterol; 48mg. calcium; 1mg. iron; 20mg. magnesium; 160mg. potassium; 52mg. sodium; trace zinc.

Whole Grains & Pastas For Light Macrobiotic Eating

The essence of macrobiotic eating is based on cooked whole grains as the way of life to health. Originally this was interpreted almost entirely in terms of brown rice, but today other grains are also recognized for their efficient protein, high complex carbohydrates and fiber as primary health supports. Whole grain variety is now widely available in many convenient and viable cooking uses to make a healthy diet more interesting. Whole grains and pastas are wonderful in salads, both cold and hot, (where raw veggies are added to, and heated by hot grains), baked casseroles, pasta mixes, and hearty soups.
The following recipes offer a selection to try in each area.

We have found that a **whole grain blend** is much more interesting and tasty than any single grain alone. A blend of grains and seeds tastes nuttier, and chewier. It cooks easier, with more definition and less stickiness, and the variety of the nutrients is enhanced. We make up a large batch of mixed grains, (see page 647 for recipe) and keep it in a cannister for ready use.

For the best flavor, *dry roast grains in the cooking pan for about 5 minutes until fragrant, before adding water or stock.* **It makes a delicious difference.**

There is a key watchword for whole grain pastas - the less you can cook them the better. **Cook just to al dente.** Have your sauce ready, then cook the pasta at the last minute so it won't be sticky and starchy. Especially with delicate, light oriental pastas - you must stay with them the entire few minutes of cooking. Keep testing for perfect doneness. Then drain, and immediately coat with a little oil or your sauce.

165   BASIC MACROBIOTIC VINEGAR RICE

For 6 cups of cooked rice:

♣Soak 2 CUPS BROWN or BASMATI RICE in 2 $1/2$ CUPS COLD WATER in a large pan for about 30 minutes. Add a 2-inch SQUARE of DRIED KOMBU or WAKAME. Bring to a rapid boil. Cover, reduce heat to medium and cook for 10 minutes until water is absorbed.
♣Reduce heat to low and simmer for 5 more minutes to dry and separate grains. Let rest for 5 minutes. Remove cover. Discard sea vegetable and pour on **VINEGAR DRESSING** below. Cool slightly.

VINEGAR DRESSING
♣Combine in a pan, and bring to a boil
$1/4$ CUP BROWN RICE VINEGAR
3 TBS. HONEY
2 teasp. SEA SALT
2 TBS. MIRIN (OPT.)

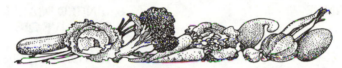

Macrobiotic Grain & Vegetable Salads
High fiber, high protein, high complex carbohydrates, low-fat, low sodium, low cholesterol, dairy free, great taste.
What more could you ask.

166   SUMMER SALAD WITH BULGUR & TOMATOES

For 4 large salads:

♣Soak $1/2$ CUP BULGUR in water or stock for 15 minutes. Drain and press out excess water.
♣Slice $1/2$ CUP WATER CHESTNUTS or a little FRESH DAIKON RADISH.
♣Chop $1/2$ CUP SCALLIONS OR LEEKS.
♣Sauté bulgar, chestnuts and scallions briefly in 2 teasp. OLIVE OIL until aromatic, about 5 minutes.
♣Remove from heat and set aside.

♣Add 1 PEELED CUCUMBER, cubed and 1 TOMATO, cubed.

♣Mix the dressing and toss to coat grains and vegetables
3 TBS. OLIVE OIL
3 TBS. LEMON JUICE
$1/2$ teasp. DRY THYME or TARRAGON
$1/4$ teasp. SESAME SALT or GREAT 28 MIX (page 645)
$1/4$ teasp. PEPPER or LEMON PEPPER (page 643)
♣Snip fresh mint leaves on top. Chill before serving.

Nutritional analysis including dressing: per serving; 186 calories; 3gm. protein; 22gm. carbos; 6gm. fiber; 10gm. fats; 0 cholesterol; 33mg. calcium; 1mg. iron; 46mg. magnesium; 313mg. potass.; 66mg. sod.; 1mg. zinc.

167 WILD RICE WINTER SALAD

For 4 salads:

♣Toast in a dry pan ³/₄ CUP WILD RICE, or MIXED WILD and BROWN RICE until fragrant.
♣Add 1¹/₂ CUPS WATER or LIGHT STOCK. Cover and cook on low heat until liquid is absorbed. Put in salad bowl.
♣Put pan back on heat and add ¹/₂ CUP CHOPPED FILBERTS or WALNUTS, and ¹/₂ teasp. SESAME or SEASONING SALT. Toast for 10 minutes until browned and aromatic.

♣Soak in the JUICE OF 1 ORANGE and add to rice
¹/₃ CUP RAISINS
1 TART APPLE, chopped
1 FENNEL BULB or 1 CELERY STALK, chopped

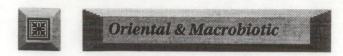

♣Make a **LEMON /ORANGE VINAIGRETTE** and toss with rice mixture

GRATED PEEL of 1 ORANGE	3 MINCED SCALLIONS
4 TBS. ORANGE JUICE	5 TBS. OLIVE OIL
2 TBS. LEMON JUICE	1 TB. CHOPPED FRESH CILANTRO
2 teasp. BALSAMIC VINEGAR	1 TB. TOASTED SESAME OIL
¹/₂ teasp. GREAT 28 MIX (Page 645)	1 TB. CHOPPED CHIVES
¹/₄ teasp. GROUND FENNEL or ANISE	1 teasp. TARRAGON

♣Top salad with toasted nuts and serve.

Nutritional analysis including dressing: per serving; 497 calories; 6gm. protein; 54gm. carbohydrate; 5gm. fiber; 30mgm. fats; 0 cholesterol; 79mg. calcium; 2mg. iron; 109 magnesium; 470mg. potassium; 126mg. sodium.

168 TUNA CASSEROLE SALAD WITH BROWN RICE OR PASTA

For 4 salads:

♣Steam 1 CUP GREEN PEAS and 1 CUP THIN SLICED GREEN ONIONS together until bright green.
♣Pick up steamer, and dump peas and onions into a salad bowl. Set aside.

♣Add to steamer and cook 2 CUPS FRENCH CUT GREEN BEANS covered until bright green.
♣Add to salad bowl with peas and onions.

♣Add to salad bowl Mix together and pour over

2 CUPS CUBED TOMATOES	JUICE OF ONE LEMON
1 CUP COOKED BROWN RICE	2 TBS. OLIVE OIL
2 TBS. FRESH CHOPPED PARSLEY OR BASIL	1 TB. SAFFLOWER OIL
ONE 7-OZ. CAN WATER PACKED TUNA	

♣Mix and toss all together.

Nutritional analysis: per serving; 278 calories; 17gm. protein; 28gm. carbohydrates; 6gm. fiber; 11gm. fats; 23mg. cholesterol; 53mg. calcium; 3mg. iron; 73mg. magnesium; 624mg. potassium; 164mg. sodium; 1mg. zinc.

169   BASMATI & PEPPERS HOT SALAD

For 6 large salads:

♣Cook 1/2 CUP WILD RICE in 2 CUPS WATER with 2 teasp. SEA SALT for 1 hour. Drain. Set aside.
♣Sauté 1 LARGE CHOPPED RED ONION in 2 TBS. OIL and 2 TBS. TAMARI until soft and aromatic.
♣Bring 4 CUPS VEGETABLE or ONION STOCK to boil in a large pot.

♣Put in a 2-qt. baking dish
2 CUPS BROWN or WHITE BASMATI RICE
1 GREEN BELL PEPPER chopped
1 RED BELL PEPPER chopped
and the SAUTÉED ONIONS

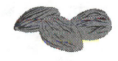

♣Pour hot stock over. Cover, bake at 375° for 25 minutes. Stir in cooked wild rice.
♣Fluff and serve warm with **HONEY ITALIAN DRESSING:**

♣Mix, pour over and toss with salad

1/2 CUP OLIVE OIL   1 teasp. HONEY
3 TBS. LEMON JUICE   1/2 teasp. ITALIAN SEASONING
1 teasp. SPIKE or SEASONING SALT (page 643)

Nutritional analysis with dressing: per serving; 454 calories; 7gm. protein; 66gm. carbohydrate; 4gm. fiber; 18gm. fats; 0 cholesterol; 40mg. calcium; 2mg. iron; 121mg. magnesium; 295mg. potassium; 249 mg. sodium; 2mg. zinc.

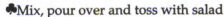

170   ALMONDS & GREEN RICE SALAD

For 6 large salads:

♣Toast 1/3 CUP SLICED or SLIVERED ALMONDS in a pan or the oven.

♣Pan roast 1 CUP BROWN RICE until fragrant. Add 2 CUPS WATER. Bring to a rapid boil. Cover, reduce heat and simmer until water is absorbed, about 30 minutes. Fluff with a fork and chill.

♣Wash and chop fine
6 CUPS SPINACH or ROMAINE LEAVES, or a mix of both
1/2 SMALL BUNCH GREEN ONIONS
♣Mix greens and onion with chilled rice.
♣Add and mix in 2 TBS. SOY BACON BITS. Season with LEMON PEPPER and SEASONING SALT.

♣Mix the **ALMOND DRESSING** and pour over:
5 TBS. OIL
1/4 CUP BALSAMIC VINEGAR
1 TB. HONEY or 2 teasp. FRUCTOSE.
1 TB. DIJON MUSTARD
1/8 teasp. PURE ALMOND EXTRACT (optional to heighten flavor)

171   HOT QUINOA & WILD RICE SALAD

Quinoa is a delicious, ancient South American grain, newly discovered as a source of high grade protein.
For 6 salads

♣Toast 1 CUP WILD RICE in a dry pan until aromatic. Add 3¹/₂ CUPS BOILING WATER. Cover and simmer for 30 minutes.
♣Add ¹/₂ CUP QUINOA. Cover and simmer 10 to 15 minutes. Drain and fluff with fork. Cover and chill while you make the rest of the salad.

♣Toast ¹/₂ CUP FILBERTS or WALNUTS in a pan or the oven until brown.

♣In a skillet sauté 1 CHOPPED ONION in 1 to 2 TBS. OIL for 5 minutes.
♣Add 1 CHOPPED TART APPLE and sauté until light brown and aromatic, about 3 minutes.

♣Add chilled wild rice mix to skillet and toss to heat and coat. Remove from heat, place in salad bowl and top with nuts. Serve with LEMON/ORANGE DRESSING:

♣Mix together

¹/₂ CUP ORANGE or PINEAPPLE/ORANGE JUICE	2 TBS. LEMON JUICE
¹/₃ CUP CURRANTS	¹/₂ teasp. ANISE SEED
5 TBS. OIL	¹/₄ teasp. POWDERED GINGER

Nutritional analysis: per serving; 343 calories; 6gm. protein; 45gm. carbohydrate; 6mg. fiber; 16gm. fats; 0 cholesterol; 46mg. calcium; 2mg. iron; 103mg. magnesium; 288mg. potassium; 10mg. sodium; 1mg. zinc.

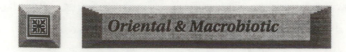

172   MILLET & MUSHROOM SALAD

For 6 salads:

♣Roast millet in a dry pan for 3 to 5 minutes before adding liquid for best flavor. For 2 CUPS COOKED MILLET use about ¹/₂ to ²/₃ CUP MILLET and 1¹/₂ to 1³/₄ CUP WATER or LIGHT STOCK. Fluff and set aside or chill while you fix the veggies.

♣Soak 6 to 8 BLACK SHIITAKE MUSHROOMS in water until soft. Slice in small julienne discarding stems. <u>Save soaking water.</u>
♣Add 2 TBS. DRIED SNIPPED WAKAME or DULSE, and 4 GREEN ONIONS to mushroom soaking water to soften and marinate.

♣Slice 1 CUP BUTTON MUSHROOMS or CHANTERELLES. Sauté briefly in 1 TB. OIL until mushrooms start to give back their juice, about 5 to 7 minutes.

♣Add to millet and toss to mix

2 CUP CHOPPED TOMATOES	2 TBS. OLIVE OIL
PINCHES SESAME SALT and PEPPER	2 teasp. LEMON JUICE

♣Drain sea veggies and onions and add. Toss and serve.

173 MILLET SALAD WITH WAKAME

For 4 salads:

♣Roast 1 CUP MILLET in a dry pan until aromatic. Add 2¹/₂ CUPS WATER and cover. Cook 25 minutes.
♣Remove from heat and fluff.
♣Snip ¹/₂ CUP WAKAME PIECES into hot water. Blanch 3 minutes. Remove with a slotted spoon.
♣Keep water hot and dice in
¹/₂ CUP CARROTS
¹/₄ CUP CELERY
¹/₃ CUP DAIKON or RED RADISH
♣Blanch 5 minutes and drain. Season with LEMON PEPPER.

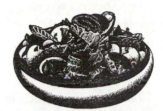

♣Add
¹/₂ CUP SNIPPED FRESH PARSLEY
¹/₂ CUP DICED CUCUMBER
A HANDFUL of DRY ROASTED PEANUTS
♣Toss all together with millet, and serve on lettuce with a SESAME MISO DRESSING:

♣For 1¹/₂ cups dressing, blender blend

A SCANT ¹/₂ CUP OIL	1 TB. LIGHT MISO
1 TB. TOASTED SESAME OIL	¹/₂ teasp. VEGGIE SALT or SPIKE
2 TBS. BROWN RICE VINEGAR	3 TBS. SESAME SEEDS TOASTED
1 TB. LEMON JUICE	DASHES CAYENNE or HOT SAUCE

174 COUSCOUS SALAD

Couscous is a low-fat, quick-cooking grain of African origin. It has an adaptable, mild nutty flavor.
For 6 salads:

♣Pour 1 CUP BOILING WATER over 1 CUP COUSCOUS in a bowl. Add a PINCH of SEA SALT, and let soak for 15 minutes until water is absorbed. Place in a steamer basket with small holes or line with cheesecloth. Steam for 15 minutes until tender. Fluff with a fork. Add 2 TBS. OIL and toss through.

♣Soak ¹/₂ CUP RAISINS in ³/₄ CUP WATER for 10 minutes. Drain, and set aside.
♣Toast ¹/₂ CUP PINE NUTS, SUNFLOWER SEEDS or SLICED ALMONDS in the oven until golden.

♣Bring ¹/₄ CUP LIGHT STOCK or WATER and a PINCH OF SALT to a boil in a skillet.
♣Add and simmer for 5 to 7 minutes until color changes
2 CUPS SLICED CELERY
2 CUPS CARROTS, julienned
¹/₂ teasp GROUND GINGER
1 teasp. DRIED MINT
♣Toss together with couscous and nuts or seeds, and let rest for 30 minutes before serving.

Nutritional analysis: per serving; 260 calories; 7gm. protein; 38gm. carbohydrate; 9 gm. fiber; 11gm. fats; 0 cholesterol; 63mg. calcium; 2 mg. iron; 98mg. magnesium; 518mg. potassium; 113mg. sodium; 1mg. zinc.

175 GOURMET GRAINS & VEGETABLES SALAD

For 4 salads:

♣Dry roast 1 CUP GOURMET GRAINS BLEND (Page 647) til fragrant.

♣Bring 2 CUPS WATER or LIGHT STOCK to a boil, add grains, cover, reduce heat and steam for 25-30 minutes until liquid is absorbed. Fluff and chill.

♣Sauté briefly in 1 TB. oil about 2 minutes
1/2 CUP CHOPPED MUSHROOMS
1/2 CUP CUBED TOFU
1/2 CUP MIXED GREEN, RED OR YELLOW BELL PEPPERS, chopped
1/4 CUP GREEN ONIONS, chopped

♣Add 1 SMALL CAN SLICED WATER CHESTNUTS, 1/2 CUP DICED CELERY, 1/4 CUP CHOPPED PARSLEY, and 1 SMALL CHOPPED TOMATO. Immediately remove from heat, mix with **DIJON DRESSING.** Toss and serve.

DIJON DRESSING:
♣Mix together

1/3 CUP OIL
1/4 CUP TAMARI

3 TBS. BASMATI VINEGAR
2 teasp. DIJON MUSTARD

♣Add HERB SALT and BLACK PEPPER to taste.

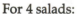

176 GOURMET GRAINS HOT PILAF SALAD

For 4 salads:

♣Dry roast 1 CUP GOURMET GRAINS BLEND (page 647) in a pan until aromatic.
♣Bring 2 1/4 CUPS ONION or VEGETABLE BROTH to a boil.

♣Sauté in 2 TBS. OIL for 5 minutes
1 ONION chopped
1 CARROT chopped
SESAME SALT and PEPPER to taste

3/4 teasp. DRY BASIL
3/4 teasp. DRY OREGANO
1 CLOVE MINCED GARLIC

♣Mix with grains. Pour stock over. Cover. Reduce heat and simmer 25 minutes. Drain. Chill. Make a simple VINAIGRETTE DRESSING and pour over.

♣Mix together
5 TBS. OIL
5 TBS. BALSAMIC or TARRAGON VINEGAR
1 TB. MUSTARD
1/2 teasp. DRY TARRAGON or CHERVIL or SAVORY

Nutritional analysis: per serving: 268 calories; 5gm. protein; 32gm. carbohydrate; 6gm. fiber; 14gm. fats; 0 cholesterol; 53mg. calcium; 2mg. iron; 65mg. magnesium; 274mg. potassium; 246mg. sodium; 1mg. zinc.

Hearty Grain One-dish Meals

The recipes in this section are packed with a wealth of concentrated nutrition. For someone following the cleansing/ rebuilding part of a healing diet, these dishes are quite enough for a meal by themselves, or simply accompanied by a light salad. Most whole grains may be used interchangeably for variety and individual preference. Whole grains are low-fat, mineral and protein-rich, and dairy free.

177   COUSCOUS & RED LENTILS

A delicious low fat, high protein whole-meal dish.
For 6 servings:

♣Bring 1¼ CUPS WATER to a boil. Add 1 CUP COUSCOUS, 2 TBS. BUTTER or OIL and ¹/₂ teasp. SEA SALT. Stir, cover and remove from heat. Allow to stand for 5 minutes. Fluff with a fork.

♣Sauté for 5 minutes in 2 teasp. OIL or BROTH
¹/₂ CUP CHOPPED LEEKS (white parts only)
¹/₄ CUP CHOPPED CELERY LEAVES

♣Add and stir in
2 CUPS WATER with 1 VEGETABLE BOUILLON CUBE
1 CUP RED LENTILS   DASHES CAYENNE or PAPRIKA
1 TB. TOMATO PASTE   1 teasp. TAMARI
1 teasp. RED WINE or BASMATI VINEGAR   1 teasp. GARLIC/LEMON SEASONING

♣Reduce heat, cover and simmer for 20 minutes.

Nutritional analysis: per serving; 238 calories; 12gm. protein; 38gm. carbohydrate; 9gm. fiber; 5gm. fats; 10mg. cholesterol; 40mg. calcium; 4mg. iron; 79mg. magnesium; 446mg. potassium; 203mg. sodium; 1mg. zinc.

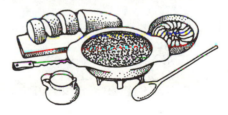

178   OATS & ALMONDS PILAF

For 2 servings:

♣Toast ¹/₂ CUP SLICED ALMONDS in the oven until golden (10 minutes at 325°) Stir and shake often.

♣Sauté 1 ONION IN RINGS and 1 CLOVE GARLIC, MINCED in 2 teasp. OIL. Add 1 CUP OATS and sauté until aromatic and browning.

♣Add 1³/₄ CUP ONION BROTH. Bring to a boil. Cover and simmer 15 to 20 minutes until liquid is absorbed.
♣Remove from heat. Fluff and mix in 3 TBS. CHOPPED FRESH PARSLEY and half of the toasted nuts.

♣Top with more chopped parsley and the rest of the nuts.

Nutritional analysis: per serving; 339 calories; 12gm. protein; 37mg. carbohydrate; 8gm. fiber; 17gm. fats; 0 cholesterol; 116mg. calcium; 3mg. iron; 141mg. magnesium; 432mg. potassium; 133mg. sodium; 2mg. zinc.

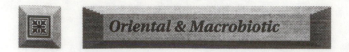
179   RICE PASTA WITH ROAST PEPPERS & DRIED TOMATOES

Orzo rice pasta is fairly new to American tastes. Quick and easy cooking are making it a fast favorite.
For 4 servings:

♣Bring a large pot of water to a rapid boil. Add 1 TB. SEA SALT and 1 LB. ORZO (rice pasta). Cook stirring for 6 minutes. Drain and set aside.

♣Sauté in 6 TBS. OLIVE OIL or LIGHT STOCK until soft, about three minutes
3 CLOVES MINCED GARLIC
6 CHOPPED SHALLOTS

♣Add
1/4 CUP SLIVERED DRIED TOMATOES in oil   1 teasp. BLACK PEPPER
1 1/2 CUPS CHICKEN or ONION STOCK   1 teasp. SEA SALT
♣Add 1 CUP CHOPPED FRESH BASIL. Add orzo and stir til stock is absorbed.
♣Add 1 JAR ROASTED BELL PEPPERS, chopped.
♣Increase heat to high and boil until reduced by half, 3 to 5 minutes. Remove from heat, put in serving dish, and top with 1 CUP SOY PARMESAN.

180   BROWN RICE & GREENS CLASSIC

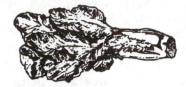

Have everything ready before you start to cook this dish. It goes fast.
For 6 main dish servings:

♣Toast 1/2 CUP CHOPPED WALNUTS and 2 TBS. SESAME SEEDS in the oven.
♣Have ready 4 CUPS COOKED BROWN RICE.

♣Shred or fine chop
1 CUP ROMAINE LETTUCE   SLICE 1 ONION
1 CUP CHINESE NAPPA CABBAGE   DICE 1 CARROT
1 CUP WASHED SPINACH LEAVES
1 CUP BOK CHOY STEMS and LEAVES

♣Preheat a large wok. Add and heat until fragrant
3 to 4 TBS. OIL
1/2 teasp. FRESH MINCED GINGER or 1 CLOVE MINCED GARLIC
♣Add the carrots and onion and sauté for about 5 minutes.
♣Add the greens and toss just until color changes.
♣Add 1 1/2 CUPS BEAN SPROUTS or SUNFLOWER SPROUTS. Toss to coat and heat.
♣Add brown rice and mix all together.

♣Turn off heat. Make a well in the center and add 2 EGGS. Toss for 3 minutes until hot and set. Turn onto large serving platter. Top with walnuts, sesame seeds, sesame salt, and 1 TB. TAMARI.

Nutritional analysis: per serving; 307 calories; 9gm. protein; 37gm. carbohydrate; 5gm. fiber; 14gm. fat; 71mg. cholesterol; 98mg. calcium; 2mg. iron; 105mg. magnesium; 362mg. potassium; 75mg. sodium; 2mg. zinc.

181 BROWN RICE PILAF PLUS

This is a macrobiotic staple dish. This is delicious fixed on the range, but is lighter and fluffier from the oven.
For 4 main course servings:

♣Toast 1/2 CUP SLICED ALMONDS and 1 TB. SESAME SEEDS until golden, 5 min.

♣Sauté in a pan in 2 TBS. OIL til aromatic, about 5 to 7 minutes
1 SMALL SLICED ONION
2 SHALLOTS or 1 CLOVE GARLIC, CHOPPED
1 TB. SOY BACON BITS

♣Add 1 STALK CELERY with leaves, 1 CUP BROWN RICE or WHOLE GRAIN MIX, and 1/4 CUP WILD
RICE. Mix and toss until shiny and hot.

♣ Add spices
1/4 teasp. GROUND GINGER   1/2 teasp. LEMON PEEL
1/2 teasp. SESAME SALT   1/4 teasp. PEPPER

♣ Add 2 1/4 CUPS WATER or LIGHT STOCK. Bring to a boil. Cover and simmer until liquid is absorbed;
or turn into a casserole. Add water or stock and cover tightly. Bake at 350° for 1 hour.

♣ Top with snipped PARSLEY and PAPRIKA. Scatter nuts and seeds over top.

Nutritional analysis: per serving; 273 calories; 7gm. protein; 39gm. carbohydrates; 3gm. fiber; 10gm. fats; 0 cholesterol; 58mg. calcium; 2mg. iron; 11mg. magnesium; 234mg. potassium; 124mg. sodium; 1mg. zinc.

182 COUSCOUS WITH STEAMED VEGGIES & SPROUTS

*This is a delicious variation on the macrobiotic staple of brown rice and vegetables. It is lighter, and less dense on the
system.*
For 4 meal-size servings:

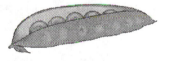

♣ Steam together until tender
2 CUPS FROZEN or FRESH CORN KERNELS
2 CUPS DICED CARROTS
♣ Add 2 CUPS FROZEN PEAS for the last 1 minute of steaming, and cook just until color changes.
♣ Bring 3 CUPS CHICKEN or ONION STOCK to a boil with 1 teasp. SEA SALT.
♣ Add 2 CUPS COUSCOUS. Remove from heat. Cover and let stand for 5 minutes. Fluff with fork.

♣ Stir in
1/4 CUP CHOPPED GREEN ONIONS
1 CUP CHOPPED FRESH PARSLEY

♣ Put couscous mix on a serving platter. Surround with vegetables. Sprinkle with 2 TBS. PARMESAN or
SOY PARMESAN, and 2 HANDFULS ALFALA SPROUTS.

183   BULGUR SHEPHERDS PIE

For 8 serving size squares:

♣Soak 1¹/₂ CUPS BULGUR in water for 15 minutes. Drain and press excess water out.
♣Boil 4 to 5 POTATOES (enough for 3 cups mashed) until soft. Mash potatoes.
♣Sauté 3 CUPS CHOPPED ONION and 2 CLOVES GARLIC in 2 TBS. OIL or ONION BROTH.

♣Add
1 teasp. DRY BASIL (or 2 TBS. FRESH CHOPPED)
¹/₂ teasp. NUTMEG
¹/₂ teasp. GROUND CUMIN
1 teasp. SESAME SALT
¹/₂ teasp. PEPPER
♣Stir to blend. Sprinkle on 3 TBS. WHOLE WHEAT FLOUR.

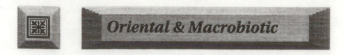

♣Mix 3 TBS. FRESH CHOPPED PARSLEY and 3 TBS. CHOPPED SCALLIONS into mashed potatoes.
♣Combine bulgur and potatoes together. Spread <u>half</u> on bottom of a lecithin sprayed 9 x 13" pan.
♣Top with onion mix. Sprinkle on ¹/₂ CUP TOASTED CHOPPED ALMONDS or PINE NUTS.
♣Spread on rest of potatoes to cover. Sprinkle with a 1 TB. ITALIAN DRESSING or VINAIGRETTE just to moisten the top. Bake at 400∞ for 45 minutes until edges turn golden.

Nutritional analysis: per serving; 251 calories; 7gm. protein; 45gm. carbohydrates; 9gm. fiber; 6gm. fats; 0 cholesterol; 51mg. calcium; 1mg. iron; 92mg. magnesium; 565mg. potassium; 80mg. sodium; 1mg. zinc.

184   CURRIED BASMATI

For 6 servings:

♣Put 2 CUPS BASMATI RICE in a pan with 2 CUPS VEGEX or ONION BROTH. Let sit for an hour.
♣Mix 2 to 2¹/₂ TBS. CURRY POWDER in 2 TBS. broth to paste consistency. Set aside.

♣Heat 1¹/₂ TBS. OIL over high heat for 1 minute. Add and cook for 1 minute until golden
1 TB. FRESH MINCED GINGER
1 CLOVE GARLIC, minced
♣Stir in curry paste, simmer 15 minutes and remove from heat. Set aside, covered.

♣Heat 2 TBS. OIL for 1 minute until hot and sauté 2 CHOPPED ONIONS for seven minutes.
♣Raise heat and sauté until brown and aromatic, 8 minutes. Season with salt and add to Basmati. Bring to a rapid boil and cook for 3 minutes. Reduce heat to low and cook until tender-firm, 8 to 10 minutes.

♣While rice is cooking, add ¹/₂ TB. OIL to a small skillet and sauté quickly
¹/₂ GREEN BELL PEPPER diced
¹/₂ RED OR YELLOW BELL PEPPER diced
¹/₄ CUP MINCED CILANTRO
♣Put curried rice on a serving platter and surround with tender-crisp vegetables.

185   FANCY COUSCOUS RING WITH GOLDEN PEPPER SAUCE

This is a company-style recipes that is actually very quick and easy.
For 8 servings:

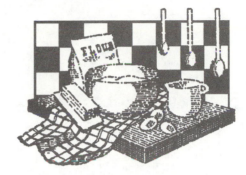

♣Marinate the **GOLDEN PEPPER & ONION SAUCE** first.

♣Mix together and put into a bowl
1/2 CUP CHOPPED ONION
1/2 CUP YELLOW BELL PEPPER

♣Combine in a pan and bring to a boil
1/4 CUP WATER
1/4 CUP RED WINE VINEGAR
1/4 CUP OLIVE OIL
2 DASHES HOT PEPPER SAUCE
1 teasp. HONEY
♣Let cook for 3 minutes and pour over peppers and onions. Cover and chill.

♣Meanwhile, bring 2$1/2$ to 3 CUPS WATER to a boil. Add ONE 12 OZ. PACKAGE COUSCOUS and 4 TBS. BUTTER or OIL. Cover, remove from heat and let sit for 10 minutes. Fluff with a fork. Set aside.

♣Drain peppers and onions. Add 1 CUP FINE DICED CHERRY TOMATOES to sauce and season.
♣Mix into couscous. Add 1 CUP HOMEMADE or BOTTLED NATURAL SALSA.
♣Put in a lecithin-sprayed ring mold, smooth top and chill well.

♣Before serving, bring 6 CUPS WATER to boil with 1 teasp. SEASONING SALT (pg. 643), or GREAT 28 MIX (pg. 645).
♣Barely blanch 1 CUP CHOPPED BROCCOLI just until color changes.
♣Remove with slotted spoon, and add 1 CUP CHOPPED CAULIFLOWER.
♣Blanch for 7 minutes, remove with slotted spoon, and add 1 CUP RED CHOPPED ONION.
♣Cook for 7 minutes to crunchy tender.

♣Unmold couscous ring onto a plate and fill with broccoli, cauliflower and onion.

Nutritional analusis: per serving with sauce; 256 calories; 7gm. protein; 39gm. carbos; 11gm. fiber; 10gm. fats; 15mg. cholesterol; 37mg. calcium; 2mg. iron; 84mg. magnesium; 415mg. potassium; 46mg. sodium; 1mg. zinc.

$\mathcal{D}$reams are what you trade your days for.

Wine was created
from the beginning to
make men joyful,
not to make men drunk.
Wine enjoyed in moderation
is a pleasure of the soul
and the heart.

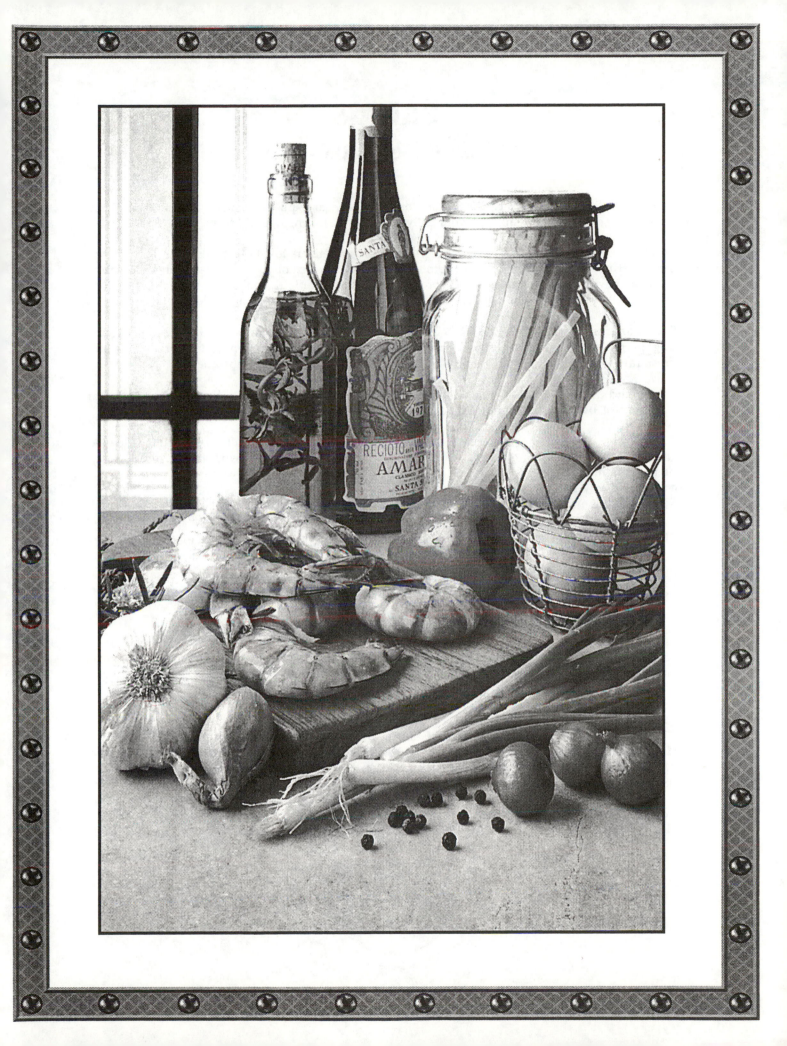

Salads
Hot & Cold

A fresh salad every day is a cardinal point for health, a vital requisite for body cleansing and healing. Even when fasting or cleansing,, your daily salad can be taken, in liquid form.

Salads can be hot or cold. They can be anything from appetizers to whole meals, in infinite combinations that provide high soluble fiber, protein, and complex carbohydrates. Greens and vegetables are delicious with cooked grains, such as brown rice, millet or bulgur, cooked or marinated legumes, such as lentils, green beans, or a gourmet bean mix, and cooked vegetable or whole grain pastas.

Salads are full of water for good body elimintion. High liquid content means light, but satisfying eating, perfect for weight loss. Rich chlorophyllins from greens have proven healing properties, and as fresh raw food, the nutrients, vitamins and minerals in a salad are easily absorbed.

Salads and all fresh foods take a longer time to eat than cooked foods. They are mainstays for weight control, by giving your body time to signal satisfaction before you overeat.

A major essential for a <u>healthy</u> salad is the dressing, which can be all too *un*healthy if it is loaded with high fats and salty condiments. All the salads in this book are made with low-fat and low salt contents in mind.

For a healthy, low-fat, low salt dressing:
- Use only polyunsaturated or mono-unsaturated vegetable oils, canola, olive or Omega-3 flax oil. Keep opened bottles refrigerated to avoid rancidity.
- Use a good vinegar, such as balsamic, champagne or tarragon vinegar. Apple cider vinegar is especially good for cleansing and alkalizing.
- Use sesame salt, herb salt, sea vegetable salt, or a vegetable seasoning instead of table salt.
- Dress your salads with a light touch. One to 3 tablespoons of dressing per salad, to keep fats, sodium and cholesterol low.

You can do just about anything with a salad. Almost any fresh food combination can be made into a successful salad with the refreshing bite of a good vinaigrette. Salads can supply almost every nutritional need. The essential idea is to find the freshest, finest ingredients available lightest food form. The recipe selection in this chapter is extensive, because I believe that salads are the basis of healthful eating. You can choose from:

SIMPLE CLEANSING SALADS APPETIZER SALADS MARINATED SALADS PASTA SALADS LAYERED SALADS FRUIT SALADS HIGH PROTEIN SALADS RICE and GRAIN SALADS CHICKEN and TURKEY SALADS HOT SALADS WHOLE MEAL SALADS FANCY COMPANY SALADS SPECIAL SALAD DRESSINGS

Other good salads are included in almost every recipe section of this book. Just check out the **INDEX By Recipe Type** when you want a new delicious salad.

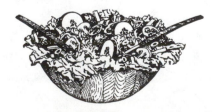

Simple Cleansing Salads

These are bright, zippy, refreshing salads that may be used for a fast or cleanse,
but are also good for "spring body cleaning" when you just want to eat less food.

186 FIREBIRD

I used to take this salad down to the beach in a big wooden bowl, and eat it watching the sun set into the ocean. It is
a good pre-fasting salad, and always reminds me of those meditation, contemplative days.
For 2 salads:

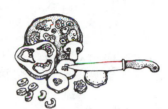

♣Toss together
1 CUP FRESH ALFALFA or SUNFLOWER SPROUTS
2 CUPS GRATED CARROTS
1 CUP MINCED CELERY

♣Make the dressing. Mix
1/4 CUP LIGHT OIL
3 TBS. TOMATO JUICE (such as KNUDSEN'S VERY VEGGIE -SPICY)
2 TBS. LIME JUICE
1 teasp. SESAME SALT
♣Pour over salad just before eating.

Nutritional analysis: per serving; 316 calories; 3gm. protein; 16gm. carbohydrate; 5gm. fiber; 28gm. fat; 0 cholesterol;
68mg. calcium; 1mg. iron; 34mg. magnesium; 611mg. potassium; 627mg. sodium; trace zinc.

187 CASABLANCA SALAD

Desert climates demand very light hydrating foods. We were served a version of this salad at almost every meal dur-
ing our stay in North Africa.
For 6 salads

♣Mix and toss together
1 LARGE EUROPEAN CUCUMBER, SLICED
4 FRESH TOMATOES IN WEDGES
4 GREEN ONIONS, SLICED
1/3 CUP FRESH CHOPPED MINT LEAVES

♣Make the dressing. Mix
1/4 CUP OLIVE OIL
1/4 CUP LIME JUICE
2 TBS. TARRAGON or BASMATI VINEGAR
♣Pour over salad. Stir gently and cover. Let chill in the fridge to blend.

Nutritional analysis: per serving; 123 calories; 2gm. protein; 10gm. carbohydrate; 3gm. fiber; 9gm. fat; 0 cholesterol;
32mg. calcium; 1mg. iron; 23mg. magnesium; 370mg. potassium; 13mg. sodium; trace zinc.

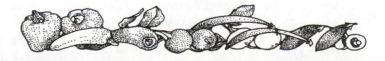

188   PERFECT BALANCE SALAD

For 6 salads:

Mix and chill
1 CUP PLAIN LOW-FAT YOGURT
2 TBS. LIGHT MAYONNAISE
3 TBS. LEMON JUICE
1¹/₂ teasp. CURRY POWDER
¹/₄ teasp. GROUND GINGER

♣Combine in a large bowl
1 EUROPEAN CUCUMBER, thin sliced
2 GREEN ONIONS thin sliced
¹/₂ CUP RAISINS
1 TART RED APPLE cored, quartered,
    wedged and cut in thin slices

♣Mix all together gently. Make ahead, cover and chill all day if possible.
♣Shred 1 quart of BOSTON LETTUCE LEAF LETTUCE and SPINACH LEAVES. Divide on salad plates.
♣Mound with salad mix and season with SEA SALT and PEPPER.

Nutritional analysis: per serving; 192 calories; 5gm. protein; 31gm. carbohydrates; 4gm. fiber; 7mg. cholesterol; 1 gm. fat; 167mg. calcium; 50mg. magnesium; 664mg. potassium; 236mg. sodium; 1mg. zinc.

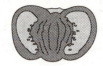

189   APPLE, SPROUT & CARROT SALAD

For 4 salads:

♣Combine in a bowl
2 CUPS MIXED SPICY SPROUTS
2 CARROTS, shredded
1 STALK CELERY, sliced
1 GRANNY SMITH APPLE, cored and shredded
♣Top with 1 TB. TOASTED SESAME SEEDS.

♣Combine the dressing and pour over
2 TBS. LIME JUICE
¹/₄ teasp. GARLIC/LEMON SEASONING
¹/₂ TB. TAMARI
1 to 2 TBS. OIL

190   FRESH TOMATOES WITH GINGER BASIL VINAIGRETTE

Enough for 8 salads:

♣Make the vinaigrette. (This dressing is also quite good on a rice salad.) Whisk in a bowl to combine
¹/₂ CUP SALAD OIL
¹/₄ CUP TARRAGON VINEGAR
1 TB. LEMON JUICE
1 TB. FRESH MINCED GINGER
2 TBS. FRESH CHOPPED BASIL LEAVES
2 TBS. CHOPPED GREEN ONIONS

¹/₂ teasp. CHINESE 5 SPICE POWDER
¹/₄ teasp. DRY CHINESE MUSTARD
¹/₂ teasp. SESAME SALT
¹/₂ teasp. BLACK PEPPER

♣Assemble overlapping tomato slices on large lettuce leaves, and pour dressing over.

Nutritional analysis: per 1-oz. serving; 125 calories; 1 gm. protein; 1 gm. carbohydrate; trace fiber; 13gm. fats; 0 cholesterol; 12mg. calcium; 3mg. magnesium; 36mg. potassium; 138mg. sodium; trace zinc.

Appetizer Salads

These are small first-course-size refreshing salads - perfect for stimulating a healthy appetite.

191 ZUCCHINI CARPACCIO

The key to this authentic Italian salad is the paper thin slices of zucchini. A food processor works the best for making these kinds of slices, or a very sure hand with a paring knife.
For 4 small salads:

♣ Cover small salad plates with tart greens such as ARUGULA, ENDIVE or RADICCHIO (All of these grow well in California kitchen gardens. Our radicchio comes back every year as a volunteer).
♣ Top greens with SUNFLOWER SPROUTS or WATERCRESS LEAVES.
♣ Slice 4 TENDER ZUCCHINI PAPER THIN and divide between salad plates.
♣ Sprinkle on a few drops of OLIVE OIL per salad, some grated SOY or REGULAR PARMESAN, or provolone cheese, and BLACK PEPPER.

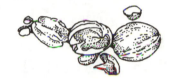

192 ROASTED WALNUTS WITH FETA CHEESE

For 2 appetizer salads:

♣ Pan roast ³/₄ CUP WALNUT PIECES in 2 teasp. OIL until fragrant; (or oven roast at 275∞ for 45 min.)

♣ Whisk the dressing in a bowl
1 TB. RED WINE VINEGAR
1 TB. DIJON MUSTARD
PINCHES of SEA SALT and PEPPER

♣ Divide 4 CUPS LOOSELY PACKED GREENS onto salad plates. Sprinkle with ¹/₃ CUP CRUMBLED FETA CHEESE. Top with dressing and walnuts.

193 SPINACH & ARTICHOKE SALAD

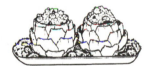

For 4 small salads:

♣ Wash and stem 1 SMALL BUNCH SPINACH LEAVES. Dry on paper towels.
♣ Drain and rinse 1 JAR (11oz.) WATER-PACKED ARTICHOKE HEARTS.
♣ Peel and crumble 2 HARD BOILED EGGS.
♣ Coarsely chop 10-12 BLACK OLIVES or 10-12 WHOLE WATERCHESTNUTS.
♣ Slice 4 LARGE MUSHROOMS.
♣ Combine all in a salad bowl.
♣ Toss with 1 TB. SOY BACON BITS, COARSE GROUND PEPPER, 1 TB. LEMON JUICE and sprinkles of OLIVE OIL.

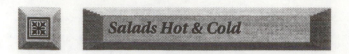

194 RED ONIONS & TOMATOES WITH MOZZARELLA CHUNKS

For 4 salads:

♣Sauté $1/2$ CUP RED ONION SLICES in 1 TB. OIL or BROTH until just fragrant.
♣Toss in a bowl with
8 OZ. MOZZARELLA CHEESE, in cubes $1/2$ teasp. DRY THYME
1 TB. RED WINE or BALSAMIC VINEGAR $1/4$ teasp BLACK PEPPER
$1/2$ teasp. CHILI SAUCE $1/2$ teasp. DRY OREGANO
♣Soak for 2 to 3 hours.
♣Slice three TOMATOES into thin slices on individual salad plates.
♣Sprinkle with FRESH CHOPPED CILANTRO. Top with cheese and onion mix; drizzle with OLIVE OIL.

Nutritional analysis: per serving: 220 calories; 16gm. protein; 9gm. carbohydrate; 2gm. fiber; 13gm. fat; 29mg. cholesterol; 432mg. calcium; 1mg. iron; 29mg. magnesium; 313mg. potassium; 321mg. sodium; 2mg. zinc.

195 FRESH VEGETABLE SALAD WITH SAFFRON & GINGER

For 4 salads:

♣Mix together in a bowl and chill while you make the SAFFRON/GINGER SAUCE
$1/2$ LB. CARROTS, shredded
1 SMALL HEAD GREEN CABBAGE, shredded
1 RED or YELLOW BELL PEPPER in thin slivers

♣Make the sauce in a bowl. Mix $1/4$ teasp. SAFFRON THREADS and 1 teasp. CURRY POWDER in 1 TB. water until it turns orange. Add
$1/4$ CUP LIGHT OIL   3 TBS. FRESH MINCED GINGER
$1/4$ CUP WHITE WINE VINEGAR $1/2$ teasp. SEA SALT
1 JALAPEÑO CHILI, seeded and minced $1/4$ teasp. PEPPER
♣Pour over vegetables. Mix, toss, cover and chill for several hours before serving.

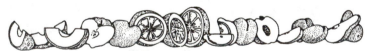

Fruit Salads

For good food combining, serve fruit salads as appetizers before the meal, or as a full meal lunch or brunch alone.

STRAWBERRY MAYONNAISE
Starting with the top, this is an excellent all purpose topping for any fruit salad.
For $1^{1}/4$ cups:

♣Whirl in the blender and chill for an hour before serving.
$1/2$ CUP LIGHT MAYONNAISE   2 TBS. HONEY
$3/4$ CUP FRESH SLICED STRAWBERRIES $1/2$ teasp. LEMON JUICE

196   RED & GREEN SALAD

For 6 salads:

♣Pan roast 1 CUP WALNUTS in 2 teasp. OIL until fragrant.

♣Toss 1 LARGE DELICIOUS APPLE **and** 1 LARGE GRANNY SMITH APPLE cored and chunked together in a large bowl.
♣Add 1 HEAD SHREDDED LETTUCE, 2 RIBS SLICED CELERY, and 2 SLICED GREEN ONIONS.

♣Mix together and pour over, the **HONEY/YOGURT DRESSING:**

1/3 CUP YOGURT CHEESE	2 TBS. HONEY
SESAME SALT and PEPPER	2 TBS. WATER

Nutritional analysis: per serving with dressing: 203 calories; 5gm. protein; 23gm. carbohydrate; 4gm. fiber; 11gm. fat; 1mg. cholesterol; 79mg. calcium; 1mg. iron; 44mg. magnesium; 384mg. potassium; 1mg. zinc.

197   PEARS & CHEVRE SALAD WITH TOASTED WALNUTS

For 8 salads:

♣Roast 1/2 CUP WALNUT PIECES in the oven or in a skillet with 1 teasp. OIL until fragrant.

♣Whisk the dressing together

1/2 CUP WALNUT or SALAD OIL	1 TB. RED WINE VINEGAR
1 CLOVE MINCED GARLIC	1/4 teasp. SEA SALT
PINCHES of WHITE PEPPER	

♣Toss 2 TORN HEADS BIBB or BOSTON LETTUCE and 2 TORN BUNCHES ARUGULA or ROMAINE LETTUCE together in a large bowl and divide onto salad plates.
♣Chunk 1/2 LB. MILD GOAT CHEESE (CHEVRE), FETA or BRIE and divide in center of greens.
♣Stem, core and thin slice 3 RIPE PEARS and place around cheese. Pour dressing over.

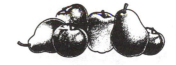

198   LIGHT WALDORF SALAD

For 4 salads:

♣Mix and toss all together.

2 DICED TART APPLES	1/4 CUP PLAIN YOGURT
1 CUP DICED CELERY	2 TBS. LIGHT MAYONNAISE
1 CUP SLICED RED FLAME GRAPES	1/2 teasp. SWEET HOT MUSTARD
1/2 CUP TOASTED WALNUTS	2 TBS. LEMON JUICE

Nutritional analysis: per serving; 202 calories; 3gm. protein; 23gm. carbohydrate; 3gm. fiber; 10gm. fat; 3mg. cholesterol; 61mg. calcium; 1mg. iron; 34mg. magnesium; 348mg. potassium; 75mg. sodium; trace zinc.

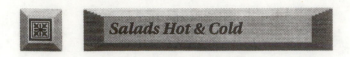
199   THAI PAPAYA SALAD

This sweet and hot salad combines unusual ingredients in a tangy sauce that uniquely pulls it all together. The recipe comes from the South Pacific islands where seafood and fruit are plentiful all year round.
For 6 salads:

♣Roast ³/₄ CUP PINE NUTS in the oven or a dry skillet until golden. Set aside.

♣Sauté 1 CLOVE MINCED GARLIC and 2 teasp. MINCED FRESH GINGER in 2 TBS. OIL in a hot skillet until fragrant.
♣Add 1 LB. BITE SIZE SCALLOPS and toss until opaque, about 2 minutes. Remove to a plate and cool.

♣Shake vigorously in a jar to combine, and chill while you assemble the salad.
3 TBS. LIME JUICE
2 TBS. HONEY   ¹/₂ teasp. ORIENTAL CHILI SAUCE
1 TB. SOY SAUCE   2 MINCED SCALLIONS
1 TB. MINCED CILANTRO
♣Peel, seed and thin-slice 1¹/₂ RIPE PAPAYAS. Peel and chop 1 RIPE KIWI. Peel, seed and dice 1 SMALL CUCUMBER. Toss together fruits and scallops, and all but 2 TBS. of the pine nuts.
♣Divide onto greens covered salad plates, spoon on dressing, and sprinkle with rest of pine nuts.

Nutritional analysis: per serving with dressing: 230 calories; 7gm. protein; 14gm. carbohydrates; 4gm. fiber; 17gm. fat; 25mg. cholesterol; 189mg. calcium; 1mg. iron; 27mg. magnesium; 404mg. potassium; 390mg. sodium.

Marinated Salads

Marinades add robustness to salad ingredients - and they are a boon to time-pressed, busy people, because they keep food so beautifully. Just make these salads when you have some time, and chill them for later.

200   RED ONION, GREEN ONION MARINADE

This is good for button mushrooms, French cut or Italian green beans, or the Gourmet Bean Mix on page 647.
For 2 to 4 salads, about ³/₄ cup:

♣Blender blend the marinade
1 TB. DIJON MUSTARD
1 TB. CHOPPED RED ONION
2 TBS. CHOPPED GREEN ONION
3 TBS. TARRAGON VINEGAR
6 TBS. OLIVE OIL
1 TB. CHOPPED FRESH RED or GREEN BASIL (in season) or 1 teasp. DRY BASIL
♣Toss with 2 CUPS WHOLE BUTTON MUSHROOMS, **or** 2 CUPS lightly cooked FRENCH CUT OR ITALIAN GREEN BEANS, **or** 2 CUPS COOKED MIXED LEGUMES.

♣The marinade "cold cooks" and tenderizes the vegetables.

Nutritional analysis: per serving for the marinade; 187 calories; trace protein; 2gm. carbohydrate; trace fiber; 20gm. fat; 0 cholesterol; 13mg. calcium; trace iron; 4mg. magnesium; 40mg. potassium; 49mg. sodium.

201   LEMON MUSHROOMS

These mushrooms are absolutely delectable. Use a mix of gourmet mushrooms such as Chanterelles, Shiitakes, Enokis, and Buttons.
For 4 salads:

♣Mix the marinade

1 CUP OLIVE OIL	1 MINCED SHALLOT
1/2 CUP WHITE WINE	1/2 teasp. BLACK PEPPER
1/4 CUP FRESH LEMON JUICE	1 teasp. DRY OREGANO

♣Toss with 20 to 24 MUSHROOMS brushed and halved, and 1 SMALL SLICED RED ONION.

♣Chill, covered overnight.

♣Top with 1/3 CUP WATERCRESS LEAVES or SUNFLOWER SPROUTS.

202   BALSAMIC ONIONS

Everybody is familiar with marinated bean salads, but onions (particularly effective for healing and antibiotic qualities) also release much of their flavor and benefits in a marinade.
For 4 to 6 servings:

♣Sauté 4 SLICED RED ONIONS in 4 TBS. OIL or BROTH until aromatic, about 5 minutes.

♣Add 2 to 3 TBS. BALSAMIC VINEGAR, 1 teasp. DRY THYME, and 1/2 teasp. PEPPER.

♣Chill for at least an hour. Serve with very tart greens.

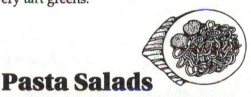

Pasta Salads

Check pasta ingredients carefully if you are on a healing or restricted diet.
There are many fine vegetable and whole grain pastas available.

203   ARTICHOKES and LINGUINE MONTEREY

This recipes sounds Italian, but actually comes from California artichoke country around Monterey , Ca.
For 4 salads:

♣Sauté until aromatic in 2 TBS. OLIVE OIL.	♣Remove from heat and toss with
1 CLOVE CHOPPED GARLIC	1/2 CUP CHOPPED TOMATO
1/2 CUP CHOPPED RED ONION	2 TBS. SLICED BLACK OLIVES
1/2 CUP CHOPPED MUSHROOMS	1 TB. LEMON JUICE
1/2 CUP WHITE WINE	

♣Bring 3 to 4-qts. salted water to a boil. Add ONE 11-OZ. JAR WATER PACKED ARTICHOKES, SLICED, and cook uncovered for 4 minutes. Remove with a slotted spoon, and add to salad. Set aside in a large bowl to chill while pasta is cooking.

♣Add 6-OZ. DRY LINGUINE to boiling artichoke water. Cook just to al dente, 5 to 7 minutes. Drain, and toss with salad ingredients. Turn onto a large platter.

♣Slice over 1 RIPE AVOCADO. Sprinkle with PARMESAN CHEESE and chill til ready to serve.

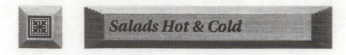

204   ADVANTAGE SALAD

The "advantages" are high quality protein, complex carbohydrates, low-fat and great taste.
For 4 salads:

♣Cook 2 CUPS MIXED VEGETABLE ELBOWS in 2-qts. boiling salted water with 1 TB. OIL added to prevent boiling over. Cook uncovered, stirring occasionally for 10 minutes until tender. Drain and toss.

♣Put pasta into a large marinating bowl with

<table>
<tr><td>1/2 CUP CHOPPED CELERY</td><td>1 GRATED CARROT</td></tr>
<tr><td>1/2 CUP LIGHTLY STEAMED GREEN PEAS</td><td>4 TBS. SOY BACON BITS</td></tr>
<tr><td>1/4 CUP SWEET PICKLE RELISH</td><td></td></tr>
</table>

<table>
<tr><td>♣Chill while you make the marinade/dressing.</td><td>♣Mix</td></tr>
<tr><td>2 CHOPPED GREEN ONIONS</td><td>1 teasp. SWEET/HOT MUSTARD</td></tr>
<tr><td>2 TBS. OLIVE OIL</td><td>1 teasp. MIXED SALAD HERBS</td></tr>
<tr><td>1/4 CUP TARRAGON VINEGAR</td><td>1 teasp. HONEY</td></tr>
</table>

♣Chill to blend flavors. Pour over salad and toss just before serving.

205   CHERRY TOMATOES AND BOWTIES

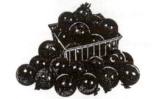

For 4 small salads:

♣Halve 2 pints of CHERRY TOMATOES into a large bowl. Snip in 1 WHOLE BUNCH OF SCALLIONS and 1 CUP FRESH PARSLEY. Toss to mix and chill while pasta is cooking.

♣Bring 2-QTS. WATER to a boil and cook 2 CUPS BOW TIES to al dente. (See How To Cook Pasta, page 225). Drain, and toss with tomato mix.
♣Divide salad onto small lettuce covered salad plates.
♣Sprinkle with PARMESAN, cubes of MOZZARELLA, and drizzles of OLIVE OIL.

♣This salad is also good with **DILL MAYONNAISE.** Omit the MOZZARELLA and OLIVE OIL, and spoon 1 to 2 TBS. dressing over each individual salad.

DILL MAYONNAISE

♣Mix in a small bowl
1/2 CUP LIGHT MAYONNAISE
1/2 CUP PLAIN LOW-FAT YOGURT
1 TB. FRESH SNIPPED DILL WEED (or 1 teasp. dry)
1 teasp. LEMON JUICE
1/2 teasp. GREAT 28 MIX (Pg. 645) or other vegetable seasoning salt

Nutritional analysis; per serving without Dill Dressing; 342 calories; 13gm. protein; 47gm. carbos; 5gm. fiber; 11gm. fat; 9 mg. chol.; 191mg. calcium; 4mg. iron; 55mg. magnesium; 493mg. potass.; 140mg. sodium; 1mg. zinc.

206   SESAME NOODLE SALAD

For 6 salads:

♣Dry roast $1/4$ CUP SESAME SEEDS in a skillet until golden. Set aside.
♣Soak 1 CUP DRIED SHIITAKE BLACK MUSHROOMS in water or broth for 30 minutes. Sliver and set aside. Reserve mushroom soaking water.

♣Bring about 3-qts. of salted water to boil in a pot. Add mushroom soaking water. Blanch 1 BUNCH BROCCOLI FLOWERETTES and PIECES 2 to 3 minutes until bright green. Remove with a slotted spoon to a bowl of ice water and chill 5 minutes.

♣Bring water to boil again and drop in 1 LB. ASPARAGUS PIECES and TOPS, and 1 CUP MUNG BEAN SPROUTS. Cook for 2 minutes until asparagus is bright green. Remove with slotted spoon to broccoli ice water. Boil and chill briefly.
♣Bring water to boil again, and cook 8 OZ. DRY CHINESE SPAGHETTI NOODLES **for $2^1/2$ minutes only** just to al dente. Drain and toss with 2 TBS. OIL. Set aside.

♣While pasta is cooking, make the dressing. Bring $1/2$ CUP CHICKEN or ONION STOCK to a boil in a saucepan. Add and stir until smooth and aromatic

$1/2$ CUP PEANUT BUTTER	$1^1/2$ teasp. ORIENTAL CHILI SAUCE
$1/4$ CUP BROWN RICE VINEGAR	$1/4$ CUP MINCED SCALLIONS
2 TBS. TAMARI	2 TBS. MINCED FRESH GINGER
1 TB. TOASTED SESAME OIL	$1/2$ GARLIC LEMON SEASONING
1 TB. SHERRY	THE RESERVED SESAME SEEDS

♣Toss the sauce with vegetables and noodles. Top with 2 TBS. MINCED CHIVES or CILANTRO, and SLIVERS of RED BELL PEPPER.

High Protein Salads Without Meat

207   NUTS & BOLTS

This salad was a regular feature of the Rainbow Kitchen, and one of the most popular.
For 4 salads:

♣Toast in a 400° oven for 7 to 10 minutes until brown
$1/2$ CUP CHOPPED ALMONDS
$1/2$ CUP CHOPPED CASHEWS

♣Mix with

1 CUP CHOPPED CELERY	$1/4$ CUP SNIPPED PARSLEY
$1/4$ CUP CHOPPED BELL PEPPER	$1/4$ CUP SNIPPED GREEN ONIONS

♣Top the salad with one of the following protein-rich dressings.

ALMOND BUTTER SAUCE

For 3 to 4 cups:

♣Blend to good dressing consistency in the blender

1/2 CUP ALMOND BUTTER
2 TBS. TAMARI
1 TB. SOY BACON BITS

1/2 teasp. BLACK PEPPER
1/2 teasp. DRY MIXED SALAD HERBS
1 TB. OIL

♣Pour over salad and sprinkle on TOASTED SUNFLOWER SEEDS and ALFALFA SPROUTS.

TOASTED ALMOND MAYONNAISE

For 2 cups:

♣Toast 3/4 cup ALMONDS in a 350° oven til browned, about 15 minutes. Then coarse chop *briefly* in the blender and set aside.

♣Make the mayonnaise in the blender
1 EGG
2 teasp. DIJON MUSTARD
1 TB. WHITE WINE VINEGAR
1/2 teasp. SEA SALT

♣Whirl briefly, and add 1 CUP OIL in a thin stream until mayonnaise thickens.
♣Combine with almonds, chill, and serve with salad.

208   EGG SALAD LIGHT

Eggs are an excellent protein source, and indeed all-around nutritious food. Remember that the cholesterol of the yolks that got such a bad "rap" for years is balanced by the lecithin phosphatides of the whites.
For 3 cups, about 4 servings:

♣Hard boil 6 EGGS the foolproof way. Put eggs in a pan of cold water. Bring to a boil. Immediately turn off heat and cover pan. Let eggs sit *exactly* 6 minutes. Pour off water and cover with cold water.
♣Let sit til ready to peel.
♣Mash together in a bowl

6 HARD BOILED EGGS
1 RIB CELERY with leaves
2 TBS. MINCED PARSLEY
JUICE of 1/2 FRESH LEMON
2 teasp. DIJON MUSTARD

2 TBS. LIGHT MAYONNAISE
2 TBS. PLAIN LOW FAT YOGURT
1/4 teasp. CURRY POWDER
1/4 teasp. SEASONING SALT

♣Mound into BOSTON LETTUCE CUPS, and top with DASHES of PAPRIKA.

Nutritional analysis: per serving; 169 calories; 10gm. protein; 3gm. carbohydrate; trace fiber; 9gm. fat; 322mg. cholesterol; 66mg. calcium; 15mg. magnesium; 1mg. iron; 239mg. potassium; 183mg. sodium; 1mg. zinc.

209   BLACK BEAN & CELERY SALAD

For 8 salads:

♣Rinse $1/2$ LB. DRY BLACK BEANS, and soak in cold water to cover overnight.

♣Drain and add enough cold water to cover by 2". Bring to a rapid boil. Reduce heat to low and simmer for 45 minutes. Add $1/2$ teasp. SEA SALT and cook for 45 minutes more. Drain and chill.

♣Sauté 1 SLICED RED ONION in 2 TBS. OLIVE OIL until translucent and aromatic.

♣Combine with cooked beans, 3 RIBS CHOPPED CELERY with leaves, and $1/2$ DICED GREEN BELL PEPPER in a large bowl, and toss to mix.

♣Make the dressing and toss gently with the salad
$1/3$ CUP LIGHT OIL
3 TBS. LIME JUICE and the GRATED ZEST of ONE LIME
$1/2$ teasp BLACK PEPPER
$1/2$ teasp. HERB or SEASONING SALT

Nutritional analysis: per serving; 315 calories; 11gm. protein; 31gm. carbohydrate; 11gm. fiber; 17gm. fat; 0 cholesterol; 51mg. calcium; 3mg. iron; 67mg. magnesium; 537mg. potassium; 81mg. sodium; 1mg. zinc.

210   SZECHUAN TOFU SALAD

For 6 salads:

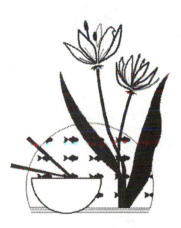

♣Make the marinade in the blender
5 or 6 FRESH BASIL LEAVES, or $1/2$ teasp. dried
$1/2$ teasp. CRUSHED DRIED HOT PEPPER, or $1/8$ teasp. SAMBAL OELEK
$1/4$ CUP GRATED FRESH GINGER
$1/4$ CUP TAMARI
$1/4$ CUP BROWN RICE VINEGAR
$1/4$ CUP SESAME OIL
3 TBS. HONEY

♣Marinate 1 LB. FRESH TOFU SLICES for 1 hour. Then brown the slices and the marinade in a skillet til flavors blend and concentrate. Pour out $1/2$ CUP MARINADE for the dressing.

♣Leave the rest in the skillet with the TOFU to toss with the following vegetable blend
$1^{1}/2$ CUPS SHREDDED GREEN or RED CABBAGE
$1^{1}/2$ CUPS GRATED CARROTS
6 CHOPPED SCALLIONS with tops

♣Wash and chop 1 HEAD ROMAINE LETTUCE. Divide onto 6 salad plates. Mound on tofu and cabbage mix. Top with crunchy CHINESE NOODLES, and pour remaining marinade over.

Nutritional analysis: per serving; 221 calories; 9gm. protein; 19gm. carbohydrate; 3gm. fiber; 14gm. fat; 0 cholesterol; 130mg. calcium; 5mg. iron; 96mg.magnesium; 439mg. potassium; 153mg. sodium; 1mg. zinc.

211   QUINOA SALAD

Quinoa is a light delicate grain - an ancient food of the Inca people. It is higher in protein than any other grain, and can be substituted for rice in many recipes.
For 4 large salads:

♣Rinse 1 CUP QUINOA in a strainer to remove bitter edge. Bring 2 CUPS WATER to a boil with 1 teasp. SEA SALT. Add Quinoa and cook over low heat until slightly chewy, about 10 minutes. Taste for doneness ♣Drain off excess water. Put in a large mixing bowl and sprinkle with 1/4 CUP CURRANTS.

♣Toast 1/4 CUP PINE NUTS for the topping in a dry skillet or the oven until golden, about 5 minutes.
♣Make the dressing and let it sit and bloom while you make the rest of the salad. Mix and whisk
1 TB. LEMON JUICE
1 teasp. GRATED LEMON ZEST
1/4 teasp. PAPRIKA   ♣Snip into the Quinoa
1/4 teasp. GROUND CUMIN   1/3 CUP RAISINS
1/4 teasp. GROUND CORIANDER   2 TBS. CHOPPED CHIVES
1 TB. CHOPPED PARSLEY   1/4 CUP MINCED CELERY
1/4 CUP CANOLA OIL
♣Add pine nuts and toss.
♣Arrange lettuce leaves on individual plates and mound salad on them. Pour dressing over and serve.

Nutritional analysis: per serving; 443 calories; 10gm. protein; 57gm. carbohydrate; 4gm fiber; 22gm. fat; 0 cholesterol; 45mg. calcium; 3mg. iron; 114mg. magnesium; 457mg. potassium; 150mg. sodium; 2mg. zinc.

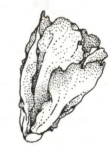

Whole Grain & Rice Salads

212   KASHA SPINACH SALAD

For 6 servings:

♣Sauté 2 CHOPPED SHALLOTS and 1 CLOVE CHOPPED GARLIC in 2 teasp. OIL for 1 minute.
♣Add 1/2 CUP KASHA (cracked wheat) and sauté for 1 more minute.
♣Sprinkle with HERB SALT and PEPPER
♣Add 1 CUP WATER. Cover, reduce heat and cook until water is absorbed, about 10 to 15 minutes. Remove from heat and fluff with a fork.

♣Add to kasha and toss to mix   ♣Whisk the simple dressing together
4-OZ. FRESH SLICED MUSHROOMS   1 TB. DIJON MUSTARD
6 CHOPPED SCALLIONS   2 TBS. TARRAGON VINEGAR
4 DICED PLUM TOMATOES   1/3 CUP OLIVE OIL
1/3 CUP WALNUT PIECES   1/4 teasp. BLACK PEPPER
3 TBS. RAISINS
♣Wash and tear 1 BUNCH FRESH SPINACH. Arrange on individual plates and top with mounds of salad. Drizzle with dressing and serve.

213   VEGETABLES WITH GOURMET GRAINS

This recipe has also become a favorite company and whole meal salad.
For 6 servings:

♣Dry roast 1 CUP GOURMET GRAINS MIX (page 647), **or** a mix of BROWN and WILD RICE in a large skillet, stirring often to keep from burning.

♣When grains are fragrant, add 2 CUPS WATER or CHICKEN or ONION BROTH and bring to a boil.

♣Cover, reduce heat and let steam for 25 minutes until water is absorbed.

♣Remove from heat, fluff, and set aside to cool while you make the veggie sauté.

♣Sauté in a large skillet in 2 TBS. OIL **and** 4 TBS. LIGHT BROTH until color changes to bright green
2 STALKS DICED CELERY with leaves
1 SLICED ZUCCHINI
1 STALK CHOPPED BROCCOLI
1 SLICED GREEN BELL PEPPER   ♣Remove from heat and toss with
1 CUP CHINESE PEA PODS, strung   3 TBS. TAMARI
1 CUP SLICED GREEN ONIONS   1 TB. HONEY
1 CUP SLICED MUSHROOMS   1 teasp. SESAME SALT
1 CAN SLICED WATER CHESTNUTS   1/2 teasp. PEPPER

♣Combine sauce and vegetables with the grains. Let rest to blend flavors for 10 minutes. Serve immediately, or chill and serve cold in LARGE LETTUCE CUPS.

Nutritional analysis: per serving; 237 calories; 6gm. protein; 42gm. carbohydrate; 5gm. fiber; 5gm. fat; 0 cholesterol; 64mg. calcium; 2mg. iron; 81mg. magnesium; 620mg. potassium; 215mg. sodium; 1mg. zinc.

214   CREAMY RICE SALAD

For 6 servings:

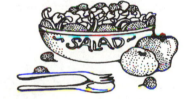

♣Use 6 OZ. MIXED BASMATI and WILD RICE. Bring 2 CUPS WATER to boil. Add rice blend and return to boil. Cover and cook over low heat until water is absorbed and rice is tender, about 40 minutes. Remove from heat , uncover and fluff. Set aside to cool while you make the salad and dressing.

♣Blanch 1 CUP FROZEN GREEN PEAS in boiling water for 3 minutes until bright green. Set aside.

♣Mix the dressing and let sit to bloom   ♣Mix the salad and toss with dressing
1/2 CUP LIGHT MAYONNAISE   1 C. HALVED CHERRY TOMATOES
1/2 CUP PLAIN YOGURT   1 CUP DICED PEELED CUCUMBER
1/2 CUP SLICED GREEN ONIONS   1/2 CUP DICED CELERY
1/4 CUP CHOPPED PARSLEY
1/4 teasp. PEPPER
1/2 teasp. SESAME SALT

♣Add peas and rice blend and toss to mix. Serve at room temperature in a large bowl lined with lettuce leaves.

Nutritional analysis: per serving; 256 calories; 5gm. protein; 30gm. carbohydrate; 3gm. fiber; 5gm. fat; 10mg. cholesterol; 69mg. calcium; 1mg. iron; 59mg. magnesium; 313mg. potassium; 167mg. sodium; 1mg. zinc.

215   MOROCCO SALAD

This salad is easy on the delicate or healing system, but still serves as a good whole grain meal.
For 4 salads:

♣Pour 1$\frac{1}{4}$ CUPS <u>BOILING</u> WATER over 1$\frac{1}{2}$ CUPS DRY COUSCOUS. Cover and let sit for 10-15 minutes until water is absorbed. Remove cover. Stir and fluff.
♣Add $\frac{1}{2}$ teasp. SEA SALT and a PINCH SAFFRON (opt.). Set aside.

♣Toast $\frac{1}{2}$ CUP SLIVERED ALMONDS in the oven until golden. Set aside.

♣Steam until tender crisp
1 CUP SLICED CARROTS   1 DICED GREEN PEPPER
1 CUP FROZEN FRENCH CUT GREEN BEANS $\frac{1}{3}$ CUP CHOPPED RED ONION
♣Drain when done and toss with the almonds and $\frac{1}{3}$ CUP CURRANTS.
♣Set aside while you make the marinade.

♣Mix in the blender
$\frac{1}{2}$ CUP OLIVE OIL
4 TBS. LEMON JUICE
$\frac{1}{2}$ teasp. LEMON PEPPER
$\frac{1}{4}$ teasp. CINNAMON
3 TBS. ORANGE JUICE
4 TBS. FRESH CHOPPED MINT (If you used saffron, omit the mint. It will cancel the saffron taste.)
2 PINCHES PAPRIKA
♣Toss with salad ingredients and couscous and chill to blend flavors.

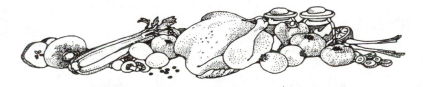

Turkey & Chicken Salads

Chicken and turkey are low fat meats, and can make any salad a satisfying protein-rich meal.

216   LIGHT CHICKEN & MUSHROOM SALAD

For 8 salads:

♣Combine marinade ingredients
4 THIN SLICED SCALLIONS
THE JUICE of ONE LEMON
$\frac{1}{3}$ CUP + 2 TBS. OLIVE OIL
2 TBS CHOPPED FRESH CILANTRO
1 teasp. SESAME SALT
$\frac{1}{4}$ teasp. PEPPER

♣Marinate the following for 1 hour
8-OZ. SLICED MUSHROOMS
6 CUPS COOKED SLICED CHICKEN
1 SMALL HEAD CHINESE CABBAGE,
   shredded

♣Mound in lettuce cups or on salad plates lined with watercress.

217 SESAME CHICKEN SALAD WITH PEA PODS

For 6 small salads:

♣Blanch $1/2$ LB. STRUNG SNOW PEAS and $1/4$ CUP SLICED GREEN ONIONS in boiling water until bright green. Rinse under cold water to set color and stop cooking. Set aside.

♣Toast 2 TBS. SESAME SEEDS in a skillet until golden. Toss 2 teasp. of the seeds with the snow peas.

♣Add $1/4$ CUP OIL to remaining sesame seeds and sauté until fragrant with
2 CLOVES MINCED GARLIC
3 TBS. LEMON JUICE
$1^1/2$ TBS. TAMARI
$1^1/2$ TBS. BROWN RICE VINEGAR
1 TB. FRESH MINCED GINGER

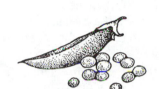

♣Add and toss to coat
3 CUPS COOKED SHREDDED CHICKEN BREAST
1 CUP SLICED CELERY with leaves
$1/3$ CUP FRESH CHOPPED CILANTRO LEAVES
♣Remove from heat and chill. Serve on greens.

Nutritional analysis: per serving; 246 calories; 24gm. protein; 6gm. carbohydrate; 2gm. fiber; 14gm. fat; 59gm. cholesterol; 46mg. calcium; 2mg. iron; 46mg. magnesium; 370mg. potassium; 119mg. sodium; 1mg. zinc.

218 TURKEY ALMOND SALAD

This is a nice "reminder" salad. It gives you the taste of holiday turkey and stuffing without the density.
For 4 salads:

♣Toast in a 350∞ oven
1 TB. CHOPPED SHALLOTS
$1/2$ CUP SLIVERED ALMONDS until golden
$1/2$ CUP SEASONED WHOLE GRAIN BREAD CUBES

♣Mix dressing and chill while you make the salad.
4 teasp. TAMARI
$1/3$ CUP BROWN RICE VINEGAR
$1/3$ CUP LIGHT OIL
1 TB. SOY BACON BITS
$1/2$ teasp. BLACK PEPPER

♣Mix the salad ingredients
2 CUPS COOKED DICED TURKEY
1 CUP CELERY, SLICED

♣Toss with roasted shallots, bread cubes and almonds.

♣Toss everything with the dressing and serve on shredded ROMAINE LETTUCE.

Nutritional analysis: per serving; 377 calories; 26gm. protein; 9gm. carbohydrate; 3gm. fiber; 27gm. fats; 48mg. cholesterol; 84mg. calcium; 3mg. iron; 77mg. magnesium; 526mg. potassium; 178mg. sodium; 2mg. zinc.

219   SPICY CHICKEN SALAD WITH SZECHUAN SAUCE

This is nice as a hot side dish with a puffy soufflé, a mixed vegetable stew or a whole grain casserole.
For 8 small salads:

♣Steam/braise 2 WHOLE CHICKEN BREASTS in a wok or other steamer until firm and white. Skin, bone, shred lengthwise, and put in a mixing bowl.

♣Toss 1 HEAD SHREDDED ROMAINE with 1 LB. MUNG BEAN or SUNFLOWER SPROUTS. Divide between individual salad plates.

♣Slice in thin julienne
1 CARROT
1 CUCUMBER, peeled
4 GREEN ONIONS
♣Mix with chicken shreds and arrange on top of romaine. Top with snipped CILANTRO LEAVES.

♣Mix the dressing in the blender. Pour over salad and serve.
3 TBS. PEANUT BUTTER
1/3 CUP SZECHUAN SAUCE, HOISIN SAUCE, or HOT HICKORY BARBECUE SAUCE
3 TBS. OIL
1 TB. CHILI OIL
1 CUP CHICKEN BROTH

Nutritional analysis: per serving; 221 calories; 22gm. protein; 9gm. carbohydrate; 4gm. fiber; 11gm. fat; 47mg. cholesterol; 52mg. calcium; 2mg. iron; 48mg. magnesium; 527mg. potassium; 139mg. sodium; 1mg. zinc.

220   VERY LOW-FAT CHINESE CHICKEN SALAD

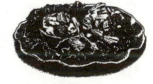

For 6 salads:

♣Simmer 2 WHOLE CHICKEN BREASTS in <u>SEASONED</u> BROTH for 1 hour until tender. Skin, bone and cut into bite size pieces in a large bowl. Pour the following marinade over and chill for 1 hour.

♣Mix the marinade
1 TB. SOY BACON BITS   1/2 teasp. PEPPER
1 TB. SOVEX SMOKED YEAST   1/4 teasp. DRY MUSTARD
2 TBS. BROWN RICE VINEGAR   2 TBS. TAMARI
1 TB. CHIVES   1 teasp. ORANGE ZEST
1/2 CUP OIL

♣Chop 1 BUNCH BROCCOLI in CHINESE RESTAURANT style. (Cut off ends of each stalk to make 5" stems. Slit <u>lengthwise.</u>) Cook in boiling salted water until broccoli turns a bright green.
♣Drain and chill with marinating chicken pieces.

♣Mix the salad
3 CUPS SPINACH or MIXED TART GREENS   2 SLICED SCALLIONS
2 TBS. SLICED DAIKON WHITE RADISH   1/2 CUP DICED CELERY

♣Pile into a big salad bowl. Remove chicken and broccoli from the marinade and pour remaining liquid over the greens. Toss to mix.

♣Arrange broccoli with *stems to the center* in a ring over the top of the greens. Fill the ring with the chicken. Sprinkle HARD BOILED EGG CRUMBLES or CRUNCHY CHINESE NOODLES over top.

Nutritional analysis: per serving; 282 calories; 27gm. protein; 7gm. carbohydrate; 3gm. fiber; 10gm. fats; 63mg. cholesterol; 78mg. calcium; 3mg. iron; 67mg. magnesium; 564mg. potassium; 184mg. sodium; 1mg. zinc.

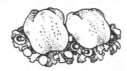

221 OLD FASHIONED SOUTHERN CHICKEN SALAD

I grew up with a version of this salad that was served on hot summer days. The fat and calorie content is much reduced in this recipe.
For 6 salads:

♣Put the stock ingredients into a large pot with water to cover by 2 inches and bring to a boil.
1 SMALL ONION chunked
1 SMALL CARROT, chopped
$1/2$ CUP CELERY LEAVES
$1/4$ CUP PARSLEY LEAVES
1 teasp. SEA SALT
10 WHOLE PEPPERCORNS

♣Add 2 WHOLE CHICKEN BREASTS and simmer for 30 to 45 minutes until tender. Remove skin and bones and cube meat. Put in a large bowl to chill with
2 SLICED HARD COOKED EGGS
$1/2$ CUP CHOPPED SCALLIONS
$1/2$ CUP CHOPPED CELERY
2 TBS. LEMON JUICE.
♣Chill while you make the BOILED DRESSING.

♣Heat 2 teasp. OIL in a saucepan. Add 2 teasp. UNBLEACHED FLOUR and roux until bubbly.
♣Add and cook until aromatic
$1/2$ teasp. ZEST (pg. 643), SPIKE or other seasoning salt
$1/2$ teasp. DRY MUSTARD
$1/4$ teasp. BLACK PEPPER
$1 1/2$ TBS. HONEY
$1/4$ CUP WHITE WINE VINEGAR
2 TBS. SHERRY
2 TBS. WATER

♣Whisk until mixture boils and thickens. Remove from heat. Stir a little dressing into 1 BEATEN EGG to warm it, then pour back into the dressing and whisk smooth. Let cool. Toss with the salad to coat.
♣Serve warm or chilled on torn greens.

Nutritional analysis: per serving; 214 calories; 26gm. protein; 10gm. carbohydrate; 1gm. fiber; 7gm. fats; 164mg. cholesterol; 57mg. calcium; 3mg. iron; 32mg. magnesium; 349mg. potassium; 250mg. sodium; 1mg. zinc.

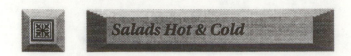

Layered Salads

These salads are some of my favorites and we have them often.
Make them in a large clear straight-sided bowl for the best effect, allowing the multicolored layers to show through.

222   MOTHER'S SUNDAY SALAD

Our big meal of the week was on Sunday after church, and often as not, this salad was part of it.
For 6 to 8 servings:

♣Shred HEAD LETTUCE to completely cover the bottom of the bowl (about $1/2$ head).
♣Cover with $3/4$ CUP CHOPPED CELERY.
♣Cover with 1 CAN SLICED WATER CHESTNUTS.
♣Cover with about 8-OZ. TINY COOKED SHRIMP, **or** $1/2$ CHOPPED RED ONION.
♣Cover with $1/2$ CUP CHOPPED BELL PEPPER.

♣Briefly steam a 10 OZ. BOX of FROZEN GREEN PEAS until color changes. Layer over bell pepper.
♣Sprinkle on 2 teasp. FRUCTOSE.
♣Frost with LIGHT MAYONNAISE to cover.
♣Top with a heavy layer of ROMANO CHEESE.
♣Cover with plastic wrap. Chill 8 to 10 hours.
♣Top with 2 CRUMBLED HARD BOILED EGGS, TOMATO WEDGES, and SNIPPED PARSLEY.

223   SEVEN LAYER TOFU SALAD

For 10 servings:

♣Heat the TOFU MARINADE in a saucepan.

$1/3$ CUP OIL	1 TB. DRY TARRAGON
$2/3$ CUP WHITE WINE VINEGAR	1 TB. SOY BACON BITS
1 teasp. BLACK PEPPER	1 TB. SHERRY

♣Marinate 1 LB. TOFU cut in strips, and $1/2$ CUP RED ONION SLICES for 1 hour. Then sauté right in the marinade until aromatic.

♣Assemble the layers in a 3-qt. clear salad bowl.
♣Cover the bottom with 3 CUPS TORN SPINACH LEAVES.
♣Cover with CHOPPED BUTTER LETTUCE.
♣Cover with 2 CUPS HALVED CHERRY TOMATOES.
♣Cover with 1 CUCUMBER, peeled and sliced in circles.
♣Cover with the TOFU and ONIONS.
♣Cover with 2 CUPS SLICED CARROTS.
♣Cover with $1/2$ CUP SLICED BLACK OLIVES.
♣Top with crunchy CHINESE NOODLES or MOZARRELLA CHEESE CUBES.

Nutritional analysis: per serving; 146 calories; 5gm. protein; 9gm. carbohydrate; 3gm. fiber; 10gm. fats; 0 cholesterol; 93mg. calcium; 4mg. iron; 75mg. magnesium; 413mg. potassium; 84mg. sodium; trace zinc.

224   LAYERED CHICKEN SALAD

For 6 servings:

♣Shake dressing ingredients together in a jar. Let sit to blend while you make the salad.
♣Chill before serving.

1/3 CUP OIL
1/4 CUP TARRAGON VINEGAR
PINCHES of SESAME SALT, BLACK PEPPER and NUTMEG

1/2 teasp. GROUND CUMIN
1 teasp. CHILI POWDER

♣Shave 1/2 HEAD ICEBERG LETTUCE and cover bottom of a large clear salad bowl.
♣Cover with 1 SMALL BUNCH OF SPINACH washed and torn.
♣Cover with 2 LARGE TOMATOES, chopped.
♣Cover with 1 1/2 CUPS DICED COOKED CHICKEN or TURKEY.
♣Cover with 1/2 CUP GRATED CHEDDAR or SWISS CHEESE.
♣Cover with 1/3 CUP FRESH CHOPPED PARSLEY.
♣Cover with 1/2 cup STEAMED GREEN PEAS.
♣Cover with 3 GREEN ONIONS, chopped.
♣Top with 1/3 CUP TOASTED CHOPPED PECANS. Pour dressing over.

Nutritional analysis: per serving; 277 calories; 15gm. protein; 8gm. carbohydrate; 3gm. fiber; 21gm. fats; 36mg. cholesterol; 116mg. calcium; 2mg. iron; 49mg. magnesium; 443mg. potassium; 112mg. sodium; 1mg. zinc.

Hot Salads

These salads use vegetables and other ingredients that impart more intense flavor and texture when served hot. They are good for winter eating, side dishes and brunch/lunches.

225   HOT BAKED POTATO SALAD

For 6 salads:

♣Cube 3 BIG RED POTATOES in bite size pieces. Steam until tender.
♣Hard boil 4 EGGS. Peel under cool running water.
♣Stir-fry in 2 TBS. OIL til aromatic

1 ONION chopped
1/4 CUP SOY BACON BITS
1 teasp. SESAME SALT
1/2 teasp. PEPPER

♣Add to a mixing bowl
1/2 CUP CUBED MILD CHEDDAR
1/2 CUP LIGHT MAYO
2 teasp. SWEET HOT MUSTARD
1/4 teasp. NUTMEG

♣Remove from heat and set aside.
♣Combine everything together and serve right away.

Nutritional analysis: per serving; 285 calories; 10gm. protein; 26gm. carbo.; 3gm. fiber; 11gm. fats; 156mg. cholesterol; 116mg. calcium; 3mg. iron; 47mg. magnesium; 537mg. potassium; 278mg. sodium; 1mg. zinc.

226   HOT BROCCOLI SALAD

For 8 servings:

♣Trim and stem TWO BUNCHES of FRESH BROCCOLI. Chop in florets. Steam 5 minutes until tender.

♣Whisk together

2 TBS. LEMON JUICE

1/2 teasp. DRY MUSTARD

2 TBS.OLIVE OIL

♣Toss with broccoli to coat.

3/4 teasp. SEA SALT

1/4 teasp. PEPPER

4 DASHES HOT SAUCE

♣Skillet roast 1/4 CUP PINE NUTS or SLIVERED ALMONDS until brown. Remove from pan and mix with broccoli. Heat 2 TBS. LIGHT OIL in the skillet and sauté 1/2 SMALL RED ONION in until very brown.

♣Toss with broccoli and serve.

Nutritional analysis: per serving; 154 calories; 7gm. protein; 10gm. cxarbohydrate; 5 gm. fiber; 12gm. fats; 0 cholesterol; 78mg. calcium; 2mg. iron; 61mg. magnesium; 562mg. potassium; 230mg. sodium; 1mg. zinc.

227   HOT DEVILED EGG SALAD

For 6 salads:

♣Sauté 1/2 CUP SLICED RED ONION in 2 TBS. BUTTER until translucent.

♣Add and sauté briefly, tossing to coat about 5 minutes

8-OZ. MUSHROOMS sliced

1 LARGE STALK BROCCOLI, chopped

2 RED POTATOES sliced thin

1/2 teasp. DILL WEED

1/2 teasp. SEA SALT

1/2 teasp. PEPPER

♣Mix in a bowl

2 CHOPPED HARD BOILED EGGS

1/2 CUP SWEET RELISH

11/2 CUPS GRATED CHEESE

1 teasp. DRY MUSTARD

♣Assemble the salad. Spread half of the vegetable mix in a buttered casserole. Top with half of the egg mix. Repeat, and pour the **YOGURT & WHITE WINE DRESSING** on top.

♣Mix to blend

1/4 CUP PLAIN LOW FAT YOGURT

2 TBS. WHITE WINE

2 TBS. WATER

1/4 CUP LIGHT MAYONNAISE

♣Dust top with PAPRIKA. Cover and heat through for 30 minutes. Serve warm on a bed of greens.

Nutritional analysis: per serving; 295 calories; 11gm. protein; 27gm. carbos.; 3gm. fiber; 12gm. fats; 101mg. cholesterol; 194mg. calcium; 2mg. iron; 41mg. magnesium; 616mg. potassium; 361mg. sodium; 1mg. zinc.

228   MUSHROOM MELT WITH HERBS

For 4 servings:

♣Sauté quickly in 1 TB. BUTTER and 1 TB. OIL until tender

1 CLOVE MINCED GARLIC	1/2 teasp. DRY OREGANO
1/2 CUP SLICED ONION	1/2 teasp. THYME
1 1/2 CUPS MUSHROOMS, sliced	1 1/2 teasp. ROSEMARY

♣Add 1/4 CUP WHITE WINE and stir in. Remove from heat, and cover mushrooms with GRATED MOZ-ZARELLA. Cover pan and let melt slightly. Serve on individual salad plates on a bed of torn spicy greens.

❋

229   SPINACH SALAD WITH HOT "BACON" DRESSING

A salad bar favorite without the meat or saturated fat.
For 4 servings

♣Wash, drain, dry, and tear 1 BUNCH SPINACH LEAVES. Set aside.

♣Dry roast 3 TBS. SOY BACON BITS in a skillet until fragrant.

♣Add and sauté briefly to blend the dressing

4 TBS. OIL	1/2 teasp. HONEY
4 TBS. RED WINE VINEGAR	1 teasp. SESAME SALT
2 TBS. LEMON JUICE	1/2 teasp. BLACK PEPPER

♣Pour over spinach and toss to coat.

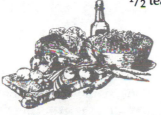

Whole Meal Salads

These salads give you lots of nutrition packed into one bowl. They are perfect for meals-in-a-hurry and outdoor eating. (Why does food seem to taste better outside?) So get a big bowl and a fork, pour on a little dressing, prop your feet up, and enjoy a delicious sunset, or a midday break with a salad.

230   TURKEY COBB SALAD

For 4 meal size salads:

♣Mix all together

1/3 CUP TOASTED ALMONDS or CRISP CHINESE NOODLES
1/2 LB. COOKED TURKEY in matchstick slices

1 HEAD SHREDDED ROMAINE	2 HARD BOILED EGGS, sliced
1 CUP WATERCRESS or SUNFLOWER SPROUTS	1 AVOCADO sliced
4-OZ. GRATED LOW-FAT CHEDDAR CHEESE	LARGE TOMATOES, chopped

♣Top with the following **CREAMY MUSTARD DRESSING:**

❋

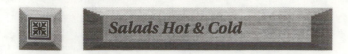

CREAMY MUSTARD DRESSING

For 1 cup:

♣Whisk together

2 TBS. DIJON MUSTARD

$^1/_4$ CUP WHITE WINE

$^1/_2$ CUP OIL

$^1/_4$ CUP PLAIN LOW-FAT YOGURT

$^1/_2$ teasp. BLACK PEPPER

$^1/_4$ teasp. DRY ROSEMARY

♣Spoon over salad. Sprinkle with toasted sourdough croutons.

�֎

231   THE SUPER BOWL

For 6 servings:

♣Rub a large salad bowl with the cut side of a garlic clove. Chop and add to the bowl

1 CUP SPINACH LEAVES, washed, drained and dried

1 CUP CELERY with leaves

1 SMALL HEAD OF BUTTER LETTUCE

1 SMALL HEAD OF ICEBERG LETTUCE

1 CUCUMBER, peeled

1 SMALL HEAD CAULIFLOWER in FLOWERETTES

2 CUPS MIXED SPROUTS

3 RED RADISHES

$^1/_4$ CUP FRESH PARSLEY LEAVES

4 LARGE TOMATOES

1 BELL PEPPER IN RINGS

2 SHREDDED CARROTS

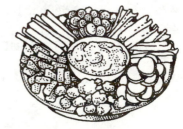

♣Toss and mix all. Top with toasted croutons, sunflower seeds or sliced almonds.

♣Pour over the following **NATURAL FRENCH DRESSING.**

Nutritional analysis: per serving; 58 calories; 3gm. protein; 12gm. carbohydrate; 5gm. fiber; trace fats; 9% calories from fats; 58mg. calcium; 2mg. iron; 37mg. magnesium; 615mg. potassium; 62mg. sodium; trace zinc.

✖

NATURAL TOMATO FRENCH DRESSING

For 2 cups:

♣Mix and shake in a covered jar

1 CUP TOMATO JUICE

$^1/_2$ CUP WHITE WINE VINEGAR

$^1/_3$ CUP SALAD OIL

2 TBS. MINCED GREEN ONION

2 TBS. HONEY

1 CHOPPED HARD BOILED EGG

1 teasp. SESAME SALT

$^1/_2$ teasp. PEPPER

Options to add:

1 teasp. MIXED SALAD HERBS

Nutritional analysis: per serving; 97 calories; trace protein; 7gm. carbohydrate; trace fiber; 8gm. fats; 0 cholesterol; 7mg. calcium; trace iron; 5mg. magnesium; 92mg. potassium; 91mg. sodium; trace zinc.

232   GARDEN HARVEST WITH SHARP VINAIGRETTE

For 6 salads:

♣Mix the vinaigrette, and let chill to blend while you make the salad.
1/2 CUP LIGHT OIL
1/4 CUP TARRAGON VINEGAR
1/4 teasp. HOT PEPPER SAUCE
2 MINCED SHALLOTS
2 TBS. DIJON MUSTARD
1/2 teasp. SESAME SALT
1/4 teasp. PEPPER

♣Make the salad. For half the salad, choose from a mix of the following greens, or whatever is available in your garden at the moment.
ROMAINE
BUTTER LETTUCE
ARUGULA or RADICCHIO
ICEBERG LETTUCE
RED LEAF LETTUCE
GREEN LEAF LETTUCE

♣For the other half of the salad, choose from the following
AVOCADO SLICES
WATER PACKED SLICED ARTICHOKE HEARTS
SLICED GREEN ONIONS
SLICED ROMA or CHERRY TOMATOES
SLICED PEELED CUCUMBER
SLICED DAIKON RADISH
SLICED BUTTON MUSHROOMS

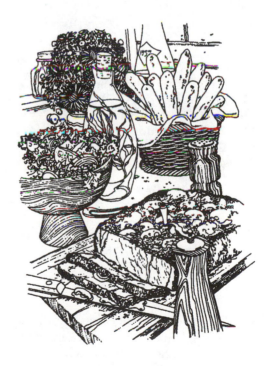

♣For the toppings, choose from the following:
GRATED LOW-FAT CHEESE
SOY BACON BITS
SNAPPED FRESH PEA PODS
SUNFLOWER or ALFALFA SPROUTS
TOASTED SUNFLOWER SEEDS
TOASTED PINE NUTS
TOASTED WALNUT PIECES
♣Pour dressing over. Toss and enjoy.

Nutritional analysis: per serving; 269 calories;
6gm. protein; 13gm. carbohydrate; 8gm. fiber;
23gm. fats; o cholesterol; 63mg. calcium; 3mg. iron;
83mg. magnesium; 610mg. potassium; 145mg. sodium;
1mg. zinc.

233 MIXED MATCHSTICK SALAD

For 8 salads:
♣Cover big dinner-size plates with BOSTON OR BIBB LETTUCE LEAVES.

♣Cut into matchstick julienne pieces and arrange on lettuce
2 LARGE CARROTS
2 PEELED CUCUMBERS   1 SMALL PEELED JICAMA
2 STALKS CELERY   1 LARGE GREEN BELL PEPPER

♣Mix the dressing and pour over
1/2 CUP PLAIN YOGURT   2 TBS. CHOPPED GREEN OLIVES
1/2 CUP LIGHT MAYONNAISE   1 TBS. SNIPPED CHIVES
1/4 CUP SWEET PICKLE RELISH   4 TBS. LEMON JUICE
1/4 CUP SNIPPED PARSLEY   1 teasp. SESAME SALT
2 TBS. DIJON MUSTARD   1/2 teasp. PEPPER
1/2 teasp. DRY TARRAGON
♣Top salad with HARD BOILED EGG SLICES or LOW-FAT FARMER CHEESE CHUNKS.

�֍

234 CRUNCHY COLESLAW WITH HOMEMADE MAYONNAISE

For 6 large servings:

♣Core and shred 1 HEAD GREEN CABBAGE in a food processor
Put in a large salad bowl and add
1 LARGE RED BELL PEPPER, sliced   1 teasp. DILL WEED
2 STALKS CELERY, sliced   4 TBS. WHITE WINE VINEGAR
4 CARROTS shredded   2 TBS. LEMON JUICE
1/2 CUP TOASTED WALNUTS   1 TBS. FRUCTOSE
1/2 CUP RAISINS

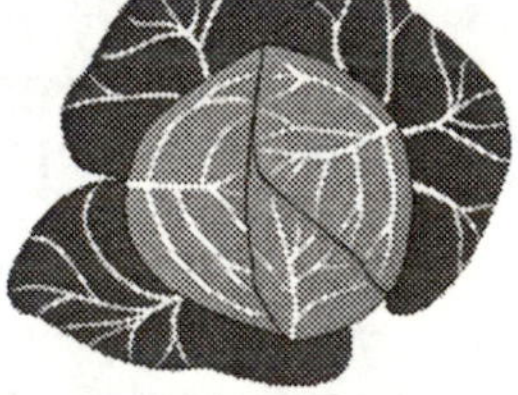

♣Mix and toss gently to coat. Cover and chill while you make the mayonnaise.

♣Enough for 2 cups: Blend in the blender
2 TBS. WHITE WINE VINEGAR   1/4 teasp. SEA SALT
2 TBS. LEMON JUICE   1/2 teasp. DRY MUSTARD
1 EGG   Optional - 1 SLICED AVOCADO

♣With the blender still going, pour 1 1/4 CUPS OIL in a slow steady stream through the hole in the blender cap, until mayonnaise thickens and turns creamy. There is definitely a taste difference from store-bought mayonnaise when you have the time to make it.
♣Add 1/2 CUP to COLE SLAW and toss to coat.

Nutritional analysis: per serving; 253 calories; 4gm. protein; 25gm. carbohydrate; 5gm. fiber; 17gm. fats; 8mg. cholesterol; 74mg. calcium; 1mg. iron; 41mg. magnesium; 575mg. potassium; 69mg. sodium; trace zinc.

✖

Fancy Company Salads

These salads have gourmet flair, are all lightly vegetarian, but pleasing to lots of different tastes.

235   CHICKEN SALAD IN A SOURDOUGH BOAT

This is an excellent choice for your contribution to a pot luck dinner or shower party.
Enough for 6 to 8 full salads, or 12 appetizer salads:

♣Serve this stunner in a ROUND WHOLE WHEAT SOUR DOUGH BREAD SHELL. Slice off the top, scoop out the middle, leaving about 1/2" crust on bottom and sides. (Cube the middle for croutons and save.) Put on a baking pan and toast to crisp in a 325° oven, about 10 minutes.
♣Remove and fill with the chicken salad.

♣Mix together
3 CUPS BITE-SIZE BONED, SKINNED, COOKED CHICKEN BREAST
1 CAN DRAINED, SLICED WATER CHESTNUTS
2 teasp. MINCED FRESH CILANTRO
2 teasp. MINCED FRESH GINGER
2 teasp. CURRY POWDER
3 TBS. MIRIN or SAKE
1 CUP LOW-FAT PLAIN YOGURT
1/2 CUP CHOPPED GREEN ONIONS
SALT and PEPPER to taste
♣Cover and chill for 6 to 8 hours.

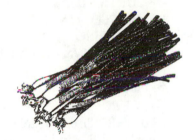

♣String and stem 1/2 LB. EDIBLE PEA PODS. Blanch in rapidly boiling water until bright green, about 2 minutes. Drain, and rinse with cold water to set color. Arrange peas in bread shell.
♣Pile salad on top. Garnish with cilantro leaves.

236   DOUBLE PEA & ALMOND SALAD

Enough for 4 small salads:

♣Blanch in rapidly boiling water until color turns bright green, 1 1/2 CUPS FROZEN PEAS and 1 1/2 CUPS STEMMED and STRUNG FRESH PEA PODS. Rinse in cold water and set aside.

♣Make the dressing
2 TBS. CHOPPED PARSLEY   1 teasp. LEMON JUICE
2 TBS. LIGHT MAYONNAISE   1/2 teasp. SESAME SALT
4 TBS. PLAIN YOGURT   1/2 teasp. BLACK PEPPER
2 TBS. FRESH SNIPPED CHIVES
♣Toss peas with dressing. Top with TOASTED SLIVERED ALMONDS and heap onto a bed of greens.

Nutritional analysis: per serving; 175 calories; 8gm. protein; 18gm. carbohydrate; 7gm. fiber; 5gm. fats; 4mg. cholesterol; 101mg. calcium; 3mg. iron; 60mg. magnesium; 394mg. potassium; 100mg. sodium; 1mg. zinc.

237   WATER CHESTNUTS & MUSHROOMS WITH CHINESE SAUCE

For 4 salads:

♣Mix the marinade
2 TBS. OIL
2 TBS. LEMON JUICE
1 teasp. HONEY
1 teasp. SHERRY or MIRIN
1/2 teasp. GRATED GINGER
1/2 teasp. SESAME SALT

♣Pour over
 2 CUPS FRESH MUSHROOMS, sliced
 1 CAN WATER CHESTNUTS, sliced
♣Toss and chill to blend flavors.

♣Make the **CHINESE SAUCE.** This sauce is good cold or hot - cold on salads, hot on steamed veggies.

♣Cook in the top of a double boiler over hot water until just thickened, about 10 minutes
3 EGGS
2 TBS. UNBLEACHED FLOUR
1/3 CUP HONEY
1 CHOPPED SHALLOT
1/3 CUP LEMON JUICE
1/3 CUP BROWN RICE VINEGAR

♣Remove from heat. Stir in
1 1/2 CUPS PLAIN LOW-FAT YOGURT
1 TB. SHERRY or MIRIN
♣Return to fire and heat just barely through, stirring until smooth. Chill in the fridge.
♣Drain excess marinade from mushrooms and mound on SUNFLOWER SPROUTS or CHOPPED FRESH SPINACH.
♣Spoon dollops of Chinese Sauce on top.

238   LIGHT CAESAR SALAD

For 6 individual salads:

♣Make the CROUTONS. Brush 3 SLICES of WHOLE GRAIN BREAD with OLIVE OIL. Cut in cubes and sauté in a skillet for 5 to 8 minutes until golden. Set aside.

♣Rinse, dry, and tear 1 HEAD ROMAINE LETTUCE. Leave loosely wrapped in paper towels.

♣Mix the dressing *in the salad serving bowl.*
6 TBS. OLIVE OIL
2 TBS. CHOPPED GREEN ONION
1 TB. DIJON MUSTARD
1 teasp. WHITE WORCESTERSHIRE SAUCE

1 EGG
4 TBS. LEMON JUICE
4 TBS. GRATED PARMESAN

♣Mix until frothy. Add romaine leaves and toss just to coat.
♣Sprinkle on croutons and toss. Grind on 1 teasp. COARSE BLACK PEPPER.
♣Top with a HANDFUL of ALFALFA or SUNFLOWER SPROUTS.

Everything You Ever Wanted In A Salad Dressing

These are some of the best and brightest when you want a change of pace.

ORIENTAL ORANGE

This one is a good choice for rice salads, as a marinade for chicken or barbecued prawns, or as a sauce for stir-fries.
For 1$^1/_2$ cups: Serve hot or cold.

♣Sauté in a small pan until aromatic
1 teasp. FRESH GRATED GINGER
2 TBS. OIL
$^1/_4$ teasp. LEMON/GARLIC SEASONING
1 teasp. FRUCTOSE

♣Add and let bubble until blended
4 TBS. TAMARI
4 TBS. LEMON JUICE
2 TBS. MIRIN OR SHERRY
$^3/_4$ CUP ORANGE JUICE
$^1/_3$ CUP OIL

Nutritional analysis: per serving; 170 calories; trace protein; 4gm. carbohydrate; trace fiber; 13gm. fats; o cholesterol; 5mg. calcium; trace iron; 7mg. magnesium; 66mg. potassium; 120mg. sodium; trace zinc.

BEST ITALIAN

For 1$^1/_2$ cups:
♣Blend in the blender
$^1/_2$ CUP OLIVE OIL
$^1/_2$ CUP LIGHT SALAD OIL
2 TBS. PARMESAN
$^1/_2$ teasp. SESAME SALT
1$^1/_2$ teasp. DRY MUSTARD
2 TBS. FRESH CHOPPED BASIL, or 1$^1/_2$ teasp. DRY

1$^1/_2$ teasp. DRY OREGANO
2 teasp. HONEY
$^1/_4$ teasp. PAPRIKA
$^1/_3$ CUP RED WINE VINEGAR
2 TBS. LEMON JUICE

Nutritional analysis: per serving; 287 calories; 1gm. protein; 3gm. carbohydrate; trace fiber; 30gm. fats; 1mg. cholesterol; 37mg. calcium; trace iron; 5mg. magnesium; 44mg. potassium; 100mg. sodium; trace zinc.

OIL FREE BLEU CHEESE DRESSING

For 3 cups:

♣Blend in the blender until smooth
$^1/_4$ teasp. LEMON GARLIC SEASONING
$^1/_4$ CUP WHITE WINE
1 CUP PLAIN YOGURT
$^1/_2$ CUP LIGHT MAYONNAISE

$^1/_4$ CUP SOUR CREAM
$^1/_2$ teasp. PEPPER
$^1/_2$ teasp. SESAME SALT

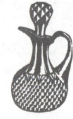
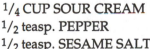
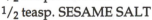

♣Remove to a bowl and add 6-OZ. CRUMBLED BLEU CHEESE.
♣Chill to blend flavors.

SWEET & SOUR FRENCH

For 1½ cups:

♣Blend in the blender until smooth

¾ CUP OIL

¼ CUP WHITE WINE VINEGAR

¼ CUP SHERRY

2 TBS. FRUCTOSE

½ teasp. CELERY SEED ground

½ teasp. PAPRIKA

½ teasp. DRY MUSTARD

1 teasp. DRY BASIL

1 teasp. ONION POWDER

1 teasp. GRATED LEMON ZEST

1 tsp. LEMON/GARLIC SEASONING

Nutritional analysis: per serving; 281 calories; trace protein; 7gm. carbohydrate; trace fiber; 27gm. fats; 0 cholesterol; 13mg. calcium; trace iron; 5mg. magnesium; 46mg. potassium; 66mg. sodium; trace zinc.

CALIFORNIA GUACAMOLE DRESSING

For 1½ cups:

♣Blend in the blender until smooth

1 SLICED AVOCADO

½ SLICED RED ONION

JUICE of ½ LEMON

¼ CUP LIGHT SALSA

3 TBS. OIL

2 TBS. CIDER VINEGAR

½ teasp. LEMON PEPPER

♣Pour into a bowl and chop in ONE TOMATO.

ELLIOT'S THOUSAND ISLAND

This is my husband's favorite.
For 1½ cups:

♣Mix in a bowl until smooth

1 CUP LIGHT MAYONNAISE

2 TBS. CIDER VINEGAR

¼ CUP KETCHUP

1 teasp. FRUCTOSE

½ teasp. SESAME SALT

¼ teasp. PEPPER

¼ teasp. DRY MUSTARD

2 TBS. SWEET PICKLE RELISH

RASPBERRY VINAIGRETTE

For 1½ cups:

♣Whisk in a bowl to blend

5 TBS. RASPBERRY VINEGAR

½ CUP SALAD OIL

2 TBS. MINCED TOASTED SHALLOTS

1 teasp. DIJON MUSTARD

1 teasp. HONEY

¼ teasp. BLACK PEPPER

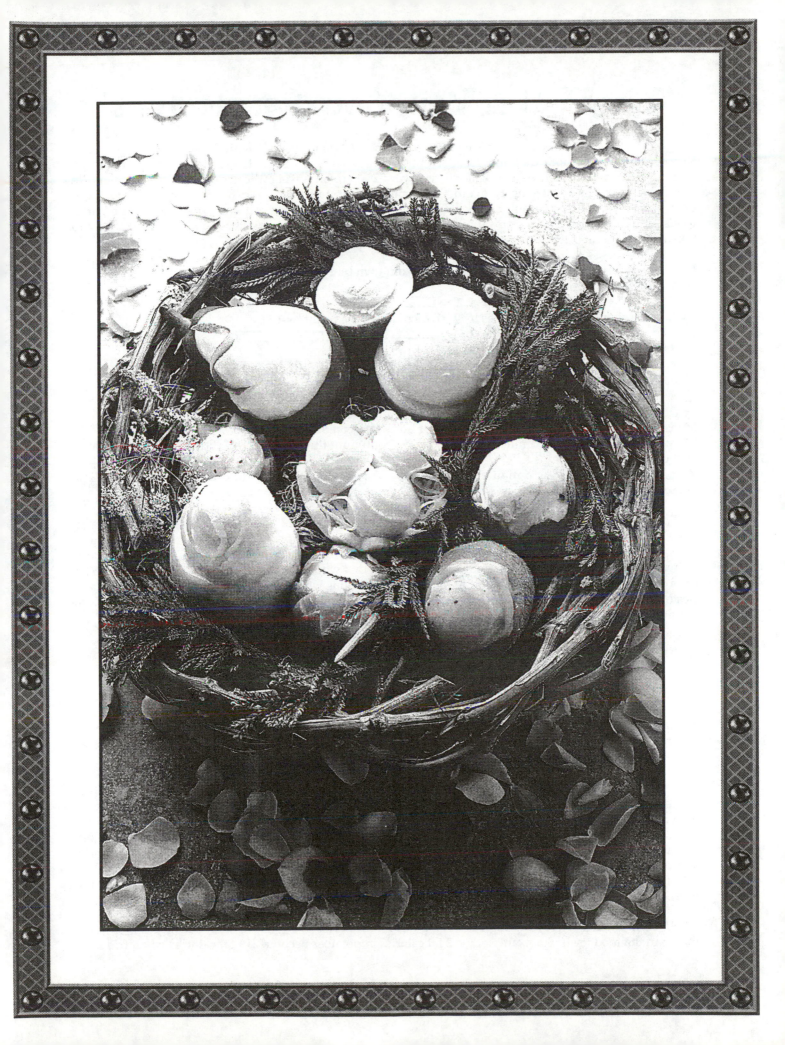

Low-Fat & Very Low-Fat Recipes

The recipes in this chapter can help *de-fat* your life style with flavor.
Keeping fats low in both diet and bloodstream is a necessity for health, longevity and weight control. Most of us know this, since most Americans (over 52%) are on a weight loss or health-related diet. We are already consciously trying to avoid fats, especially saturated fats, and "empty calorie" foods. Yet, even when we think we aren't eating much fat, it is hidden in processed and commercially prepared foods, in hydrogenated oils, tropical oils, or cottenseed oil. Fat in these foods is so high that it is easy to take in as many fat calories as a stick of butter a day!

Here is a quick formula chart for determining your own body fat percentage:
1. Divide your weight by 2.2.

$$\underline{\hspace{3cm}} \div 2.2 = \boxed{\hspace{4cm}}$$

2. Multiply your height in inches by 2.54, then divide the result by 100.

$$\underline{\hspace{2cm}} \times 2.54 = \underline{\hspace{2cm}} \div 100 = \boxed{\hspace{4cm}}$$

3. Multiply the result of step two by itself.

$$\underline{\hspace{2cm}} \times \underline{\hspace{2cm}} = \boxed{\hspace{4cm}}$$

4. Divide the result of step one by the result of step three.

$$\underline{\hspace{2cm}} \div \underline{\hspace{2cm}} = \boxed{\hspace{4cm}}$$

Measure your results against the standards of body fat percentage for adults:
<u>Men</u>: **essential fat,** 5%; optimum health, 10 to 25%; optimum fitness, 12 to 18%; athlete, 5 to 13%; obese, 25% or more.
<u>Women</u>: **essential** fat, 8%; optimum health, 18 to 30%; optimum fitness, 16 to 25%; athlete, 12 to 22%; obese, 30% or more.

For a **low-fat** to **very low-fat** diet, fat calories should be 16 to 23% of total calorie intake. Sex, age, bone structure, activity level, metabolic rate, and general health all play a part in determining optimum daily fat calories, but based on an average of 2000 total calories a day, a low-fat diet would mean about 44 grams of fat, or 396 fat calories a day. A <u>very</u> low fat diet would mean about 32 grams of fat, or 286 fat calories a day. It should be noted that many weight-conscious women do not even come near 2000 calories of food per day; people 45 years or older should consciously undereat from the diet of their youth to maintain the best health.

In this book, low-fat recipes contain less than 9 grams of fat per serving; very low-fat recipes contain less than 5 grams per serving.

Fats are not all bad. Unsaturated, naturally occurring fats, such as those in whole grains, fresh vegetables, seafoods, beans, seeds, and low-fat dairy products, are our greatest source of energy and fuel. They play an integral role in the production of prostaglandins, hormones that regulate body functions at the molecular level. "Good" fats assist the body in utilizing B vitamins, help transport the fat soluble A, D, E, and K vitamins, elevate calcium levels in the blood, and activate necessary bile flow.

Too much saturated fat, in the form of fried and fast foods, pasteurized dairy products, and refined, processed foods, is at the heart of many health problems. Reducing this kind of dietary fat is a good way to avoid and correct bad health conditions. The biggest saturated fat-calorie culprits, butter, certain oils, margarine, cream, mayonnaise, sausage, gravy, and prepared sandwich meats, are more than 90% fat. Cream cheese, red meats, and salad dressings are more than 80% fat. Hard cheeses, nuts, half and half, and potato chips are more than 70% fat. Ice cream, eggs, cream soups, and sweet pastries are more than 60% fat. Pies, doughnuts, french fries, cakes, and corn chips are more than 50% fat. Cookies, whole milk, most crackers and snack foods are more than 40% fat.

All **fried foods are very high in fat.** Frying raises fat calories in <u>any</u> food, often over 100% <u>more</u> than the fat in the food itself. For example, the 2 fat calories in potatoes become **219 fat calories when fried.**

This LOW FAT chapter is dedicated to "light hearted" cooking. It is large and comprehensive so that you can satisfy many favorite food areas with low-fat combinations. The emphasis is on low-fat recipes where it is easy to get a lot of fat quickly, such as:
🍃APPETIZERS 🍃SOUTH-OF-THE-BORDER SNACKS 🍃SANDWICHES 🍃BAKED GOODIES 🍃COOKING IN CLAY 🍃PASTAS 🍃PIZZAS 🍃QUICHES 🍃SAUCES & DRESSINGS 🍃TREATS and DESSERTS 🍃

☛ Four motivating reasons to lower the fat in your diet:

#1) Dietary fat becomes body fat. Saturated food fat is most common cause of excess body fat than sugary carbohydrates or even vegetable oils. Overweight is **_not_** a result of total calorie intake. Fatter people actually tend to eat **fewer** calories. But it takes more energy to convert carbohydrates to body fat than to convert dietary fat to body fat. Fatty foods actually **_do_** go straight from your mouth to your thighs. They are also more likely to be stored there. Carbohydrate calories are hardly ever stored as fat.

#2) Fat consumption is linked to cancer. Ovarian, breast, cervical, and colon cancer are especially linked to a high-fat diet.

#3) Saturated fat increases blood cholesterol levels. Body cholesterol itself is not a fat, even though it is found in combination with fatty acids. Dietary cholesterol is found only in animal foods, including dairy products. Plant foods, except for tropical oils, do not contain dietary cholesterol. Saturated fat has the strongest influence on blood cholesterol because it affects liver function. The liver is less able to remove it normally from the bloodstream, and thus allows it to accumulate on the artery walls.

#4) Toxins accumulate in body fat. Pollution studies recently done at UCLA indicate that environmental poisons and toxins accumulate in the fatty tissues. Food animals were found to be "bio-concentraters" of pollutants, where pesticides, sprays and toxins build up over a lifetime. Vegetables and plant foods may contain these chemical toxins, but the levels are low compared to those in animals. The human body stores toxins in fatty tissue. Reducing dietary fat, and the resultant shedding of excess pounds also gets rid of many accumulated chemical poisons.

Techniques to lower the fat and lighten up your favorite dishes:

1) Instead of pan frying, braise food in water or stock, then deglaze the pan with wine or water to retain the flavorful bits for a sauce. Steam or sauté in a little oil, broth, white wine or sauce. Steam or blanch vegetables to crunchy tenderness. Roast or poach poultry, fish and seafood in broth, wine, or an herb sauce. Oven fry small pieces of food like meatballs, by rolling them in a healthy coating and arranging on a baking sheet with enough space between to let moisture evaporate quickly. Brown well in a 400° to 500° oven.

2) Instead of deep fat frying, broil one to two minutes in the oven to sear in juices, then bake for a nice crispy crust.

3) Instead of milk, use a yogurt, white wine and water mix, to give a delicious gourmet flavor without the fat calories or dairy sensitivity.

4) Instead of full fat cheeses, use farmer or feta cheese, skim, low-fat and no-fat cheese, or soy cheese.

5) Instead of sour cream, cream cheese or ricotta, use yogurt cheese, kefir cheese, low-fat cottage cheese, or soy cheese, cream cheese style.

6) Instead of butter and rich sauces, season with herbs and spices.

7) Instead of ice cream or sherbet with 8 to 10% milkfat, use plain or frozen yogurt.

8) Instead of greasing baking pans, use a Lecithin no-stick spray, such as PAM.

9) Fill in with water instead of fat. Fat makes sauces and dressings taste smooth and elegant, but you can easily replace some or all of it with slightly thickened water and eliminate the fat calories.

☛*Note: The fat grams listed in the **Nutritional Analyses** for this chapter include saturated fats, mono-unsaturated fats, and poly-unsaturated fats.*

Low-Fat Dips, Snacks & Appetizers

239 GARDEN SHRIMP DIP

For 2¹/₂ cups:

♣Combine in a bowl

³/₄ CUP PLAIN LOW FAT YOGURT

³/₄ CUP LIGHT MAYONNAISE

2 TBS. CHOPPED CHIVES

6 to 7-OZ. COOKED SHRIMP PIECES

¹/₄ CUP CHOPPED BELL PEPPER

¹/₄ CUP CHOPPED CUCUMBER

♣Chill to blend flavors.

♣This is especially good on hard-toasted rye cocktail rounds.

Nutritional analysis: per serving on 2 rye rounds; 87 calories;; 3gm. protein; 4gm. carbohydrate; trace fiber; 2gm. fats; 19mg. cholesterol; 9% fats; 83mg. sodium.

240 LOW-FAT CLAM DIP

A perennial favorite. This is also good with cooked crab pieces, or 1 TB. soy bacon bits and parmesan.
For approx. 1¹/₂ cups:

♣Mix and mash together

ONE 7-OZ. CAN MINCED CLAMS. Drain and save clam juice.

ONE 8-OZ. CARTON KEFIR CHEESE, or 8 OZ. YOGURT CHEESE, or SOY CREAM CHEESE

2 TBS. LEMON JUICE

1 teasp. WORCESTERSHIRE SAUCE

¹/₄ teasp. SESAME SALT

¹/₄ teasp. BLACK PEPPER

2 TBS. FRESH CHOPPED PARSLEY

♣Add enough reserved clam liquid for good dip consistency.

♣Chill to blend flavors and serve with crisp PITA or BAGEL CHIPS.

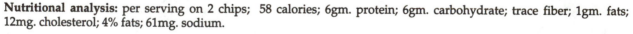

Nutritional analysis: per serving on 2 chips; 58 calories; 6gm. protein; 6gm. carbohydrate; trace fiber; 1gm. fats; 12mg. cholesterol; 4% fats; 61mg. sodium.

241 MEDITERRANEAN SPINACH DIP FOR CRUDITÉS

For 1¹/₃ cups:

♣Blender blend until fine chopped

1 BUNCH FRESH SPINACH, washed, chopped

1 CUP PLAIN LOW-FAT YOGURT

1 GREEN ONION, chopped

¹/₂ teasp. DILL WEED

Nutritional analysis: per serving of 4 tablespoons; 31 calories; 3gm. protein; 4gm. carbohydrate; 1gm. fiber; trace fats; 3% fats; 49mg. sodium.

242   HOT SALMON SPREAD

For twelve 2-oz. servings: Preheat oven to 400°.

♣Blender blend all ingredients
8-OZ. LOW-FAT NEUFCHATEL, YOGURT CHEESE or SOY CREAM CHEESE
2 TBS. FRESH CHOPPED PARSLEY
2 CHOPPED GREEN ONIONS with tops
DASHES of WORCESTERSHIRE and HOT PEPPER SAUCE
ONE 7-OZ. CAN or 7-OZ. FRESH BONELESS SALMON
1/2 CUP SLICED MUSHROOMS
♣Spray a small oven-safe mold with lecithin spray. Line with waxed paper and spray the paper.
♣Pack in the paté and bake til puffy and brown. Serve with toasted rye rounds or raw vegetables.

Nutritional analysis: per serving of 2 rye rounds; 58 calories; 5gm. protein; 6gm. carbohydrate; trace fiber; 1gm. fats; 10mg. cholesterol; 4% fats; 86mg. sodium.

243   LOW-FAT HOT TUNA PATÉ

For 1¹/₄ cups:

♣Mix in a bowl, and spoon into lecithin-sprayed ramekins

1 CAN WATER-PACKED TUNA, drained   1 teasp LEMON JUICE
1 TB. DIJON MUSTARD   1/4 teasp. PEPPER
1 TB. CAPERS or SWEET RELISH drained 1 TB. MINCED PARSLEY
♣Heat at 325° for 40 minutes until brown on top.
♣Spread on crackers or toasted rye rounds.

Nutritional analysis: per serving of 2 rye rounds; 74 calories; 9gm. protein; 7gm. carbohydrate; 1gm. fiber; 1gm. fats; 4% fats; 236mg. sodium.

244   EGGPLANT DELIGHT

The lowly eggplant is finally coming into its own as a great flavor base and for its nutritious composition.
Enough for 6 to 8 people:

♣Peel and slice 1 LARGE EGGPLANT. Sprinkle with salt and let drain in a colander to remove bitterness and excess water, about 45 minutes.
♣Sauté eggplant in 1/4 CUP OLIVE OIL and 1/4 CUP ONION BROTH in a skillet until golden.
♣Drain eggplant on paper towels.
♣Mix in 2 CUPS PLAIN YOGURT, YOGURT CHEESE, or SOY CREAM CHEESE
1/2 CUP CHOPPED FRESH TOMATOES
1 teasp. CHOPPED DRY MINT
1/2 CUP CHOPPED FRESH PARSLEY
1/2 teasp. PEPPER
♣Cover and chill to blend flavors.

245   SMOKY EGG DIP
An oldy but goody.
Makes about 1¹/₃ cups:

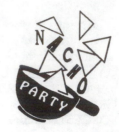

♣Mix and mash with a fork to good dip consistency.
2 HARD BOILED EGGS
1 CUP LOW-FAT COTTAGE CHEESE
2 TBS. SWEET RELISH
¹/₂ teasp. DIJON MUSTARD
¹/₄ teasp. NATURAL LIQUID SMOKE

Nutritional analysis: per serving; 60 calories; 7gm. protein; 3gm. carbohydrate; trace fiber; 2gm. fats; 72mg. cholesterol; 9% fats; 215mg. sodium.

246   TWO VERY GOOD TOFU DIPS

Each recipemakes about 1¹/₂ cups:

1
♣Mix and mash together
2 CUBES TOFU
¹/₃ CUP PLAIN LOW-FAT YOGURT
2 teasp. MUSTARD
¹/₃ CUP SWEET PICKLE RELISH
¹/₂ teasp. SESAME SALT
¹/₄ CUP CHOPPED TOMATO
¹/₄ CUP CHOPPED CELERY
2 TBS. CHOPPED CHIVES
1 HARD BOILED EGG, mashed

2
♣Mix and mash together
2 CUBES TOFU
¹/₄ CUP PLAIN LOW-FAT YOGURT
1 teasp. TAMARI
¹/₃ CUP CHOPPED CELERY
¹/₂ teasp. HERB or VEGETABLE SALT
2 CHOPPED GREEN ONIONS
¹/₄ CUP TOASTED SUN SEEDS

Representative nutritional analysis: per serving; 54 calories; 4gm. protein; 5gm. carbohydrate; trace fiber; 2gm. fats; 9% fats; 27mg. cholesterol; 151mg. sodium.

247   GREAT 28 DIP & SPREAD
Great 28 Mix has been used regularly since the days of the Rainbow Kitchen for every imaginable kind of dipper. We still sample with it for Country Store customers to taste new crackers or chips. They usually want to buy the dip along with the snack!
or about 1 cup:

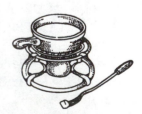

Mix 1 to 2 teasp. **GREAT 28 MIX**   (page 645) with your favorite dip or spread base
CUBES OF TOFU **or**
CARTON KEFIR CHEESE (my favorite) **or**
DY CREAM CHEESE **or**
CUP OF LOW-FAT YOGURT or YOGURT CHEESE
•Add 1 TB. LIGHT MAYONNAISE for extra richness if desired.

248 FRESH STRAWBERRIES & FIGS APPETIZER

A lovely, refreshing <u>no-fat</u> opener to a romantic dinner for two.
For 2 people:

♣Toss together gently

1 PINT HALVED FRESH STRAWBERRIES
2 TBS. SHREDDED FRESH BASIL LEAVES

3 QUARTERED FRESH FIGS
2 teasp. BALSAMIC VINEGAR

♣Serve on small hors d'oeuvres plates with a decorative toothpick.

Nutritional analysis: per serving; 45 calories; 1gm. protein; 11gm. carbohydrate; 3gm. fiber; 0 fats; 0 cholesterol; 0% calories from fat; 2mg. sodium.

249 LOW-FAT SAVORY POPCORN TREATS

Popcorn is a healthy, nutritious snack. Make 4-qts. popcorn in an air popper for the lowest fat results. Use only a small amount of oil for pan popping.
For 8 cups: Preheat oven to 350°.

♣Mix ¼ CUP GRATED PARMESAN CHEESE, or SOY PARMESAN
1 TB. CHICKEN or VEGETABLE BOUILLON GRANULES
1 teasp. LEMON/GARLIC or HERB SEASONING SALT
1 EGG WHITE, whipped to soft peaks with a pinch of CREAM OF TARTER

♣Quickly toss egg white with popcorn so it doesn't deflate and pour into baking pans. Bake until crisp and dry, about 10 to 15 minutes, stirring often.

Nutritional analysis: per serving; 45 calories; 3gm. protein; 6gm. carbohydrate; 1gm. fiber; 1gm. fats; 1mg. cholesterol; 3.5% fats; 143mg. sodium.

250 BAKED SWEET POTATO CHIPS

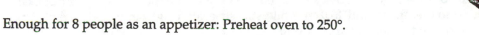

Enough for 8 people as an appetizer: Preheat oven to 250°.

♣Slice 4 LARGE PEELED SWEET POTATOES or YAMS <u>very</u> thin. Rinse in cold water. Drain and dry on paper towels. Put in a large bowl and toss with
½ teasp. SEA SALT
½ teasp. WHITE PEPPER
1 teasp. FRUCTOSE or 2 teasp. DATE SUGAR (Opt.)
3 TBS. OIL

♣Layer in a large <u>oven-proof</u> skillet. Mound slightly in center. Pour in any liquid from the mixing bowl.
♣Cover with foil. Bake for 1 hour until tender.
♣Serve right from the skillet, topped with thin strips of FRESH LEMON PEEL and MINT SPRIGS.

Nutritional analysis: per serving; 123 calories; 2gm. protein; 21gm. carbohydrate; 2gm. fiber; 3gm. fats; 0 cholesterol; 13% fats; 53mg. sodium.

251   LOW-FAT STUFFED MUSHROOMS

For 6 servings:

♣Brush and stem 1/2 LB. LARGE STUFFING MUSHROOMS. Chop stems and sauté them briefly in 1 TB. BUTTER with 2 TBS. SOY BACON BITS until aromatic.
♣Remove from heat and add
1 EGG
1/2 teasp. CELERY SALT
1 TB. WHITE WINE
1/2 teasp. CARRAWAY SEED
2 teasp. *DRIED MINCED* ONION
1/2 CUP BREAD CRUMBS
♣Let mixture sit for a few minutes to absorb flavors. Fill caps. Drizzle with a little melted butter or oil if desired, and bake in a shallow dish at 350° for 15 minutes until brown on top.

252   DILL FINGER CREPES WITH SPICY SHRIMP FILLING
These are unusual, but delicious appetizers, with very low-fat calories.
For 8 crepe appetizers:

♣Make the crepes. Mix and let stand 20 minutes
1/2 CUP UNBLEACHED or WHOLE WHEAT PASTRY FLOUR
2 EGG WHITES, beaten until foamy
1/2 CUP PLAIN SPARKLING MINERAL WATER
2 TBS. MINCED CHIVES
2 teasp. DILL WEED
1/4 teasp. BLACK PEPPER

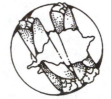

♣Heat a griddle or teflon skillet to *moderately hot*. When a drop of water on the skillet sizzles, ladle on a small amount of batter. Spread to make a thin crepe about 2 or 3" across. Cook until holes appear in the batter. Turn immediately and cook until golden. Stack between pieces of wax paper until all are done, and fill when cool. (These can be made ahead and frozen while still separated by the waxed paper. Wrap tightly, and thaw while still wrapped so they won't dry out.)

♣Make the filling.
♣Sauté 1/2 LB. TINY SHRIMP in a little oil until just pink.
♣Add 2 TBS. white wine and toss for 1 minute until shrimp is coated. Remove with a slotted spoon.
♣Add 1 TB. OIL to the pan, and sauté the following until aromatic and moisture is almost evaporated
1 teasp. WHITE WORCESTERSHIRE SAUCE
1 teasp. DIJON MUSTARD
PINCHES of GINGER POWDER, TARRAGON, CHILI POWDER and BLACK PEPPER
2 MINCED MUSHROOMS
♣Mix shrimp with mushroom sauce for filling.
♣Divide between the 8 small crepes. Roll crepes. Put seam side down in a shallow baking dish and heat in a 350° oven until browned. Top each with snips of parsley leaves and a shake of sea salt.

Nutritional analysis: per serving; 82 calories; 8gm. protein; 6gm. carbohydrate; 1gm. fiber; 2gm. fats; 44mg. cholesterol; 9% fats; 71mg. sodium.

253 DEVILED CLAM TOASTS

For 8 appetizer toasts: Preheat oven to 400°.

♣Quarter 2 PIECES of WHOLE GRAIN BREAD. Toast squares on a baking sheet in the oven.
♣Sauté 1 CLOVE MINCED GARLIC in 2 TBS. OIL until aromatic
♣Add 1 TB. WHOLE WHEAT FLOUR and roux for a minute until frothy.
♣Add

1 CAN MINCED CLAMS and JUICE
1/2 CUP SEASONED BREAD CRUMBS
2 teasp. WORCESTERSHIRE SAUCE
1 TB. CHOPPED PARSLEY
1 teasp. DIJON MUSTARD
1/2 teasp. LEMON PEPPER

♣Stir and let bubble briefly, then pile on toast squares and bake until hot and bubbly. Sprinkle with pinches of parmesan if desired.

Nutritional analysis: per serving; 81 calories; 5gm. protein; 9gm. carbohydrates; 1gm. fiber; 2.5gm. fats; 9mg. cholesterol; 11% fats; 141mg. sodium.

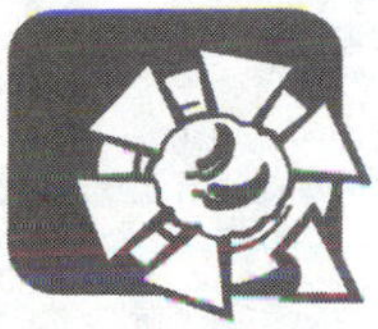

Low Fat South-Of-The-Border Snacks

Just about everybody likes spicy Mexican snacks, but they often have a justified reputation for being high in saturated fat and hard on digestion. The unusual versions here don't have either of those problems. You can enjoy this healthy Mexican food guilt free.

Tortillas have an undeserved reputation in our society as junk food. Like popcorn, they are made of corn, a nutritious whole grain. **LIME TORTILLAS** are even better. Here is the authentic restaurant recipe from the bar at the Red Onion in Puerta Vallarta, Mex. Use them with the following salsa or in any of the healthy Mexican food snacks in this chapter.

For 2-qts. of tortilla chips:

♣Dip 12 CORN TORTILLAS in water and let drain. Season with SEA SALT and SQUEEZED LIME JUICE. Stack and cut in 8 wedges. Arrange in a single layer on 3 baking sheets.
♣Bake at 500° for 4 minutes. Turn with tongs and bake until brown and crispy, for 2 to 3 minutes.

254 CHERRY TOMATO SALSA FOR TORTILLA CHIPS

For about 2 cups:

♣Pulse-chop all ingredients coarsely in the blender so there are still recognizeable chunks.

2 PINTS CHERRY TOMATOES
1 CHOPPED SHALLOT
1 CHOPPED GREEN ONION
2 SERRANO CHILIES seeded, and minced
2 TBS. FRESH MINCED CILANTRO
1 TB. TARRAGON VINEGAR
2 teasp. LIME JUICE
1/2 teasp. SEA SALT

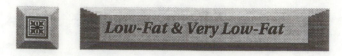

255   LOW FAT HOT TACOS

For 6 tacos:
♣Toast taco shells in the oven until crisp.

♣Mix 1 CUBE TOFU with 2 to 3 TBS. NATURE BURGER, TOFU BURGER, or FALAFEL MIX. Sauté in 1 TB. OIL in a skillet until brown and crumbly. Spoon about 1 TB. in each taco shell.

♣Mix in a bowl
2 TBS. CHOPPED BLACK OLIVES   1 TOMATO, chopped
4 TBS. GRATED LOW-FAT CHEDDAR or JACK   1/2 RED ONION, chopped
♣Divide filling between tacos. Broil briefly to melt cheese, and top with some SHAVED LETTUCE or AL-FALFA SPROUTS, and a drizzle of SALSA.

256   BOCADILLOS CON QUESO

These were the first "nachos" we ever served regularly in the Rainbow Kitchen. We made them fresh in the morning, and heated a few at a time to serve with or before an order. They were very popular.
For about 24 nachos:

♣Cut 3 LARGE FRESH FLOUR TORTILLAS in 8 wedges each. Put on a baking sheet and drizzle a little OLIVE OIL over each wedge. Toast in the oven until light gold and crisp.
♣Cut 4-OZ. LOW-FAT JALAPEÑO JACK CHEESE or SOY JALAPEÑO JACK into thin slices, and then into wedges the same size as the tortilla wedges. Top each wedge with a cheese wedge.
♣Mix in a bowl
1 TOMATO peeled and chopped, 6 to 8 BLACK OLIVES, sliced, and 2 to 3 MINCED SCALLIONS.
♣Sprinkle a little over each tortilla wedge. Bake at 375° about 8 minutes til cheese bubbles. Put on a serving plate and top each with a small dollop of PLAIN YOGURT mixed with a little SALSA, or a little drizzle of salsa by itself.

Nutritional analysis: per wedge serving; 59 calories; 3gm. protein; 9gm. carbohydrate; 1gm. fiber; 1.5gm. fats; 3mg. cholesterol; 24% calories from fats; 42mg. sodium.

*Speaking of salsas, the best ones for you and your stomach are usually the ones you make yourself.
I make this one up in a jar just like salad dressing and then use it as needed.
It is good, can be as mild or hot as you like, and keeps a long time.*

HOMEMADE SALSA FRESCA

This salsa is also good over a Guacomole salad on shaved lettuce.
For about 2 cups:

♣Combine all ingredients in a bowl. Let stand for 30 minutes to let flavors blend.
1 CHUNKED PEELED TOMATO
1/2 CUP MIXED CHOPPED GREEN and RED ONIONS
4 HOT CHILIS, roasted, peeled and chopped, or ONE 4-OZ. CAN GREEN CHILIS, chopped and drained
1/2 teasp. GARLIC/LEMON SEASONING

257　SOFT SEAFOOD TACOS WITH CITRUS SALSA

For 6 people; 2 tacos each:

♣Sauté 1 CLOVE MINCED GARLIC and 1 CHOPPED RED ONION in 2 TBS. OLIVE OIL until brown.
♣Add 1 LARGE CHOPPED TOMATO and 1 LB. COOKED CHOPPED SEAFOOD, such as SALAD SHRIMP, SCALLOPS or CRAB MEAT and sauté for 8 to 10 minutes until aromatic.
♣While taco filling is cooking, wrap 12 CORN TORTILLAS in foil and warm in a 350° oven for 10 minutes. Remove, and while still warm, spoon in some seafood filling. Top with CITRUS SALSA:

♣Mix together in a bowl
1/2 CUP CHOPPED CUCUMBER	1 teasp. GRATED LIME ZEST
1 FRESH JALAPEÑO CHILI seeded, minced	3 TBS. LIME JUICE
1 CUP CANNED CRUSHED PINEAPPLE	2 TBS. MINCED FRESH CILANTRO

♣Season with SALT AND PEPPER to taste.

258　BABY SHRIMP TOSTADAS

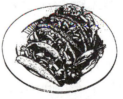

For 24 tostada chip rounds:

♣Bring 4 cups water to a boil. Add 1 teasp. VEGETABLE SALT and 1 TB. CIDER VINEGAR.
♣Boil 24 MEDIUM SHRIMP just until pink, about 1 minute. Drain.
♣Mix and mash in a bowl
1/2 SMALL RIPE AVOCADO	1 TB. CHOPPED RED ONION
3 TBS. LIGHT MAYONNAISE or KEFIR CHEESE	2 TBS. LEMON JUICE
1 GREEN JALAPEÑO CHILI, chopped	1 TB. FRESH CHOPPED CILANTRO
1 teasp. LEMON/GARLIC SEASONING	

♣Divide between 24 Tostada chip rounds Top each with a shrimp. Broil 1 minute. Serve hot.

259　TOSTADA FIESTA

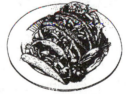

For 4 regular size corn tortillas:

♣Toast tortillas on a baking sheet until crisp.
♣Top with a mixture of
1 CUP REFRIED BEANS (instant mix is fine)	4 TBS. SALSA
1 SMALL RED ONION, sliced	3 TBS. SLICED BLACK OLIVES
1 CHOPPED TOMATO	PINCHES CHILI POWDER

♣Add 4 TBS. GRATED JACK CHEESE or SOY JACK CHEESE, or JALAPEÑO JACK CHEESE.
♣Toast to melt cheese and heat beans. Top with SHAVED LETTUCE and/or ALFALFA SPROUTS.

Nutritional analysis: per serving; 143 calories; 7gm. protein; 23gm. carbohydrate; 8gm. fiber; 3gm. fats; 4mg. cholesterol; 13% fats; 313mg. sodium.

Low Fat Sandwiches

Sandwiches can be satisfying and healthy, like salads in whole grain bread. It's a shame that they have a reputation as junk food. There is a complete chapter on these convenient, all-in-one meals; here are three light sandwiches that fit into a low-fat diet.

260   PIZZA POUCHES

For 4 sandwich pouches:

♣Mix the filling in a bowl and sauté briefly in 1 TB. OLIVE OIL in a small skillet to release flavors:
¹/₂ CUP COOKED FALAFELS crumbled **or** TOFU BURGER **or** GRAIN BURGER, crumbled
¹/₄ CUP CHOPPED ZUCCHINI or MUSHROOMS

2 TBS. CHOPPED RED ONION	2 TBS. CHOPPED BLACK OLIVES
1 CHOPPED TOMATO	2 TBS. CHOPPED GREEN PEPPER

♣Fill split pita bread pockets, or pile onto half a chapati and fold over. Top each sandwich with 1 TB. PIZZA or TOMATO SAUCE and 1 TB. GRATED LOW-FAT CHEESE. Toast to melt cheese in a 350° oven.
♣Remove and top with MIXED SPROUTS if desired.

Nutritional analysis: per serving; 175 calories; 6gm. protein; 25gm. carbohydrate; 3gm. fiber; 6gm. fats; 4mg. cholesterol; 26% fats; 81mg. sodium.

261   FRUIT 'N' FIBER TORTILLA SANDWICHES

For 2 sandwiches: Preheat a heavy skillet or griddle.

♣Soften two whole wheat flour tortillas on the skillet or griddle. Top each with a SLICE of LOW-FAT MOZZARELLA or FARMER CHEESE. Spread cheese with 1 teasp. JAM or FRUIT BUTTER, and top with 1 MORE SLICE of CHEESE. Fold up bottom, fold in sides, and roll snugly to secure top flap. Arrange seam side down, and grill over medium heat til tortillas are brown and cheese melts - 4 minutes per side.

262   ROLLED SHRIMP SANDWICHES

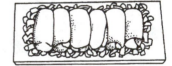

For 8 rolls: 2 per person

♣Cook ¹/₂ CUP BROWN RICE in 1¹/₄ CUP WATER, covered, for 20 minutes. Uncover, fluff, and cool.
♣Make the vinegar shrimp filling. Mix together and add to the rice
3-OZ. TINY COOKED SHRIMP

2 TBS. CAPERS or SWEET RELISH, drained	1 teasp. FRUCTOSE or 2 teasp. HONEY
2 TBS. BROWN RICE VINEGAR	2 teasp. GRATED LEMON ZEST

♣Dip 8 LARGE ROMAINE LETTUCE LEAVES in boiling water until limp, then immediately into ice water until cold. Lay on paper towels to dry. Divide filling between leaves. Fold sides over, and roll from stem end, tucking in edges as you go to make a packet. Chill before serving.

Nutritional analysis: per serving; 132 calories; 7gm. protein; 24gm. carbohydrate; 1gm. fiber; 1gm. fats; 41mg. cholesterol; 8% fats; 106mg. sodium.

Low Fat Breads & Baked Goodies

Breads and pastries are an area where many people find it difficult to lower fats. Favorite foods often fall into this category. However, by making a few changes in the way you bake, fats can indeed be kept low, and you won't be deprived of the good familiar tastes.

Make sure you are using only whole grain flours when you bake. It makes a big difference not only in matabolic activity and body assimilation, but in higher nutrition and fiber.

A mixture of whole grain flours is a better choice for lightness and complex flavor than whole wheat flour alone. See page 647 for a reliable flour blend that may be used for any of the breads and muffins in this book, or as inspiration to blend your own baking mix. Also see the SPECIAL INGREDIENTS SECTION for descriptions and properties of whole grains and flours.

263   VERY LIGHT POPOVERS

These are wonderful little "carriers" for almost anything. Eat them plain with a little kefir cheese, or use as the base for miniature low-fat pot pies, or just fill with some steamed veggies and dress with a low-fat sauce. The fat content is much less than a pie or other pastry crust.
For 6 popovers: Preheat oven to 425°.

♣Preheat popover pan, or individual small pyrex custard cups that can take and hold high heat. Leave in the oven until just before use.

♣Blend in the blender to the consistency of cream
1 CUP UNBLEACHED FLOUR
PINCH SEA SALT
3 EGGS
1/2 CUP PLAIN YOGURT
1/2 CUP WATER
♣Fill **hot** popover cups <u>half full</u>. Bake 2 minutes. Reduce heat to 325° and bake 15 to 20 minutes more until golden and fully puffed.

Nutritional analysis: per serving;109 calories; 7gm. protein; 13gm. carbohydrate; 1gm. fiber; 3gm. fats; 108mg. cholesterol; 13% fats; 38mg. sodium.

264   NO-FAT MUFFINS

For 12 muffins: Preheat oven to 400°.

♣Mix together
1 1/2 CUPS WHOLE WHEAT FLOUR
1 CUP OAT BRAN
2 TBS. WHEAT GERM
2 1/2 teasp. BAKING POWDER
1/4 teasp. SEA SALT

♣Add to dry mix just to moisten
2 EGG WHITES beaten to foamy
2 TBS. HONEY
1 1/2 CUPS APPLE JUICE
1/4 teasp. CINNAMON

♣Line a 12 cup muffin tin with cupcake papers. Fill 2/3 full and bake 30 minutes until a toothpick poked into the center comes out clean. Remove and cool.

265   DONA'S LOW FAT CORN BREAD

Dona has been with our company for many years. At one point she owned a restaurant of her own and she has contributed several recipes from that time. She is now a full time nutritional consultant. Occasionally, when we have a "pot luck" party, Dona brings this corn bread, right in the skillet! Delicious.
For 12 pieces: Preheat oven to 425°. Preheat pan or iron skillet while you mix ingredients.

♣Mix in the blender
2 EGGS
$1/4$ CUP OIL
$3/4$ CUP PLAIN LOW FAT YOGURT
$3/4$ CUP WATER
2 TBS. FRUCTOSE or HONEY

♣Combine just to moisten with
1 CUP UNBLEACHED FLOUR
2 TBS. WHEAT GERM
$1 1/2$ CUPS YELLOW CORNMEAL
4 teasp. BAKING POWDER
$1/2$ teasp. SEA SALT

♣Pour into a lecithin-sprayed 9 x 9" pan or cast iron skillet and bake 15 to 20 minutes until crusty.

266   SOUTHERN CORN & RICE MUFFINS

This is an old oldy, from my Atlanta days. I can hardly read the writing on the card any more. But the muffins were very good, so I was delighted when the nutritional analysis showed that they were also low in fat.
For 12 muffins: Preheat oven to 400°.

♣Mix everything just to moisten. Mixing too much toughens the batter.
1 CUP YELLOW CORNMEAL
1 TB. BAKING POWDER
$3/4$ teasp. SEA SALT
1 CUP COOKED SHORT GRAIN BROWN RICE
2 TBS. MELTED BUTTER

2 TBS. HONEY
1 TB. MAPLE SYRUP or MOLASSES
2 EGGS
$7/8$ CUP LOW-FAT MILK

♣Pour into lecithin-sprayed muffin cups and bake for 20 minutes until a toothpick comes out clean.

Nutritional analysis: per serving; 113 calories; 3gm. protein; 17gm. carbohydrates; 1gm. fiber; 3gm. fats; 41mg. cholesterol; 13% fats; 111mg. sodium.

267   LEMON YOGURT MUFFINS

For 12 muffins: Preheat oven to 375°.

♣Mix together very lightly
5 TBS. HONEY
3 TBS. BUTTER
1 CUP PLAIN LOW-FAT YOGURT
1 EGG
$1/4$ CUP LEMON JUICE

$1/2$ teasp. GRATED LEMON RIND
2 CUPS WHOLE GRAIN FLOUR MIX
$1/2$ CUP CHOPPED PECANS
2 teasp. BAKING SODA
PINCH NUTMEG

♣Fill lecithin-sprayed or paper-lined muffin cups, and bake for 25 minutes until golden and a toothpick inserted in a muffin comes out clean.

Clay Cookery - A New/Old Way to Lower Fat

Cooking in clay pots has been a healthy, nutritious and delicious way to cook poultry, fish and vegetables since early Roman times. Clay cookers are enjoying a renaissance today because of their ability to cook food in its natural juices for maximum flavor, without extra fats or liquids, while preserving vitamins and minerals. Clay pots also impart a wonderful outdoor flavor to foods, and a browning capability like an outside grill.

There are two easy essentials for maximum benefits from these pots. 1)They must be soaked in water for 15 to 20 minutes before adding the food. The clay absorbs the water and the heat from the the oven heats this water first, causing an immediate flush of steam to seal in the natural food flavors. 2)They must also begin baking in a cold oven, because they are unfired, and thus vulnerable to sudden temperature changes. But these are small differences, and the nutritional cooking, low-fat benefits are worth it. If you are on a healing diet, clay cooking could be a delicious answer. The following recipes represent a small sampling of the possibilities.

268   OVEN STIR FRY

Clay cooking and poultry seem to be made for each other, blending seasonings harmoniously in the style of almost any cuisine - as in this Chinese chicken blend. Use a 2 to 3-quart cooker.

For 6 servings: Soak bottom and top of clay cooker in water to cover for 15 minutes before use.

♣Soak 8 DRIED BLACK SHIITAKE MUSHROOMS in water til soft; sliver and discard woody stems.

♣Layer in the cooker in order
4-OZ. SLICED BUTTON MUSHROOMS
THE SLIVERED BLACK MUSHROOMS
ONE 8-OZ. CAN SLICED BAMBOO SHOOTS
3 SKINNED, BONED, SLICED CHICKEN BREASTS

♣Combine and pour over chicken
2/3 CUP CHICKEN BROTH
2 TBS. ARROWROOT or KUZU
1/4 CUP SOY SAUCE
1/2 teasp. FRUCTOSE
1/2 teasp. SESAME SALT
1/2 teasp. GROUND GINGER

♣Cover cooker and place in a cold oven. Set oven to 400° and bake, stirring once until chicken is tender, 45 minutes. Pan roast 3/4 CUP CASHEWS in 1 teasp. oil, or oven roast 10 minutes until brown.
♣Stem and string 6 to 8 OZ. FRESH CHINESE PEA PODS. Slice 4 GREEN ONIONS with tops.
♣Lay on top of chicken in the cooker.
♣Turn off oven. Cover cooker and return to the oven for 5 minutes, just to gently steam peas and onions. Remove and sprinkle with cashews.

269   WINE-SCENTED MUSHROOMS

This dish can be elegant as well as healthy when you use a delicate mushroom mix.

For 6 servings: Soak bottom and top of clay cooker in water to cover for 15 minutes before use.

♣Mix together 2 CUPS FRESH WHOLE GRAIN BREAD CRUMBS and 1/2 CUP OLIVE OIL.
♣Slice 1 LB. MIXED MUSHROOMS; choose from OYSTER, CHANTERELLE, BUTTON, PORCINI and SHIITAKE. Place half in the cooker and season with salt and pepper. Top with *half of the crumbs and olive oil mix.* Drizzle with 2 TBS. WHITE WINE. Top with rest of mushrooms, seasonings and 2 MORE TBS. WHITE WINE. Place covered cooker into a cold oven. Set oven to 425° and bake until mushrooms are tender, about 25 minutes.
♣Sprinkle on rest of crumbs, and bake uncovered until browned, about 10 minutes.

270   PERFECT SHRIMP JAMBALAYA

A clay cooker can also be a slow cooker, for easy, authentic one pot meals.
For 8 servings: Soak bottom and top of clay cooker in water to cover for 15 minutes before use.

♣Combine in the cooker

1 CUP RAW BROWN RICE	1/2 teasp. SEA SALT
1 LARGE ONION, fine chopped	1/2 teasp. CHILI POWDER
1 CLOVE GARLIC, minced	1/4 teasp. DRY THYME
1 CUP RAW OYSTERS, chopped	1/4 teasp. NUTMEG
1/4 CUP FRESH PARSLEY, minced	2 PINCHES CAYENNE PEPPER

♣Stir in ONE 16 OZ. CAN PEELED ROMA TOMATOES WITH JUICE, ONE 14-OZ. CAN CHICKEN BROTH, and ONE 8 OZ. CAN TOMATO SAUCE. (Or use equivalent amounts of fresh ingredients.)

♣Top with a BAY LEAF, and place cooker in a cold oven. Set oven to 450∞ and bake, stirring occasionally for 45 minutes, until rice is just tender.

♣Top rice with 1 LB. RAW, PEELED SHRIMP and bake covered until shrimp is firm and pink, about 10 minutes. Serve hot in shallow soup bowls with sourdough bread and vegetable relishes.

Nutritional analysis: per serving; 203 calories; 17gm. protein; 27gm. carbohydrate; 2gm. fiber; 3gm fats; 103mg. cholesterol; 13% fats; 298mg. sodium.

271   AUHENTIC SAFFRON RICE

A traditional Northern Italian dish, done in foolproof style.
For 4 servings: Soak bottom and top of clay cooker in water to cover for 15 minutes before use.

♣Combine in the cooker
1 CUP BROWN RICE or GOURMET GRAIN MIX (page 647)
8 to 10 SHALLOTS, fine chopped
2 CLOVES GARLIC, minced
1/4 teasp. SEA SALT
2 PINCHES WHITE PEPPER
1 PINCH DRIED SAFFRON THREADS
14 OZ. canned or homemade CHICKEN BROTH (Vegetable broth or onion broth may also be used.)
1/4 CUP WHITE WINE or WATER
2 TBS. OLIVE OIL

♣Place covered cooker in a cold oven. Set oven to 425° and bake until rice is tender, 45 to 50 minutes.
♣Sprinkle with PARMESAN or SOY PARMESAN CHEESE, and serve hot.

Nutritional analysis: per serving; 249 calories; 5gm. protein; 43gm. carbohydrate; 2gm. fiber; 5gm. fats; 1mg. cholesterol; 19% calories from fats; 225mg. sodium.

Note: The recipes in this section are just a tiny sample of clay cooking capabilities. You can also bake breads, prepare soups and healthier desserts. We use ours frequently, and recommend it as a good tool for lowering the fat in your cooking.

Low Fat Pasta

Whole grain and vegetable pastas are amazingly low in fat. Many are made only with the grain itself and water. Nutritional analyses of these pastas show minimal fat content, anywhere from trace amounts up to 2 grams per serving for those containing eggs. Ninety-nine percent of the fat in a pasta dish comes from the sauce. This section offers tasty pasta sauces without the high fats. If you like pasta, you can finally lose the guilt. Please review the PERFECT PASTA TIPS on page 225 before you start, so the recipe will be everything you want it to be.

272   PASTA WITH FRESH BASIL & TOMATOES

For 8 servings:

♣ Put 3 QUARTS WATER on to boil with a little salt. When you see a rolling boil, add 2 CUPS DRY WHOLE GRAIN or EGG PASTA SHELLS. Cook 12 to 15 minutes to *al dente*.
♣ Drain and toss with 2 teasp. OLIVE OIL to separate.

♣ While the pasta is cooking, sauté briefly in a skillet in 2 TBS. OIL until fragrant
2 LBS. FRESH ROMA TOMATOES, chopped
1/2 CUP SCALLIONS, chopped
1 1/2 CUPS FRESH BASIL LEAVES, minced
♣ Pour onto pasta. Toss and lift with two forks. Top with GRATED PARMESAN or MOZZARELLA.

Nutritional analysis: per serving; 153 calories; 5gm. protein; 26gm. carbohydrate; 3gm. fiber; 3.5gm. fats; trace cholesterol; 15% fats; 30mg. sodium.

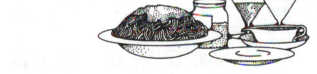

273   PASTA MOLTO VERDE

For 6 servings:

♣ Put 3 QUARTS WATER on to boil with a little salt. When you see a rolling boil, add 8 OZ. DRY SPINACH NOODLES and cook to al dente, about 5 to 7 minutes.
♣ Drain and toss with 2 teasp. OLIVE OIL to separate.

♣ While noodles are cooking, toss in skillet with 2 TBS. OLIVE OIL for two minutes to coat
1 LB. CHOPPED SPINACH, ROMAINE and CHARD LEAVES
1/4 CUP FRESH CHOPPED PARSLEY
1/3 CUP CHOPPED GREEN ONION
♣ Remove from heat and toss with hot pasta.

♣ Mix the sauce. Toss with pasta, and serve hot.
1/2 teasp. GARLIC/LEMON SEASONING   1/4 CUP GRATED PARMESAN
3/4 CUP PLAIN LOW-FAT YOGURT   1/2 teasp. DRY TARRAGON

Nutritional analysis: per serving; 233 calories; 10gm. protein; 34gm. carbohydrate; 5gm. fiber; 6gm. fats; 4mg. cholesterol; 25% fats; 148mg. sodium.

274   HOT PASTA VERDE SALAD

For 4 large salads:

♣Blanch 1 CUP SNOW PEAS, stemmed and strung, 1 CUP FROZEN PEAS, and 1 CUP ASPARAGUS PIECES in boiling water for three minutes until color changes to bright green. Remove with a slotted spoon and keep water boiling.

♣Add 1 CUP DRY SPINACH PASTA SHELLS and cook to *al dente*, about 6 to 7 minutes. Drain pasta.
♣Toss with 2 teasp. OLIVE OIL to separate.

♣Mix with vegetables together in a bowl with **CREAMY HERB DRESSING:**

1/4 CUP LIGHT MAYONNAISE	1/2 teasp. DRY BASIL
1/3 CUP PLAIN LOW-FAT YOGURT	1/2 teasp. DRY TARRAGON
1 TB. CHOPPED CHIVES	

Nutritional analysis: per serving; 261 calories; 8gm. protein; 30gm. carbohydrate; 4gm. fiber; 5gm. fats; 8mg. cholesterol; 20% fats; 81mg. sodium.

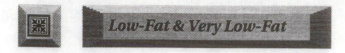

275   LOW-FAT CANNELLONI

Cannelloni is part of an Italian food lover's heaven, but it is traditionally full of fat. This recipe changes that.
For 8 cannelloni rolls, (2 per person): Preheat oven to 450°.

♣Combine in a 9 x 13" pan and bake until onion browns and liquid evaporates, about 15 minutes

1 LARGE ONION, chopped	
1 CLOVE GARLIC, minced	2 TBS. WATER
1 teasp. OLIVE OIL	2 TBS. RED WINE

♣Remove from oven, add 1/4 CUP WATER or WINE and scrape browned bits free. Return to oven and bake for 8 more minutes to intensify flavors.

♣Chunk up 3/4 LB. BONED, SKINNED CHICKEN BREAST, and 3/4 LB. SKINNED TURKEY BREAST FILET and scatter in the pan. Bake for 10 minutes until white in the center. Remove and set aside.

♣Whirl half of the poultry mix, 1/2 CUP PARMESAN and 4-OZ. LOW-FAT RICOTTA in the blender.
♣Scrape into a bowl and repeat. Season with NUTMEG and SALT.
♣Mix in 1 EGG, 2 TB. BREAD CRUMBS, and 2 TBS. RED WINE. Cover and chill.

♣Lay 8 LARGE CHINESE EGG ROLL WRAPPERS flat on a baking sheet, and divide filling among them, placing it along one edge. Roll to enclose filling. Set seam side down. Cover and chill.

Make the two sauces:

♣For the **YOGURT SAUCE,** melt 1 TB. BUTTER and 1 TB. OIL in a saucepan.
♣Add 1 1/2 TBS. WHOLE WHEAT FLOUR and stir until toasted and browning. Remove from heat and mix in 1 CUP PLAIN LOW-FAT YOGURT and 1 CUP CHICKEN or ONION BROTH.
♣Stir to a boil, and cook until sauce is reduced to 1 1/2 cups, about 20 minutes.

♣For the TOMATO SAUCE, lay 2 LBS. HALVED ROMA TOMATOES skin side down on a baking pan.

♣Bake at 450° until juices evaporate, leaving a dark brown residue. Remove and add to the pan, 1 CUP CHICKEN or VEGETABLE BROTH and 1 TB. BALSAMIC VINEGAR. Scrape up browned bits.

♣Whirl in the blender until pureed. Then cook in a small saucepan for 30 minutes to intensify flavors. Stir in 1/2 CUP CHOPPED FRESH BASIL or 2 teasp. DRY.

♣Pour some of each sauce into two 7 x 10" baking pans. Swirl to make a marble effect. Set cannellonis onto the sauce, leaving about 1/2" between. Bake uncovered at 425° until hot, about 10 minutes.

Nutritional analysis: per serving; 266 calories; 28gm. protein; 20gm. carbohydrate; 3gm. fiber; 8gm. fats; 90mg. cholesterol; 27% fats; 204mg. sodium.

❋

The next two sauces are the lowest fat sauces we can find. Both are still delicious. You will never miss the fat.

LOW FAT MARINARA SAUCE FOR PASTA

For 2¹/₂ cups:

♣Sauté 2 CLOVES MINCED GARLIC in 2 TBS. OLIVE OIL or ONION BROTH until aromatic.

♣Add and sauté until color changes and vegetables soften
1 YELLOW ONION, chopped
1 CARROT chopped

1 STALK CELERY, chopped
1 GREEN PEPPER, chopped

♣Stir in and braise until soft
2 CHOPPED TOMATOES
2 TBS. TOMATO PASTE
1 teasp. HONEY

♣Remove from heat and add
1 CUP CHOPPED FRESH CILANTRO
1/4 teasp. CRUSHED FENNEL SEED
1 teasp. DRY BASIL or 1 TB. FRESH

Nutritional analysis: per serving; 43 calories; 1gm. protein; 10gm. carbohydrate; 2gm. fiber; trace fats; 0 cholesterol; 2% fats; 25mg. sodium.

VERY LOW FAT FRESH TOMATO WINE SAUCE

For about 3 cups:

♣Sauté in 2 TBS. OIL or ONION BROTH until vegetables are fragrant, about 7 minutes
1 CLOVE GARLIC, minced
1 SMALL ONION, chopped
3 to 4 LARGE TOMATOES, chopped
1/2 BELL PEPPER chopped, any color

1/2 CARROT, chopped
1/2 teasp. DRY BASIL
1/2 teasp. DRY THYME

♣Add and simmer until stock reduces by about 1/3
1 CUP WHITE WINE
2 CUPS WATER
1/2 teasp. VEGETABLE SEASONING SALT

1 teasp. HONEY
1/4 teasp. BLACK PEPPER

Nutritional analysis: per serving; 43 calories; 1gm. protein; 7gm. carbohydrate; 1gm. fiber; trace fats; 0 cholesterol; 3% fats; 24mg. sodium.

❋

More Light Italian - Pizzas

Contrary to popular opinion, and lots of what passes for Italian food in America, much Italian cooking is light, low fat and easy - leagues apart from the usual idea of greasy, heavy food. On our honeymoon in Italy, both my husband and I fell in love all over again with Italian cooking. And both of us lost weight on the trip.

The pizzas were incredibly light, and we were struck by the differences in Italian pizzas with their thin, yeast-free semolina crusts, <u>lightly</u> strewn with buffalo milk mozzarella and aromatic vegetable soffrito toppings, as opposed to the heavy American use of spiced meats, double cheese, few vegetables, and thick doughy crusts.

The recipes in this section have true light, delicious Italian taste - without the guilt or health problems.

HOW TO MAKE AN INCREDIBLY LIGHT PIZZA

✿**THE CRUST -** This is the real thing - quick and crisp. They don't come any better. The dough can be made ahead, frozen, and thawed to use. But it's so easy, you might as well just do it when you make the pizza. It only takes 5 minutes and you'll have it fresh.

♣Mix together to make a dough;

1 CUP SEMOLINA FLOUR

1/3 CUP HOT WATER

1 TB. OLIVE OIL

1 teasp. BAKING POWDER

1/2 teasp. SEA SALT

♣Knead dough a few turns until elastic. Let it sit, covered in plastic wrap for 15 minutes, (or make it several hours ahead if you like). Roll or pat out into a 7 or 8" circle.

♣**Heat a *cast iron skillet until hot*.** Test a little piece of dough in the skillet when you think it's ready. Bubbles should appear on the underside in *45 seconds*. Lay in a dough circle, and cook on <u>one side only</u> to dark brown, about 3 minutes. Remove from skillet to a plate and strew on 1/3 CUP MOZZARELLA CHUNKS (or any soft low-fat melting cheese that let the flavors of the veggies come through).

✿**THE TOPPING -** Included below are several delicious toppings to try. Each one makes enough for <u>two crusts</u>. Toppings go on *top of the cheese* for intensfied, seasoned vegetable taste.

♣Use about 1/2 cup topping per pizza crust. Drop dollops and spoonfuls all over the pizza. Drizzle with OLIVE OIL and return pizza to the <u>hot</u> iron skillet. <u>Cover</u>, and cook about 2 minutes more until cheese melts and vegetables are hot. Try it - almost fool proof - and low-fat too!

WATCHWORDS FOR WONDERFUL LOW-FAT PIZZAS:

☛Make sure vegetables aren't too wet or too heavy.

☛Be generous with seasonings, light on cheeses.

☛Keep sun-dried tomatoes, semolina flour, water-packed artichokes, and pesto-in-a-tube on hand. Good ingredients are hard to find.

☛Use the freshest low-fat mozzarella cheese and the best olive oil you can find.

✺

276   AUTHENTIC VERDE TOPPING

♣Chop about 1 CUP FRESH WELL-RINSED GREENS FOR EACH PIZZA. Use SPINACH, ROMAINE, CHARD or other tangy greens.

♣Sauté in 2 TBS. OLIVE OIL for 2 minutes until aromatic

DASHES OF HOT SAUCE

2 teasp. PESTO PASTE

1/4 teasp. crushed FENNEL SEED

PINCHES of SEA SALT and PEPPER

♣Add greens to skillet, remove immediately from heat and let them wilt in the seasonings.

✺

277   ZUCCHINI & SUN-DRIED TOMATOES TOPPING

♣Slice 3 SMALL ZUCCHINI in rounds. Sprinkle with salt and let sit for 5 minutes in a colander to release moisture and bitterness. Drain and <u>press out moisture.</u>
♣Slice 4 SUN-DRIED TOMATOES PACKED IN OIL, or sliver 2 FRESH TOMATOES
♣Pour packing oil from the jar in a skillet and sauté the tomatoes with 1 CLOVE MINCED GARLIC and DROPS OF HOT PEPPER SAUCE.
♣Add zucchini and sauté rapidly for 3 minutes. Season and remove from heat. Add 2 TBS. FRESH CHOPPED BASIL, or 2 teasp. DRY BASIL, and 1/4 teasp. GROUND FENNEL SEED. Mixture should be very aromatic.

278   SCALLIONS & BLACK OLIVES SCENTED WITH ROSEMARY

This pizza is wonderful with FETA CHEESE instead of mozzarella. Use about 3 TBS. per pizza.

♣Sauté in 2 TBS. OLIVE OIL for 5 to 10 minutes until fragrant
6 CHOPPED SCALLION WHITES (save chopped green parts for topping)
2 SPRIGS FRESH or 1 teasp. DRY ROSEMARY
1 or 2 BAY LEAVES
2 TBS. HOT WATER
♣Discard bay leaf and rosemary. Sprinkle with PINCHES of BLACK PEPPER, SEA SALT, reserved SCALLION TOPS, and 2 TBS. CHOPPED BLACK OLIVES.

279   ARTICHOKE HEARTS SAUCE

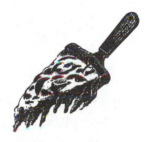

♣Sauté in 2 TBS. OLIVE OIL
1 teasp. GARLIC/LEMON SEASONING
1/4 teasp. DRY THYME
PINCHES of SEA SALT AND PEPPER
ONE 8-OZ. JAR ARTICHOKE HEARTS packed in water, chopped
♣Squeeze on the JUICE FROM HALF A LEMON and 1 TB. WHITE WINE.

Steam for 3 minutes, covered. Remove from heat and top with 1/4 CUP FRESH PARSLEY.

280   PESTO PIZZA

♣Toast 3 TBS. PINE NUTS in the oven until golden.
♣Blend them in the blender with
1 CUP PACKED FRESH BASIL LEAVES (Use only fresh leaves for this)
1/2 CUP GRATED PARMESAN
1/4 CUP OLIVE OIL
PINCHES SESAME SALT, PEPPER, and OREGANO

Representative nutritional analysis: per serving of 224 grams; 92 calories; 5gm. protein; 19gm. carbohydrate; 6gm. fiber; 1gm. fats; 0 cholesterol; 8% fats; 29mg. sodium.

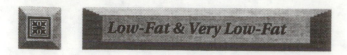

Low Fat Quiches

Most of us love quiches. They are perfect casual company food. But all the cream, butter and eggs weighs you and your circulation down. Traditional quiche recipes make it hard to stay away from fat. This section presents quiches with slightly restructured recipes, for low-fat eating. The good taste remains, the high fats don't.

☞**THE CRUST -** This is the main change. Lots of fat comes from a traditional stand-up-alone quiche crust. The three on this page keep the fat low, and present a whole new platform for quiches.
☞*Note: You can grind up almost any vegetable casserole leftovers in the blender or food processor, re-season, add a little butter or oil, and press the mixture into a quiche pan. Bake at 375° for 10 minutes to set the layer and you have an instant quiche crust.*

281   VEGETABLE QUICHE CRUST

♣Grate all vegetables in a blender, food processor or salad shooter and combine.
2 CUPS DICED ZUCCHINI
1/2 CUP DICED CARROTS
1/2 CUP PEELED DICED PARSNIPS or FRESH DAIKON RADISH
♣Salt the vegetables, and let stand about 5 minutes. Squeeze out excess moisture.
♣Mix vegetables with 2 TBS. OIL and 1/3 CUP WHOLE GRAIN FLOUR MIX. (See page 647.)
♣Press into a lecithin-sprayed quiche pan. Brush with a little more oil, and bake for about 30 minutes at 375°. Cool and fill.

282   MASHED POTATO CRUST

♣Sauté 1/2 CUP CHOPPED ONION in 2 TBS. OIL with PINCHES of SEA SALT and PEPPER.
♣Boil 2 LARGE POTATOES until tender. Mash and mix with onions.
♣Sculpt the mixture into a lecithin-sprayed quiche dish to form a high crust. Brush with a little oil and bake at 375° for about 40 minutes until set and crusty. Remove, cool and fill.

283   WHOLE GRAIN & SEED CRUST

Just plain crackers layed in a single layer on the quiche pan make a lovely crust. Drizzle with oil, or spread with butter if desired, and toast briefly before filling.

♣Mix together
1 CUP WHOLE GRAIN BREAD CRUMBS
1/4 CUP WHOLE WHEAT FLOUR   1/4 CUP MELTED BUTTER
1/2 CUP WHEAT GERM   1/4 teasp. SEA SALT
1/2 CUP SESAME SEEDS   PINCHES of ITALIAN HERBS
♣Press into a lecithin-sprayed quiche pan and bake at 350° for 10 minutes. Cool and fill.

Representative nutritional analysis: per serving; 109 calories; 4gm. protein; 11gm. carbohydrates; 2gm. fiber; 6gm. fats; 7mg. cholesterol; 28% fats; 114mg. sodium.

✦**THE FILLINGS** - The ones given here are different, delicious and unusual. Let the filling *just set*, so it will be very tender when you take it out of the oven. Remember that the interior keeps on cooking even after you remove it from the oven.

283   RUSSIAN SWEET CHEESE FILLING

♣Mix together

16 OZ. LOW-FAT COTTAGE CHEESE

2 EGGS

4 TBS. HONEY

2 TBS. LOW-FAT YOGURT

$^1/_4$ CUP RAISINS

$^1/_3$ CUP CHOPPED WALNUTS

1 teasp. CARDAMOM POWDER

$^1/_4$ teasp. NUTMEG

♣Put in a whole grain crust, or thin unbaked crust. Bake at 375° for 1 to 20 minutes until crust browns.

Nutritional analysis: per serving without the shell; 163 gm.; 137 calories; 10gm. protein; 16gm. carbohydrate; 1gm. fiber; 5gm. fats; 56mg. cholesterol; 22% fats; 248mg. sodium.

284   ORIENTAL VEGETABLE FILLING

♣Soak 4 BLACK SHIITAKE MUSHROOMS until soft. Sliver and discard woody stems

♣Mix in the blender.

3 EGGS

1 CUP LOW-FAT YOGURT

$^1/_2$ CUP COTTAGE CHEESE

$^1/_2$ teasp. SESAME SALT

$^1/_4$ teasp. BLACK PEPPER

4 TBS. WATER

♣Pour into a whole grain crust and add

One handful SUNFLOWER SPROUTS

THE BLACK MUSHROOMS

$^1/_2$ CUP WATER CHESTNUTS, sliced

$^1/_2$ CUP SLICED BOK CHOY

$^1/_2$ teasp. GROUND GINGER

♣Bake at 450° for 10 minutes - then at 350° for 20 minutes, until filling is just firm. Let sit for 5 minutes and serve hot.

Nurtritional analysis; per serving without the shell; 68 calories; 5gm. protein; 7gm. carbohydrate; 1gm. fiber; 2gm. fats; 82mg. cholesterol; 9% fats; 88mg. sodium.

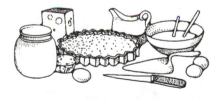

285   FRESH TOMATO BASIL FILLING

Preheat oven to 400°.

♣Sprinkle 2 TBS. SOY BACON BITS onto a whole grain crust.

♣Sauté in 2 TBS. OIL until aromatic

1 RED ONION, chopped

4 TOMATOES, chopped

$^1/_4$ CUP PACKED FRESH CHOPPED BASIL

SEA SALT and PEPPER

♣Spoon into shell. Cover with GRATED LOW-FAT MOZZARELLA CHEESE. Bake for 15 minutes until cheese melts and quiche is fragrant.

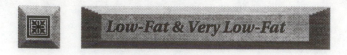

286   PROVENCE FILLING

♣Sprinkle 3 TBS. PARMESAN CHEESE or SOY PARMESAN onto a potato or vegetable crust.

♣Sauté in 2 TBS. OLIVE OIL or ONION BROTH until aromatic
2 CUPS CHOPPED ONION
1 CLOVE MINCED GARLIC
PINCHES SEA SALT and HERBS DE PROVENCE

♣Spread onion mix on quiche shell. Scatter 3 TBS. CHOPPED BLACK OLIVES on top.

♣Mix together and pour over filling
4 EGGS   1 TB. WHOLE WHEAT FLOUR
1/2 CUP LOW-FAT YOGURT   1/4 teasp. DRY MUSTARD
1/2 CUP WHITE WINE

♣Sprinkle with 2 TBS. PARMESAN or SOY PARMESAN. Decorate with TOMATO SLICES on top.

♣Bake at 375° for 40 minutes until *just set*.

Nutritional analysis: per serving; 86 calories; 5gm. protein; 6gm. carbohydrates; 1gm. fiber; 3gm. fats; 108mg. cholesterol; 14% fats; 107mg. sodium.

287   VERY LOW-FAT ITALIAN VEGETABLE FILLING

♣Use a pre-baked potato shell, or no shell. Sprinkle shell or quiche pan with 1 TB. SOY BACON BITS and GARLIC/LEMON SEASONING.

♣Sauté 1 CLOVE GARLIC and 1 CHOPPED ONION in 1 TB. OLIVE OIL until aromatic

♣Add and sauté 2 minutes   ♣Mix and pour over vegetables
1 ZUCCHINI, sliced thin   2 EGGS
1 RED BELL PEPPER, diced   2 TBS. PLAIN LOW-FAT YOGURT
PINCHES OF ITALIAN HERBS and PEPPER   2 TBS. SNIPPED PARSLEY

♣Add onion/zucchini mix to quiche shell or pan.

♣Sprinkle with 2 TBS. GRATED PARMESAN. Bake at 375° until just set, about 30 minutes.

Nutritional analysis: per serving; 40 calories; 3gm. protein; 4gm. carbohydrate; trace fiber; 2gm. fats; 54mg. cholesterol; 16% fats; 31mg. sodium.

288   ENGLISH LEEK AND MUSTARD TART

♣Preheat oven to 375°. Sprinkle a RYE CRISP CRACKER CRUST with LOW-FAT CHEDDAR CHEESE to cover a 9" tart pan.

♣Sauté 1 LB. LEEKS, white parts, sliced in rings in 2 TBS. OIL, or 3 TBS. ONION BROTH until soft.

♣Add 1/2 CUP WHITE WINE, and simmer for 10 minutes.

♣Sprinkle with 1/2 teasp. SESAME SALT and 1/4 teasp. PEPPER.

♣Scrape into quiche shell.

♣Beat the sauce until smooth
1/2 CUP PLAIN YOGURT
1/2 CUP LIGHT CREME FRAICHE
2 1/2 TBS. DIJON MUSTARD
3 OZ. CRUMBLED FETA OR GOAT CHEESE
♣Pour over quiche. Scatter on 2 TBS. CHIVES and 2 TBS. CHEESE CRUMBLES.
♣Bake until top is firm and golden, about 30 minutes. Let sit for 5 minutes and slice.

Nutritional analysis: per serving for the filling; 120 calories; 4gm. protein; 11gm. carbohydrates; 1gm. fiber; 5gm. fats; 23mg. cholesterol; 40% calories from fats; 139mg. sodium.

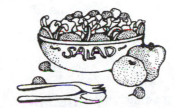

Low-Fat Salad Dressings & Sauces

It's hard to get any other way - the refreshing taste of oil, vinegar and herb dressings, complementing the greens and vegetables of a fresh salad. But the oil amounts in most dressings supply too much fat for a low-fat diet.
A real solution without the loss of taste is to use a <u>lot less</u> oil and more vinegar to escape the fat. You get the same gratifying taste - but in a more delicate way. Or use no oil at all. Instead puree tomato or lemon juice with plain low fat yogurt. Use low-fat yogurt, low fat cheeses and light mayonnaise in place of full fat ingredients. To lower fat in a bottled dressing, mix it with equal parts of plain low-fat yogurt, lemon juice or your favorite vinegar.

VERY LOW FAT DRESSING OR VEGGIE DIP

For about 2 cups:

♣Measure and blend all ingredients in the blender. Whirl until smooth.
1/2 CUP LOW FAT COTTAGE CHEESE
1/2 CUP LOW FAT YOGURT or KEFIR CHEESE
1 teasp. DIJON MUSTARD
2 SCALLIONS, chopped
1 TB. SALAD OIL
1 to 2 teasp. LEMON JUICE
PINCHES of SEA SALT and BLACK PEPPER
DASHES of HOT PEPPER SAUCE

♣**Optional additions:**
1 SMALL TOMATO
1 teasp. DRY BASIL
2 TBS. SWEET PICKLE RELISH

Nutritional analysis: per serving; 72 calories; 5gm. protein; 3gm. carbohydrates; trace fiber; 4gm. fats; 3mg. cholesterol; 18% fats; 206mg. sodium.

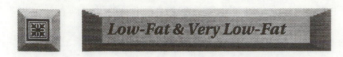

TWO LOW OIL VINAIGRETTE DRESSINGS
You can mix either of these with kefir cheese, soy cream cheese, or yogurt cheese for vegetable or chip dips.
About 3/4 cup each:

VINAIGRETTE #1

♣Mix by hand in a dressing pitcher and serve
2 TBS. LIGHT OIL
2 TBS. BALSAMIC VINEGAR
2 TBS. SPARKLING WATER
2 TBS. LIME JUICE

1 TB. DIJON MUSTARD
2 TBS. MINCED GREEN ONION
1 TB. CHIVES
1/2 teasp. WHITE PEPPER

VINAIGRETTE #2

♣Mix by hand in a dressing pitcher and serve
2/3 CUP WHITE WINE VINEGAR or RASPBERRY VINEGAR
2 to 3 TBS. FRESH CHOPPED HERBS of your choice
3 TBS. OLIVE OIL
1/2 teasp. SEASONING SALT

1/2 teasp. DRY MUSTARD
DASH PAPRIKA

❈

HOT & SOUR SALAD DRESSING

For about 1 1/2 cups:

♣Sauté 3 TBS. SOY BACON BITS in 3 TBS. OIL or until aromatic.
♣Sprinkle on 1 TB. WHOLE WHEAT FLOUR and stir until oil and flour combine and bubble.
♣In a measuring cup, combine 1/3 CUP BROWN RICE VINEGAR and enough water to make 1 cup.
♣Add and stir til dissolved
2 teasp. HONEY
1 teasp. SESAME SALT
1 teasp. DRY MUSTARD
♣Beat 1 EGG in a bowl and gradually add vinegar mix. Pour over mixture in the hot skillet, and cook over low heat, stirring for several minutes until thickened. Pour over salad greens. Toss and serve.

❈

KIWI NO OIL DRESSING
Perfect for greens with feta cheese crumbles and toasted walnuts.
For 1 cup:

♣Blend in the blender
2 KIWIS, peeled
2 TBS. WHITE GRAPE JUICE
SALT and PEPPER to taste

1 teasp. FRUCTOSE
2 teasp. LIME JUICE

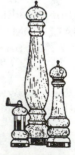

❈

NO OIL SHALLOT DRESSING

For 1 cup:

♣Mix together in a bowl

2/3 CUP WATER

1 teasp. ARROWROOT

1 TB. DIJON MUSTARD

1/4 CUP CHOPPED SHALLOTS

1/4 CUP BALSAMIC VINEGAR

♣Bring to a boil in a saucepan. Simmer until fragrant.

GREEK LEMON DRESSING

For about 1 cup:

♣Blend all ingredients in the blender

1/4 CUP OLIVE OIL

1/2 CUP FRESH LEMON JUICE

2 CLOVES MINCED GARLIC

1 teasp. DIJON MUSTARD

1 teasp. GROUND CORIANDER

1 teasp. SESAME SALT

1 TB. TOASTED SESAME SEEDS

1/2 teasp. CRACKED BLACK PEPPER

Nutritional analysis: per serving; 59 calories; trace protein; 2gm. carbohydrates; trace fiber; 6gm. fats; 0 cholesterol; 28% fats; 130mg. sodium.

YOGURT CHEESE SAUCE & DIP FOR VEGETABLES

Also good choice for baked potatoes, broiled fish, rice crackers, and chips.

For 3 cups, about 8 servings:

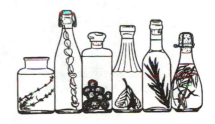

♣Mix all in the blender until green, and chill to intensify flavors

1/2 CUP YOGURT CHEESE (See page 392 for how to make)

2 TBS LOW-FAT MAYONNAISE

1 teasp. LEMON ZEST

1/2 teasp. GARLIC/LEMON SEASONING

2 TBS. CHOPPED FRESH CILANTRO or PARSLEY

Nutritional analysis: per serving; 86 calories; 3gm. protein; 4gm. carbohydrates; trace fiber; 2gm. fats; 7mg. cholesterol; 9% fats; 37mg. sodium.

LOW OIL MUSHROOM SAUCE

For 2 servings:

♣Heat 2 TBS. OLIVE OIL in a skillet with 2 CLOVES MINCED GARLIC. Add 1 LB. SLICED MUSHROOMS. Cook until mushrooms release their liquid, and liquid evaporates.

♣Add and cook til fragrant

1/3 CUP WHITE WINE

1/4 CUP CHOPPED PARSLEY

1/2 teasp. GREAT 28 MIX

1/4 TEASP. BLACK PEPPER

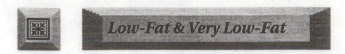

Sweet & Low Desserts and Treats

Desserts can be fudgy, chewy, creamy, crusty, sweet and gooey - and still be low in fat and nutritious.

289   CRUSTY HONEY ALMOND CREAM

For 1 8 x 8" square pan:

♣ Soften 1 TB. UNFLAVORED GELATIN in $1/2$ CUP LOW-FAT MILK, or $1/4$ CUP PLAIN LOW-FAT YOGURT and $1/4$ CUP WATER.

♣ Combine $11/2$ CUPS LOW-FAT MILK, or 1 CUP PLAIN LOW-FAT YOGURT and $1/2$ CUP WATER in the top of a double boiler.

♣ Add
2 EGG YOLKS
PINCH SEA SALT
$1/4$ teasp. VANILLA

♣ Cook custard gently until mixture coats a spoon. Remove from heat and add gelatin mixture. Stir to blend, then chill til custard begins to set.

♣ Whip 2 EGG WHITES to stiff peaks. Add 4 TBS. HONEY and $1/4$ teasp. NATURAL ALMOND EXTRACT. Whip until well blended. Fold into gelatin mixture, and turn into a square pan that has been rinsed in cold water.

♣ Mix and sprinkle over top
$11/2$ CUP TOASTED WHEAT GERM
$1/4$ CUP TOASTED SLICED ALMONDS

♣ Chill until firm, and cut in squares.

Nutritional analysis: per serving; 122 calories; 7gm. protein; 15gm. carbohydrates; 2gm. fiber; 4gm. fats; 37mg. cholesterol; 17% fats; 42mg. sodium.

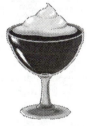

290   INSTANT STRAWBERRY MOUSSE

For 4 people:

♣ Briefly heat $1/2$ CUP PURE MAPLE SYRUP
♣ Blend 2 CUPS FROZEN UNSWEETENED STRAWBERRIES in the blender with half of the syrup.
♣ Add 1 teasp. VANILLA and the rest of syrup and blend until smooth
♣ Beat 2 EGG WHITES in a bowl with a PINCH of CREAM OF TARTER until stiff.
♣ Pour cold strawberry purée over the whites and quickly fold in. Mound into mousse cups and garnish with fresh strawberry halves.

Nutritional analysis: per serving; 135 calories; 2gm. protein; 33gm. carbohydrates; 2gm. fiber; trace fats; 0 cholesterol; 1% fats; 33mg. sodium.

291   LIGHT ORANGE SOUFFLÉ

For 6 servings: Preheat oven to 375°.

♣Make the soufflé in the top of a double boiler over hot water. Blend until thick and creamy
4 EGG YOLKS
1/2 CUP FRUCTOSE

♣Stir in
1/4 CUP UNBLEACHED FLOUR
1 CUP PLAIN LOW-FAT YOGURT
1/2 CUP WATER
GRATED ZEST FROM ONE ORANGE
♣Cook over low heat stirring, until mixture boils. Let cool, stirring gently every few minutes.
♣Add 1/2 CUP ORANGE JUICE

♣Fold in 6 EGG WHITES WHIPPED STIFF with a PINCH of CREAM OF TARTER.
♣Turn into a lecithin-sprayed 2-qt. straight-sided soufflé dish. Bake for 30 minutes until light and puffy.

♣While soufflé is baking, make the sauce. Combine in a sauce pan, and heat until well blended, stirring
2 CUPS RASPBERRIES
3 TBS. SUGAR-FREE RASPBERRY JELLY
2 TBS. ORANGE JUICE
♣Chill and pour over cold soufflé.

Nutritional analysis: per serving; 215 calories; 8gm. protein; 36gm. carbohydrates; 3gm. fiber; 4gm. fats; 144mg. cholesterol; 17% fats; 76mg. sodium.

292   QUICK PINEAPPLE BRUNCH CAKE

For 12 servings:

♣Mix into a runny batter
11/2 CUPS UNBLEACHED FLOUR
2 teasp. BAKING POWDER
1/4 teasp. SEA SALT
1 CUP HONEY
2 EGGS
3 TBS. OIL
3/4 CUP PINEAPPLE JUICE
♣Pour into a lecithin-sprayed 9" square pan. Sprinkle with cinnamon, nutmeg, and 4 TBS. BROWN SUGAR or TURBINADO SUGAR to caramelize.
♣Bake for 30 minutes until just set and a toothpick tester comes out clean.

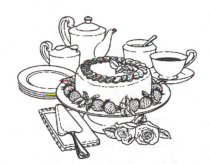

Nutritional analysis: per serving; 200 calories; 4gm. protein; 38gm. carbohydrates; 1gm. fiber; 5gm. fats; 35mg. cholesterol; 22% fats; 59mg. sodium.

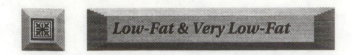

Cheesecakes are the essence of indulgence. The three here let you gratify your soul without guilt.

293   VERY LOW-FAT CHERRY CHEESECAKE

This is so rich, you can hardly believe that it only has one gram of fat.

♣Make the filling in a double boiler. Dissolve 2 TBS. PLAIN GELATIN in $1/2$ CUP WATER
♣Add and stir until well blended
2 CUPS LOW-FAT YOGURT
4 TBS. CHERRY JUICE from a package of THAWED FROZEN CHERRIES
4 CUPS LOW-FAT COTTAGE CHEESE
1 teasp. ALMOND EXTRACT

♣Beat well until mixture is smooth. Then chill in the fridge. When mixture begins to thicken, add 1 carton of KEFIR CHEESE, 8-OZ. NEUFCHATEL or 8-OZ. SOY CREAM CHEESE, and 2 TBS. LEMON JUICE.
♣Beat very well again to blend smooth, to the consistency of thick whipped cream.
♣Spoon into a spring form pan and chill until firm.

♣Make the topping: stir 2 MORE TBS. CHERRY JUICE from the thawed cherries with 2 TBS. ARROW-ROOT or KUZU CHUNKS until dissolved.

♣Make the CHERRY GLAZE:
♣Put the frozen CHERRIES from the package in a sauce pan on low heat with 1 CUP APPLE JUICE.
♣Gradually stir in arrowroot mixture until smooth, thickened and glossy. Remove from heat and cool.
♣To serve, release the springform sides of the cheesecake pan. Leave the bottom on the cake, and put the cake on a plate. Spoon over sauce and cut.

Nutritional analysis: per serving; 128 calories; 13gm. protein; 13gm. carbohydrates; trace fiber; 2gm. fats; 9mg. cholesterol; 9% fats; 330mg. sodium.

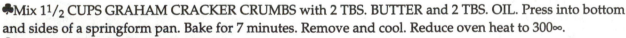

294   BERRY BERRY LOW FAT CHEESECAKE

For 10 to 12 pieces: Preheat oven to 350°.

♣Mix $1^1/2$ CUPS GRAHAM CRACKER CRUMBS with 2 TBS. BUTTER and 2 TBS. OIL. Press into bottom and sides of a springform pan. Bake for 7 minutes. Remove and cool. Reduce oven heat to 300∞.
♣Whirl the filling ingredients in the blender until very smooth

1 CUP LOW-FAT COTTAGE CHEESE	1 EGG
2 CUPS PLAIN LOW-FAT YOGURT	2 EGG WHITES
$1/3$ CUP FRUCTOSE	$1^1/2$ teasp VANILLA
1 TB. WHOLE WHEAT FLOUR	

♣Pour into crust, and bake until top feels dry when touched, and the center jiggles when shaken slightly, about 55 minutes. Let cool, and then chill for 8 hours.
♣Top with 2 CUPS WHOLE FRESH RASPBERRIES, BLACKBERRIES or BLUEBERRIES.

295   SCRUMPTIOUS PEACH CHEESECAKE

This cake is perfect with a juice-sweetened cookie crumb crust, or a macaroon cookie crust. Crumble the cookies, put them in the bottom of a cheesecake pan, and toast for 10 minutes. It is also delicious with no crust at all.

♣Make the cake. Mix together
2^1/$_2$ CUPS THIN SLICED FRESH PEACHES
^{1}/$_2$ CUP SHREDDED COCONUT
^{1}/$_4$ CUP FRUCTOSE
2 TBS. UNBLEACHED FLOUR
1 teasp. SWEET TOOTH BAKING SPICE (Page 645) **or** ^{1}/$_2$ teasp. cinnamon and ^{1}/$_2$ teasp. nutmeg
♣Turn into a lecithin-sprayed spring form pan.

♣Make the topping. Mix in the blender until very smooth
2 EGGS
12 OZ. <u>VERY FRESH</u> TOFU and 6 OZ. CREAM CHEESE or SOY CREAM CHEESE,
or 1 CARTONS of KEFIR CHEESE and ^{1}/$_2$ CARTON of PEACH YOGURT

♣Add and blend in until very smooth
^{3}/$_4$ CUP HONEY
^{1}/$_2$ teasp. CINNAMON
2 teasp. VANILLA
♣Pour over peach mixture. Do not stir, so that the integrity of the separate layers is maintained.
♣Bake at 350∞ 50 to 60 minutes until just set, and slightly wobbly in the center. Remove, cool and chill.

Nutritional analysis: per serving; 172 calories; 5gm. protein; 30gm. carbohydrates; 2gm. fiber; 4gm. fats; 36mg. cholesterol; 17% fats; 21mg. sodium.

✤ **Serve this cake with a low fat delicious custard sauce if desired.**

VANILLA CUSTARD SAUCE

This is good, hot or cold, with the cheesecake above, or over fresh fruit.
For 4 to 6 servings:

♣Whirl 2 EGGS and 1 teasp. VANILLA in the blender

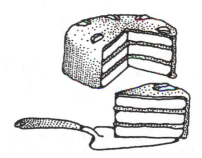

♣Heat in a saucepan almost to a boil
1 CUP LOW-FAT MILK or VANILLA KEFIR
3 TBS. FRUCTOSE

♣Remove from heat and add to the eggs in the blender in a thin stream, to warm, but not cook them.

♣Mixture should coat the back of a spoon. If it doesn't, return briefly to the saucepan, and cook gently a little longer until thickened.

Nutritional analysis: per serving; 79 calories; 4gm. protein; 10gm. carbohydrate; 0 fiber; 2gm. fats; 87mg. cholesterol; 10% fats; 50mg. sodium.

296 RAISIN GRANOLA CREAM CAKE

Makes 1 9 x 13" pan: Preheat oven to 350°.

♣Mix ingredients gently in a large bowl just til blended

1 CUP BROWN SUGAR **or** 1/2 CUP FRUCTOSE and 1/2 CUP DATE SUGAR, mixed

4 TBS. BUTTER	1 teasp. BAKING SODA
3 TBS. OIL	1 teasp. BAKING POWDER
2 EGGS	2 teasp. FIVE SPICE POWDER
2/3 CUP LOW-FAT CAPPUCINO YOGURT	1/2 CUP ORANGE JUICE
1 teasp. VANILLA	1 1/2 CUPS GRANOLA
2 CUPS WHOLE GRAIN FLOUR	1/2 CUP RAISINS

♣Turn into a lecithin-sprayed 9 x 13" pan, and bake 25 minutes until a toothpick inserted in the center comes out clean.

Nutritional analysis: per serving; 202 calories; 5gm. protein; 30gm. carbohydrates; 3gm. fiber; 8gm. fats; 31mg. cholesterol; 34% fats; 40mg. sodium.

❀Serve with **CREAMY BANANA DRIZZLE** if desired.

Makes about 2 cups:

♣Blend all ingredients in the blender until very smooth, and drizzle over dessert.
2 RIPE BANANAS
2 teasp. LEMON JUICE
2 TBS. OIL
1 teasp. VANILLA or BANANA EXTRACT
1/2 CUP HONEY
2 TBS. MAPLE SYRUP

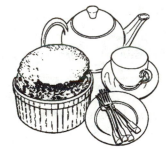

297 PUDDING PUFF

This is good by itself or with **Banana Drizzle** *above.*
For 6 servings:

♣Cream and beat together well
1 CUP LOW-FAT MILK **or** 3/4 CUP PLAIN LOW-FAT YOGURT and 1/4 CUP WATER
1/3 CUP FRUCTOSE or 1/2 CUP BROWN SUGAR
1/4 CUP UNSALTED BUTTER 3 TBS. LEMON JUICE
1 teasp. GRATED LEMON PEEL 2 TBS. WHOLE GRAIN FLOUR
2 EGG YOLKS 1/4 CUP GRAPENUTS

♣Beat 2 EGG WHITES to stiff and fold in.
♣Pour mixture into a lecithin-sprayed 1-qt. baking dish, and bake at 325° for 1 hour and 15 minutes until the top springs back when touched. **There will be cake on top and pudding on the bottom.**

298   GINGER DROP COOKIES

These are low in fat and high in fiber, too.
For 24 cookies: Preheat oven to 350°.

♣Mix together in a bowl
1/4 CUP OIL
1/2 CUP HONEY
1 TB. MOLASSES
1/2 CUP APPLE JUICE
1 EGG
1 teasp. SEA SALT

♣Mix togeher in another bowl
1 CUP RYE FLOUR
1/2 CUP OAT FLOUR
1/2 CUP OAT BRAN
2 teasp. CINNAMON
2 teasp. GINGER POWDER
1 teasp. BAKING POWDER

♣Mix wet and dry ingredients together just to moisten. Drop by spoonfuls onto lecithin-sprayed or oiled sheets. Bake for 10 minutes until edges start to brown.

Nutritional analysis: per serving; 78 calories; 2gm. protein; 13gm. carbohydrates; 1gm. fiber; 3gm. fats; 8mg. cholesterol; 14% fats; 93mg. sodium.

299   CHEESE STUFFED PEARS

For 8 pear halves: slice 4 pears lengthwise. Core to form a pocket; brush surface with lemon juice.

♣Mix cheese filling;
1/2 CUP LOW-FAT COTTAGE CHEESE or NEUFCHATEL CHEESE

1/3 CUP LOW-FAT GRATED CHEDDAR
4 OZ. YOGURT CHEESE
1/3 CUP CHOPPED WALNUTS

2 TBS. MINCED MINT or ROSEMARY
2 TBS. HONEY
1/2 teasp. SEA SALT

♣Mound filling on top of pears and smooth with a knife. Decorate with slivers of dried apricots.

Nuritional analysis: per serving; 142 calories; 6gm. protein; 17gm.\ carbohydrates; 2gm fiber; 5gm. fats; 11mg. cholesterol; 22% fats; 142mg. sodium.

300   FROZEN YOGURT BARS

For 9 pieces:

♣Freeze 2 containers of FRUIT YOGURT, any flavor or mixed flavors. Freeze 1 CUP CHOPPED FRESH FRUITS.
♣Put the frozen ingredient in a blender and add 2/3 CUP NON-FAT DRY MILK and 2 TBS. HONEY.
♣Blend until smooth. Pour into an 8" square pan. Add 1 CUP GRAPENUTS, and gently mix them in.
♣Top with ONE MORE CUP OF GRAPENUTS and press in to top.
♣FREEZE SOLID. Cut in bars. Wrap in foil to keep, and freeze until just before you want to eat them.

Nutritional analysis: per serving; 171 calories; 7gm. protein; 34gm. carbohydrates; 2gm. fiber; trace fats; 4mg. cholesterol; 4% fats; 139mg. sodium.

The person who
follows the crowd
will usually go
no farther than the crowd.

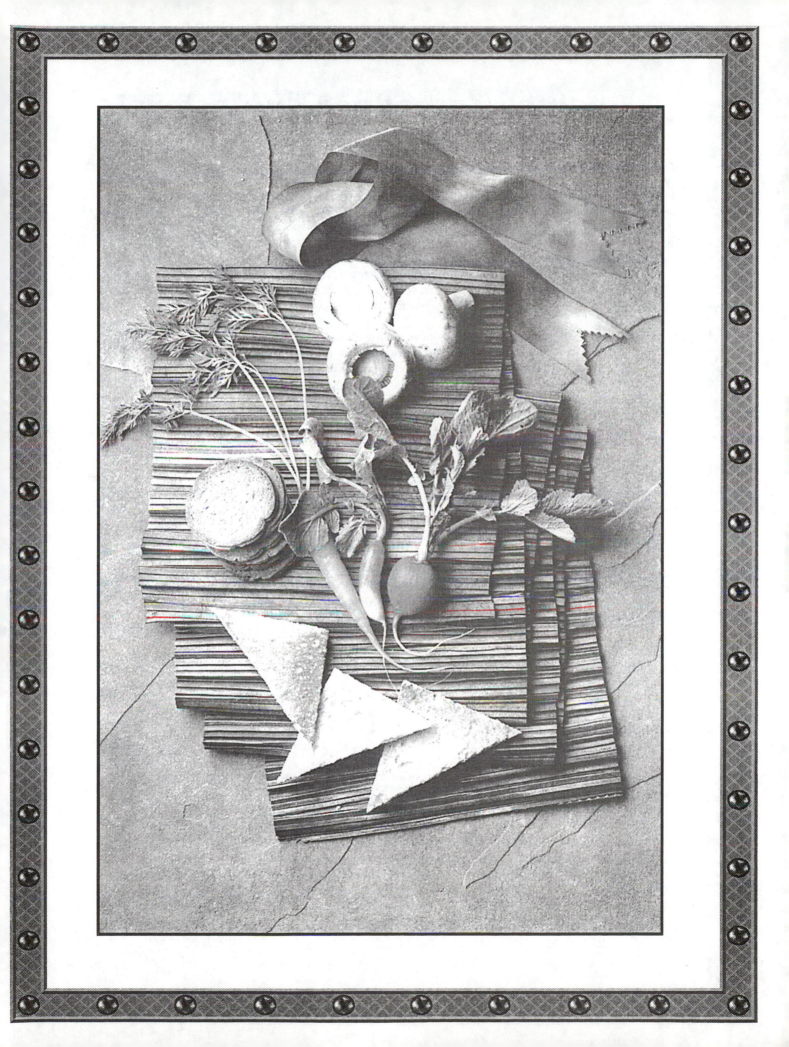

Recipes To Reduce Cholesterol

Just as there are good and bad fats in the body, so there are two kinds of cholesterol. High density lipo-protein, (HDL), or "good cholesterol," is internally manufactured in the intestinal tract and liver. It serves as raw material for cell membranes, protects nerve sheathing, plays a role in the creative process of vitamin D and sex hormones, and is beneficial to the heart and arteries by transporting cholesterol to the liver for removal as bile. Low density lipo-protein, (LDL), "bad cholesterol," is caused by dietary sources; too much saturated fat, meats and other animal foods, and low fiber, refined foods. Bad cholesterol causes harmful deposits that lodge in the blood vessels and become arterial plaque. The good health idea is to lower LDL, and increase HDL in the body. Fortunately, this is quite easy to do with awareness about the foods that promote these substances, and conscious attention to food choices and ingredients. Well-documented studies have shown, for instance, that cold water fish and seafood, containing high omega-3 oils, consistently raises HDL and lowers LDL.

While the ratio of HDL to LDL is important, the lower your total cholesterol level, the better.
**Every one percent increase in total blood cholesterol
translates into a two percent increase in heart disease risk.**

The medical world rule of thumb has been 180mg. or less for people under thirty, and 200mg. or less for people over thirty. Vegetarians find these levels quite easy to achieve, since most of the saturated fat and cholesterol in the American diet comes from animal products. Total vegans average around 125mg., and lacto-vegetarians average around 150 to 160mg.

The strongest influence on blood cholesterol levels is saturated fat, from the marbleing in red meats to the tropical coconut oil in cookies. Saturated fats affect cholesterol levels **five times more than even dietary cholesterol (LDL)**. The second most important factor is an excess of total fat calories. Excess is defined as more fat calories than are needed to maintain ideal body weight.

Most of us know by now that foods with soluble fiber help reduce harmful cholesterol. Some of these include oat, rice and other brans, peas, beans, lentils and barley, apples, prunes, guar gum, psyllium and flax seeds, carrots, leafy greens, citrus fruit, sea greens, and whole grains. The soluble fiber in these foods soaks up water in the stomach and intestines, and lowers cholesterol levels by making dietary cholesterol (LDL) unabsorbable. In addition, these foods help to regulate sugar use in the bloodstream by slowing down its absorption in the body, and they play a major part in removing toxic carcinogens. Natural plant lipids (phytosterols), such as those from olive, flax, evening primrose oil and other unsaturated vegetable oils, also emulsify and lower harmful blood fats. High chlorophyll foods, such as spirulina, chlorella, and dark leafy greens favorably metabolise fatty substances, too.

The recipes in this chapter are representative for each **low cholesterol or cholesterol lowering** area; they make good beginning examples of these foods and combinations. The section includes:
COLD WATER FISH & SEAFOOD NO CHOLESTEROL TOFU TURKEY: A LOW CHOLESTEROL MEAT BROWN RICE, WHOLE GRAINS & LEGUMES HIGH FIBER VEGETABLES

For more extensive recipes, see listings under the following chapters: FISH & SEAFOOD HIGH FIBER RECIPES COMPLEX CARBOHYDRATES FOR ENERGY SUGAR FREE SPECIALS TOFU FOR YOU SALADS HOT AND COLD DAIRY FREE COOKING

Keeping cholesterol low is easy. Keeping it low with traditional diet is a little harder. Keeping it low and delicious is a lot harder. Most of us like, and are used to, lots of eggs, butter, pasteurized dairy products and meats. **In this book, low cholesterol means 100mg. or less. Very low cholesterol means 30mg. or less.**

Animal fats and meats, fried and fast foods, sugars, refined foods, and an excessive use of salt, all contribute to a cholesterol problem. Omit them from your diet as much as possible. A pleasant glass or two of wine with dinner, however, can reduce stress and encourage good HDL production.

Cold Water Fish & Seafood

Including cold water fish in a healthy diet has become a byword of the nineties for lowering harmful cholesterol.
They are also an excellent source of absorbable ocean minerals.
These recipes demonstrate just how delicious a heart healthy diet can be.

301   SESAME FISH

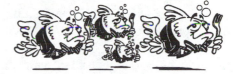

For 6 servings:

♣Rinse 2 LBS. WHITE FISH FILETS ABOUT 1 " thick, and cut in 6 serving pieces. Season with SESAME SALT and PEPPER. Dust with UNBLEACHED or WHOLE GRAIN FLOUR.

♣Mix $1/2$ CUP WHOLE GRAIN BREAD CRUMBS and 4 TBS. PAN ROASTED SESAME SEEDS.

♣Separately mix 1 EGG and 2 TBS. WATER or WHITE WINE. Dip fish pieces in egg mix, then in crumb mix to coat well.
♣Cover the bottom of a shallow baking dish with OLIVE OIL. Lay fish pieces in a single layer, and bake at 350∞ for 10 minutes until fish is firm and white.

♣Make a simple sauce, and spoon over fish when serving. Mix $1/4$ CUP FRESH CHOPPED PARSLEY, $1/4$ CUP LEMON JUICE, $1/2$ CUP CHOPPED GREEN ONIONS.

Nutritional analysis: per serving; 244 calories; 32gm. protein; 8gm. carbohydrate; 2gm. fiber; 8gm. fats; 98mg. cholesterol; 58mg. calcium; 2mg. iron; 85mg. magnesium; 667mg. potassium; 221mg. sodium.

302   SHARK LIGHT

Several types of shark meat are now readily available in fish markets. Shark is a delicious cold water fish with a meaty texture good for grilling or broiling. The light Italian touch of fresh tomato sauce balances it perfectly.
For 4 to 6 servings:

♣This recipe is good broiled or baked.
♣If you are broiling, brush the shark steaks all over with OLIVE OIL. Broil 5 to 7 minutes on each side, and pour the sauce over to serve.
♣If you are baking, preheat oven to 400° and place $1 1/2$ - 2 LBS SHARK STEAKS in a shallow baking dish in a single layer. Brush all over with OLIVE OIL.

♣Make the sauce in the blender. Whirl 2 CHOPPED GREEN ONIONS, 2 MINCED SHALLOTS, $1/4$ CUP FRESH CHOPPED PARSLEY, 1 TB. FRESH MINCED BASIL (or 1 teasp. dry), 1 LARGE FRESH CHOPPED TOMATO, and 3 TBS. LEMON JUICE.

♣Pour over fish. Sprinkle on $1/4$ CUP SLICED BLACK OLIVES.
♣Cover and bake for 15 minutes.

Nutritional analysis: per serving; 270 calories; 34gm. protein; 6gm. carbohydrates; 1gm. fiber; 11gm. fats; 66mg. cholesterol; 41mg. calcium; 2mg. iron; 58mg. magnesium; 672mg. potassium; 2mg. zinc; 199mg. sodium.

303   KING CRAB PASTA SALAD

This recipe works well with both king crab legs and fresh lump crabmeat.
For 4 people:

♣Make the dressing and chill.

¹/₄ CUP LIGHT MAYONNAISE   2 TBS. GRATED PARMESAN
¹/₄ CUP PLAIN LOW-FAT YOGURT   ¹/₄ CUP SNIPPED CHIVES

♣Bring 3 to 4-qts. salted water to a boil, and add 2 CUPS WHOLE GRAIN or VEGETABLE PASTA (VEGETABLE ELBOWS, BOWTIES, or SESAME SHELLS). Cook just to *al dente. (See pasta instructions page 225.)* Drain and toss with 1 TB. OLIVE OIL to keep separated.

♣Sauté 8 OZ. KING CRAB LEG CHUNKS or LUMP CRABMEAT in 1 TB. LIGHT OIL. Toss just until opaque and whitened, about 5 or 6 minutes. Remove from pan with a slotted spoon, and set aside.
♣Add 1 more TB. oil to the sauté pan, heat and sauté until color changes, 1 CUP CHOPPED BROC-COLI FLORETS, ¹/₂ CUP CHOPPED RED BELL PEPPER, and ¹/₄ CUP MINCED GREEN ONIONS.
♣Remove from heat. Mix and toss with crabmeat and pasta.
♣Add ¹/₂ CUP CHOPPED FRESH TOMATO and toss. Add chilled dressing and toss. Serve immediately. The warm salad, and the cold dressing are wonderful together.

Nutritional analysis: per serving; 400 calories; 21gm. protein; 43gm. carbohydrate; 7gm. fiber; 12gm. fats; 45mg. cholesterol; 131mg. calcium; 2mg. iron; 84mg. magnesium; 481mg. potassium; 262mg. sodium; 4mg. zinc.

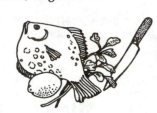

304   QUICK CALIFORNIA ROUGHY

For 4 people: Preheat oven to 350°.

♣Rinse 1 LB. ORANGE ROUGHY FILETS and pat dry. Arrange in an oiled shallow baking pan and season with SALT and LEMON PEPPER. Spread on ¹/₂ CUP LEMON YOGURT, and sprinkle with 2 CHOPPED SCALLIONS. Bake for 12 to 18 minutes until fish is just opaque.
♣Squeeze on 1 WEDGED LEMON and sprinkle with SEA SALT.

305   MUSTARD/DILL SAUCE FOR BROILED SALMON

Salmon is the most important cold water fish for high Omega-3 oils. It can be fixed in many delicious ways.

♣Enough sauce for 6 broiled or grilled salmon filets:
♣Blend sauce in the blender, and let sit for 20 minutes to meld flavors.
3 TB. BROWN SUGAR or 2 TBS. FRUCTOSE
1 TB. DIJON MUSTARD
3 TBS. SHERRY
1 CLOVE MINCED GARLIC
2 TBS FRESH CHOPPED DILL WEED, or 2 teasp. dry dill
♣While the blender is on, add ¹/₂ CUP OLIVE OIL in a thin stream until sauce thickens.

306 TERIYAKI SALMON

For 4 servings:

♣Marinate 4 SALMON STEAKS in the following sauce for 1 hour. Mix
2 TBS. TAMARI
2 TBS. SHERRY
2 TBS. WHITE WINE
2 CLOVES MINCED GARLIC
1 teasp. MIRIN
1 teasp. BROWN RICE VINEGAR

♣Reserve marinade. Place fish in a single layer on a steamer rack over simmering water. (A wok and rack are excellent for this.) Cover and steam for about 6 minutes. Remove to a serving plate.

♣Heat reserved marinade in a saucepan until aromatic. Remove from heat.
♣Dissolve 1 teasp. KUZU chunks or 1 teasp. arrowroot in 1 TB. water. Add to marinade and heat briefly until thickened and glossy.
♣Pour over salmon, and snip on 2 to 3 scallions with tops.

Nutritional analysis: per serving; 229 calories; 24gm. protein; 3gm. carbohydrates; trace fiber; 11gm. fats; 74mg. cholesterol; 35mg. calcium; 1mg. iron; 39mg. magnesium; 502mg. potassium; 143mg. sodium; trace zinc.

307 SALMON & RICE LOAF

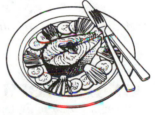

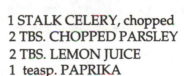

For 6 servings:

♣Mix the loaf ingredients together in a bowl
1 LB. FRESH, FROZEN or CANNED SALMON FILETS
1/4 CUP WHEAT GERM
1 CUP COOKED BROWN RICE
1/2 CUP WHOLE WHEAT BREAD CRUMBS
2 EGG WHITES beaten to frothy
2 LEEKS, white parts only, sliced

1 STALK CELERY, chopped
2 TBS. CHOPPED PARSLEY
2 TBS. LEMON JUICE
1 teasp. PAPRIKA

♣Moisten with juice from the canned salmon, or 1/2 CUP WHITE WINE for good consistency.

♣Smooth into a lecithin-sprayed loaf pan. Bake at 350° for 40 minutes until light brown. Let stand for 10 minutes while you make the sauce. Turn out onto a greens-covered serving plate.
♣Slice to serve. Top slices with a **LEMON SAUCE**.

♣Heat 1 CUP CHICKEN BROTH and 1/2 teasp. GARLIC/LEMON SEASONING to boiling in a saucepan.
♣Dissolve 1 1/2 teasp. ARROWROOT in 2 TBS. WATER and whisk in.
♣Remove from heat and whisk in 1 CUP PLAIN LOW-FAT YOGURT and 1 TB. LEMON JUICE.

Nutritional analysis: per serving; 261 calories; 22gm. protein; 22gm. carbohydrates; 3gm. fiber; 9gm. fats; 52mg. cholesterol; 126mg. calcium; 2mg. iron; 73mg. magnesium; 585mg. potassium; 142mg. sodium; 1mg. zinc.

308 SALMON & FRESH VEGETABLE SAUCE

For 6 salmon steaks:

♣Rinse steaks and pat dry. Sprinkle with 1¹/₂ teasp. GRATED LIME ZEST and ³/₄ teasp. WHITE PEPPER.
♣Heat I CUP WATER or LIGHT BROTH in a heavy skillet over high heat. Add salmon pieces in a single layer and cook for 45 seconds. Turn and cook for 45 seconds more. Remove pan from heat and let sit, covered for 2 to 3 minutes.
♣Transfer salmon with a spatula to a serving plate and keep warm while you make the sauce.

♣Make the sauce with cooking juices from the salmon. Sauté in 2 TB. OLIVE OIL in a skillet with
6 THIN SLICED RED RADISHES or FRESH SLICED DAIKON RADISH (about 1 cup)
3 PLUM TOMATOES diced
1 ZUCCHINI diced
3 TBS. MINCED CHIVES
³/₄ teasp. HERB SALT
♣Stir and toss quickly for 1 minute only. Bring to a boil for 1 minute and spoon over salmon steaks.

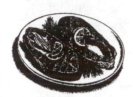

No Cholesterol Tofu

*Tofu is high in protein, minerals and soluble fiber, and low in saturated fat. It is hearty and satisfying.
Adding tofu to your diet is a good way to lower cholesterol.*

309   MARINATED TOFU
This is a basic, very simple way to fix tofu. The flavor of fresh tofu is light and delicate by itself; perfect for a spicy marinade or sauce. This one is an old favorite of mine. Eat it as is for a quick lunch or snack, or use in a salad with vegetables, or as a side dish with rice, or in a sandwich.

For a one pound tub; 4 serving cakes:

♣Cube 1 LB. TOFU. Blanch in boiling water for a few minutes to firm.
♣Mix the marinade
1 TB. FRESH GRATED GINGER   1 TB. SESAME OIL
2 TBS. SHERRY   ¹/₂ teasp. FRUCTOSE
¹/₄ CUP TAMARI   1 teasp. TOASTED SESAME SEEDS
2 TBS. BROWN RICE VINEGAR   ¹/₂ teasp. SEA VEGGIES SUPREME MIX
1 TB. SESAME OIL   2 TBS. WATER if needed
DASHES HOT PEPPER SAUCE or ORIENTAL BARBECUE SAUCE
♣Marinate tofu cubes for 1 hour or longer in the fridge.

Nutritional analysis: per serving; 142 calories; 10gm. protein; 5 gm. carbohydrates; 1gm. fiber; 9gm. fats; 0 cholesterol; 125mg. calcium; 6mg. iron; 126mg. magnesium; 189mg. potassium; 185mg. sodium; 1mg. zinc.

310   BROWN RICE & TOFU

The protein complementarity of brown rice and tofu together is particularly good for a healing diet.
For 8 servings:

♣Soak 6 TO 8 DRIED BLACK SHIITAKE MUSHROOMS in water to cover. Sliver when soft and set aside. Reserve soaking water.

♣Dry roast $1^1/_3$ BROWN RICE in a pan, and then cook in $2^1/_2$ CUPS WATER, for 4 cups cooked.

♣Sauté 2 CAKES CUBED TOFU in 2 TBS. OIL in a skillet, and add to rice.

♣Add 1 TB. OIL to skillet and sauté until onions are translucent and spices are aromatic

1 ONION, chopped
2 CLOVES GARLIC, chopped
1 teasp. CUMIN POWDER
$1/_4$ teasp. NATURAL LIQUID SMOKE

1 teasp. BREWER'S YEAST FLAKES
$1/_2$ teasp. SESAME SALT
$1/_4$ teasp. BLACK PEPPER

♣Add and sauté until color changes

2 CARROTS, chopped
2 STALKS CELERY, chopped
1 GREEN BELL PEPPER, chopped

2 ZUCCHINI, chopped
THE SHIITAKE MUSHROOMS

♣Add mushroom soaking water and steam/braise for 5 minutes. Vegetables should be just *tender crisp, not* completely cooked.

♣ Stir in 6-OZ. GRATED LOW-FAT CHEDDAR.

♣Combine mixture with rice and tofu. Season with HERB SALT. Put in a greased casserole, cover with foil and bake at 350° for 30 minutes. Uncover and bake until bubbly for 15 minutes.

Nutritional analysis: per serving; 289 calories; 11gm. protein; 33gm. carbohydrates; 4gm. fiber; 9gm. fats; 22mg. cholesterol; 215mg. calcium; 3mg. iron; 99mg. magnesium; 389mg. potassium; 117mg. sodium; 2mg. zinc.

311   SWEET & SOUR TOFU WITH VEGGIES

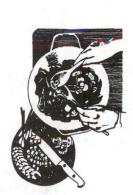

For 6 people:

♣Cube 2 CAKES TOFU into a bowl.

♣Mix the marinade, pour over tofu and let sit for 20 minutes.

4 TBS. BROWN SUGAR
6 TBS. BROWN RICE VINEGAR
$1^1/_2$ teasp. GRATED FRESH GINGER DASHES HOT CHILI OIL

3 TBS. TAMARI
$1/_4$ CUP KETCHUP

♣Heat 2 TBS. OIL in a wok and sauté until aromatic

3 CUPS SLICED YELLOW and RED ONIONS
1 TB. GRATED GINGER
2 CARROTS, SLICED IN JULIENNE

8 OZ. FRENCH CUT GREEN BEANS
1 BELL PEPPER IN JULIENNE SLICES
4 CUPS ZUCCHINI ROUNDS

♣Toss briefly to coat. Turn down heat. Cover wok, and simmer until just tender crisp, about 5 minutes.

♣Add $3/_4$ CUP PINEAPPLE CHUNKS and the DRAINED TOFU, and toss.

♣Dissolve 1 TB. ARROWROOT POWDER or KUZU CHUNKS into $1/_2$ cup PINEAPPLE JUICE. Add to veggie/tofu mix. Toss until glossy for 4 minutes. Shake on drops of HOT CHILI OIL and serve.

312   TOFU NUT LOAF

This dish is also good as a baked stuffing, fragrantly calling people to the kitchen while it's baking,
For 6 to 8 servings:

♣Toast 1 CUP CHOPPED WALNUTS, 1 CUP CHOPPED CASHEWS AND ¼ CUP SESAME SEEDS in a 350° oven until cashews are golden. Leave oven on.

♣Sauté in 3 TBS. OIL and ¼ CUP ONION BROTH until translucent and aromatic
1½ CUPS CHOPPED ONION
1 CUP CHOPPED CELERY with leaves
½ CHOPPED RED BELL PEPPER

♣Remove vegetables to a bowl with a slotted spoon, and add 1 TUB MASHED TOFU and 2 CUPS COOKED MILLET or BULGUR to the skillet.
♣Toss and sizzle for a few minutes. Add to nuts to grain mix and toss. Remove from heat.

♣Beat together, and stir into grain mix

3 EGGS	¼ teasp. GROUND ROSEMARY
½ teasp. BLACK PEPPER	¼ teasp. SAVORY
1 teasp. SESAME SALT	¼ teasp. DRY THYME
¼ teasp. GROUND SAGE	1 TB. DRY PARSLEY FLAKES

♣Mix all ingredients together and put in a lecithin-sprayed loaf pan. Bake for 40 minutes until set.

Nutritional analysis: per serving; 428 calories; 15gm. protein; 28gm. carbohydrate; 4gm. fiber; 30gm. fats; 79mg. cholesterol; 116mg. calcium; 5mg. iron; 180mg. magnesium; 429mg. potassium; 3mg. zinc.

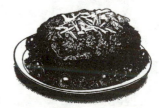

313   TEX-MEX CHILI & TOFU DOME

For 6 servings: Preheat oven to 350°.

♣Sauté for 10 minutes in 2 TBS. OLIVE OIL and 2 TBS.RED WINE until aromatic

1 RED ONION, chopped	
1 RED BELL PEPPER, chopped	1 teasp. SEA SALT
4 GARLIC CLOVES, chopped	2 teasp. DRY OREGANO
2 JALAPEÑO PEPPERS, minced	2 TEASP. CUMIN POWDER
2 TBS. CHILI POWDER	2 PINCHES THYME LEAVES

♣Add 1 28 OZ. CAN PEELED ITALIAN TOMATOES, drained. Cook for 10 minutes more.

♣Combine 1 LB. GROUND TURKEY and 1 LB. FROZEN TOFU, thawed, squeezed out and crumbled. Add to vegetables with 1 CUP WHOLE GRAIN BREAD CRUMBS, 2 EGGS, and 1 CUP CORN KERNELS.

♣Transfer to a shallow baking dish and pat into a dome. Bake for 1 hour. Remove, pour off excess juices, and grate on 8 OZ. SOY CHEESE CHEDDAR STYLE to cover dome.

Turkey - A Low Cholesterol Meat

If you are reducing your red meat intake, turkey can be a good "transition" meat. It is low in cholesterol and saturated fat, but has plenty of flavor and texture. Light meat from both turkey and chicken is much leaner than dark meat. **It contains <u>less than half</u> the fat of dark meat.** *Light meat also has 20% less calories and 10% more protein than dark meat. Buy free-run turkeys if possible, that have not been given hormones or anti-biotics. Avoid buying pre-basted turkeys. Most have been injected with saturated or partially hydrogenated oils, which raise cholesterol levels, and treated with artificial colorings.*

314   ROAST TURKEY SOUTHERN STYLE

I grew up in the South, where this time-tested favorite has been around a long time. But the "new South" eats much lighter now, and this recipe has been changed to reflect that new way of eating. The taste is still there, but the saturated fats and dense stuffing are not.
Preheat oven to 325°.

♣ Use a TURKEY ROAST (the all-white-meat ones are lower in fat). Rub all over with a paste of 2 TBS. ORANGE LIQUEUR, 1 TB. HONEY, 1 teasp. PAPRIKA, and 2 teasp. SEA SALT.
♣ Roast in a shallow open pan, 25 minutes per pound, until tender and juices run clear. Scatter 1/2 CUP CHOPPED ONIONS around the turkey so they can roast along with it and be ready for the gravy.

♣ Prepare the STUFFING in a separate dish. Make up one pound of TOFU BURGER or GRAIN BURGER MIX from a box. Crumble and sauté in a little BUTTER until browned and and crisp. Remove to a mixing bowl.
♣ Add 2 TBS. BUTTER or CHICKEN BROTH to the hot skillet, and sauté 1 1/2 CUPS CHOPPED ONION and 1/2 CUP CHOPPED CELERY for 5 minutes. Add to mixing bowl with the tofu burger.

♣ Add and mix well

4 CUPS CRUMBLED CORNBREAD	1/4 CUP FRESH CHOPPED PARSLEY
1 1/2 CUPS CHOPPED PECANS	1/2 teasp. DRY THYME
1/4 CUP SHERRY	1/4 teasp. NUTMEG
1/4 CUP PLAIN LOW-FAT YOGURT	1/4 teasp. BLACK PEPPER

♣ Spoon into a lecithin-sprayed casserole. Put in 325° oven with the turkey, the last 45 minutes of roasting and bake until firm and crisp on top.
♣ Remove turkey and dressing when done, and let rest while you make the low-fat pan sauce.

Nutritional analysis: per serving w/ gravy; 492 calories; 52gm. protein; 24gm. carbo.; 5gm. fiber; 20gm. fats; 101mg. cholest.; 110mg. calcium; 5mg. iron; 113mg. magnesium; 742mg. potassium; 396mg. sodium; 5mg. zinc.

TURKEY PAN SAUCE

♣ Put turkey on a carving/serving plate. Scrape drippings into a saucepan (or use the roasting pan on low heat). Sprinkle with 3 to 4 TBS. WHOLE WHEAT FLOUR, and roux, stirring and scraping up browned bits into the sauce until everything is bubbly and well blended, 3 minutes.
♣ Add 1/2 CUP PLAIN LOW-FAT YOGURT and 1/2 cup water. Heat stirring, until bubbly and thickened.
♣ Add 1 CUP CHICKEN STOCK and 1/4 CUP WHITE WINE. Bring to a boil and season with 1 teasp. SEA SALT and PEPPER to taste.

315   SPLIT PEA SOUP WITH TURKEY WEINERS

For 8 servings:

♣Bring 4 CUPS WATER to a boil, and add
2 CUPS QUICK COOKING SPLIT PEAS
4 CUPS CHICKEN or TURKEY STOCK
2 CHUNKED YELLOW ONIONS

3 STALKS CHOPPED CELERY
1 teasp. SEA SALT
1/2 teasp. BLACK PEPPER

♣Simmer, partially covered over low heat for 2 hours. Cool slightly. Purée in the blender until smooth.

♣Return to the soup pot, and add 1 PKG. TURKEY WEINERS, sliced in rounds. (Get the ones from the natural food store that don't have fillers or preservatives.) Heat through for 5 minutes and serve.

316   TURKEY & BROWN RICE IN THE CLAY COOKER

See the LOW-FAT RECIPES chapter for more about these great low-fat cooking tools.

For 6 servings:

♣Chop 6 CLOVES GARLIC and 4 TBS. FRESH GINGER in the blender. Add 2 3/4 CUP WATER or LIGHT BROTH, 1 teasp. SEA SALT, 1 teasp. PEPPER, 1/4 teasp. HOT PEPPER SAUCE. Set aside.
♣Soak both top and bottom of a clay cooker in water for 15 minutes. Put in 2 to 3 LBS. TURKEY BREAST PIECES WITH BONE and put in a cold oven. Turn oven to 400° and cook for 10 minutes.
♣Add 3 ONIONS, minced, and 1 teasp. CUMIN POWDER and cook til onions brown. Turn oven to 425°.
♣Add 1 CUP BROWN RICE, the ginger/garlic/water mix in the blender, and 1/2 CUP DRIED TOMATO PIECES. ♣Cover and bake for 45 minutes until tender.
♣Remove from the oven and add 1 CUP FROZEN GREEN PEAS at the last minute. Let steam covered for 3 minutes. Remove turkey meat from the bone before serving.

Nutritional analysis: per serving; 342 calories; 49gm. protein; 22gm. carbohydrate; 4gm. fiber; 5gm. fats; 92mg. cholesterol; 68mg. calcium; 3mg. iron; 80mg. magnesium; 760mg. potassium; 167mg. sodium; 4mg. zinc.

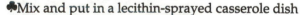

317   EASY TURKEY TETRAZZINI
The perfect one dish "leftovers" meal.
For 4 people: Preheat oven to 350°.

♣Mix and put in a lecithin-sprayed casserole dish
3 CUPS DICED COOKED TURKEY
4 CUPS COOKED CHINESE NOODLES
1 RED ONION, chopped
8 OZ. MUSHROOMS, chopped
1/2 CUP GRATED PARMESAN or SOY PARMESAN

1 CUP TURKEY or CHICKEN STOCK
1/2 CUP FRESH CHOPPED PARSLEY
1 CUP LOW-FAT COTTAGE CHEESE
2 TBS. LEMON JUICE
2 EGGS

♣Season with 1 teasp. SEA SALT and 1/2 teasp. PEPPER. Sprinkle with PAPRIKA, MORE PARMESAN and CRUNCHY CHINESE NOODLES if desired. Bake for 40 minutes. Mmmm good.

318   TURKEY IN THE STRAW

This is a favorite with kids - kind of like Turkey Sloppy Joes.
For 6 servings:

♣Sauté in a pot <u>without oil or butter</u> for 10 minutes
1 LB. GROUND TURKEY
1 STALK CHOPPED CELERY
1 SMALL ONION, chopped
1/2 GREEN PEPPER, chopped
1 teasp. SEA SALT and 1/4 teasp. BLACK PEPPER

♣Add and simmer uncovered for 1 hours
ONE 6 OZ. CAN TOMATO PASTE
4 TBS. CATSUP
1 teasp. WORCESTERSHIRE SAUCE
DASHES HOT PEPPER SAUCE
1 CUP WATER

♣Serve over crisp corn chips and top with GRATED LOW FAT CHEDDAR or SOY CHEDDAR.

Nutritional analysis: per serving; 291 calories; 20gm. protein; 18gm. carbohydrates; 3gm. fiber; 15gm. fats; 50mg. cholesterol; 89mg. calcium; 3mg. iron; 48mg. magnesium; 574mg. potassium; 263mg. sodium; 3mg. zinc.

319   TURKEY TACOS

For 12 tacos:

♣Sauté 1 CLOVE MINCED GARLIC in 1 TB. OIL for 3 minutes. Add and sauté for for 10 minutes
8 OZ. UNCOOKED TURKEY BREAST STRIPS
1 CHOPPED RED ONION
1/2 teasp. GROUND CUMIN
1/2 teasp. DRY OREGANO
PINCHES of SEA SALT and PEPPER

♣Remove from heat and add
2 TOMATOES, diced
1 CUP SHREDDED LETTUCE
1/3 CUP FRESH CILANTRO, chopped

320   TURKEY CHOW MEIN CASSEROLE

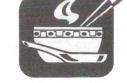

For 4 to 6 servings: Preheat ooven to 350°.

♣Sauté 1 LB. GROUND TURKEY and 3 SMALL SLICED ONIONS in 2 TBS. OIL until brown and crumbly, (<u>or</u> use 2 to 3 cups of cooked left-over turkey, cubed. Do not sauté. Add right before baking).
♣Add and sauté for 5 more minutes
3 STALKS CHOPPED CELERY
1 CUP SLICED MUSHROOMS

♣Add 2 1/2 CUPS CREAM OF MUSHROOM <u>SAUCE</u> made from MAYACAMAS CREAM OF MUSH-ROOM SOUP MIX, or leftover turkey gravy with 2 TBS. SOY SAUCE added.
♣Add and mix in
2 TBS. SHERRY or MIRIN
1 CUP OVEN TOASTED CASHEWS
1 SMALL CAN CRISP CHOW MEIN NOODLES (reserve some for topping)
♣Turn into a casserole, and bake for 45 minutes until bubbly. Top with reserved noodles.

Whole Grains, Brown Rice & Legumes For Soluble Fiber

When awareness about high blood fats first became known by the general public, whole grain muffins became the first food of choice for reducing them. They remain a delicious, healthy means of keeping cholesterol down.

321   BUCKWHEAT & BRAN MUFFINS

For 16 muffins: Preheat oven to 400°. Line muffin cups with papers, or spray with lecithin spray.

♣Stir the wet ingredients together
1/4 cup APPLE JUICE
1/2 CUP SUGAR-FREE APPLESAUCE
1/4 CUP PLAIN LOW-FAT YOGURT
2 EGG WHITES
1 CUP FAVORITE BRAN CEREAL
2 teasp. SWEET TOOTH MIX (Pg. 645)

♣Mix the dry ingredients
1 CUP WHOLE WHEAT PASTRY FLOUR
1/2 CUP BUCKWHEAT FLOUR
3 TBS. FRUCTOSE
1 TB. BAKING POWDER
1 teasp. BAKING SODA

♣Bake for 15 to 18 minutes until a toothpick inserted in the center comes out clean.

Nutritional analysis: per muffin; 66 calories; 3gm. protein; 15gm. carbohydrates; 3gm. fiber; trace fats; trace cholesterol; 58mg. calcium; 1mg. iron; 35mg. magnesium; 328mg. potassium; 84mg. sodium; 1mg. zinc.

322   FRUIT & OAT SCONES

These have the true old Scottish recipe taste, but with healthier ingredients.
For 8 scones: Preheat oven to 400°.

♣Mix dry ingredients
1 3/4 CUPS WHOLE GRAIN FLOUR MIX
3/4 CUP ROLLED OATS
3/4 CUP DATE SUGAR
2 teasp. BAKING POWDER
1/2 teasp. BAKING SODA
 1/4 CUP CHOPPED DRIED FIGS

♣Mix wet ingredients together
1/2 CUP OIL
2 TBS. MAPLE SYRUP
2 EGGS
1/4 CUP CHOPPED WALNUTS
1/3 CUP CURRANTS

♣Stir all together until evenly moistened. Scrape dough onto a lightly floured board and knead 4 or 5 times. Then place dough on a lecithin-sprayed baking sheet and pat into a 9" round.
♣Cut into 8 wedges with a sharp knife dipped in flour, and leave in place to bake.

♣Brush with EGG WHITE beaten to frothy. Bake for 25 minutes until top is golden brown. Serve warm.

Nutritional analysis: per serving; 334 calories; 8gm. protein; 47gm. carbohydrate; 5gm. fiber; 14gm. fats; 53mg. cholesterol; 104mg. calcium; 2mg. iron; 62mg. magnesium; 664mg. potassium; 32mg. sodium; 1mg. zinc.

323   CARROT 'N' HONEY MUFFINS

For 8 big muffins: Preheat oven to 350°. Line muffin cups with papers, or spray with lecithin spray.

♣Beat together wet ingredients
1/3 CUP HONEY
2 CUPS GRATED CARROTS
1 CHOPPED APPLE
2 TBS. MAPLE SYRUP
6 EGG WHITES
1 SCANT CUP CANOLA OIL
1 teasp. VANILLA

♣Mix together dry ingredients
1/2 CUP ROLLED OATS
1/2 CUP OAT FLOUR
2 CUPS WH. WHEAT PASTRY FLOUR
1/2 CUP CHOPPED WALNUTS
1/2 CUP RAISINS
2 teasp. CINNAMON
1 teasp. NUTMEG

♣Mix all ingredients together gently. Fill muffin cups. Bake for 25 minutes until a toothpick inserted in the center comes out clean.

Nutritional analysis: per muffin; 346 calories; 7gm. protein; 36gm. carbohydrates; 4gm. fiber; 20gm. fats; 0 cholesterol; 39mg. calcium; 2mg. iron; 52mg. magnesium; 360mg. potassium; 37mg. sodium; 1mg. zinc.

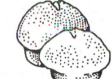

324   BLUEBERRY CORNMEAL MUFFINS

For 12 muffins: Preheat oven to 425°. Line muffin cups with papers, and oil the upper rim.

♣Mix all ingredients together gently, just so streakes of flour remain
1 1/2 CUPS UNBLEACHED FLOUR
1/2 CUP YELLOW CORNMEAL
1/4 CUP FRUCTOSE
1 TB. BAKING POWDER
1 teasp. BAKING SODA
1/4 teasp. SEA SALT

1/2 CUP PLAIN LOW-FAT YOGURT
1/2 CUP WATER
3 EGGS
4 TBS. OIL
1 1/2 CUPS (1/2 PINT) BLUEBERRIES

♣Place muffin tin in the middle of the oven and reduce heat to 400∞. Bake for 20 to 25 minutes til light gold. Serve warm with honey.

325   BASMATI BARCELONA

The soluble fiber from brown rice and beans can also play a major role in lowering cholesterol.
For 6 servings:

♣Sauté in 4 TBS OLIVE OIL until fragrant
3 CUPS COOKED BASMATI RICE
6 to 8 CHOPPED SCALLIONS
3 STALKS CHOPPED CELERY
1 CHOPPED RED or YELLOW BELL PEPPER
1 TB. TAMARI

♣Add and toss to blend
4 OZ. CAN CHOPPED GREEN CHILIS
1 SM. CAN GREEN OLIVES, sliced
3 FRESH CHOPPED TOMATOES
1 teasp. DRY OREGANO
1/2 teasp. GROUND CUMIN

♣Put mixture into a shallow baking dish. Stick corn chips points down all around the mixture. Sprinkle 3 TBS. CHEDDAR over top and bake for 10 minutes at 350° until cheese just melts.

326   BLACK BEAN SOUP WITH VEGGIES

For 8 servings:

♣Bring to a boil in a large kettle. Cover and simmer 2^1/$_2$ hours until beans are soft.
1^1/$_2$ CUPS BLACK TURTLE BEANS
1^1/$_2$ QTS VEGETABLE BROTH
1 TB. OIL

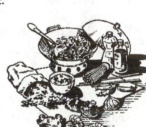

♣Heat 1 TB. OIL or 2 TBS. ONION BROTH in a skillet. Then sauté briefly until aromatic
1 SLICED CARROT
1 CHOPPED ONION   1 teasp. HONEY MUSTARD
1 CHUNKED POTATO ^{1}/$_4$ teasp. SAVORY
2 STALKS CHOPPED CELERY ^{1}/$_2$ teasp. PEPPER
1 teasp. DRY OREGANO   2 teasp. HERB SALT or GREAT 28 MIX
♣Remove from heat. Add to beans in the <u>last hour</u> of cooking.

♣When beans are tender and soup is ready, add
2 TBS. BLUSH WINE
JUICE OF 1 LEMON
THIN LEMON SLICES ON TOP

Nutritional analysis: per serving; 155 calories; 7gm. protein; 27gm. carbohydrate; 7gm. fiber; 2gm fats; 0 cholesterol; 45mg. calcium; 2mg. iron; 62mg. magnesium; 469mg. potassium; 247mg. sodium; 1mg. zinc.

327   MANY TREASURE RICE SALAD

For 4 servings:

♣Toast ^{3}/$_4$ CUP SLIVERED ALMONDS in the oven until golden.
♣Soak 6 DRY SHIITAKE MUSHROOMS in water until soft. Slice and discard woody stems.
♣Cook 1 CUP GOURMET GRAIN BLEND or BASMATI RICE until tender. Add 1 TB. BROWN RICE VINEGAR and let stand while you make the rest of the salad.

♣Sauté in 2 TBS. OIL until aromatic   ♣Add and sauté for 5 minutes
3 GREEN ONIONS   THE SHIITAKE MUSHROOMS
2 LEEKS SLICED, white parts only   1 RED BELL PEPPER, sliced thin
1 TB. GRATED FRESH GINGER   1 CUP BAMBOO SHOOTS or MUNG BEAN
                                                                          SPROUTS
♣Add rice and almonds and heat through. Remove from heat and let rest.

♣Make a large cup of BUTTER LETTUCE LEAVES, and fill with salad mixture; <u>or</u> roll up in 12-16 large ROMAINE LETTUCE leaves and put 3 to 4 on each salad plate

Nutritional analysis: per serving; 369 calories; 10mg. protein; 54gm. carbohydrate; 8gm. fiber; 14gm. fats; 0 cholesterol; 105mg. calcium; 3mg. iron; 152g. magnesium; 554mg. potassium; 23mg. sodium; 2mg.zinc.

High Fiber Vegetables

328 SAIGON GADO GADO

We know several guys who were in Vietnam during the war years. Gado Gado was a favorite thing to order during R & R in Saigon. They say this tastes like the real thing.
For 4 people:

♣Steam in a wok or other steamer for 8 or 9 minutes
2 CARROTS, sliced
2 CAKES OF TOFU in strips
1 CUP FRENCH CUT GREEN BEANS

♣Add and steam for 5 more minutes
1 SMALL ZUCCHIN,I sliced
1 CUP GREEN CABBAGE in julienne

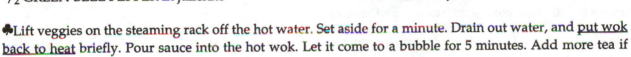

♣Make the sauce while veggies are steaming, so it will be ready when they are. Mix
$1/2$ CUP BLACK TEA
$1/4$ CUP PEANUT BUTTER
2 MINCED SHALLOTS
DASHES OF HOT PEPPER SAUCE
$1/2$ GREEN BELL PEPPER in julienne

2 TBS. MALT SYRUP or HONEY
1 TB. TAMARI
2 CHOPPED GREEN ONIONS
1 TB. LEMON JUICE

♣Lift veggies on the steaming rack off the hot water. Set aside for a minute. Drain out water, and put wok back to heat briefly. Pour sauce into the hot wok. Let it come to a bubble for 5 minutes. Add more tea if necessary.

♣Add vegetables back to wok with 1 CUP MUNG BEAN SPROUTS. Cook just to heat through, about 3 minutes. Serve over brown rice.

Nutritional analysis: per serving; 231 calories; 12gm. protein; 27gm. carbohydrate; 5gm. fiber; 11gm. fats; 0 cholesterol; 118mg. calcium; 5mg. iron; 119mg. magnesium; 658mg. potassium; 73mg. sodium; 1mg. zinc.

329 SPAGHETTI SQUASH SALAD

Spaghetti squash is a favorite in our family. Not only is it extremely low in calories and fat free, but it takes almost any savory sauce beautifully. It can be used with any pasta sauce easily and successfully.
For 4 servings:

♣Bake a $2^{1}/_{2}$ LB. SPAGHETTI SQUASH in a 350° oven on a baking pan for 30 minutes. Turn once and pierce shell with fork. Cut squash in half lengthwise and scoop out seeds. Return to the oven and bake for 30 more minutes until strands separate easily. Pull out strands with a fork into a bowl.

♣Add to the bowl and mix gently
1 CUP LOW-FAT PLAIN YOGURT
1 TB. FRUCTOSE
1 TB. CUMIN SEEDS ($1/2$ teasp. CUMIN POWDER)

1 TB. MINCED PARSLEY
2 teasp. MINCED FRESH BASIL
$1/4$ CUP CHOPPED WALNUTS

Nutritional analysis: per serving; 166 calories; 6gm. protein; 24gm. carbohydrates; 7gm. fiber; 6gm. fats; 3mg. cholesterol; 176mg. calcium; 2mg. iron; 54mg. magnesium; 474mg. potassium; 65mg. sodium; amg. zinc.

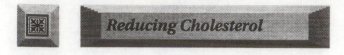
330   EASY ITALIAN POTATOES

Potatoes are high fiber, low fat foods, and work well with almost any seasoning.
For 6 servings: Preheat oven to 400°.

♣Slice 6 CUPS of BABY RED or WHITE NEW POTATOES. Mix with $1/3$ CUP CHOPPED ONION and 1 CUP of your favorite BOTTLED ITALIAN DRESSING.

♣Spoon into a shallow round pan. Cover tightly with foil. Bake 45 minutes until tender.

Nutritional analysis: perserving; 244 calories; 5gm. protein; 53gm. carbohydrate; 5gm. fiber; 2gm. fats; 1mg. cholesterol; 22mg. calcium; 3mg. iron; 56mg. magnesium; 861mg. potassium; 174mg. sodium; 1mg. zinc.

331   TWICE BAKED BROCCOLI POTATOES

For 4 potato halves:

♣Bake 2 LARGE RUSSET POTATOES at 400° until soft. Scoop out insides into a bowl and mash. Put shells in a shallow baking dish or pan and reserve.

♣Steam about $1 1/2$ CUPS CHOPPED BROCCOLI FLORETS and UPPER STEMS until color changes.
♣Drain and divide between potato shells.

♣Heat 2 TBS. OIL in a saucepan. Add 2 TBS. WHOLE WHEAT FLOUR and roux, stirring until blended.
♣Add and cook until bubbly and thickened

$3/4$ CUP PLAIN YOGURT	$1/2$ teasp. SESAME SALT
$1/4$ CUP WATER	1 teasp. TAMARI
$1/2$ CUP GRATED CHEDDAR	$1/4$ teasp. NUTMEG
1 teasp. SWEET MUSTARD	DASHES OF PAPRIKA

♣Mix with reserved potato meat for the filling. Spoon on top of broccoli, mounding as high as you can.
♣Sprinkle with a little more grated cheese if desired and bake at 350∞ for 15 minutes. Then run under the broiler for 30 seconds until brown and crusty.

Nutritional analysis: per serving; 304 calories; 11gm. protein; 39gm. carbohydrate; 4gm. fiber; 10gm. fats; 17mg. cholesterol; 213mg. calcium; 2mg. iron; 61mg. magnesium; 783mg. potassium; 1mg. zinc.

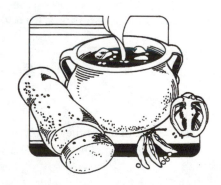

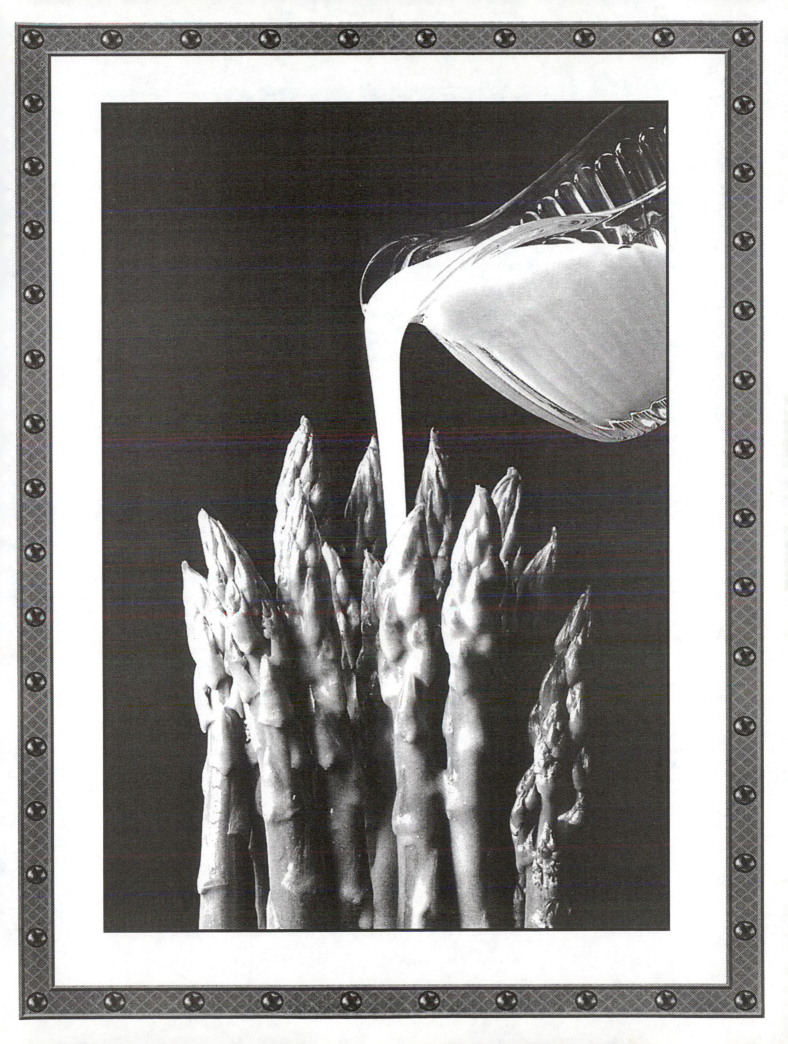

Dairy Free Cooking

For almost 25% of Americans, dairy intolerance can cause allergic reactions, poor digestion, and abnormal mucous build-up in the body. The human system in general does not easily process cow's milk, cream, ice cream or hard cheese. Our bodies tend to throw off excess from dairy foods, causing cumulative strain on eliminative organs, and system clogging as the unused matter turns to mucous. Dairy foods can interfere with the cleansing/healing process because of density and high saturated fats. Even people with no noticeable sensitivity to dairy products report a rise in energy when they stop using them as a main part of their diet. Because of high dairy fats, reduced intake usually means effective weight loss, and reduced blood pressure and cholesterol levels. In addition, women do not handle dairy products as well as men; their systems back up more easily. Many female problems, such as fibrous growths, bladder, and kidney ailments can be improved by avoiding dairy foods.
Contrary to advertising, dairy products are not even the most desirable source of calcium. Absorbability is poor because of pasteurizing, processing, high fat content, and unbalanced relationship with phosphorus. In tests with animals, calves given their own mother's milk that had first been pasteurized, didn't live six weeks. Hormone residues and additives from current cattle-raising practices, also indicate that calcium and other minerals are incompletely absorbed. Other foods, such as vegetables, nuts, seeds, fish and sea vegetables contain calcium that is much easier to assimilate. Soy cheese, tofu, soy milk, and nut milks can all be used successfully in place of dairy products. Kefir and yogurt, which although made from milk, are usually free of the assimilation problems of dairy products. Unless lactose intolerance is very severe, neither of these foods causes allergic reactions, and they are beneficial to the healing process because of the friendly bacteria cultures they add to the digestive tract.

Dairy foods should be avoided during a cleansing diet. In building and maintenance diets, consider most dairy products as wonderful for taste, but questionable for premium nutrition. A little is fine - a lot is not. Rich quality can still be achieved without cream, milk, butter, eggs or cheese. A small change in cooking habits and point of view are all it takes - mostly a matter of not having these products around the house, and substituting dairy-free alternatives in your favorite recipes. Soon you won't feel deprived at all. Just remember the easy weight you'll lose by not eating saturated dairy fats.

When you *do* opt for dairy foods, purchase low-fat or non-fat products; buy goat's milk, or raw milk and cheeses instead of pasteurized. Whole and full fat dairy foods are clearly not good if there is lactose intolerance or if you are on a mucous cleansing diet. There is a world of difference in taste. Raw, fresh cream cheese is light years ahead of commercial brands with gums, fillers and thickeners. Raw mozzarella, farmer cheese, ricotta and cheddar are also notably superior in taste to pasteurized cheeses or cheese foods with high salts and additives. Low-fat, raw cheeses also provide immediately usable protein, with a proper calcium/phosphorus/sodium ratio.

The dairy free recipes in this section emphasize the areas of diet where the creaminess and richness of dairy products are traditional and hard to omit.
❧DAIRY FREE APPETIZERS & HORS D'OEUVRES ❧NON-DAIRY DIPS & SPREADS ❧RICH NON-DAIRY SALAD TOPPINGS ❧DAIRY FREE SAUCES & GRAVIES ❧CREAMY SOUPS WITHOUT THE CREAM ❧NON-DAIRY DESSERTS ❧DAIRY FREE SWEET BAKING ❧

About Dairy Options - Alternatives To Milk, Cream, Eggs, and Cheese

❦Almond Milk - use one to one in place of milk in baked recipes, sauces or gravies. For 1 cup almond milk, blend in the blender until very smooth: 1 teasp. almond butter, 1 teasp. honey, 1 cup water.

❦Yogurt - a good intesinal cleanser and laxative, yogurt helps balance and replace friendly flora in the G.I. tract. Yogurt is dairy in origin, but the culturing process makes it a live food, and beneficial for health. There are several easy alternatives, cup for cup, as a replacement for milk in recipes: $1/2$ cup plain yogurt, mixed with $1/2$ cup water, broth, white wine, or sparkling water for lightness and consistency. For baking needs where special richness is desired, or for whipped cream consistency, whip $1/3$ the amount of heavy cream called for in the recipe, and fold in $2/3$ non-fat plain yogurt.

❦**Yogurt Cheese** - easy to make, much lighter in fat and calories than sour cream or cream cheese, but with the same richness and consistency. **Here's how to make it:**
Use a piece of cheesecloth or a sieve-like plastic funnel, (available from kitchen catalogs or hardware stores). Simply spoon in as much plain yogurt as you want (usually use about 16 oz.) and hang the cheesecloth over the sink faucet, or put the funnel over a large glass. It takes about 14 to 16 hours for the whey to drain out (whey is delicious used as part of the liquid in soups and stews), and voila! you have yogurt cheese. Stored in a covered container in the refrigerator, it will keep for 2 to 3 weeks.

❦**Kefir** - a cultured food made by adding kefir grains (naturally formed milk proteins), available at health food stores, to milk and letting it incubate overnight at room temperature to milkshake consistency. Kefir has 350mg. of calcium per cup. Use the plain flavor cup for cup as a replacement for whole milk, buttermilk or half and half; the fruit flavors may be used in sweet baked dishes.

❦**Kefir Cheese** - an excellent replacement for sour cream or cream cheese in dips and other recipes, kefir cheese is low in fat and calories, and has a slight tangy-rich flavor that really enhances snack foods. Use it cup for cup in place of sour cream, cottage cheese, cream cheese or ricotta.

❦**Soy Milk** - nutritious, versatile, smooth and delicious, soy milk is vegetable-based, lactose/cholesterol free, with unsaturated or poly-unsaturated fat. Studies show that using soy milk in your diet can help reduce serum cholesterol. Soymilk contains less calcium and calories than milk, and more protein and iron. It adds a slight rise to baked goods. Use it cup for cup as a milk replacement in cooking; plain flavor for savory dishes, vanilla for sweet dishes or on cereal.

❦**Soy Cheese** - made from soy milk, this non-dairy cheese is free of lactose and cholesterol. The small amount of calcium caseinate (a milk protein) added allows it to melt. Mozzarella, cheddar, jack and cream cheese types are available. Use it cup for cup in place of any low-fat or regular cheese.

❦**Soy Ice Cream, Frozen Desserts and Soy Yogurt** - now available in a variety of flavors. **Soy mayonnaise** has also finally been developed with the taste and consistency of dairy mayonnaise.

❦**Tofu** - a white, digestible curd made from soybeans, tofu is one of the best replacements for dairy foods, in texture, taste, and nutritional content. It is high in protein, low in fat and contains no cholesterol. It is available in several varieties, is extremely versatile, and may be used in place of eggs, sour cream, cheese and cottage cheese. See the **TOFU FOR YOU section on page 502 in this book for more information and recipes.**

❦**Miso** - a good dairy substitute in macrobiotic and cleansing/alkalizing diets. Light chickpea miso mixed with vegetable or onion stock is a tasty replacement for milk and seasonings.

❦**Lecithin** - a soy product, low in fat and cholesterol that helps thicken and emulsify ingredients without using dairy foods. It can make many recipes extra rich and smooth. Add a tablespoon of lecithin granules to a sauce, custard dessert or homemade ice-y dessert.

❦**Sesame Tahini** - a rich, smooth, creamy product made from ground sesame seeds. Tahini may be used in place of cream or sour cream in dips, sauces and gravies. Mixed with water to milk consistency, use it as a high protein milk substitute in baking. It is an excellent complement to greens and salad ingredients. Mix tahini with oil and other ingredients for salad toppings.

About Low-Fat Cottage Cheese - a low-fat, cultured dairy product, cottage cheese is beneficial for those with only slight lactose intolerance, and is a good substitute for ricotta, commercial cream cheese, and processed cottage cheese foods that are full of chemicals. Mix with non-fat or low-fat plain yogurt to add the richness of cream or sour cream to recipes without the fat.

⚜

About Butter - Surprise! Butter is okay in moderation. Although butter is a saturated fat, it is relatively stable and the body can use it in small amounts for energy. Its make-up, like that of raw cream, is a whole and balanced food, used by the body better than its separate components might indicate. When butter is needed, use raw, unsalted butter, never margarine, pasteurized butter or shortening. Don't let butter get hot enough to sizzle or smoke. If less saturation is desired, use clarified butter. Simply melt the butter. Skim off the top foam. Remove from heat. Let rest a few minutes, and spoon off the clear butter for use. Discard whey solids that settle to the bottom of the pan.
High quality **vegetable oil** may almost always be substituted for butter without loss of taste in a sauté or stir-fry. **Soy margarine** is an acceptable vegetarian alternative for baking.

⚜

About Eggs - More good news! "Eggsperts" are finally realizing what many of us in the whole foods world have long known. Although high in cholesterol, eggs are also high in balancing lecithins and phosphatides, **and do not increase the risk of atherosclerosis.** Nutrition-rich fertile eggs from free-run-and-scratch chickens are a perfect food. The difference in fertile eggs and the products from commercial egg factories is remarkable; the yolk color is brighter, the flavor definitely fresher, and the workability in recipes better. The distinction is particularly noticeable in poached and baked eggs, where the yolks firm up and rise higher. Many health food stores stock locally supplied fresh eggs. Eggs should be lightly cooked for the best nutrition, preferably poached, soft-boiled, or baked, never fried. As concentrated protein, use them with discretion.
Egg Replacer Mix made from potato starch and tapioca flour is a viable substitue for baking needs.

Tofu may be used in place of eggs in quick breads, cakes, custard-based dishes and quiches.

Flax seeds and water mixed can replace eggs in quick breads, pancakes and muffins. Use $1/4$ cup flax seeds to $3/4$ cup water. Whirl in the blender until <u>thoroughly</u> crushed, and add to batter in place of 3 eggs. Flax seeds are healthful in them selves as a source of soluble and insoluble fiber, and an aid to regularity. They are also rich in lignans. High levels of lignans in the digestive tract have been associated with the reduced risk of colon and breast cancer.

⚜

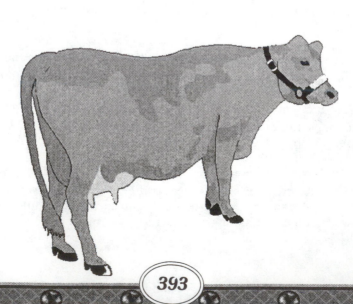

Dairy Free Appetizers & Hors D'oeuvres

Appetizers and snacks without cheese or dairy-rich fillings seems almost like a contradiction in terms.
A small sampling is offered in this section to give you inspiration in the right direction. We have served
these recipes many times to compliments, even at gatherings where no one had a problem with dairy foods.

332   ITALIAN TOMATO TOAST

For 6 to 8 servings: Preheat oven to 350°.

♣Slice 1 LOAF of ITALIAN LONG BREAD in 1/4" slices. Lay on a lecithin-sprayed baking sheet and drizzle 4 TBS. OLIVE OIL over the slices. Toast in the oven for 10 minutes. Leave oven on.

♣Line a shallow baking dish with <u>half</u> the slices. Patch any empty spaces with bits of toast. Slice 4 LARGE TOMATOES and arrange overlapped on top. Drizzle with 2 TBS. OLIVE OIL. Season with SEA SALT, PEPPER and a PINCH OF FRUCTOSE. Top with 2 TBS. MINCED PARSLEY. Cover with the rest of the toast. Drizzle with 2 TBS. OLIVE OIL.

♣Toast 2 WHOLE WHEAT ENGLISH MUFFINS or equivalent slices SOURDOUGH BREAD in the oven; or use equivalent SEASONED BREAD CRUMBS. Crumb in the blender with 6 TBS. SOY PARMESAN CHEESE, and scatter over dish. Bake uncovered for 45 minutes until light brown.
♣Then cover with foil and bake for 15 minutes until soft.

Nutritional analysis: per serving; 248 calories; 5gm. protein; 21gm. carbohydrate; 2gm. fiber; 16gm. fats; 2mg. cholesterol; 106mg. calcium; 2mg. iron; 26mg. magnesium; 329mg. potassium; 270mg. sodium; trace zinc.

333   FRESH HERB EGGPLANT ROLLS

Even people who have never liked eggplant (like my husband), like this.
For 8 to 10 appetizer servings: Preheat oven to 375°.

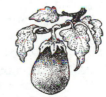

♣Trim, stem and peel a large eggplant. Cut in quarters, and then into 8ths for 32 slices 1/8" thick.

♣Mix 3 TBS. OLIVE OIL with 2 teasp. GARLIC/LEMON SEASONING. Brush on 3 baking pans. Lay on eggplant slices in a single layer. Brush with remaining oil and bake until soft and brown, about 10 to 12 minutes. Do not let scorch. Loosen with a spatula and let cool on the baking pan.

♣Mix in a small bowl
1 TB. OLIVE OIL
8 OZ. SOY MOZZARELLA, cut in 32 two inch pieces   2 teasp. FRESH or DRY ROSEMARY
3 TBS. FRESH CHOPPED BASIL (1 teasp. DRY)   2 teasp. FRESH OREGANO (1/2 teasp. DRY)

♣Place a piece of cheese on the narrow end of the eggplant slice. Roll to enclose. Place seam side down on an ovenproof platter. Season lightly and heat just before serving.

Nutritional analysis: per serving; 116 calories; 2gm. protein; 3gm. carbohydrate; 11gm. fats; 0 cholesterol; 40mg. calcium; 1mg. iron; 26mg. magnesium; 104mg. potassium; 3mg. sodium; trace zinc.

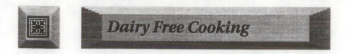

334　SULTAN'S PURSES

For 60 steamed pouches:

♣Soak 4 to 6 DRIED BLACK MUSHROOMS to soften. Sliver and set aside. Reserve soaking water.
♣Trim white and green parts from a LARGE BUNCH OF SCALLIONS separately.
♣Set aside $1/4$ CUP CHOPPED GREEN PARTS for topping.

♣Bring 2 CUPS WATER to a rapid boil. Add $1/4$ teasp. BAKING SODA and the SCALLION PARTS and blanch until bright green, 2 minutes. Drain and rinse under cold water. Cut into matchsticks.

♣Blend the filling in the blender to a savory paste
8 OZ.　TINY COOKED SHRIMP
1 teasp. TAMARI
$1^1/_2$ teasp. FRUCTOSE
1 EGG WHITE (opt.)
$1^1/_2$ teasp. FRESH GRATED GINGER
1 TB. WHITE or RICE WINE

2 TBS. ARROWROOT or KUZU
1 teasp. SESAME SALT (GOMASHIO)
$1^1/_2$ teasp. TOASTED SESAME OIL
$1^1/_2$ TBS. PEANUT OIL
$1/4$ teasp. GROUND PEPPER

♣Turn into a bowl, add $1/4$ CUP DICED WATER CHESTNUTS and $1/4$ CUP FROZEN GREEN PEAS. Mix lightly, and chill.

♣Purchase and separate 60 skins from a package of won ton wrappers. Put about 1 teaspoon of filling in the center of each. Draw the four points of the sides together, seal edges with water, and twist the top to form a drawstring "purse." Chill while steaming water is coming to a boil.
♣Use a large steamer or wok with a steaming rack, and bring an inch of water to a boil. Lay lettuce leaves on the rack, and put purses in a single layer on the leaves. Steam for 10 minutes. Transfer to a lettuce-lined serving plate. Sprinkle with reserved scallions.

♣Mix 3 TBS. DRY MUSTARD or CHINESE HOT MUSTARD POWDER in a bowl with $1^1/_2$ teasp. HOT PEPPER SAUCE and enough water to make a dip for the tops of the purses.

Nutritional analysis: per pouch; 75 calories; 5gm. protein; 9gm. carbohydrates; 1gm. fiber; 3gm. fats; 29mg. cholesterol; 20mg. calcium; 2mg. iron; 51mg. magnesium; 153mg. potassium; 120mg. sodium; trace zinc.

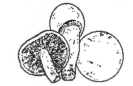

335　SHERRY MUSHROOMS ON RYE

For 8 to 10 servings:

♣Heat 6 TBS. OLIVE OIL and 1 teasp. GARLIC/LEMON SEASONING in a skillet until hot. Add $3/4$ CUP CHOPPED RED ONIONS (ONE SMALL) and sauté until translucent.
♣Add $1^1/_2$ LBS. BUTTON MUSHROOMS and toss until they stop producing liquid, about 20 minutes.
♣Add $3/4$ CUP SHERRY or VERMOUTH, some DASHES of SESAME SALT and WHITE PEPPER, and simmer until liquid evaporates, about 10 minutes
♣Serve hot on TOASTED RYE COCKTAIL ROUNDS.

336   WHITE BEAN PATÉ WITH HERBS

♣Blend everything in the blender
2 CUPS COOKED WHITE BEANS
$1/2$ teasp. **each:** <u>DRY</u> BASIL, THYME, DILL WEED, TARRAGON
1 teasp. GARLIC/LEMON SEASONING or 2 CLOVES GARLIC, minced
$1/2$ CUP PEELED DICED SHALLOTS

$1^1/2$ TB. <u>FRESH</u> MINCED GARDEN HERBS	1 teasp. DIJON MUSTARD
1 TB. CAPERS	$1/4$ teasp. NUTMEG
1 TB. SESAME TAHINI	$1/2$ teasp. WHITE PEPPER
2 TBS. FRESH SNIPPED PARSLEY	$1/2$ teasp. SEASONING SALT

♣Add DASHES of HOT PEPPER SAUCE to taste. Transfer to a serving dish. Snip on more fresh herbs to cover the top. Chill briefly and serve.

Nutritional analysis: per 2 oz. serving; 86 calories; 5gm. protein; 14gm. carbohydrates; 4gm. fiber; 1gm. fats; 0 cholesterol; 51mg. calcium; 2mg. iron; 43mg. magnesium; 274mg. potassium; 70mg. sodium; 1mg. zinc.

337   DAIRY FREE MUSHROOM PATÉ

For 1 cup; 4 servings:

♣Soak 1-OZ. BLACK SHIITAKE MUSHROOMS in water until soft. Sliver and discard woody stems.
♣Mix with 5-OZ. CHOPPED BUTTON MUSHROOMS and $1/3$ CUP MINCED ONION.
♣Sauté the mixture in 2 to 3 TBS. OIL for 15 minutes until softened.
♣Add 1 TB. SHERRY, $1/2$ CARTON KEFIR CHEESE or SOY CREAM CHEESE or 1 CAKE TOFU CRUMBLED, and $1/4$ CUP CHOPPED FRESH PARSLEY.
♣Whirl in the blender if a smooth paté is desired, or pack into a thick crock. Chill overnight or longer (it just gets better if covered well, up to a week). Use cocktail knives to spread on toasted rye rounds.

Nutritional analysis: per serving; 124 calories; 4gm. protein; 10gm. carbohydrates; 4gm. fiber; 8gm. fats; 0 cholesterol; 41mg. calcium; 2mg. iron; 46mg. magnesium; 523mg. potassium; 1mg. zinc.

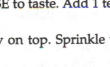

338   JALAPEÑO POTATO BITES

♣Cut SMALL RED POTATOES in half and steam until tender. Scoop out some of the meat from the cut side to leave a shell for filling.
♣Mix potato meat with SOY BACON BITS and GRATED SOY JALAPEÑO CHEESE to taste. Add 1 teasp. WORCESTERSHIRE SAUCE and $1/4$ teasp. BLACK PEPPER.
♣Stuff potato shells. Arrange on a baking sheet and broil until brown and crispy on top. Sprinkle with PAPRIKA and serve with toothpicks.

Nutritional analysis: per 2 "bite" serving; 166 calories; 3gm. protein; 22gm. carbohydrate; 2gm. fiber; 7gm. fats; 0 cholesterol; 26mg. calcium; 2mg. iron; 40mg. magnesium; 382mg. potassium; 43mg. sodium; trace zinc.

Creamy Dairy Free Dips & Spreads

This section shows how to successfully substitute dairy free products in your favorite dip and spread recipes, without depriving yourself of their creamy richness. The decision to omit dairy just means thinking in terms of soy cheeses or tofu in place of cheeses, and yogurt, yogurt cheese or kefir cheese in place of sour cream, cream cheese or cottage cheese. If a total vegan diet is desired, sesame tahini, tofu, avocados and ground nuts or nut milk may be used to replace dairy foods, while still offering richness and good taste.

339   TRIPLE HOT TOFU GUACAMOLE

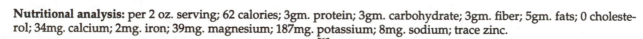

For about 8 servings:

♣ Mash all together in a bowl
1 LARGE AVOCADO, peeled and seeded
1 teasp. ONION POWDER
1 teasp. CHILI POWDER
1/4 teasp. HOT SAUCE or SAMBAL OELEK (Found in oriental food stores. Very very hot)
2 TBS. LEMON JUICE
1 SMALL CHOPPED TOMATO
1/4 teasp. PAPRIKA
2 CAKES MASHED TOFU
♣ Serve with spicy rice chips, tamari chips or vegetable crackers.

Nutritional analysis: per 2 oz. serving; 62 calories; 3gm. protein; 3gm. carbohydrate; 3gm. fiber; 5gm. fats; 0 cholesterol; 34mg. calcium; 2mg. iron; 39mg. magnesium; 187mg. potassium; 8mg. sodium; trace zinc.

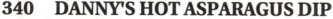

340   DANNY'S HOT ASPARAGUS DIP

This creation is a simple delight from a former produce manager at The Country Store Natural Foods who used to wax poetic when the first organic asparagus of the season appeared.
For 2 to 3 servings:

♣ Sauté 1 SMALL CHOPPED RED ONION to soften and bring up the sweetness.
♣ Steam 1 BUNCH ASPARAGUS lightly. Chop and blender blend with ONE 8-OZ. CARTON KEFIR CHEESE, 1/2 teasp. SESAME SALT and THE ONIONS until smooth.

341   SURPRISE DIP AND SPREAD

The base of this dip is pureed vegetables - excellent for those with dairy sensitivities. Every combination is surprisingly different, and almost every combination works. If you liked it yesterday as a soup or salad or casserole, you will like it as a dip today. Leftover lentil, black bean or pea soup are especially good.

♣Take *any* left-over salad and dressing, <u>or</u> leftover steamed veggies and sauce, <u>or</u> the last serving of a vegetable casserole, <u>or</u> the remains of yesterday's vegetable soup, and puree it in the blender. Sometimes that's all there is to it; a delicious raw veggie or cracker spread just as it is.
♣If it needs more spice, add something for richness, such as favorite SPICES and HERBS, a CUBE of TOFU, an AVOCADO, a LITTLE SESAME TAHINI, or KEFIR CHEESE.

342   GINGER DIP WITH TOFU

Makes about 2 cups:

♣Blender blend and chill to let flavors bloom. Serve with 6 cups sliced, chunked raw vegetables.

1 LB. CREAMY SOFT TOFU
1/4 CUP CHOPPED GREEN ONION
1/2 teasp. GARLIC/LEMON SEASONING

1 TB. TOASTED SESAME OIL
2 TBS. TAMARI
PINCH CAYENNE

343   THREE STAR DIP FOR RAW VEGETABLES

This is very versatile, kind of like a citrus guacamole. It can be made hot or mild to taste.
Makes about 3 cups:

♣Blender blend

1 AVOCADO, seeded and chopped
1 GRAPEFRUIT, seeded and sectioned
1 TOMATO, seeded and chopped
1 TB. MINCED FRESH HERBS of your choice

1/2 teasp. CHILI POWDER
1 teasp. SESAME SALT
1/4 teasp. PEPPER

Nutritional analysis: per 2 oz. serving; 53 calories; 1gm. protein; 5gm. carbohydrate; 3gm. fiber; 4gm. fats; 0 cholesterol; 9mg. calcium; trace iron; 15mg. magnesium; 223mg. potassium; 93mg. sodium; trace zinc.

344   NUT BUTTER DELIGHT

This is a stiff spread; delicious on raw celery sticks or apple crescents. It is best served chilled.
For 2 cups:

♣Toast in the oven until golden and aromatic

3 TBS. SUNFLOWER SEEDS
3 TBS. SESAME SEEDS
4 TBS. CASHEWS

♣Grind in the blender until buttery with

1 CUP PEANUT BUTTER
1/2 CUP SESAME TAHINI

345   TOFU TAHINI DIP

For 1 cup:

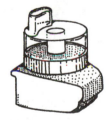

♣Blender blend everything together

2 TBS. BALSAMIC or RASPBERRY VINEGAR
2 TBS. WHITE WINE
1 GREEN ONION, chopped
1/2 CUP FRESH MINCED PARSLEY
1 CUBE TOFU
1/4 CUP SESAME TAHINI

1 teasp. TOASTED SESAME OIL
1 TB. TAMARI
1 TB. LEMON JUICE
1/2 teasp. SESAME SALT
1/4 teasp. BLACK PEPPER
1/4 teasp. PAPRIKA

Nutritional analysis: per 2 oz. serving; 136 calories; 6gm. protein; 5gm. carbohydrate; 2gm. fiber; 11gm. fats; 0 cholesterol; 67mg. calcium; 3mg. iron; 89mg. magnesium; 180mg. potassium; 143mg. sodium; 2mg. zinc.

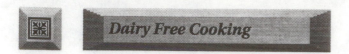

346   HOT GREEN BEAN & POTATO PUREE

For 6 servings: Preheat oven to 450°.

♣ Cook 1 LB. RED or WHITE DICED POTATOES in boiling salted water for 10 minutes.
♣ Add 1 LB. FROZEN GREEN BEANS, partially cover pot, and cook for 7 to 10 minutes more. Drain.
♣ Puree in the blender with 5 TBS. OIL or BUTTER, and NUTMEG, SALT and PEPPER to taste.
♣ Scrape into a lecithin-sprayed gratin dish. Bake for 15 minutes until a skin forms on the top, and puree is heated through. Serve immediately with crackers or rye rounds.

✳

347   NUTTY TOFU SPREAD

This recipe is very different; good with dunkers or by itself. Pack it into individual oiled scalloped shells and chill. Serve in the shell with crackers or toast, or unmold onto large lettuce leaves, and top with sesame seeds.
About 1 1/2 cups, for 4 to 6 people:

♣ Mix in the blender to a paste

1/2 carton KEFIR CHEESE	1 TB. HONEY
2 CUBES TOFU	1 TB. MINCED PARSLEY
3 TBS. ALMOND BUTTER	2 TBS. TOASTED SESAME SEEDS
1 teasp. VANILLA or ALMOND EXTRACT	

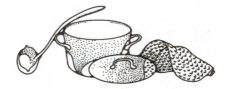

Cream Soups Without The Cream

Hearty cream soups often get their richness from the fats in dairy foods, with taste that is hard to forget.
The soups in this section are creamy and satisfying without the dairy. You'll never miss it.

348   "CREAM" OF ASPARAGUS SOUP

For 4 servings:

♣ Cut off woody bottom stems and slice 1 BUNCH (about 1 LB.) FRESH ASPARAGUS. Blanch in hot water until color changes to bright green. Drain and rinse in cold water.
♣ Heat 4 TBS. OIL and add 4 TBS. WHOLE GRAIN FLOUR in a soup pot. Roux and stir until well blended and aromatic. Add 1 CUP CHICKEN or ONION STOCK and blend well.
♣ Place asparagus pieces except tops in the blender and whirl briefly with 1/3 CUP WHITE WINE.
♣ Add to the soup pot. Add 2 MORE CUPS STOCK and heat until blended. Add in 1 TB. mixed herbs to taste such as THYME, ROSEMARY or BASIL. Season with HERB SALT and PEPPER. Top with reserved asparagus tops and serve.

Nutritional analysis: per 1 cup serving; 156 calories; 10gm. carbohydrate; 4gm. protein; 2gm. fiber; 11gm. fats; 0 cholesterol; 48mg. calcium; 1mg. iron; 33mg. magnesium; 381mg. potassium; 179mg. sodium; 1mg. zinc.

✳

349 ONION ALMOND CREAM

For 6 servings:

♣Sauté 4 or 5 CHOPPED ONIONS in 3 TBS. OIL or BROTH until aromatic. Add 1¹/₂ CUP CHOPPED ALMONDS and sauté til both are browned, about 20 minutes. Puree in the blender until creamy.
♣Pour into a soup pot and add 7 CUPS ONION STOCK or *RICH BROWN STOCK* (page 652) and 1 CUP WHITE WINE. Cover and cook over low heat for 20 minutes. Season with SALT and PEPPER.

♣Place a SLICE OF TOAST on the bottom of each soup plate. Sprinkle with grated SOY MOZARRELLA CHEESE. Pour soup over and serve.

Nutritional analysis: per serving; 231 calories; 6gm. protein; 15gm. carbohydrate; 4gm. fiber; 15gm. fats; 1mg. cholesterol; 110mg. calcium; 1mg. iron; 79mg. magnesium; 317mg. potassium; 201mg. sodium; 1mg. zinc.

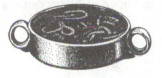

350 CREAMY TOMATO ONION

For 8 servings:

♣Sauté 2 CUPS CHOPPED ONION in 2 TBS. OIL in a large soup pot for 5 minutes until aromatic.
♣Add 1 CUP CHOPPED CARROTS and 1 CUP CHOPPED CELERY and sauté for 5 more minutes.
♣Whirl a few seconds in the blender with 1 CUP TOMATO JUICE.
♣Pour back into soup pot and add

3 more CUPS TOMATO JUICE	3 TBS. ONION BROTH POWDER
1 CUP WHITE WINE	2 TBS. TAMARI
1 CUP WATER	¹/₄ CUP ALMOND BUTTER

♣Heat and stir occasionally about 10 to 15 minutes. Serve tasty hot.

Nutritional analysis: per serving; 148 calories; 3gm. protein; 13gm. carbohydrates; 3gm. fiber; 8gm. fats; 0 cholesterol; 56mg. calcium; 1mg. iron; 50mg. magnesium; 512mg. potassium; 77mg. sodium; trace zinc.

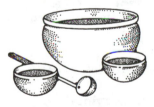

351 CREAMY BROCCOLI SOUP

For 4 servings:

♣Add 1 BUNCH CHOPPED BROCCOLI and 1 SMALL CHOPPED ONION to 3 CUPS BOILING WATER. Simmer for 5 minutes. Remove vegetables with a slotted spoon and put into a blender.
♣Add 1 teasp. TARRAGON, 2 VEGETABLE BOUILLON CUBES (**or** 2 teasp. vegetable or onion broth mix), ¹/₂ teasp. SAVORY, and ¹/₄ teasp. CHERVIL. Whirl briefly, and return to pot.

♣Put 1 CUP OVEN TOASTED CASHEWS in the blender with ¹/₂ cup of the soup and blend briefly.
♣Add back to soup. Stir to blend. Cover and simmer gently for 5 minutes.
♣Serve with a few cashews sprinkled on top.

352   SESAME MUSHROOM SOUP
This soup is rich in non-dairy protein.
For 6 servings:

♣Sauté briefly in 2 TBS. OIL until fragrant
1 LARGE CHOPPED ONION
1 teasp. grated FRESH GINGER ROOT
1/2 teasp. DRY BASIL (or 1 TB. FRESH MINCED)
PINCH CAYENNE

♣Add and sauté for 7 to 10 minutes
 3 STALKS SLICED CELERY
 2 CUPS SLICED MUSHROOMS
 1/2 teasp. SESAME or HERB SALT
 1/4 teasp. BLACK PEPPER

♣Add and simmer about 15 to 20 minutes
4 CUPS CHOPPED TOMATOES
1/2 CUP VEGETABLE STOCK
1/2 WHITE WINE

3 TBS. PEANUT BUTTER
2 TBS. SESAME TAHINI

♣Add 1 CAKE TOFU in 1/2" dice, and simmer 5 minutes.

♣Serve hot with a little dry or fresh cilantro sprinkled on top.

Dairy Free Sauces & Gravies

It's often hard to imagine some sauces without the dairy products that give them creaminess. But almond or cashew milk, or yogurt or kefir are easy to substitute, and still get all the good taste you want.

ALMOND OR CASHEW NUT MILK
Almond milk is a rich, non-dairy liquid that may be used as a base for cream soups, sauces, gravies and protein drinks. Use it in baking for cakes and other desserts, including cheesecakes. It makes any recipe rich.

♣Put 1 CUP ALMONDS (toasted or raw) in the blender with 2 to 4 CUPS WATER, depending on how thick you want the liquid, (milk, half and half, or cream consistency). Add 1 teasp. honey, and whirl.

Nutritional analysis: per serving; 215 calories; 7gm. protein; 8gm. carbohydrate; 4gm. fiber; 18gm. fat; 0 cholesterol; 97mg. calcium; 1mg. iron; 106mg. magnesium; 260mg. potassium; 7mg. sodium; 1mg. zinc.

ALMOND MILK GRAVY

For four 5oz. servings:

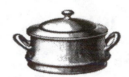

♣Pureé in the blender until smooth
2 CUPS WATER
1 CUP CHOPPED ALMONDS
2 TBS. SNIPPED FRESH PARSLEY
1 TB. CHOPPED CELERY
1/2 teasp. CHOPPED DRIED ONION

2 TBS. WHOLE WHEAT FLOUR
1/4 teasp. ONION POWDER
 2 TBS. OIL
1/4 teasp. TAMARI

♣Pour into a pan and cook, stirring over medium heat until thick and creamy.

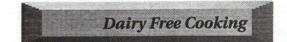
353   DEFINITELY GOURMET MUSHROOM SAUCE

For this recipe, the more exotic the mushrooms, the better the sauce.
For 2 cups:

♣Soak 6 BLACK DRY SHIITAKE MUSHROOMS in WATER or WHITE WINE. Slice into thin strips; discard woody stems and reserve soaking liquid.

♣Mix with 1/2 package FRESH ENOKI MUSHROOMS (or 1/3 of a can) with tough stems removed.

♣Add 4 to 6 FRESH THIN-SLICED CHANTERELLES or BUTTON MUSHROOMS.

♣Put 1/2 CUP MUSHROOM SOAKING LIQUID in a saucepan. Bring to a boil and add 1 MINCED ONION, 1/2 DICED RED BELL PEPPER, 1 teasp. TAMARI, 1/4 teasp. ROSEMARY and 1/4 teasp. GARLIC GRANULES. Cover, reduce heat and cook 15 minutes. Uncover and cook to evaporate liquid. Continue cooking until onions brown and are aromatic.

♣Add 2 TBS. BALSAMIC VINEGAR to the pan. Stir, scraping up brown bits. Puree in the blender using more of the soaking water for consistency. Return to the saucepan. Add mushrooms and rest of soaking water. Simmer for 30 minutes until sauce is reduced to half to intensify flavor.

Nutritional analysis: per serving; 22 calories; 1 gm. protein; 5gm. carbohydrate; 2gm. fiber; trace fats; 0 cholesterol; 7mg. calcium; trace iron; 8mg. magnesium; 32mg. potassium; 9mg. sodium; trace zinc.

354   CREAMY KEFIR CHEESE SAUCE FOR STEAMED VEGGIES

Makes about 2 1/2 cups:

♣Blender blend until creamy

1/2 CUP LEMON JUICE	4 TBS. SESAME SEEDS
1 CARTON KEFIR CHEESE	6 TBS. HONEY
4 TBS. BRAGG'S LIQUID AMINOS or VEGEX BROTH	1 1/2 teasp. SESAME SALT

Nutritional analysis: per serving; 159 calories; 4gm. protein; 26gm. carbohydrate; 6gm. fats; 5mg. cholesterol; 71mg. calcium; 1mg. iron; 36mg. magnesium; 150mg. potassium; 240mg. sodium; 1mg. zinc.

355   LEMON SESAME SAUCE

This sauce is excellent for chicken salads, turkey breast slices, roast yams or potatoes, and a good choice for a strict diet to control candida albicans.
For 1 cup:

♣Whisk all ingredients together.

1 TB. HONEY	1/4 CUP LEMON JUICE
1/4 CUP WATER, WHITE WINE or CHICKEN BROTH	1/2 teasp. SEA SALT
1/2 CUP SESAME TAHINI	1/2 teasp. LEMON JUICE

Nutritional analysis: per serving; 203 calories; 5gm. protein; 11gm. carbohydrate; 3gm. fiber; 0 cholesterol; 46mg. calcium; 1mg. iron; 108mg. magnesium; 163mg. potassium; 286mg. sodium; 3mg. zinc.

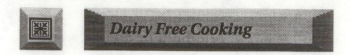

356 TOFU OR TEMPEH PASTA SAUCE
This sauce is for those of you who love meaty spaghetti sauces.
For about 4 cups:

♣Shake 8 OZ. FIRM TOFU or TEMPEH in a bag with 1/2 CUP FLOUR, SALT and PEPPER to coat.
♣Brown in 2 TBS. OLIVE OIL. Remove with a slotted spoon and set aside.

♣Keep skillet hot and sauté until aromatic
2 LARGE CHOPPED ONIONS
2 CLOVES MINCED GARLIC
1 teasp. DRY BASIL

♣Add and sauté for 5 minutes
1 CHOPPED GREEN PEPPER
1 CHOPPED RED PEPPER
4 OZ. SLICED MUSHROOMS

♣Add tofu or tempeh cubes back to the skillet. Then add ONE 28-OZ. CAN ROMA STYLE TOMATOES with juice, 1 TB. HONEY, 1/2 teasp. TARRAGON, and 1/2 teasp. OREGANO. Bring to a boil.
♣Reduce heat. Cover and simmer 10 minutes. Uncover and simmer 10 minutes. Season again.
♣Serve over spaghetti or rotelli.

Nutritional analysis: per serving; 101 calories; 5gm. protein; 14gm. carbohydrate; 3gm. fiber; 3gm. fats; 0 cholesterol; 67mg. calcium; 3mg. iron; 54mg. magnesium; 377mg. potassium; 66mg. sodium; trace zinc.

357 COLD CUCUMBER SAUCE
This is delicious over cold seafood such as salmon or prawns; a lovely change from cocktail sauce.
For 6 servings:

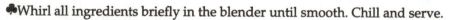

♣Whirl all ingredients briefly in the blender until smooth. Chill and serve.
2 CUCUMBERS, peeled and chunked
4 to 6 GREEN ONIONS sliced
1/4 CUP PLAIN YOGURT
1 TB. DILL WEED
1/4 teasp. LEMON PEPPER

2 TBS. FRESH PARSLEY, minced
1 TB. FRESH MINT, minced
1 teasp. TARRAGON VINEGAR
1/4 teasp. CELERY SEED
1/4 teasp. HERB SEASONING

Nutritional analysis: per 2 oz.serving; 25 calories; 1gm. protein; 5gm. carbohydrate; 2gm. fiber; trace fats; 0 cholesterol; 54mg. calcium; 1mg. iron; 18mg. magnesium; 233mg. potassium; 14mg. sodium; trace zinc.

358 SPINACH TOFU TOPPING WITH FRESH BASIL
Use this chlorophyll-rich sauce on rice, pasta or steamed vegetables.
For 8 servings:

♣Steam 1 BUNCH WASHED STEMMED SPINACH LEAVES and 2 LOOSELY PACKED CUPS WASHED STEMMED BASIL LEAVES briefly until *just wilted* and color changes to bright green.
♣Add 1 teasp. LEMON/GARLIC SEASONING, and 1 teasp. TAMARI. Toss to coat leaves.
♣Blender blend 1 LB. CUBED TOFU and 1/2 CUP SESAME TAHINI until smooth. Add spinach mixture and blend until creamy. Reheat briefly. Serve hot topped with 2 TBS. TOASTED SESAME SEEDS.

359 PARSLEY ALMOND PESTO

This is a delicate pesto for pasta or rice, and especially for new, steamed or baked potatoes. Unlike basil pestos, the ingredients are always in season!
Enough for 6 servings:

♣Blend everything in the blender

1 CUP FRESH CHOPPED PARSLEY

1/2 CUP TOASTED CHOPPED ALMONDS

1/4 teasp. LEMON HERB SEASONING

1/2 CUP OLIVE OIL

2 TBS. LEMON JUICE

1/4 teasp. WHITE PEPPER

Nutritional analysis: per 2 oz. serving; 164 calories; trace protein; 1gm. carbohydrates; trace fiber; 17gm. fats; 0 cholesterol; 14mg. calcium; 1mg. iron; 5mg. magnesium; 62mg. potassium; 9mg. sodium; trace zinc.

Creamy Rich Salad Toppings

Your salads will love these dairy free dressings; and so will your taste buds and your bathroom scale.

360 TAHINI POPPY SEED DRESSING

For 6 servings:

♣Blend to smooth in the blender

4 TBS. SESAME TAHINI

1 TB. LEMON JUICE

2 TBS. HONEY

2 TBS. POPPY SEEDS

1/2 teasp. BLACK PEPPER

1/2 teasp. GRATED ORANGE PEEL

1 teasp. TAMARI

1/4 teasp. NUTMEG

♣Fill to 1 cup with SALAD OIL and blend until combined.

Nutritional anaylsis: per 2 oz.serving; 203 calories; 3 gm. protein; 10gm. carbohydrate; 2gm. fiber; 17gm. fats; 0 cholesterol; 41mg. calcium; 1mg. iron; 41mg. magnesium; 106mg. potassium; 15mg. sodium; 1mg. zinc.

361 TARRAGON SALAD CREAM

For about 6 servings:

3 CUBES SOFT TOFU (about 12 oz.)

1/4 CUP OLIVE OIL

1/4 CUP TARRAGON VINEGAR

1 teasp. DRY TARRAGON.

1/4 teasp. BLACK PEPPER

1 GREEN ONION, CHOPPED

1 TB. HONEY

Nutrirional analysis: per 2 oz.serving; 102 calories; 4gm. protein; 4gm. carbohydrate; trace fiber; 9gm. fats; 0 cholesterol; 49mg. calcium; 2mg. iron; 45mg. magnesium; 72mg. potassium; 4mg. sodium; trace zinc.

362   CREAMY GREEN DRESSING

For about 2 cups:

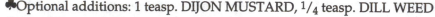

♣Whirl briefly to blend in the blender

³/₄ CUP OIL
2 TBS. TARRAGON VINEGAR (or lemon juice)
2 CHOPPED GREEN ONIONS
6 to 8 SPINACH or ROMAINE LEAVES
2 TBS. FRESH MINCED PARSLEY

¹/₄ teasp. DRY BASIL
¹/₄ teasp. MARJORAM
¹/₂ teasp. SESAME SALT
1 teasp. HONEY
¹/₄ teasp. GROUND PEPPER

♣Optional additions: 1 teasp. DIJON MUSTARD, ¹/₄ teasp. DILL WEED
♣Add slowly while blending ¹/₂ CUP PLAIN YOGURT and ¹/₄ CUP WATER until dressing thickens. Chill to blend flavors before serving.

Nutritional analysis: per 2 oz. serving; 196 calories; 1 gm. protein; 3gm. carbohydrate; trace fiber; 20gm. fats; trace cholesterol; 39mg. calcium; trace iron; 10mg. magnesium; 95mg. potassium; 55mg. sodium; trace zinc.

363   ALMOND TOMATO FRENCH

For 1¹/₂ cups:

♣Toast 3 to 4 TBS. CHOPPED ALMONDS in the oven or a skillet. Blend in the blender with
1 CUP CHOPPED TOMATOES

¹/₂ CUP OLIVE OIL
¹/₄ CUP SALAD OIL
2 TBS. BALSAMIC VINEGAR
2 TBS. CHOPPED FRESH PARSLEY
1¹/₂ TBS. HONEY

1 TBS. TAMARI
2 TBS. LEMON JUICE
1¹/₂ teasp. DRY BASIL
PINCH DILL WEED
¹/₂ teasp. HERB SEASONING

Nutritional analysis: per 2 oz. serving; 218 calories; 1gm. protein; 6gm. carbohydrate; 1gm. fiber; 22gm. fats; 0 cholesterol; 18mg. calcium; trace iron; 14mg. magnesium; 103mg. potassium; 32mg. sodium; trace zinc.

364   SWEET TAHINI CREAM FOR FRESH FRUIT

Fresh fruit and cream just seem to go together. This version offers the hint of sesame seeds.
Makes 1 pint:

♣Whirl in the blender until creamy
²/₃ CUP PLAIN YOGURT
3 TBS. HONEY

1 teasp. VANILLA
JUICE of 1 LIME
♣Fill to the 2 CUP MARK with SESAME TAHINI. Add more honey if you like it very sweet.

Nutritional analysis: per 2 oz. serving; 188 calories; 5gm. protein; 13gm. carbohydrate; 2gm. fiber; 14gm. fats; 1mg. cholesterol; 70mg. calcium; 1mg. iron; 92mg. magnesium; 170mg. potassium; 15mg. aodium; 3mg. zinc.

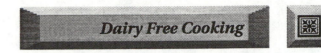

365   BEST CREAMY TOMATO

A good choice for salads, open face sandwiches or baked tofu. Tastes like a gourmet Thousand Island dressing.
For 3 cups:

♣Blender blend everything until *very* creamy

1/3 CUP SUN SEEDS or DICED ALMONDS, toasted
2 CUPS CHOPPED FRESH TOMATOES
3/4 CUP OLIVE OIL
3/4 CUP SALAD OIL
1/4 CUP BALSAMIC VINEGAR
1/3 CUP FRESH CHOPPED PARSLEY
4 TBS. FRESH CHOPPED (or 1 TB. DRY BASIL)
1 TB. CHOPPED DRY ONION
   (or 1/2 teasp. ONION POWDER)

3 TBS. HONEY
2 TBS. TAMARI
1 GREEN ONION, chopped
1 teasp. TARRAGON
1/4 teasp. DILL WEED
1 teasp. HERB or VEGETABLE SALT
JUICE of 1 LEMON or LIME

♣Thin with WHITE WINE. Pour into a serving container, and add 1 TB. SWEET PICKLE RELISH.

Nutritional analysis: per 2 oz. serving; 221 calories; 1gm. protein; 7gm. carbohydrates; 1gm. fiber; 22gm. fats; 0 cholesterol; 17mg. calcium; 1mg. iron; 17mg. magnesium; 116mg. potassium; 39mg. sodium; trace zinc.

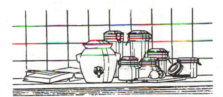

Dairy Free Sweet Baking

Dairy free baking can still have plenty of richness and taste. It's just a matter of easy adjustment to alternative ingredients. The recipes here are for inspiration, to give you an idea of how to substitute in your own favorites.

366   KATE'S OATMEAL COOKIES

These were devised by a young helper in the beginning days of the Rainbow Kitchen. She has long grown and changed, but her cookies have stood the test of time.
For about 4 dozen: Preheat oven to 350°.

♣Mix 1/2 CUP OIL, 1/2 CUP HONEY, and 3 TBS. SESAME TAHINI (or 2 TBS. YOGURT mixed with 1 TB. WATER) in a large bowl til well blended.
♣Add to wet ingredients and mix just to moisten

1 1/4 CUPS OATS
1 1/2 CUPS WHOLE WHEAT PASTRY FLOUR
1/2 CUP RASINS

1 teasp. BAKING POWDER
1/4 teasp. BAKING SODA
1/2 teasp. NUTMEG
1 teasp. CINNAMON

♣Drop onto lecithin-sprayed baking sheets. Sprinkle each with SESAME SEEDS and flatten with a fork dipped in cold water so it won't stick. Bake for 8 minutes until golden brown.

Nutritional analysis: per 2 cookie serving; 132 calories; 3gm. protein; 16gm. carbohydrate; 2gm. fiber; 7gm. fats; 0 cholesterol; 23mg. calcium; 1mg. iron; 29mg. magnesium; 153mg. potassium; 7mg. sodium; trace zinc.

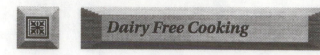

367　SWEET SAVORY SCONES

For 8 scones: Preheat oven to 425°.

♣Mix all ingredients until just moistened
1¹/₂ CUP GOURMET FLOUR MIX (¹/₂ CUP EACH OAT, RICE AND RYE FLOUR).
¹/₂ CUP WHOLE WHEAT FLOUR

2 teasp. BAKING POWDER   1 teasp. DRY SAVORY
2 TBS. FRUCTOSE or HONEY   ¹/₂ teasp. SEA SALT
¹/₄ CUP OIL   ¹/₂ teasp. BAKING SODA
¹/₂ CUP CURRANTS (better than raisins here)
¹/₂ CUP YOGURT mixed with ¹/₄ CUP WATER or ³/₄ CUP PLAIN KEFIR or ³/₄ CUP SOY MILK

♣Turn dough onto floured board and knead JUST 12 TURNS. Pat into a round on a greased baking sheet. Score into 8 wedges with a knife. Bake until browned, about 25 to 30 minutes.

Nutritional analysis: per serving; 205 calories; 6gm. protein; 30gm. carbohydrate; 3gm. fiber; 8gm. fats; 0 cholesterol; 104mg. calcium; 1mg. iron; 45mg. magnesium; 543mg. potassium; 167mg. sodium; 1mg. zinc.

✳

368　MIDGET PEANUT BUTTER COOKIES

A favorite of one of the chefs in the Rainbow Kitchen. She could make them lightening fast.
For 36 cookies: Preheat oven to 350°.

♣Mix all ingredients and drop onto greased baking sheets.
¹/₄ CUP OIL   ¹/₂ CUP PEANUT BUTTER
¹/₂ CUP HONEY   ¹/₄ CUP WHOLE GRAIN GRANOLA
2 TBS. MAPLE SYRUP   1 teasp. VANILLA
1¹/₄ CUP WHOLE WHEAT PASTRY FLOUR
♣Flatten each cookie with a fork dipped in cold water and bake for about 10 minutes.

Nutritional analysis: per cookie; 68 calories; 2gm. protein; 8gm. carbohydrate; 1gm. fiber; 3gm. fats; 0 cholesterol; 5mg. calcium; trace iron; 12mg. magnesium; 65mg. potassium; 12mg. sodium; trace zinc.

✳

369　SESAME OATMEAL COOKIES

For 12 cookies: Preheat oven to 350°.

♣Stir together until well blended.
¹/₂ CUP HONEY   1¹/₂ CUP OATMEAL
¹/₂ CUP WALNUT PIECES   ¹/₂ teasp. CINNAMON
6 TBS. SESAME TAHINI   ¹/₄ teasp. NUTMEG
♣Drop teaspoonfuls on lecithin-sprayed baking sheets. Bake for 10 minutes til edges are brown. Cool.

✳

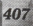

370   OATMEAL RAISIN WHEELS

For 18 cookies: Preheat oven to 375°.

♣Mix together to make a stiff dough
1/2 CUP ROASTED PEANUTS or ALMONDS, chopped
2 CUPS CHOPPED DATES
2 CUPS RAISINS
1 CUP ROLLED OATS
1/2 CUP ALMOND or PEANUT BUTTER
1/2 CUP WHOLE WHEAT PASTRY FLOUR
1/2 CUP TOASTED WHEAT GERM

4 TBS. OIL
2 TBS. WATER or FRUIT JUICE
1 teasp. VANILLA
2 teasp. SWEET TOOTH BAKING MIX
   (or 1 teasp. cinnamon, 1/2 teasp. nutmeg
   and 1/2 teasp. ginger powder)

♣Process some of the dough in a food processor or blender; then mix back in so cookies will hold together, but still have nice chewy chunks. Bake about 15 minutes until brown, and crusty around the edges.

Nutritional analysis: per 2 cookie serving; 244 calories; 5gm. protein; 39gm. carbohydrate; 5gm. fiber; 10gm. fats; 0 cholesterol; 52mg. calcium; 2mg. iron; 67mg. magnesium; 409mg. potassium; 4mg. sodium; 1mg. zinc.

Creamy Dairy Free Desserts

These desserts are guaranteed creamy and delicious without dairy products; rich and satisfying without the fat.

371   CHEESECAKE WITHOUT THE CHEESE

This cake is rich in absorbable calcium; an added bonus to good taste. Top with fresh sliced drained fruits for a spectacular dessert.
For 8 to 10 servings: Preheat oven to 350°.

♣Crush about 15 GRAHAM CRACKERS and mix with 3 TBS. ALMOND BUTTER, SESAME TAHINI or HONEY for the crust. Press into a lecithin-sprayed spring form-pan and sprinkle with CINNAMON.
♣Chill crust while you mix the filling ingredients.

♣Crumble about 3 1/2 LBS. VERY FRESH TOFU into a bowl. Add 2/3 CUP VANILLA SOY MILK, 1/4 CUP SESAME TAHINI, 3/4 CUP MAPLE SYRUP, 2 TBS. LEMON JUICE and 2 teasp. VANILLA.
♣(Add 2 EGGS if your diet and system can tolerate them. If not they can be easily omitted. Taste will not suffer, only lightness.)

♣Pour into a blender and blend until absolutely smooth. Pour into the chilled springform crust, smooth the top and bake until filling sets and begins to turn golden. Remove and cool on a rack. Cover and chill.
♣Arrange drained FRESH FRUITS on top in an artistic pattern.

Nutritional analysis: per serving; 372 calories; 20gm. protein; 37gm. carbohydrate; 4gm. fiber; 19gm. fats; 0 cholesterol; 273mg. calcium; 12mg. iron; 264mg. magnesium; 438mg. potassium; 104mg. sodium; 3mg. zinc.

372   LEMON TOFU CHEESECAKE

The lemon version is also excellent, and it makes up beautifully without a crust, for even less fat calories.
For 6 servings: Preheat oven to 350°.

♣Blend in a blender until very smooth

ONE 8-OZ. CARTON LEMON YOGURT   2 TBS. LEMON JUICE
1/2 CUP HONEY   1/4 CUP OIL
1 teasp. GRATED LEMON RIND   1 1/2 teasp. VANILLA
1 1/2 LBS "VERY FRESH" TOFU

♣Pour into individual cups or a straight-sided casserole dish, and bake for 40 minutes until set.
♣Top with 1 1/2 CUPS FRESH CHOPPED FRUITS and some fresh snipped MINT LEAVES.

♣Or top with this all-natural, showy **FRUIT GLAZE**:
♣Puree 1 CUP FRESH FRUITS, such as raspberries, peaches or apricots, in the blender. Add 2 to 3 teasp. HONEY, 2 TBS. KUZU or ARROWROOT dissolved in 3 TBS. WATER and 1 TB. LEMON JUICE. Blend well. Pour into a saucepan and bring to a boil. Simmer until glaze thickens and clears, about 1 minute.
♣Spoon over cheesecake immediately, then either chill, or serve at room temperature.

373   FRESH PEACH COBBLER WITH GRAPENUTS TOPPING

For 8 servings: Preheat oven to 350°.

♣Mix and put in a 8 x 11 x 2 1/2" lecithin-sprayed pan   ♣Mix topping and sprinkle over to cover
8 FRESH SLICED PEACHES   1/2 CUPS GRAPENUTS CEREAL
2 1/2 TBS. TAPIOCA GRANULES   1/2 CUP CHOPPED PECANS
1/4 CUP HONEY   2 TBS. MAPLE SYRUP
1/4 CUP ORANGE JUICE 2 TBS. SWEET TOOTH BAKING MIX
♣Bake for 40 minutes til browned, bubbly and aromatic.

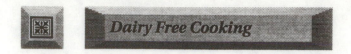

374   CLASSIC HASTY PUDDING CAKE

For 6 old fashioned servings: Preheat oven to 350°.

♣Make the hot molasses sauce. Combine 1/3 CUP MOLASSES, 1/3 CUP HONEY, and 1/3 CUP WATER in a saucepan. Bring to a boil and set aside.
♣Mix together until smooth

1 CUP WHOLE GRAIN FLOUR   1 1/2 teasp. VANILLA
1/3 CUP VANILLA SOY MILK or ALMOND MILK   1/2 teasp. BAKING POWDER
1/4 CUP HONEY   1/2 teasp. BAKING SODA
1/4 CUP OIL   1/3 CUP RAISINS

♣Pour into an oiled casserole. Sprinkle on a few more raisins. Pour hot molasses syrup over top and bake about 40 minutes. Serve warm.

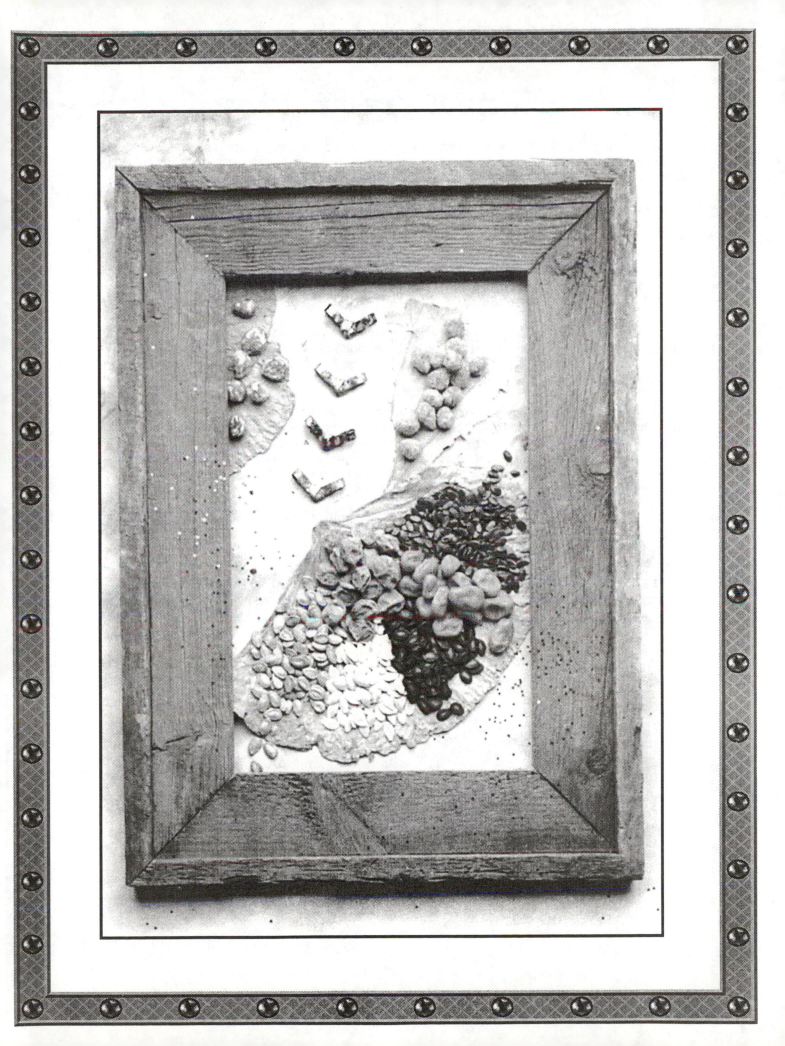

Wheat Free Baking

Wheat and gluten sensitivity are common problems in today's allergic, immune deficient, chronic fatigue conditions. These protein intolerances are not only caused by diet and environmental circumstances, but through inheritance as well.

Growing research on pesticides and chemical fertilizers used in agri-business, has shown that the human body is affected by these things in the way we use and absorb wheat and gluten. Chronic headaches, moodiness and depression are usually the first stages of sensitivity. When sugar and wheat are combined, as they are in many things we eat, the problems are often aggravated, because the carbohydrate in the wheat cannot be fully digested. (This is true even with <u>whole</u> wheat products; refined wheat flour causes additional problems). The poorly digested carbohydrates are then attacked by bacteria in the intestines, and contribute to gas and loose bowels.

If you suspect a wheat or gluten sensitivity problem, begin by eliminating these foods from your diet. During the initial stages of healing, it is recommended to stick fairly close to the recipes in this section. All are wheat and gluten free. The grains used are **brown rice, amaranth, buckwheat, quinoa, oats, millet and corn**.

It is also a good idea to eat at home during this time, preparing your food from scratch, so that you can completely control its contents. The gluten-containing grains - wheat, barley, bulgur and rye - appear in a wide variety of restaurant and pre-prepared food products, including such items as ice cream, candies, salad dressings, meats, soups, sauces and condiments - foods you might not suspect. There is no way you can effectively know or control everything you are eating away from home. Even very small amounts of gluten may initiate an allergic reaction.

The good news is that wheat free baking isn't very difficult. There are many other good grains to choose from. The recipe categories include:

&**WHEAT FREE PIE, QUICHE and TART CRUSTS; HEALTHY FILLINGS TO GO IN THEM** & **WHEAT FREE MUFFINS and BREADS** &**PANCAKES and SPOONBREADS** &**WHEAT FREE CAKES & COOKIES** &**MAIN DISHES with ALTERNATIVE GRAINS** &

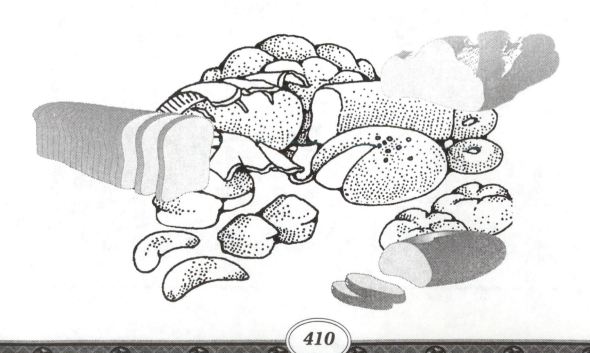

Wheat Free Pie, Quiche & Tart Crusts
&
Healthy Fillings To Go In Them

If you avoid fresh dessert and vegetable pies, tarts and quiches because of the wheat flour in the crust, there is good news in this chapter. It offers several choices for both sweet and savory fillings - all wheat free. Fill with a favorite filling, one of the healthy ones suggested here that we have already tested with the crusts.

375   SESAME OAT CRUST

This crust is excellent with creamy pies like the BANANA SOUR CREAM filling included in this chapter.
For one 10" pie: Preheat oven to 350°.

♣Make the wheat free crust. Mix and press into a pie pan

1¹/₂ CUPS OATS

1/₄ CUP TOASTED SESAME SEEDS

1/₄ CUP GROUND NUTS

1/₂ CUP RICE FLOUR 3 TBS. HONEY

1 teasp. SWEET TOOTH BAKING MIX, page 645 (or a mix of cinnamon, nutmeg and allspice)

1 TB. VANILLA

1/₂ teasp. SESAME SALT

4 TBS. MELTED BUTTER

♣Bake for 10 minutes, and cool.

Nutritional analysis: per serving; 208 calories; 5gm. protein; 23gm. carbohydrate; 3gm. fiber; 11gm. fats; 15mg. cholesterol; 34mg. calcium; 1mg. iron; 61mg. magnesium; 143mg. potassium; 47mg. sodium; 1mg. zinc.

❀

376   COCONUT CAROB CHIP CRUST

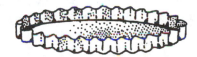

For one 8" pie:

♣Sauté 4 TBS. MELTED BUTTER and 2 CUPS SHREDDED COCONUT until golden and toasty.
♣Add 1/₂ CUP CAROB CHIPS. Press mixture into a pie plate.
♣Cool and fill.

Nutritional analysis: per serving; 233 calories; 2gm. protein; 11gm. carbohydrate; 3gm. fiber; 22gm. fats; 15mg. cholesterol; 10mg. calcium; 1mg. iron; 32mg. magnesium; 145mg. potassium; 10mg. sodium; trace zinc.

❀

377   MACAROON COOKIE CRUST

This crust is very rich, but absolutely delicious with almost any fruit or cream filling, and heavenly with ice cream or frozen yogurt filling for a little splurge.

♣Crumble chewy wheat- free macaroons (those made of non-fat dry milk, sweetener, coconut and egg whites) into a pie plate.
♣Pour 3 to 4 TBS. MELTED BUTTER over and press onto the top and sides.

❀

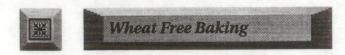

378   MIXED NUT CRUST
This crust is good for both savory and dessert fillings.

♣Mix together, pat into a pie pan and chill.
1/2 CUP FINE CHOPPED NUTS. (WALNUTS and PECANS are good for sweet fillings, CASHEWS and PEANUTS for savory fillings.)

1/2 CUP OAT FLOUR   2 TBS. MELTED BUTTER
1/2 CUP RICE FLOUR   2 TBS. OIL
1/4 CUP BUCKWHEAT FLOUR   3 to 5 TBS. COLD WATER

Nutritional analysis: per serving; 176 calories; 3gm. protein; 16gm. carbohydrate; 2gm. fiber; 11gm. fats; 7mg. cholesterol; 14mg. calcium; trace iron; 41mg. magnesium; 97mg. potassium; 2mg. sodium; trace zinc.

379   SPINACH CHARD CRUST
This crust is a good choice for quiches and vegetable or chicken pies.
For one 10" pie: Preheat oven to 375°.

♣Sauté and toss until wilted, about 3 minutes   ♣Add and mix together
1/2 BUNCH SPINACH LEAVES chopped   1/2 CUP OAT FLOUR
1/2 BUNCH CHARD LEAVES chopped   1/2 CUP RICE FLOUR
2 TBS. BUTTER   1/2 teasp. SESAME SALT
1 TB. OIL   1/2 teasp. NUTMEG
♣Pat into the bottom of an oiled pie pan. Bake for 10 minutes to set. Cool and add filling.

Nutritional analysis: per serving; 88 calories; 2gm. protein; 9gm. carbohydrate; 1gm. fiber; 5gm. fats; 7mg. cholesterol; 26mg. calcium; 1mg. iron; 39mg. magnesium; 163mg. potassium; 86mg. sodium; trace zinc.

380   SAVORY BROWN RICE CRACKER CRUST
This crust is very low-fat; good for weight control quiches.
For one 8" pie - 3 to 4 servings:

♣Crush 15 to 20 SAVORY BROWN RICE CRACKERS, (enough to make 3/4 cup).
♣Combine with 3 TBS. MELTED BUTTER or OIL, and 1/2 SMALL ZUCCHINI, minced.
♣Press into bottom and sides of pie plate, and top wih filling.

381   POPPY SEED CRUST

♣Mix together to make a dough ball
1/2 CUP OAT FLOUR   2 TBS. POPPY SEEDS
1/4 CUP BUCKWHEAT FLOUR   2 TBS. BUTTER
1/2 CUP CORNMEAL   2 1/2 to 3 TBS. ICE WATER
1/2 teasp. SEA SALT
♣Chill, roll out and pat into a pie plate. Freeze for 15 minutes before filling for best texture.

Delicious Mix & Match Fillings

382   SOUR CREAM APPLE PIE
A rich, but healthy, no-sugar apple pie. Try it with the SESAME OAT CRUST.
For 10 slices: Preheat oven to 375°.

♣Mix in a bowl

5 CUPS TART SLICED APPLES	2 TBS. ROLLED OATS
THE JUICE and GRATED RIND of 1 LEMON	1/2 teasp. CINNAMON
1/4 CUP HONEY or MAPLE SYRUP	1/4 teasp. NUTMEG

♣Mix 1 EGG and 1/2 CUP ALL NATURAL SOUR CREAM for the topping and drizzle over.

♣Pour into crust and bake for 40 minutes until bubbly.

Nutritional analysis: without crust; 97 calories; 1gm. protein; 17gm. carbohydrate; 2gm. fiber; 3gm. fats; 26mg. cholesterol; 25mg. calcium; trace iron; 7mg.magnesium; 107mg. potassium; 13mg. sodium; trace zinc.

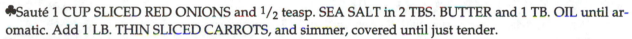

383   SWEET & SAVORY CARROT FILLING

For 8 servings: Preheat oven to 375°.

♣Sauté 1 CUP SLICED RED ONIONS and 1/2 teasp. SEA SALT in 2 TBS. BUTTER and 1 TB. OIL until aromatic. Add 1 LB. THIN SLICED CARROTS, and simmer, covered until just tender.
♣Add 1 TB. SHERRY and 1 TB. HONEY.

♣Beat together in a large bowl

1/2 CUP GRATED LOW-FAT CHEESE	1 EGG
1 1/2 CUP LOW-FAT COTTAGE CHEESE	1/4 teasp. WHITE PEPPER

♣Add carrot mixture and combine. Pour into pie shell and sprinkle with NUTMEG.
♣Bake for 15 minutes, then reduce heat and bake at 350° for 30 minutes more.

384   DRIED TOMATO FILLING

For 4 servings: Preheat oven to 350°.

♣Cover a pre-baked 9" crust with 3/4 CUP GRATED LOW FAT MOZZARELLA CHEESE, 1 GRATED ZUCCHINI, 3 MINCED GREEN ONIONS and 1/2 CUP SLIVERED DRIED TOMATOES.

♣Mix together

3 EGGS	1/4 teasp. ITALIAN SEASONING
1/2 CUP PLAIN LOW-FAT YOGURT	1/4 teasp. SESAME SALT
1/4 CUP RED WINE	1/4 CUP WATER

♣Pour over cheese and vegetables and bake for 25 minutes til set. Let stand for 5 minutes before cutting.

385 CREAMY HOT ONION FILLING

For 8 pieces: Preheat oven to 375°.

♣Sauté in 3 TBS. BUTTER or OIL til onions are translucent and fragrant

4 CUPS SLICED YELLOW ONIONS	1 teasp. DIJON MUSTARD
1 teasp. SESAME SALT	3 TBS. LEMON JUICE

♣Sprinkle on 3 TBS. OAT or BUCKWHEAT FLOUR. Stir to blend well, and add 3 TBS. WHITE WINE.

♣Beat together until smooth

1/2 CUP SOUR CREAM or KEFIR CHEESE	1 EGG
1 CUP PLAIN YOGURT	1/4 teasp. BLACK PEPPER
4 TBS. MAYONNAISE	1/3 CUP GRATED PARMESAN
2 TBS. FRESH CHOPPED PARSLEY	
2 PINCHES WASABI POWDER or 1/2 teasp. HOT SAUCE	

♣Pour into shell, and bake for 45 minutes. Sprinkle with PAPRIKA and SESAME SEEDS to serve.

Nutritional analysis: per filling serving; 191 calories; 6gm. protein; 13gm. carbohydrate; 2gm. fiber; 9gm. fats; 48mg. cholesterol; 143mg. calcium; 1mg. iron; 28mg. magnesium; 269mg. potassium; 202mg. sodium; 1mg. zinc.

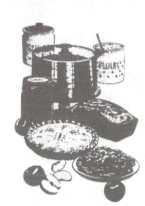

386 HONEY CHEESECAKE FILLING

A very low calorie cheesecake, perfect with the Coconut Carob Chip or Nut crusts
For 8 servings: Preheat oven to 350°.

♣Blend ingredients in the blender.

1 CUP LOW FAT COTTAGE CHEESE	3 EGGS
1 CUP PLAIN YOGURT CHEESE	1/2 CUP HONEY
1/2 CUP SOUR CREAM, or KEFIR CHEESE	1 TB. LEMON JUICE
3/4 teasp CINNAMON or SWEET TOOTH baking mix	1 1/2 teasp. VANILLA

♣Pour into prepared crust and bake for 40 minutes. Cool and chill for 2 hours.

Nutritional analysis: per filling serving; 166 calories; 8gm. protein; 22gm. carbohydrate; trace fiber; 5gm. fats; 89mg. cholesterol; 110mg. calcium; trace iron; 12mg. magnesium; 163mg. potassium; 158mg. sodium; 1mg. zinc.

387 LOW-FAT ITALIAN SAVORY FILLING

For 4 servings: Pre heat oven to 350°.

♣Beat together in a bowl

1/2 CUP SHREDDED LOW-FAT MOZZARELLA	1/4 teasp. ITALIAN SEASONING
1/4 CUP PLAIN LOW-FAT YOGURT	1/4 teasp. SEA SALT
1/2 TOMATO, chopped	1/4 teasp. NUTMEG

♣Pour into a rye cracker or other prepared crust. Bake for 30 minutes until set.

388   CRANBERRY JAM FILLING

This filling is excellent atop the almond nut crust. It can be a dessert showpiece, so press the crust into a spring form pan, and remove the sides when chilled and set. We have made this with a HONEY CUSTARD CREME top layer, and also plain with just the glossy top. Both ways are very rich and very good.
For 10 small slices: Preheat oven to 350°.

♣Cook 4 CUPS FRESH CRANBERRIES and 1 CUP ORANGE HONEY until berries pop, about 30 minutes. ♣Set a strainer over a bowl. Pour in berries, and let cool.

♣Return strained juice to the pan, and blend in 2 teasp. ARROWROOT or KUZU CHUNKS for high gloss. Stir; bring to a rolling boil. Add 1/2 CUP SUGAR-FREE RASPBERRY JAM and stir until melted.

♣Mix in berries and pour into crust. Bake until crust is browned, about 20 to 30 minutes. Remove and cool. Loosen crust with a long spatula from sides. Chill for two hours before serving, or while you make the CUSTARD TOPPING.

♣Whisk together 2 EGG YOLKS, 3 TBS. HONEY and a PINCH of SEA SALT in the top pan of a double boiler over hot water.
♣Gently heat 1 CUP RAW MILK or 1 CUP VANILLA KEFIR. Pour slowly into egg yolk mix and whisk. Place pan over hot water and stir with a wooden spoon til custard coats the back of the spoon. Remove from heat, and add 2 TBS. SHERRY or 1 teasp. ALMOND or VANILLA EXTRACT. Smooth over cranberries. Chill again to set. Remove sides of spring form pan and serve.

Wheat Free Cakes & Cookies

389   WHEAT FREE CARROT NUT CAKE

For 12 slices: Pre heat oven to 350°.

Beat and blend til fluffy
5 EGG YOLKS
3 TBS. FRUCTOSE
1/3 CUP HONEY

1/4 teasp. SEA SALT
1 teasp. ALMOND EXTRACT

♣Process 2 CARROTS, 8-OZ. WHOLE ALMONDS and 1/3 CUP ROLLED OATS through a salad shooter or food processor, and stir into egg mixture.
♣Beat 5 EGG WHITES TO STIFF PEAKS, and fold into cake.

♣Bake in an oiled spring form pan for about 1 hour until cake springs back when touched. Cool in pan and then remove sides.

Nutritional analysis: per serving; 197 calories; 7gm.protein; 17gm. carbohydrate; 3gm. fiber; 12gm. fats; 88mg. cholesterol; 66mg. calcium; 1mg. iron; 63mg. magnesium; 215mg. potassium; 76mg. sodium; 1mg. zinc.

390   FRESH FRUIT WHEEL on a GIANT WHEAT-FREE COOKIE

Both kids and guests love this when it appears. Use it as a dessert palette for your imagination. Arrange the fruits in expressive patterns.
For 10 pieces: Preheat oven to 325°.

♣Combine dry cookie ingredients
1/2 CUP CHOPPED NUTS
1/3 CUP AMARANTH FLOUR
1/3 CUP OAT FLOUR
1/3 CUP RICE FLOUR
1 TB. RUMFORD'S BAKING POWDER
1 CUP CHOPPED DATES

♣Blender blend wet cookie ingredients
1/3 CUP HEATED LIQUID HONEY
1/4 CUP HEATED BUTTER
1/3 CUP HEATED ORANGE JUICE
2 TBS. FROZEN O. J. CONCENTRATE
2 teasp. VANILLA
2 EGGS

♣Mix wet and dry ingredients together, and pour the whole thing onto a lecithin-sprayed round pizza pan with a lip. Spread batter to the edges. Bake for 5 minutes at 325°, then turn down oven to 300° and bake for 10 more minutes. Watch closely to avoid burning. Remove when center is springy.
♣Cool completely before topping.

♣Blend the topping in the blender.
2 CUPS LOW-FAT COTTAGE CHEESE
2 TBS. MAPLE SYRUP
2 TBS. HONEY
3 TBS. YOGURT CHEESE OR CREAM CHEESE

2 teasp. GRATED LEMON PEEL
1 teasp. GRATED ORANGE PEEL
1 teasp. LEMON EXTRACT

♣Spread on top of cooled crust. Top with seasonal FRESH SLICED or CHOPPED FRUITS, such as raspberries, peaches, kiwi, blueberries and nectarines in artful patterns.

※

391   WHEAT FREE RAISIN SPICE COOKIES

For 24 to 30 pieces: Preheat oven to 400°.

♣Combine dry ingredients in a bowl
1/4 CUP BUCKWHEAT FLOUR
1/4 CUP AMARANTH or RICE FLOUR
1 1/2 CUPS ROLLED OATS
1 TB. CINNAMON
1 teasp. BAKING POWDER
1 teasp. BAKING SODA

♣Combine wet ingredients together
1/2 CUP APPLESAUCE
1/2 CUP APPLE JUICE CONCENTRATE
1 teasp. VANILLA
1/2 CUP RAISINS
1/4 CUP CHOPPED DATES
1 1/2 teasp. NUTMEG
1/2 teasp. ALLSPICE

♣Mix all together. Beat 2 EGG WHITES to soft peaks and fold in. Drop by heaping tablespoons onto lecithin-sprayed baking sheets. Bake 12 to 15 minutes.
♣Leave in the <u>turned-off</u> oven to cool and harden. Remove from baking sheets.

Nutritional analysis: per cookie; 59 calories; 2gm. protein; 13gm. carbohydrate; 1gm. fiber; trace fats; 0 cholesterol; 20mg. calcium; 1mg. iron; 15mg. magnesium; 138mg. potassium; 24mg. sodium; trace zinc.

※

392   NO WHEAT, NO SUGAR, NO BAKE FRUITCAKE

This cake is truly feasting on the raw.
For 10 pieces:

♣Combine in a large bowl
3 CUPS FINE GRAHAM CRACKER CRUMBS
3 teasp. GRATED ORANGE PEEL
1 1/2 teasp. GRATED LEMON PEEL
1/2 teasp. GINGER
1/2 teasp. ALLSPICE
1 teasp. SWEET TOOTH BAKING MIX (pg. 645)
   or 1/2 teasp. **each** CINNAMON and NUTMEG

♣Combine in another bowl
1/2 CUP SHERRY
1/4 CUP HONEY
3 TBS. LEMON JUICE
1 CUP RAISINS
1 LB. MIXED DRIED FRUITS
3 to 4-OZ. SHREDDED COCONUT

♣Combine both mixtures together to moisten. Pack firmly into a foil-lined loaf pan. Cover with foil and chill for 3 days. To serve, remove from pan, peel off foil and slice thin with a very sharp knife.

Nutritional analysis: per serving; 479 calories; 6gm. protein; 92gm. carbohydrate; 6gm. fiber; 11gm. fats; 0 cholesterol; 56mg. calcium; 3mg. iron; 55mg. magnesium; 690mg. potassium; 328mg. sodium; 1mg. zinc.

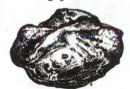

Wheat Free Breads & Muffins

Breads are usually the most difficult to either buy or make without wheat or gluten grains.
The recipes given here show you how easy it can be without loss of taste or function.

393   SWEET CORN LOAF

This low fat recipe is particularly good as a toasted breakfast bread, with sweet toppings.
For 1 loaf: Preheat oven to 350°. Place loaf pan in the oven to preheat while you mix the ingredients.

♣Stir together
2 CUPS YELLOW CORNMEAL
1/3 CUP HONEY
1 teasp. SEA SALT
1/4 CUP OAT FLOUR
1/4 CUP RICE FLOUR
2 teasp. BAKING POWDER
1 teasp. BAKING SODA

♣Mix in just to moisten
1 CUP PLAIN YOGURT
1 CUP WATER
1 TB. OIL

♣Melt 1 TB. BUTTER or OIL in a loaf pan and tip to coat bottom and sides. Return loaf pan to oven to heat. When butter or oil smokes, pour in batter. Bake for 1 hour until firm, browned and crusty.
♣Turn out on a rack to cool before slicing.

Nutritional analysis: per serving; 226 calories; 5gm. protein; 42gm. carbohydrate; 4gm. fiber; 5gm. fats; 5mg. cholesterol; 111mg. calcium; 1mg. iron; 55mg. magnesium; 404mg. potassium; 341mg. sodium; 1mg. zinc.

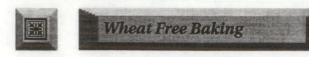

394   BROWN BATTER BREAD

For 2 loaves: Preheat oven to 350°.

♣Cream together until very smooth
1/2 CUP HONEY
3 TBS. BUTTER OR OIL
3 TBS. UNSULPHURED MOLASSES
1 CUP PLAIN YOGURT
1 CUP WATER
1 CUP RAISINS

♣Add and combine well
1 CUP CORNMEAL
1 CUP BUCKWHEAT FLOUR
1 CUP AMARANTH FLOUR
2 teasp. BAKING SODA
1 teasp. SEA SALT
1 CUP CHOPPED WALNUTS

♣Divide batter into 2 greased loaf pans, and bake for 40 minutes until centers test done with a toothpick.

Nutritional analysis: per serving; 221 calories; 5gm. protein; 37gm. carbohydrate; 3gm. fiber; 8gm. fats; 6mg. cholesterol; 71mg. calcium; 2mg. iron; 57mg. magnesium; 347mg. p[otassium; 199mg. sodium; 1mg. zinc.

395   YAM BREAD

For 2 loaves: Preheat oven to 350°.

♣Combine the dry ingredients
1 CUP BUCKWHEAT FLOUR
1 CUP AMARANTH FLOUR
1/2 CUP OAT FLOUR
1/2 CUP BROWN RICE FLOUR

1 1/2 teasp. BAKING SODA
1 teasp. GROUND GINGER
1/2 teasp. SEA SALT
1 TB. SWEET TOOTH BAKING MIX

♣Combine the wet ingredients in the blender until smooth
1/2 CUP SOFT BUTTER
1/4 CUP OIL
1/2 CUP HONEY
1/2 CUP MAPLE SYRUP
2 teasp. VANILLA

1 CUP DATE SUGAR
1/2 CUP PLAIN YOGURT
2 TBS. WATER
3 EGGS

♣Combine wet and dry ingredients. Add 1 1/2 CUPS COOKED MASHED YAMS (about 2 small).
♣Add 1 CUP CHOPPED DATES and 1 CUP CHOPPED WALNUTS and blend in.

♣Pour into 2 lecithin-sprayed loaf pans, and bake for 60 to 70 minutes until bread pulls away from the sides of the pan, and a toothpick inserted in the center comes out clean.

Nutritional analysis; per serving; 239 calories; 4gm. protein; 35gm. carbohydrates; 3gm. fiber; 10gm. fats; 37mg. cholesterol; 42mg. calcium; 1mg. iron; 39mg. magnmesium; 251mg. potassium; 83mg. sodium; 1mg. zinc.

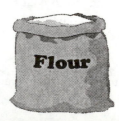

396   WHEAT FREE HERB BREAD

For 1 skillet:

♣Put 2 TBS. OIL in a 12" <u>iron</u> skillet and heat in a 425° oven while you make the bread.

Mix all ingredients and pour into the skillet

2 CUPS YELLOW CORNMEAL	3 teasp. BAKING POWDER
1/4 CUP OAT FLOUR	1/2 teasp. DRY OREGANO
1/4 CUP RICE FLOUR	1/2 teasp. SEA SALT
1/2 CUP PLAIN YOGURT	1 TB. CHIVES
1/2 CUP WATER	1/2 teasp. SAGE
2 EGGS	1/2 teasp. ROSEMARY

♣Pour into sizzling hot skillet. Bake for 20 minutes until center springs back when touched. Cut in squares, and top with a pat of butter.

Nutritional analysis: per serving; 133 calories; 4gm. protein; 21gm. carbohydrate; 3gm. fiber; 4gm. fats; 38mg. cholesterol; 80mg. calcium; 1mg. iron; 37mg. magnesium; 331mg. potassium; 111mg. sodium; 1mg. zinc.

397   WHEAT FREE APPLE MUFFINS

For 12 to 18 muffins: Preheat oven to 375°.

♣Process 7 APPLES (any kind), 3 CUPS ROLLED OATS, and 1 TB. SHERRY in a food processor leaving the apples chunky. Let stand for 5 minutes.
♣Mix in 1/2 CUP RAISINS and 1/2 CUP WALNUT PIECES. Spoon into paper-lined muffin tins, and bake for 25 minutes until firm.

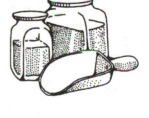

398   WHEAT FREE BREAKFAST MUFFINS

For 12 muffins: Preheat oven to 375°.

♣Mix everything together <u>just to moisten.</u>
1 CUP OF YOUR FAVORITE WHEAT FREE DRY BREAKFAST CEREAL (almost anything works)
1 CUP BUTTERMILK, or 1/2 CUP PLAIN YOGURT and 1/2 CUP WATER mixed
1/2 CUP OAT BRAN

1/4 CUP PEANUT BUTTER	1 TB. FRUCTOSE
1/4 CUP ANY FRUIT YOGURT	1/2 teasp. BAKING SODA
1 EGG	1/2 teasp. BAKING POWDER
3 TBS. MAPLE SYRUP	1 TB. OIL

♣Mix in 1/2 CUP RAISINS and 1/4 CUP CHOPPED WALNUTS. Spoon into paper-lined muffin cups, and bake for 20 to 25 minutes til a toothpick comes out clean.

399 DARK CHEWY CRANBERRY BREAD

This bread is also delicious with raisins instead of cranberries. It may be frozen for later use.
For 1 loaf: Preheat oven to 350°.

♣Sauté in 4 TBS. BUTTER and 4 TBS. OIL for 10 minutes until fragrant

1$1/2$ CUPS WHOLE FRESH CRANBERRIES	$1/2$ teasp. CINNAMON
$1/2$ CUP CHOPPED WALNUTS	$1/4$ teasp. NUTMEG

♣Remove from heat and set aside.

♣Mix together

1 CUP BUCKWHEAT FLOUR	$1/2$ teasp. SEA SALT
$3/4$ CUP AMARANTH FLOUR or RYE FLOUR	$1/2$ teasp. BAKING SODA
$1/4$ CUP OAT FLOUR	

♣Mix together

$1/2$ teasp. VANILLA	4 TBS. DATE SUGAR
$1/4$ CUP UNSULPHURED MOLASSES	2 TBS. MAPLE SYRUP
2 EGGS	

♣Combine all mixtures together. Spread into a lecithin-sprayed loaf pan, and bake for 45 to 50 minutes.

♣Cool for 10 minutes in the pan. Rap bottom of pan sharply to loosen and remove.

Nutritional analysis: 68 gm.; 182 calories; 4gm. protein; 24gm. carbohydrate; 3gm. fiber; 9gm. fats; 40mg. cholesterol; 71mg. calcium; 3mg. iron; 63mg. magnesium; 376mg. potassium; 88mg. sodium; 1mg. zinc.

400 DONA'S OAT BRAN MUFFINS

This is the recipe we give out at the Country Store when people want to know how to use oat bran.
For 9 small or 6 large muffins: Preheat oven to 400°.

♣Mix in a bowl	♣Mix in the blender
1 CUP OAT BRAN	$1/4$ CUP ANY FRUIT JUICE
1 TBS. LECITHIN GRANULES	$1/4$ CUP RAISINS
1 teasp. RUMFORD'S BAKING POWDER	1 teasp. VANILLA
1 teasp. CINNAMON	1 APPLE CORED and CHUNKED
$1/2$ teasp. SWEET HERB (STEVIA)	$1/4$ CUP CHOPPED PECANS

♣Mix wet and dry ingredients together.

♣Beat 1 EGG WHITE to stiff peaks and fold into batter.

♣Fill muffin tins lined with paper muffin cups, and bake for 15 to 20 minutes, until a toothpick inserted in the center of a muffin comes out clean.

Nutritonal analysis: per serving; 112 calories; 4gm. protein; 21gm. carbohydrate; 6gm. fiber; 4gm. fats; 0 cholesterol; 58mg. calcium; 1mg. iron; 31mg. magnesium; 347mg. potassium; 1mg. zinc.

Wheat Free Pancakes & Spoonbreads

Pancakes can often be a delicious healthy food for any meal. It's usually the fat loaded toppings we put on them that are the problem. These recipes are rich traditional ways to keep you wheat free.

401 ALMOND BUTTER PANCAKES

For 9 to 10 pancakes: Preheat griddle to medium hot.

♣Combine just to moisten

1/4 CUP OAT FLOUR	1 TB. FRUCTOSE (opt.)
1 CUP BUCKWHEAT FLOUR	3 TBS. OIL
1 EGG	2 TBS. ALMOND BUTTER
1/2 CUP PLAIN LOW-FAT YOGURT	1/2 teasp. SEA SALT
1/2 CUP WATER	DROPS ALMOND EXTRACT
	1/2 teasp. VANILLA

♣Cook on a sizzling griddle brushed with oil. Use 3 TBS. of the batter for each pancake, to make 4" circles.

♣Cook until bubbles appear, then turn and brown on the bottom.

♣Top with MAPLE SYRUP or this rich ALMOND BUTTER TOPPING:

♣Mix and melt 1/2 CUP ALMOND BUTTER, 1/2 CUP BUTTER, 3 teasp. HONEY and DROPS of ALMOND EXTRACT. Stir until smooth and fragrant.

Nutritional analysis: per serving <u>with</u> topping; 264 calories; 5gm. protein; 15gm. carbohydrate; 2gm. fiber; 21gm. fats; 46mg. cholesterol; 65mg. calcium; 1mg. iron; 57mg. magnesium; 187mg. potassium; 120mg. sodium.

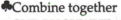

402 PUFFY VEGETABLE PANCAKES

For 16 pancakes: Preheat griddle to medium hot.

♣Combine together	♣Combine together
1 CUP BUCKWHEAT FLOUR	3 EGGS
1/4 CUP OAT FLOUR	1 CUP PLAIN YOGURT
2 TBS. AMARANTH FLOUR	1 CUP WATER
1 TB. BAKING POWDER	1/4 CUP MELTED BUTTER
1/2 teasp. SEA SALT	2 teasp. HONEY

♣Combine both mixtures together and set aside.

♣Sauté in 1 TB. OIL in a small skillet for 3 to 4 minutes

2 STALKS CELERY, minced	1 ONION, chopped
1/2 GREEN BELL PEPPER, minced	2 SMALL CARROTS, sliced

♣Remove from heat and set aside.

♣Combine all ingredients together. Beat 3 EGG WHITES TO STIFF PEAKS, and fold into batter.

♣When water beads on the griddle, ladle on 3 to 4 pancakes. Turn when bubbles appear on the surface, and cook 1 minute more. (*no longer, or they will be tough*).

♣Serve with a light mushroom or cheese sauce. (See index for suggestions.)

403   REAL COUNTRY SKILLET CORN BREAD

Make this in a cast iron skillet for best results.
For 1 skillet: Preheat oven to 375°.

♣Heat 2 TBS. OIL in an iron skillet; sauté til translucent
1/2 CUP CHOPPED ONION
2 CLOVES MINCED GARLIC

♣Add
1 CUP SALSA or TOMATO SAUCE
1 CUP CHOPPED BELL PEPPERS
    or 1 CUP CORN KERNALS

♣Remove from heat and add 1/4 CUP CHOPPED FRESH CILANTRO.

♣Mix in a separate bowl and lightly stir together
2 CUPS POLENTA or CORN BREAD MIX
1/2 CUP PLAIN YOGURT
1/4 CUP WATER
1/4 CUP LIGHT BEER or CALISTOGA WATER

2 EGGS
1/4 CUP HONEY
2 TBS. OIL

♣Pour over the vegetables in the skillet and sprinkle with JALAPEÑO or SOY JALAPEÑO CHEESE.

♣Turn oven to 325° and bake for 20 minutes until set and cheese bubbles and browns.

404   BROCCOLI PANCAKES

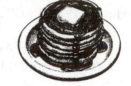

For 6 dinner pancakes: Preheat griddle to medium hot.

♣Fine chop 1 1/2 CUP BROCCOLI. Blanch in boiling water until color changes to bright green. Drain.
♣Mix together
1/2 CUP BUCKWHEAT FLOUR
1 EGG
2 TBS. PLAIN LOW-FAT YOGURT

1 teasp. BAKING POWDER
1/4 teasp. SEA SALT
2 TBS. WATER

♣Add broccoli and mix. When water beads up on the hot griddle, ladle 3 to 4 pancakes and cook until bubbles appear. Turn over, cook 1 minute and remove. Serve plain or with a mushroom sauce.

Nutritional analysis: per serving; 50 calories; 3gm. protein; 8gm. carbohydrate; 1gm. fiber; 1gm. fats; 35mg. cholesterol; 61mg. calcium; trace iron; 18mg. magnesium; 282mg. potasssium; 107mg. sodium; trace zinc.

405   VIRGINIA SPOONBREAD

For 8 servings: Preheat oven to 400°.

♣Butter a 1-qt. soufflé or 8" square pan and heat in the oven until sizzling.
♣Bring 2 CUPS COLD WATER, 1 CUP YELLOW CORNMEAL and 3/4 teasp. SEA SALT to a boil in a saucepan over high heat. Reduce heat to low and simmer for 5 minutes, stirring til stiff. Remove from heat and stir in 1 CUP COLD BUTTERMILK, 2 EGGS, and 2 TBS. BUTTER.
♣Pour batter into hot baking dish and bake 40 minutes until firm in the center and well-browned on top. Serve hot.

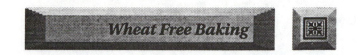

406   HERB PANCAKES

These pancakes have no wheat and no dairy products. They are good for a Candida Albicans diet.
For 16 small pancakes:

♣Combine in a large bowl

3 EGGS

1 CUP CHOPPED FRESH PARSLEY

1/2 CUP FRESH DILLWEED **or** BASIL

1/2 CUP CHOPPED GREEN ONIONS

1 teasp. HERB SALT

1/4 teasp. WHITE PEPPER

♣Cook on a sizzling griddle or skillet brushed with oil. Drop in 2 TBS. of the mixture. Make four at a time, and cook 3 minutes until golden and crispy on the edges. Serve alone or with a mushroom sauce.

407   POLENTA SPOONBREAD WITH PESTO

A light, wheat free, traditional Italian recipe.
For 6 servings: Preheat oven to 400°.

♣Add 2 CUPS BOILING WATER to 1 1/2 CUPS POLENTA and 1 teasp. SEA SALT. Cook over low heat, for 5 minutes until thick. Remove from heat. Add and beat in 4 EGG YOLKS and 1 WHOLE EGG, 1/4 CUP ROMANO CHEESE, and 2/3 CUP BASIL/GARLIC PESTO.

♣Beat 5 EGG WHITES to stiff peaks. Fold into polenta mix, and spoon the whole thing into a buttered soufflé dish. Bake for 2 minutes, and reduce oven heat to 375°. Bake for 35 to 40 minutes more.

♣Do not open oven door. This is *very light* and it will fall.

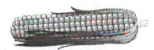

Main Dishes With Alternative Grains

408   DONA'S QUINOA PASTA SALAD

For 6 servings:

♣Rinse 2 CUPS QUINOA in a colander under running water. Place in a pan with 2 CUPS WATER.

♣Bring to a boil, reduce heat and simmer for 10 to15 minutes until water is absorbed. Drain and cool.

♣Toss with the following ingredients and chill well.

1/2 CUP CHOPPED GREEN ONION

1 CUP CHOPPED FRESH PARSLEY

1 TB. FRESH CHOPPED BASIL (1 teasp. DRY)

1 TB. CHOPPED FRESH MINT LEAVES

1 SHALLOT MINCED

1/4 CUP SLICED BLACK OLIVES

24 CHERRY TOMATOES halved

♣Whisk 1/2 CUP FRESH LEMON JUICE and 1/4 CUP OLIVE OIL together. Pour over and toss with salad. Serve on tangy lettuce leaves.

Nutritional analysis: per serving; 318 calories; 7gm. protein; 51gm. carbohydrate; 5gm. fiber; 11gm. fats; 0 cholesterol; 76mg. calcium; 3mg. iron; 114mg. magnesium; 386mg. potassium; 34mg. sodium; 2mg. zinc.

409   2 CHEESE QUIZZA

This dish is a wheat free version of a favorite from Sunset magazine - like a pizza, but different.
For 6 servings: Preheat oven to 350°.

♣Sauté 1 CHOPPED ONION in 2 TBS. OLIVE OIL for 5 minutes. Add 4 SLICED MUSHROOMS and sauté for 5 minutes.

♣Add 1/2 CUP WHITE WINE, 1 TB. FRESH CHOPPED BASIL and 1/4 teasp. BLACK PEPPER and stir until liquid evaporates. Remove from heat and set aside.

♣Combine and pour into a lecithin-sprayed quiche pan
3 EGGS
1/4 CUP BUCKWHEAT FLOUR
2 TBS. OAT FLOUR
2 TBS. PLAIN YOGURT or YOGURT CHEESE
2 TBS. WATER

♣Spoon onion mix over. Top with GRATED MOZZARELLA to cover, and bake until top is golden and jiggles slightly when moved, about 25 minutes. Let cool for 10 minutes before cutting in wedges.

Nutritional analysis: per serving; 132 calories; 7gm. protein; 8gm. carbohydrate; 1gm. fiber; 7gm. fats; 112mg. cholesterol; 101mg. calcium; 1mg. iron; 19mg. magnesium; 152mg. potassium; 84mg. sodium; 1mg. zinc.

410   CORN BREAD PIZZA

For 8 servings: Preheat oven to 375°.

♣Cut 1 1/2 to 2 LBS. ZUCCHINI in chunks and steam until tender. Puree in the blender to make 2 cups.

♣Add and mix until blended
2 1/2 CUPS YELLOW CORNMEAL   2 teasp. BAKING POWDER
2 EGGS   1 teasp. SEA SALT
2 TBS. OIL

♣Turn into a lecithin-sprayed 12 x 18" baking pan, or large pizza pan. Bake for 12 to 15 minutes until crust begins to pull away from sides.

♣While crust is baking, sauté filling ingredients briefly in OLIVE OIL until aromatic
1 LARGE ONION chopped   1 teasp. DRY OREGANO
1 teasp. CHILI POWDER   1 teasp. DRY BASIL
1 teasp. CUMIN POWDER   1/2 teasp. GROUND CORIANDER

♣Scatter 3 CHOPPED TOMATOES on top. Sprinkle with 1 1/2 CUPS JACK CHEESE or JALAPEÑO JACK and bake for 10 more minutes.

Nutritional analysis: per serving; 274 calories; 10gm. protein; 37gm. carbohydrate; 6gm. fiber; 11gm. fats; 65mg. cholesterol; 198mg. calcium; trace iron; 82mg. magmnesium; 724mg. potassium; 382mg. sodium; 1mg. zinc.

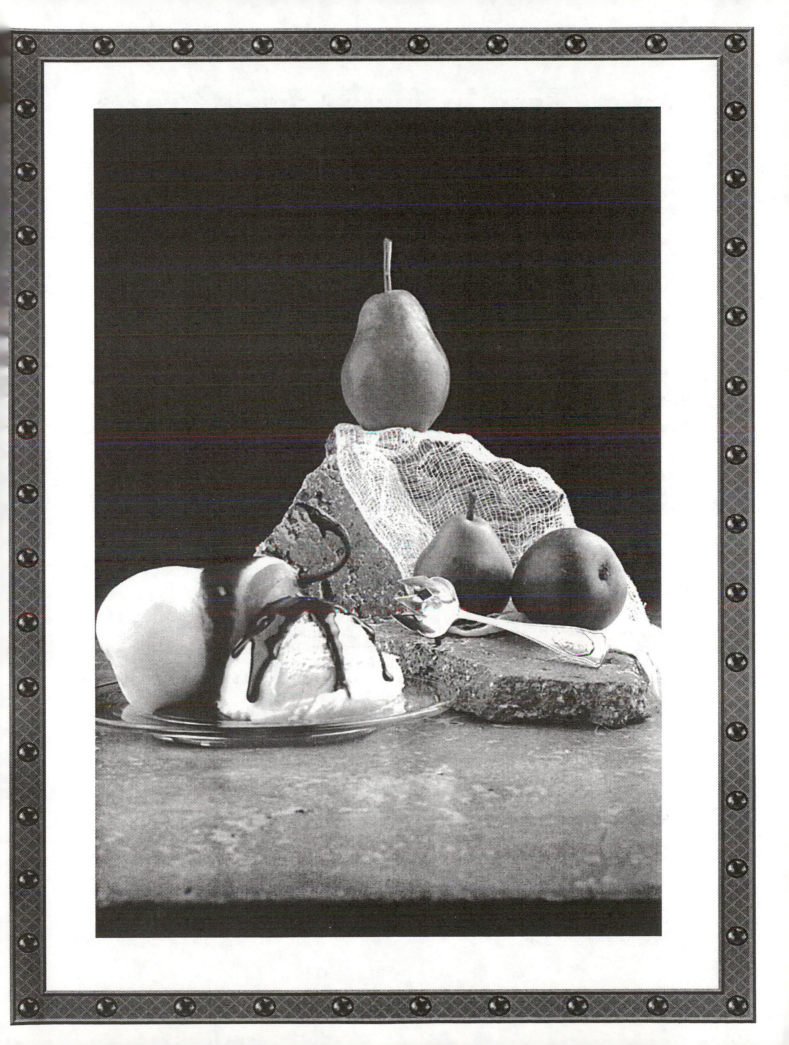

Sugar Free Specials & Sweet Treats

Sugar in America is synonymous with fun, good times and snacking. Our culture instills the powerful urge for sweetness from an early age. But in reality, refined sugar is sucrose, the ultimate naked carbohydrate - stripped of all nutritional benefits. Refined sugar includes raw, brown, natural, yellow D, sucanat, and white sugar. All can be physically addictive, and add nothing but calories to your body. Excessive sugar consumption has many detrimental effects, but the main interest for us in this section is that sugar can be a major interference in a healing program.

Regular sugar intake is known to play a negative part in a host of common illnesses: diabetes, hypoglycemia, heart disease, high cholesterol, overweight, nearsightedness, eczema, psoriasis, dermatitis, gout, indigestion, yeast infections, and tooth decay. It also favors the development of staph infection. Sugar is addictive, like a drug or alcohol. And like these substances, it affects the brain first, offering a false energy lift that eventually lets you down lower than when you started.

Sugar also plays a part in many negative psychological reactions. It is a food that we eat to "cope" in times of stress. It seems to satisfy a hole in both our palates and our psyches. In reality, it produces an over-acid condition in the body, stripping out stabilizing B vitamins. Satisfaction is the very thing you can't get from eating sugar. But as our lives move faster and faster and become more and more stressful, sugar often becomes a bigger and bigger part, pushed on us in an over-abundance of convenience foods. Too much sugar becomes harder and harder to avoid.

Excess sugar can upset mineral balances in the body. It particularly drains away calcium, overloading the body with the acid/ash residues that are responsible for much of the stiffening of joints and limbs in arthritic conditions. Sugar ties up and dissolves B vitamins in the digestive tract, so that they cannot act. Skin, nerve and digestive problems result. Sugar requires the production of insulin for metabolism - a process that promotes the storage of fat. Metabolized sugar is transformed into fat globules, and distributed over the body where the muscles are not very active, such as on the stomach, hips and chin. Every time you eat sugar, some of those calories become body fat instead of energy.

Finally, excess sugar consumption has been shown to depress immune response and the body's resistance to disease, by inhibiting the release of growth hormone. It also lowers disease control, a proven fact for those with diabetes and hypoglycemia, and now becoming known as well for people with high triglycerides and blood pressure.

The good news is that just because you follow a sugar-free diet doesn't mean you have to give up good taste or the comforts of sweetness. The recipes in this section help by satisfying the sweet need with honey, molasses, maple syrup, fruit juice or barley malt. These are naturally occurring whole foods, that can be handled and metabolized easily by the body in its regular processes.

The following chart can help you convert your favorite recipes using sugar to the correct substitutions for natural sweeteners. **Amounts are for each cup of sugar.**

Sweetener	Amount	Reduce Liquid in the Recipe
Fructose	$1/2$ cup	------------
Maple Syrup	$3/4$ cup	2 TBS.
Honey	$3/4$ cup	2 TBS.
Molasses	$1/2$ cup	------------
Barley Malt/Rice Syrup	$11/4$ cups	6 TBS.

See the *Sugar Substitutions* section, page 224 in this book for more information.

The recipes in this chapter concentrate on areas where sugar use is traditionally considered necessary. ❧SUGAR FREE COOKIES & BARS ❧CANDIES & SWEET TREATS ❧CAKES & SWEET MUFFINS ❧PIES & CHEESECAKES ❧FRUIT SWEETENED PUDDINGS, CUSTARDS & MOUSSES ❧

❧❧If you have serious blood sugar regulation problems, such as diabetes or hypoglycemia, consult the **SUGAR IMBALANCES DIET** in this book, or your healing professional, about the kind and amount of sweets your body can handle.

Sugar Free Cookies & Bars

411   CHEWY GRANOLA MACAROONS

For 4 dozen cookies: Preheat oven to 350°.

♣Beat together
2 EGGS
1 CUP MAPLE SUGAR GRANULES
2 TBS. OIL
$1^1/_2$ teasp. VANILLA
1 teasp. SEA SALT

♣Add and mix in
1 CUP SHREDDED COCONUT
$1/_4$ CUP RAISINS
1 CUP COCONUT/ALMOND
   or other GRANOLA

♣Drop spoonfuls onto greased baking sheets, and bake about 10 minutes until golden.

Nutritional analysis: per cookie; 46 calories; trace protein; 6gm. carbohydrate; trace fiber; 2gm. fats; 8mg. cholesterol; 9mg. calcium; trace iron; 6mg. manesium; 40mg. potassium; 48mg. sodium; trace zinc.

412   ALMOND BUTTER CRISPS

For 4 dozen cookies: Preheat oven to 350°.

♣Cream together
$1/_4$ CUP BUTTER
$1/_2$ CUP MAPLE SYRUP
$2/_3$ CUP ALMOND BUTTER (or GOURMET BAKING MIX page 647)

♣Add and mix in
1 teasp. BAKING POWDER
$1^1/_3$ CUPS WHOLE WHEAT PASTRY

♣Roll into balls. Drop onto oiled sheets and bake for 12 to 15 minutes until edges brown. Cool on racks.

413   CRUNCHY GRANOLA COOKIES

For 36 cookies: Preheat oven to 350°.

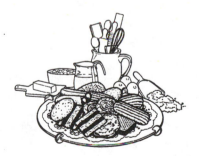

♣Mix and stir all ingredients together
6 TBS. PEANUT BUTTER
$1/_2$ CUP HONEY
1 teasp. CINNAMON
$1/_2$ CUP CAROB CHIPS
$1^1/_2$ CUPS COCONUT/ALMOND or YOUR FAVORITE GRANOLA
♣Drop onto oiled sheets, and bake for 10 minutes until edges brown.

Nutritional analysis: per cookie; 67 calories; 1gm. protein; 9gm. carbohydrate; 1gm. fiber; 4gm. fats; 0 cholesterol; 6mg. calcium; trace iron; 13mg. magnesium; 56mg. potassium; 1mg. sodium; trace zinc.

414   FROSTED LEMON TEA WAFERS

For 24 cookies: Preheat oven to 350°.

♣Mix dry ingredients together
1 CUP UNBLEACHED FLOUR
1/2 CUP SHREDDED COCONUT
1/3 CUP GROUND ALMONDS
1/4 CUP RICE FLOUR
1 teasp. BAKING POWDER
1 teasp. SWEET TOOTH BAKING MIX (pg. 645)
1/2 tesp. BAKING SODA

♣Mix wet ingredients together
1 EGG
1/2 CUP HONEY
1/4 CUP OIL
1/4 CUP MELTED BUTTER
1/4 CUP LEMON YOGURT
2 TBS. FRESH GRATED LEMON ZEST

♣Combine both sets of ingredients to make a dough. Drop onto lecithin-sprayed baking pans about 1" apart. They will spread. Bake for 10 minutes until edges are light brown.
♣Cool. Do not stack. They will get soggy.

Frost with **LEMON CREAM CHEESE FROSTING:**

♣Whip together 3 OZ. NEUFCHATEL CHEESE, 2 TBS. HONEY and 1 teasp. GRATED LEMON PEEL and frost just before serving.

Nutritional analysis: per cookie; 121 calories; 2gm. protein; 12gm. carbohydrate; 1gm. fiber; 7gm. fats; 17mg. cholesterol; 28mg. calcium; trace iron; 16mg. magnesium; 119mg. potassium; 28mg. sodium; trace zinc.

415   CAROB OAT SQUARES

Another goody from the Rainbow Kitchen years - surprisingly high in fiber, low in fat and wheat free.
For 16 squares: Preheat oven to 350∞.

♣Combine dry ingredients
3/4 CUP GRAPENUTS
3/4 CUP OAT FLOUR
1 TB. BAKING POWDER
1/2 teasp. BAKING SODA
3 TBS. CAROB POWDER
 1 TB. BUTTER

♣Heat wet ingredients. Simmer 1 minute
1/3 CUP OIL
1 TB. BARLEY MALT
1/3 CUP HONEY
2 TBS. MAPLE SYRUP
1/2 teasp. ALMOND EXTRACT

♣Mix both sets of ingredients together. Add 2 TBS. YOGURT for smoothness. Pour into a lecitnin-sprayed square pan and bake for 35 minutes.

♣Make the maple glaze while cookie base is still warm. Heat and stir in a pan until liquid and smooth.
4 teasp. MAPLE SYRUP
2 DROPS ALMOND EXTRACT
1 TB. CAROB POWDER
♣Spread thinly over warm cake. Cut in squares.

Nutritional analysis: per square; 121 calories; 1gm. protein; 17gm. carbohydrate; 1gm. fiber; 6gm. fats; 2mg. caholesterol; 59mg. calcium; 2mg. iron; 14mg. magnesium; 233mg. potassium; 42mg. sodium; trace zinc.

416 PINEAPPLE CRANBERRY BARS

For 24 bars: Preheat oven to 350°.

♣Heat $1^1/_2$ CUPS CRANBERRIES and $1^1/_2$ CUPS ORANGE JUICE in a pan until cranberries pop.

♣Beat together
4 TBS. BUTTER
CRANBERRY/ORANGE JUICE MIX
1 teasp. GRATED ORANGE ZEST
1 TB. MAPLE SYRUP (opt.)
2 EGGS

♣Stir together
$2^1/_2$ CUPS WH. WHEAT PASTRY FLOUR
2 teasp. BAKING POWDER
1 teasp. BAKING SODA
$1/_2$ teasp. CINNAMON
$1/_2$ teasp. NUTMEG

♣Mix together and stir in 1 CUP WALNUT PIECES. Spoon into an oiled 9 x 13" baking pan.

♣Top with a mixture of $3/_4$ CUP SHREDDED COCONUT and $3/_4$ CUP CRUSHED DRAINED PINEAP-PLE. Bake for 20 to 25 miutes until a knife stuck in the center comes out clean. Cool and cut.

Nutritional analysis: per bar; 122 calories; 4gm. prtoein; 12gm. carbohydrate; 2gm. fiber; 7gm. fats; 23mg. cholesterol; 36mg. calcium; 1mg. iron; 29mg. magnesium; 253mg. potassium; 25mg. sodium; trace zinc.

417 APRICOT BANANA COOKIES

For 30 cookies: Preheat oven to 350°.

♣Blend all ingredients together until well combined
4 TBS. BUTTER
$1/_3$ CUP MAPLE SYRUP
$1/_2$ OVER RIPE BANANA
$1/_4$ CUP PLAIN LOW-FAT YOGURT
1 EGG WHITE

2 CUPS ROLLED OATS
$1/_2$ CUP WH. WHEAT PASTRY FLOUR
$1/_2$ CUP OAT FLOUR
2 teasp. BAKING POWDER
$1/_2$ CUP CHOPPED DRIED APRICOTS

♣Drop onto lecithin-sprayed baking sheets and bake for 10 to 12 minutes until golden.

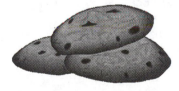

418 MONSTER OATMEAL COOKIES

For 12 cookies: Preheat oven to 350°.

♣Mix all ingredients and let sit for 10 minutes to blend
$1/_2$ CUP OIL
1 CUP HONEY
$1/_2$ CUP RAISINS
1 CUP SHREDDED COCONUT
1 CUP BLUEBERRY NUT GRANOLA
2 TBS. ORANGE JUICE

$1/_2$ CUP WH. WHEAT PASTRY FLOUR
1 CUP ROLLED OATS
1 CUP TOASTED WHEAT GERM
$1/_4$ teasp. BAKING POWDER
$1/_2$ tsp. SWEET TOOTH MIX (pg. 645)

♣Add more orange juice if necessary to moisten. Divide into 12 balls. Place on greased sheets and flatten into big cookies, (about 3 or 4 on a sheet). Bake until golden, about 15 minutes.

419   MOLASSES GINGER COOKIES

For 36 cookies: Preheat oven to 350°.

♣Combine in a pan and heat until smooth and melted
2 TBS. LEMON JUICE
1/2 teasp. BAKING SODA
1/4 CUP MOLASSES
1/4 CUP OIL
1/2 CUP HONEY
♣Remove from heat and set aside.

♣Mix together dry ingredients
2 C. GOURMET FLOUR MIX (pg. 647)
1 teasp. GROUND GINGER
1/2 teasp. SEA SALT
1/2 teasp. ALLSPICE
1/4 teasp. NUTMEG
PINCH GROUND CLOVES

♣Combine both mixtures together to make a well-mixed dough. Roll or press out into long ovals. Bake on lecithin-sprayed baking sheets for 7 to 10 minutes until brown. Cool on racks.

Nutritional analysis: per cookie; 135 calories; 5gm. protein; 28gm. carbohydrate; 3gm. fiber; 1gm. fats; 0 cholesterol; 27mg. calcium; 1mg. iron; 39mg. magnesium; 277mg. potassium; 3mg. sodium; 1mg. zinc.

♣Frost if desired with **BUTTERSCOTCH CANDY FROSTING.** This frosting holds very well, and is perfect for cookies. Cooking thickens the honey and hardens it to a candy-like substance.
♣Bring 1/3 CUP HONEY and 2 TBS. BUTTER to a simmer.
♣Simmer for 10 minutes over low heat until color just begins to darken. Remove from heat and let bubbles die. Spoon over cookies, and let harden.

420   FRUIT JUICE BARS

For 16 cookies: Preheat oven to 350°.

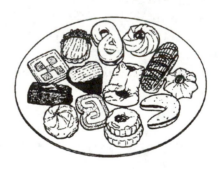

♣Blend in the blender and set aside
1 CUP PITTED CHOPPED DATES
1/2 CUPS APPLE JUICE
1/2 CUP ORANGE JUICE
3 TBS. GRATED ORANGE RIND
1 teasp. VANILLA

♣Grind 2 CUPS ROLLED OATS in the blender to a coarse meal. Stir together in a bowl with 2 CUPS WHOLE WHEAT PASTRY FLOUR and 1 TB. CINNAMON. Moisten with 1 1/2 CUPS APPLE or PEAR JUICE.

♣Press dough into a lightly oiled 8" square pan. Spread date puree on top. Bake for 35 to 45 minutes until crust is firm. Cool completely and cut in squares.

Nutritional analysis: per serving; 135 calories; 5gm. protein; 28gm. carbohydrate; 3gm. fiber; 1gm. fats; 0 cholesterol; 27mg. calcium; 1mg. iron; 39mg. magnesium; 277mg. potassium; 3mg. sodium; 1mg. zinc.

Sugar Free Candies & Sweet Treats

421   BUTTERSCOTCH COCONUT BALLS

For 8 balls:

♣Brown 1 CUP SHREDDED COCONUT in a 250° oven until light gold. Pour in a mixing bowl.

♣Brown 1 CUP NON-INSTANT MILK POWDER in a 250° oven until light gold. Pour in the bowl.

♣Add

1/2 CUP HONEY

1/2 teasp. VANILLA

2 TBS. BUTTER

♣Roll into balls and press a WHOLE NUT into each.

Nutritional analysis: per ball; 230 calories; 5gm. protein; 25gm. carbohydrate; 2gm. fiber; 13gm. fats; 9mg. cholesterol; 116mg. calcium; 1mg. iron; 31mg. magnesium; 245mg. potassium; 21mg. sodium; 1mg. zinc.

422   ALMOND BUTTER MEDJOOLS

These are super sweet and a perfect blend of tastes.
Stuffing for 8 big dates:

♣Cut open 8 BIG MEDJOOL DATES and spread apart for stuffing.

♣Mash and mix 1/2 teasp. HONEY and 1/4 CUP ALMOND BUTTER together.

♣Stuff dates and roll in 1/4 CUP SHREDDED COCONUT. Serve chilled.

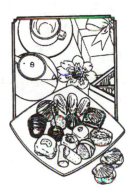

423   BEE POLLEN SURPRISE

A nice high protein little treat. Very nutritious.
For 18 pieces:

♣Heat 1 CUP HONEY and 1 CUP PEANUT BUTTER together stirring until smooth.

♣Remove from heat and mix in

2/3 CUP TOASTED COCONUT ALMOND GRANOLA

1 CUP CAROB POWDER   1/2 CUP CHOPPED NUTS

1 CUP TOASTED SUNFLOWER SEEDS   1/2 CUP SHREDDED COCONUT

1/2 CUP RAISINS.   4 TBS. BEE POLLEN GRANULES

♣Press into a lecithin-sprayed square pan. Chill and cut in squares.

Nutritional analysis: per serving; 246 calories; 7gm. protein; 30gm. carbohydrate; 5gm. fiber; 15gm. fats; 0 cholesterol; 42mg. calcium; 1mg. iron; 62mg. magnesium; 307mg. potassium; 13mg. sodium; 1mg. zinc.

424   HONEY CANDIED FRUITS

You can eat these just like they are, or use them in holiday fruit cakes, or to decorate cookies.

♣Heat 2 CUPS WATER, 1½ CUPS HONEY and 2 TBS. LEMON JUICE in a saucepan until blended.
♣Dip in your choice of fruits, such as PINEAPPLE, FIGS, APRICOTS, PEACHES, or PEARS.

♣Then dehydrate in a dehydrator or on drying screens in the sun, until rubbery and chewy, but not too dry. Candied fruit can be stored airtight in the fridge for quite a while.

425   BAKED CANDY POPCORN

For 12 servings: Preheat oven to 350°.

♣Make a big batch of POPCORN. Put in a large bowl. Add 1½ CUPS DRY ROASTED PEANUTS

♣Melt ONE STICK of BUTTER in a saucepan. Add ½ CUP HONEY, ¼ CUP MOLASSES and ½ CUP MAPLE SYRUP. Stir and simmer until bubbles form.
♣Immediately pour over popcorn and peanuts, and toss to coat.
♣Spread mixture on two lecithin-sprayed baking sheets, and bake until coating darkens, about 10 minutes. ♣Cool completely before storing, so mix won't turn soggy.

Nutritional analysis: per serving; 281 calories; 5gm. protein; 31gm. carbohydrate; 2gm. fiber; 17gm. fats; 21mg. cholesterol; 74mg. calcium; 3mg. iron; 69mg. magnesium; 372mg. potassium; 13mg. sodium; 1mg. zinc.

426   APPLE BARS

For 12 pieces: Preheat oven to 350°.

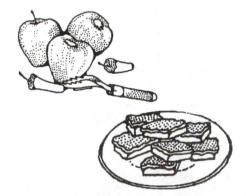

♣Blend all ingredients in a bowl
½ CUP APPLESAUCE
½ CUP APPLE JUICE
3 EGGS
4 TBS BUTTER
2 CUPS WHOLE WHEAT PASTRY FLOUR
2 teasp. BAKING POWDER
1 teasp. BAKING SODA
1½ teasp. CINNAMON
1 teasp. NUTMEG
1 CUP RAISINS
♣Press into an oiled square pan. Sprinkle with SWEET TOOTH BAKING MIX or APPLE PIE SPICE.
♣Bake for 25 minutes.

Nutritional analysis: per serving; 166 calories; 5gm. protein; 25gm. carbohydrate; 3gm. fiber; 6gm. fats; 63mg. cholesterol; 66mg. calcium; 1mg. iron; 31mg. magnesium; 440mg. potassium; 53mg. sodium; 1mg. zinc.

Sugar Free Cakes & Sweet Muffins

427 LIGHT CARROT NUT CAKE

For 12 pieces: Preheat oven to 350°.

♣Separate 6 EGGS. Beat yolks with

1 CUP GRATED CARROTS
1 CUP CHOPPED WALNUTS
1/2 CUP WHOLE WHEAT PASTRY FLOUR
1/4 CUP TOASTED WHEAT GERM
1/4 CUP GRANOLA

1/2 CUP HONEY
2 TBS. MAPLE SYRUP
1 teasp. CINNAMON
1/2 teasp. SEA SALT
1/4 teasp. NUTMEG

♣Beat WHITES to STIFF PEAKS and fold into cake. Pour into a lecithin-sprayed square baking dish, and bake for 45 minutes until very puffy and golden on top.

♣Top with dollops of **ALMOND HONEY ICING:**

♣Beat 1 EGG WHITE with 2 PINCHES CREAM OF TARTER to stiff peaks.
♣Add 1/2 CUP HONEY in a thin stream while beating.
♣Add 1/4 teasp. ALMOND EXTRACT and beat until thick and fluffy.

428 HONEY WALNUT CAKE

This is a good November/December cake with Maple Boiled Icing.
For 12 pieces: Preheat oven to 350°.

♣Mix the dry ingredients
3/4 CUP UNBLEACHED FLOUR
3/4 CUP BARLEY FLOUR
2 teasp. BAKING POWDER
1/4 teasp. BAKING SODA
1 teasp. CINNAMON
1 teasp. APPLE PIE SPICE

♣Heat wet ingredients til smooth
1/2 CUP HONEY
1/4 CUP BUTTER
1/4 CUP APPLE JUICE
2/3 CUP CHOPPED WALNUTS
2 teasp. VANILLA

♣Combine both mixtures together to make a batter.

♣Beat 4 EGG WHITES to STIFF PEAKS and fold into batter. Pour into greased 9 x 11" cake pan, and bake for 35 minutes until a toothpick inserted comes out clean.

♣Top with **MAPLE BOILED ICING:** Boil in a saucepan until large, heavy threads form from a lifted spoon.

1/2 CUP MAPLE SYRUP
3 TBS. HONEY

1/2 teasp. CREAM OF TARTER
1/4 teasp. SEA SALT

♣Beat 2 EGG WHITES to STIFF PEAKS. Add syrup and beat into whites until thick enough to spread.

429   SPICE INFUSED MUFFINS WITH MARMALADE WELLS

For 10 muffins: Preheat oven to 350°.

♣Mix dry ingredients together
1$^1/_2$ CUPS WHOLE WHEAT PASTRY FLOUR
1 CUP SLICED ALMONDS
1 teasp. BAKING POWDER
$^1/_2$ teasp. BAKING SODA
1 teasp. CINNAMON
$^1/_2$ teasp. NUTMEG
$^1/_2$ teasp. GROUND CORIANDER

♣Beat wet ingredients together
$^1/_2$ CUP HONEY
$^1/_2$ CUP BUTTERMILK
4 TBS. OIL
1 EGG
1 teasp. GRATED LEMON PEEL
$^1/_4$ teasp. GROUND ALLSPICE

♣Combine the two mixtures and stir until moistened. Fill 10 paper-lined muffin cups $^2/_3$ full. Using a tea-spoon, gently press 1 rounded teaspoon marmalade into the center of each muffin. Bake 20 minutes until golden and firm. Cool briefly in pan, then remove to racks.
♣Mix 2 TBS. DATE SUGAR and $^1/_4$ teasp. CINNAMON and dust tops of muffins.

Nutritional analysis: per serving; 230 calories; 6gm. protein; 29gm. carbohydrate; 3gm. fiber; 11gm. fats; 21mg. cho-lesterol; 78mg. calcium; 1mg. iron; 53mg. magnesium; 344mg. potassium; 42mg. sodium; 1mg. zinc.

✖

430   SWEET CARROT BABY CAKES WITH LEMON TOPPING

We made this recipe as individual cakes for the restaurant, but it works just as well baked in a 9 x 11" dish. Very moist and rich without the sugar.
For 18 muffin cakes: Preheat oven to 350°.

♣Mix together until smooth
$^3/_4$ CUP OIL
2 CUPS GRATED CARROTS
$^1/_2$ CUP ALMOND BUTTER

$^3/_4$ CUP HONEY
$^1/_4$ CUP LEMON JUICE
2 TBS. VANILLA

♣Mix dry ingredients together
2$^1/_2$ CUPS GOURMET FLOUR MIX (page 647)
1 CUP CHOPPED WALNUTS
1$^1/_2$ CUPS CURRANTS

$^1/_2$ teasp. BAKING SODA
2 teasp. BAKING POWDER
2 teasp. SWEET TOOTH BAKING MIX

♣Combine both mixtures and spoon into paper-lined or greased muffin cups. Bake for 45 minutes until springy when touched.

Top with **FRESH LEMON GLAZE.** For 2 cups:

♣Heat over low heat for 5 minutes until thickened
1 CUP HONEY
2 TBS. ARROWROOT dissolved in 2 TBS. water 1
1$^3/_4$ CUP WATER
PINCH SEA SALT

♣Remove from heat and add
2 TBS. BUTTER
$^1/_2$ teasp. LEMON JUICE
$^1/_2$ teasp. GRATED LEMON ZEST

✖

431   GLAZED PEAR CAKE

For 10 pieces: Preheat oven to 350°.

♣Separate 3 EGGS. Mix the yolks with
1 CUP OAT FLOUR
1/2 CUP BARLEY FLOUR
2 teasp. BAKING POWDER
1/2 teasp. BAKING SODA

♣Melt together
4 TBS. BUTTER
1/2 CUP MAPLE SYRUP
2 TBS. ORANGE JUICE CONCENTRATE
2 teasp. VANILLA

♣Blend the two mixtures together. Beat egg whites to stiff with a pinch of CREAM OF TARTAR. Fold into batter. Pour into a lecithin-sprayed ceramic quiche dish. Bake for 20 minutes.
♣Cool while you make the **PEAR GLAZE**:
♣Simmer 2 LARGE THIN-SLICED PEARS in a skillet with 1 CUP FROZEN APPLE JUICE CONCEN-TRATE until most of the juice is cooked off. The small remaining amount should be thick and syrupy. Arrange pears on top of the cake decoratively. Spoon juice over.

Nutritional analysis: per serving; 228 calories; 5gm. protein; 38gm. carbohydrate; 3gm. fiber; 7gm. fats; 76mg. cholesterol; 87mg. calcium; 1mg. iron; 34mg. magnesium; 533mg. potassium; 42mg. sodium; 1mg. zinc.

432   BEST SUGAR FREE GINGERBREAD

For 12 pieces: Preheat oven to 350°.

♣Sauté 3 TBS. GRATED GINGER ROOT in 5 TBS. OIL in a pan til fragrant.
♣Add 1/2 CUP HONEY and 1/2 CUP MOLASSES and heat. Remove from heat and add 1/2 CUP PLAIN YOGURT and 1 EGG.
♣Mix dry ingredients in a bowl
2 CUPS WH. WHEAT PASTRY FLOUR
1/2 teasp. SEA SALT
1/2 teasp. CINNAMON

3/4 teasp. SWEET TOOTH BAKING MIX
1 1/2 teasp. BAKING SODA
1/2 teasp. ALLSPICE

♣Combine both mixtures just to moisten. Spread into a lecithin-sprayed 8" square baking pan. Bake for 30 minutes until top is springy and a toothpick inserted in the center comes out clean.

433   SWEET ZUCCHINI MUFFINS

These are a pleasant surprise from the making to the eating.
For 12 muffins: Preheat oven to 400°.

♣Grate 1 CUP ZUCCHINI in a salad shooter or food processor and set aside.
♣Cream well in a bowl
4 TBS. OIL
3/8 CUP HONEY
2 EGGS

♣Beat in
1/3 CUP PLAIN YOGURT
2 TBS. WATER
1 teasp. VANILLA

♣Mix the dry ingredients

1 CUP UNBLEACHED FLOUR

1/2 CUP WHOLE WHEAT PASTRY FLOUR

3/8 CUP CAROB POWDER

1/2 teasp. CINNAMON

1/2 teasp. NUTMEG

1/2 teasp. BAKING SODA

♣Combine the two mixtures together gently just to moisten. Bake in paper-lined muffin cups for 15-18 minutes til a toothpick inserted in the center comes out clean.

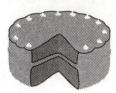

Sugar Free Pies & Cheesecakes

434   SWEET YAM PIE

The original down home southern country version. I can hear the old screen door slamming now.
For 10 pieces: Preheat oven to 325°. Try a POPPY SEED/CHEDDAR CRUST or your favorite.

♣Separate 3 EGGS.

♣Blend the filling in the blender until very smooth

4 COOKED MASHED YAMS

1/3 CUP ORANGE JUICE

1/4 CUP HONEY

1/4 CUP MAPLE SYRUP

1 1/2 teasp. GRATED ORANGE PEEL

3 TBS. BUTTER

3 EGG YOLKS

1 TB. CINNAMON

1/2 teasp. VANILLA

1/2 teasp. SEA SALT

♣Beat the 3 EGG WHITES to stiff peaks with a pinch of CREAM OF TARTAR. Fold into batter, and pour into pie shell. Garnish decoratively with pecan halves. Bake for 40 minutes until set.

Nutritional analysis: per serving; 211 calories; 3gm. protein; 39gm. carbohydrate; 3gm. fiber; 5gm. fats; 73mg. cholesterol' 55mg. calcium; 1mg. iron; 23mg. magnesium; 410mg. potassium; 135mg. sodium; trace zinc.

435   EASY HONEY WALNUT PIE

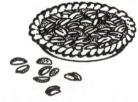

For 8 servings: Preheat oven to375°.

♣Heat and mix together in a saucepan until smooth

2/3 CUP DATE SUGAR

1 CUP HONEY

1/2 teasp. VANILLA or BLACK WALNUT EXTRACT

2 TBS. MAPLE SYRUP

PINCH SEA SALT

♣Remove from heat, and add 1 CUP CHOPPED WALNUTS. Pour into a crushed SUGAR-FREE COOKIE CRUMB and BUTTER CRUST. Bake for 10 minutes. Reduce heat to 300°, and bake for 40 minutes more. Center will *still be wobbly when done.*

Nutritional analysis: per filling serving; 278 calories; 2gm. protein; 52gm. carbohydrate; 2gm. fiber; 9gm. fats; 0 cholesterol; 26mg. calcium; 1mg. iron; 32mg. magnesium; 201mg. potassium; 31mg. sodium; trace zinc.

436 AMBROSIA CHEESECAKE

For 16 small rich servings: Preheat oven to 350°.

♣Combine 2 CUPS SWEET AMARANTH or SUGARLESS GRAHAM CRACKERS and 4 TBS. MELTED BUTTER and pat onto the bottom and part of the sides of a lecithin-sprayed springform pan. Chill until ready to fill.

♣Make the filling in the blender.
4-OZ. RAW CREAM CHEESE
3 EGGS
1 CARTON KEFIR CHEESE
1/2 CUP HONEY

♣Blend until *very* smooth
1 teasp. LEMON JUICE
2 teasp. ORANGE JUICE
1 teasp. GRATED LEMON PEEL

♣Pour into shell, and bake for *20 minutes only*. Remove from the oven and cool for 10 minutes while you make the topping. Blend the topping in the blender
1 CUP PLAIN YOGURT
2 TBS. HONEY

1 teasp. VANILLA
1 teasp. LEMON EXTRACT

♣Pour over the cake and bake for 10 to 15 more minutes. Remove, cool and chill until ready to serve. Decorate with <u>drained</u> MANDARIN ORANGE SLICES if desired.

437 ALMOND SCENTED CHEESECAKE BITES

For 24 individual cakes: Preheat oven to 300°.

♣Place 12-OZ. LOW-FAT COTTAGE CHEESE in a strainer over the sink and drain for 30 minutes.
♣Combine in a blender and process until smooth
THE COTTAGE CHEESE
3 EGGS
1/4 CUP APPLE JUICE CONCENTRATE
1/4 CUP PINEAPPLE JUICE CONCENTRATE

1 TB. WHEAT GERM
1 teasp. VANILLA
1 teasp. ALMOND EXTRACT

♣Fill paper-lined muffin tins 2/3 full with batter. Bake 35 minutes until a toothpick inserted in the center comes out clean. Cool on rack, and then chill.
♣Combine 1/3 CUP PLAIN LOW FAT YOGURT and 3 TBS. MAPLE SYRUP. Drizzle on cheesecake.

Desserts: fruit Sweetened

438 WATERMELON ICE with CAROB CHIP SEEDS

Makes about 1 qt.: Serve within 30 minutes of blending for best texture.

♣Freeze 4 CUPS WATERMELON CUBES solid. Freeze 1 small basket raspberries or strawberries (or use one half a 12 OZ. package frozen). Put in a blender and pulse until mixture resembles shaved ice. ♣Add 1/3 CUP PLAIN YOOGURT and process until smooth and creamy. Freeze for 30 minutes or longer. Mound into a serving bowl and stud with CAROB CHIPS.

439 CRANBERRY MOUSSE

This is so rich and creamy, you won't believe it doesn't have any sugar or fatty dairy products. It is a good Thanksgiving or holiday dessert choice after a heavy meal and for people trying to stick to a diet.
For 4 to 6 servings:

♣Beat in the blender until very smooth

$^1/_2$ CUP KEFIR CHEESE

$^1/_2$ teasp. SWEET TOOTH BAKING MIX

ONE 8-OZ. JAR SUGAR FREE CRANBERRY PRESERVES

2 TBS. ROSÉ WINE

2 TBS. HONEY

♣Beat 4 EGG WHITES to stiff peaks, and fold into the kefir/wine mix. Spoon into parfait glasses or mousse cups and chill overnight.

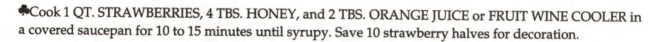

440 FRESH STRAWBERRY MOUSSE

This is also delicious with raspberries and pitted bing cherries.
For 4 to 5 servings:

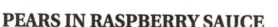

♣Separate 3 EGGS. Set each part aside in separate mixing bowls.

♣Cook 1 QT. STRAWBERRIES, 4 TBS. HONEY, and 2 TBS. ORANGE JUICE or FRUIT WINE COOLER in a covered saucepan for 10 to 15 minutes until syrupy. Save 10 strawberry halves for decoration.

♣Mix a little of the hot syrup with 3 TBS. ARROWROOT or KUZU until dissolved. Add to the reserved EGG YOLKS. Return to the strawberry mix and beat for 2 minutes til combined.

♣Beat EGG WHITES to stiff peaks with PINCH CREAM OF TARTER. Fold into strawberry mix and chill for at least 2 hours.

♣Beat 1 CUP KEFIR CHEESE with 2 to 3 TBS. MORE JUICE or WINE COOLER until light and fluffy.

♣Mix gently with chilled mousse, and chill another 2 hours. Serve in individual mousse or custard cups and top each with a strawberry half.

Nutritional analysis: per serving; 183 calories; 6gm. protein; 30gm. carbohydrate; 4gm. fiber; 5gm. fats; 134mg. cholesterol; 92mg. calcium; 1mg. iron; 25mg. magnesium; 366mg. potassium; 103mg. sodium; 1mg. zinc.

441 PEARS IN RASPBERRY SAUCE

For 4 to 6 servings: Preheat oven to 350°.

♣Slice and seed 3 RIPE PEARS and place cut side down in a baking dish.

♣Combine $^1/_4$ CUP RASPBERRY JELLY or JAM, the JUICE OF ONE ORANGE (or $^1/_2$ CUP), and 2 TBS. WHITE WINE in a bowl. Pour over pears. Cover with foil and bake for 30 minutes until pears are soft. Remove to a serving dish and spoon sauce on top.

♣Sprinkle on FRESH CHOPPED RASPBERRIES and CHOPPED ROASTED ALMONDS.

442   MOM'S APPLE CRISP

For 1 9 x 14" pan: Preheat oven to 350°.

♣Mix together in a bowl
6 TART APPLES peeled, cored and sliced
1/2 CUP HONEY
2 teasp. CINNAMON
2 teasp. LEMON JUICE
1/4 teasp. ALLSPICE

♣Mix in another bowl until crumbly
3/4 CUP WH. WHEAT PASTRY FLOUR
6 TBS. BUTTER
1/4 CUP WALNUT PIECES
1/4 teasp. SEA SALT

♣Layer half the apple mixture into the pan. Top with half of the crumble mixture. Repeat layers, making sure that topping covers all the apples. Bake for 30 minutes until apples are nearly tender. Remove and drizzle honey over top. Return to oven and bake until gooey and syrupy.

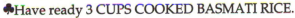

443   BASMATI CINNAMON PUDDING

The nutty flavor of the basmati rice really comes through.
For 6 to 8 servings: Preheat oven to 325°.

♣Have ready 3 CUPS COOKED BASMATI RICE.
♣Mix rice with

2 CUPS PLAIN or LEMON YOGURT
1/2 CUP WATER
1/2 CUP HONEY
5 EGGS
2 TBS. FRESH GRATED ORANGE PEEL

2 TBS. MAPLE SYRUP
1 teasp. VANILLA
1 teasp. CINNAMON
3/4 CUP RAISINS
2 TART APPLES chopped

♣Turn the entire pudding into a deep buttered baking dish, and bake for 1 hour until custard sets, and browns slightly at the edges. Stir occasionally while baking if it is looking too dry. Remove and let set for 10 minutes, while you make a quick topping.

Kids love this easy **FRUIT & JELLY TOPPING:**
♣Melt 1/2 CUP SUGAR FREE STRAWBERRY or RASPBERRY JELLY in a small saucepan. Slice in some strawberries, or a peach or nectarine, and spoon over pudding.

444   RAISIN PECAN ICE CREAM

For 6 to 8 servings:

♣Chop 2 CUPS FRUIT of your choice and 2 CUPS BANANAS. Freeze solid. Put in the blender with 1 CUP PINEAPPLE or ORANGE JUICE and blend until stiff.
♣Stir in 1 CUP RAISINS and 3/4 CUP CHOPPED PECANS. Serve immediately.

Nutritional analysis: per serving; 201 calories; 2gm. protein; 34gm. carbohydrate; 4gm. fiber; 8gm. fats; 0 cholesterol; 22mg. calcium; 1mg. iron; 36mg. magnesium; 440mg. potassium; 3mg. sodium; 1mg. zinc.

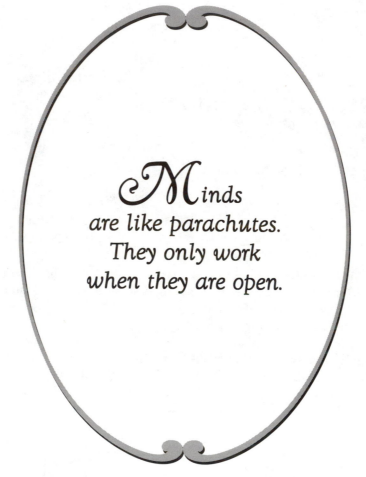

$\mathcal{M}$inds
are like parachutes.
They only work
when they are open.

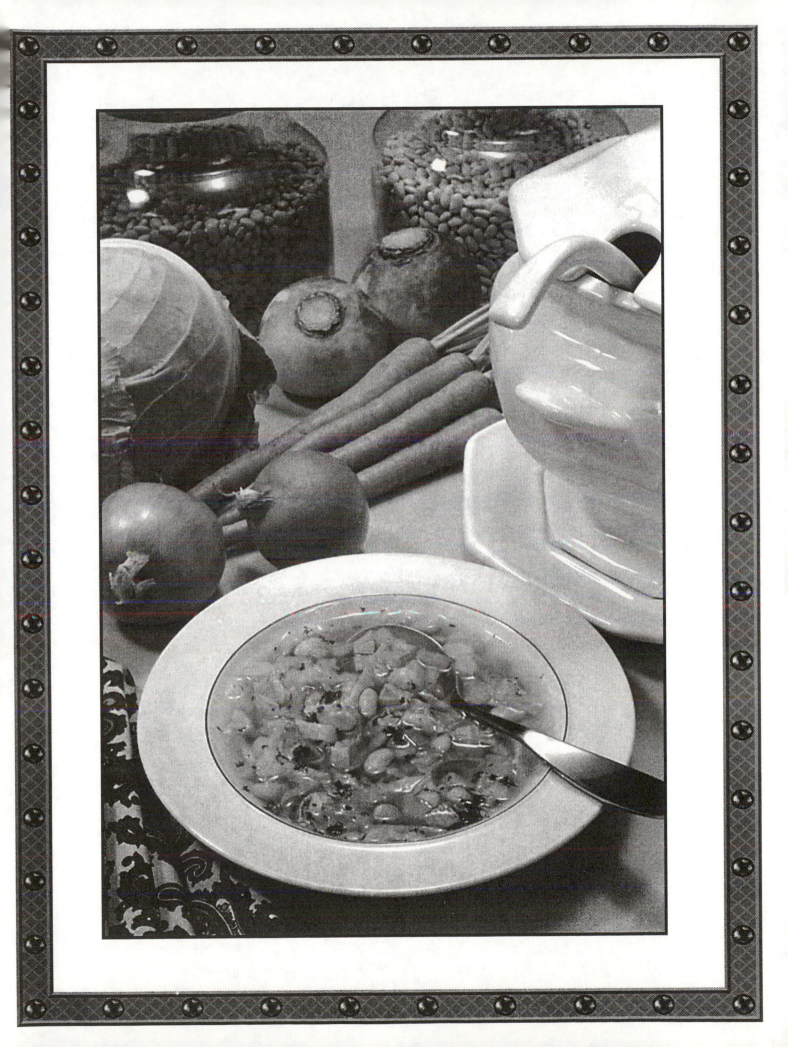

Soups
Liquid Salads

Soups are super foods for a healing diet. They can fill many uses as delicious "medicinals." They are easy-to-assimilate nutrition, a great deal like liquid salads. They may be light, vitamin-filled, clear broths that can allay hunger during a flushing and cleansing diet. Or they may be packed with high protein for faster healing, fiber and complex carbohydrates for rebuilding; yet they don't have the density of solid food that can slow things down.

Healing herbs are perfect taken in a hot, hearty broth. One might think of an herb-scented soup as a robust, healing tea. In fact, soups are the *best* medium for getting the best healing benefits from extremely pungent herbal medicinals such as garlic, (every healing tradition has a garlic type soup), or sea vegetables for iodine therapy, or hot chilis or cayenne peppers.

You can use soups hot and cold, as low-fat, low calorie, satisfying meals or snacks for taking off extra weight without feeling hungry, or toning fat-free muscle, and for keeping the circulatory system clear of clogging fats.

An aromatic, simmered foundation is essential to wonderful homemade soup taste. Today it is easy to buy delicious dry, preservative-free mixes in health food stores and gourmet groceries. But if your diet must be very low in salt, it is best to make your soups from scratch with your own vegetables and seasonings, (see page 657 for stock recipes). Canned and commercially prepared stocks, broths and bouillons may be too high in salt, and sometimes fat as well.

Make soups in a large open pot if possible. It gives the stock and ingredients room to "work," and allows the aroma to develop.

The recipe categories in this chapter include:
❧PURIFYING LIGHT BROTHS ❧LOW CALORIE, LOW-FAT SOUPS ❧HIGH PROTEIN SOUPS ❧ HIGH COMPLEX CARBOHYDRATE SOUPS ❧WHOLE MEAL SOUPS and STEWS ❧DUMPLING GOODIES FOR SOUP TOPPERS ❧

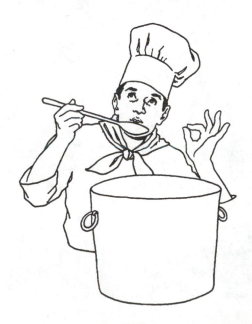

Purifying Light Broths
These soups are blood and system cleansers - good for health, delicious in taste.

445   DOUBLE MUSHROOM CONSOMMÉ
As new information about the anti-carcinogenic properties of certain mushrooms becomes available, we are adding more recipes to take advantage of their valuable healing benefits.
For 6 servings:

♣Heat 6 CUPS RICH ONION STOCK (page 652) in a large soup pot.

♣Soak 2 to 3 LARGE DRIED BLACK SHIITAKE MUSHROOMS in water to cover until soft. Sliver, discard woody stems, and add soaking water to the soup pot.
♣Slice 8-OZ. BUTTON MUSHROOMS and 3 GREEN ONIONS WITH TOPS. Add to soup pot and simmer for 45 minutes.

♣Add seasonings

2 TBS. LEMON JUICE	1 teasp. HERB SALT
2 TBS. WHITE WINE	1/2 teasp. WHITE PEPPER
1 teasp. TAMARI	1 teasp. MINCED DRY WAKAME

♣Strain for a light consommé, or eat as is with mushroom pieces.

Nutritional analysis: per serving; 35 calories; 2gm. protein; 7gm. carbohydrate; 2gm. fiber; trace fats; 0 cholesterol; 23mg. calcium; 1mg. iron; 15mg. magnesium; 243mg. potassium; 252mg. sodium; trace zinc.

446   ORIENTAL DOUBLE PEA & MUSHROOM BROTH

For 8 servings:

♣Soak 6 to 8 DRIED SHIITAKE BLACK MUSHROOMS until soft. Sliver, discard woody stems, and reserve soaking water.

♣Sort and rinse 1 CUP DRIED SPLIT PEAS.
♣Sauté in a large soup pot in 1 TB. OIL until aromatic, about 5 minutes

1 SMALL ONION	1 CARROT, thin sliced
2 TBS. FRESH MINCED GINGER	2 CUPS THIN SLICED CELERY

♣Add 6 CUPS MISO or CHICKEN BROTH, the slivered mushrooms, and the split peas. Bring to a boil, partially cover and simmer until peas are tender - about 1 1/2 hours.
♣Remove cover and add a 10-OZ. PACKAGE FROZEN PEAS. Turn off heat, and let peas heat until color changes to bright green.
♣Season with 1 teasp. HOT PEPPER SAUCE and 1 teasp. TOASTED SESAME OIL, or SZECHUAN CHILI OIL.

Nutritional analysis: per serving; 167 calories; 9gm. protein; 8gm. carbohydrate; 8gm. fiber; 3gm. fats; 0 cholesterol; 50mg. calcium; 2mg. iron; 53mg. magnesium; 530mg. potassium; 162mg. sodium; 1mg. zinc.

447   GREAT GRANDMA'S HEALING CHICKEN SOUP

Sometimes the old, traditional remedies are the best.
For 4 to 6 servings:

♣Rinse 4 to 4$^1/_2$ LBS. CHICKEN PIECES and put in a large soup pot with

5 CARROTS, quartered	3 PARSNIPS, quartered
4 LEEKS, quartered	2 WHOLE BAY LEAVES
4 CELERY RIBS in 2" lengths	1 teasp. SEA SALT
2-QTS. HOMEMADE CHICKEN STOCK	$^3/_4$ teasp. PEPPER
4 CUPS WATER	

♣Bring to a boil slowly. Reduce heat and simmer, uncovered, skimming off fat and foam until chicken is tender - about 1 hour. Strain and transfer chicken vegetables to a platter. Cover with foil.
♣Return broth to soup pot and bring to a rapid boil. Boil until liquid is reduced to 6 cups, about 30 minutes. Season again.
♣Remove bones from chicken, tear into bite size pieces, and divide the chicken and vegetables between soup bowls. Pour broth over and serve.

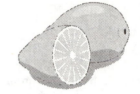

448   LIGHT LEEK, LETTUCE & LEMON SOUP

For 4 servings:

♣ Cut most of the green tops from 2 LARGE LEEKS, and slice in thin julienne.
♣ Shred $^1/_2$ HEAD ROMAINE or HEAD LETTUCE
♣ Braise lettuce and leeks in 2 TBS. OIL and 1 CUP ONION BROTH or MISO SOUP for 10 minutes.
♣ Add a 10 OZ. PKG. FROZEN GREEN PEAS, and steam for 1 to 2 minutes until color is bright green. Remove from heat. Add 1 teasp. SEA SALT, $^1/_4$ teasp. WHITE PEPPER, 4 FRESH MINT LEAVES and 2 teasp. LEMON JUICE.
♣ Pureé in the blender until smooth. Add 2 SCOOPS PLAIN YOGURT if desired, and pureé again.

449   GREEN BROTH

For 6 servings:

♣ Sauté in 1 TB. OIL til aromatic - 5 minutes
1/4 CUP MINCED LEEKS
1/2 CUP MINCED GREEN ONIONS
2 TBS. MINCED SHALLOTS
1/4 CUP MINCED CELERY
♣ Sprinkle with 1 TB. WHOLE WHEAT FLOUR and toss to coat.

♣ Add and toss just to wilt - 1 minute
1 CUP FINELY CHOPPED GREENS
   (spinach, chard, endive, romaine, etc.)
1/4 CUP MINCED FRESH PARSLEY
1/4 CUP MINCED WATERCRESS

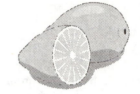

♣ Bring 4 CUPS VEGETABLE STOCK or MISO SOUP to a boil. Add vegetables and 1 TB. LEMON JUICE, $^1/_2$ teasp. SESAME SALT or HERB SALT, and $^1/_4$ teasp. WHITE PEPPER.
♣ Heat just through, and garnish with very thin SLICES of DAIKON WHITE RADISH.

Low Calorie, Low Fat Soups
Soups are a wonderful way to keep your middle little.

450 FRESH TOMATO BASIL SOUP
A prime summertime taste.
For 4 to 6 servings:

♣Sauté in 2 TBS. BUTTER or OIL until fragrant - 5 minutes.
♣Add 1 CLOVE MINCED GARLIC, 1 FRESH ZUCCHINI, chopped, 1 CUP CHOPPED ONION, and 1 GREEN BELL PEPPER, chopped. Sauté for 3 minutes.

♣Add 4 CUPS ONION or VEGETABLE STOCK, and bring to a quick boil. Reduce heat to a simmer.
♣Add ³/₄ CUP WHITE or ROSÉ WINE and 2 or 3 LARGE FRESH CHOPPED TOMATOES.
♣Simmer for 20 minutes.

♣Add 4 MINCED SCALLIONS, ¹/₂ CUP CHOPPED FRESH BASIL and ¹/₂ teasp. WHITE PEPPER and heat for 5 more minutes until basil is aromatic.

♣Serve as is, or place 2 spoonfuls of cooked brown rice in each soup bowl, and pour soup over. Sprinkle with a little Parmesan cheese if desired.

Nutritional analysis: per serving; 74 calories; 1gm. protein; 7gm. carbohydrate; 2gm. fiber; 3gm. fats; 7mg. cholesterol; 31mg. calcium; 1mg. iron; 21mg. magnesium; 283mg. potassium; 80mg. sodium; trace zinc.

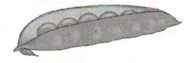

451 SWEET PEA & FRESH MINT SOUP

For 8 servings:

♣Sauté 2 CUPS CHOPPED YELLOW ONIONS in 3 TBS. BUTTER or OIL until aromatic and translucent.

♣Add 3 CUPS VEGETABLE STOCK or BOUILLON. Bring to a boil, reduce heat and simmer for 10 minutes. Remove from heat and cool slightly.

♣Chop 1 SMALL HEAD ROMAINE or 1 SMALL BUNCH SPINACH very fine. Add half to the soup.

♣CHOP 2 CUPS FRESH MINT LEAVES very fine, and add half to the soup.

♣Blender blend soup with 1 CUP PLAIN YOGURT. Whirl until smooth. Return to soup pot and heat.

♣Add 1 10-OZ. PACKAGE FRESH FROZEN PEAS and heat soup until peas turn a bright green.
♣Add rest of romaine and mint leaves. Stir in and season with HERB SALT and WHITE PEPPER.

Nutritional analysis: per serving; 98 calories; 5gm. protein; 13gm. carbohydrates; 4gm. fiber; 4gm. fats; 9mg. cholesterol; 107mg. calcium; 2mg. iron; 37mg. magnesium; 359mg. potassium; 139mg. sodium; 1mg. zinc.

452   WHITE GAZPACHO

This soup is a traditional summer favorite.
For 6 servings:

♣Peel and chop 1 LONG EUROPEAN CUCUMBER.
2 CUPS PLAIN LOW-FAT YOGURT
2 TBS. LEMON JUICE

♣Blend in the blender until smooth with
1/4 teasp. GARLIC/LEMON SEASONING
1/2 CUP ONION BROTH

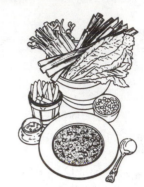

♣Add to soup pot with
1 1/2 MORE CUPS ONION BROTH
1/2 CUP WHITE WINE
1/2 CUP WATER
♣ Stir and heat til combined and smooth. Remove from heat.

♣Top with
2 TBS. FRESH CHOPPED CILANTRO
2 TBS. CHOPPED GREEN ONION
1 TB. FRESH CHOPPED BASIL
♣Chill in the fridge for 1 to 2 hours.

Nutritional analysis: per serving; 75 calories; 5gm. protein; 9gm. carbohydrate; 1gm. fiber; 1gm. fats; 5mg. cholesterol; 158mg. calcium; trace iron; 26mg. magnesium; 332mg. potassium; 81mg. sodium; 1mg. zinc.

453   GREENS & HERBS SOUP

For 8 people:

♣In a large soup pot, sauté in 3 TBS. OIL until translucent
1 ONION CHOPPED
1 CLOVE GARLIC, MINCED

♣Add and sauté for 5 minutes
1 STALK CHOPPED CELERY

♣ Add 1 CUP LIGHT VEGETABLE STOCK (pg. 652) and heat to a simmer.
♣ Add 1 FINELY CHOPPED HEAD ROMAINE LETTUCE and 1 16-OZ. BAG FRESH FROZEN PEAS
and steam braise for 2 minutes just until color changes.
♣ Remove from heat. Let cool slightly and puré in the blender until smooth.
♣ Return to soup pot. Add 5 MORE CUPS of LIGHT STOCK.
Bring to a simmer just to heat and add
1/2 teasp. GREAT 28 SEASONING MIX (Page 645)
1/2 teasp. DRY BASIL (or 1 TB. FRESH)
1/4 teasp. THYME
1/4 teasp. SAVORY
1/4 teasp. WHITE PEPPER

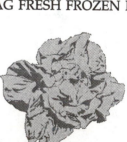

♣ Remove from heat and top with 2 handfuls of CRUNCHY CHINESE NOODLES to serve.

Nutritional analysis: per serving; 123 calories; 4gm. protein; 15gm. carbohydrate; 4gm. fiber; 5gm. fats; 0 cholesterol; 38mg. calcium; 2mg. iron; 25mg. magnesium; 207mg. potassium; 182mg. sodium; 1mg. zinc.

454   NEW POTATOES WITH TOMATOES, BASIL & LEEKS
Definitely gourmet fare.
For 8 large soup bowls:

♣Sauté briefly in a large soup pot for 4 to 5 minutes
2 TBS. BUTTER or OIL
2 LARGE SLICED LEEKS (mostly white parts)

1 teasp. THYME
1/2 teasp. LEMON/GARLIC SEASONING

♣Add 1/2 CUP WATER, 1 1/2 LBS. CHUNKED POTATOES, and 1 teasp. SEA SALT.
♣Cover pot and simmer for 5 minutes

♣Add 6 1/2 CUPS MORE WATER, and bring to a boil. Lower heat and simmer, covered, until potatoes are tender. Remove from heat. Cool slightly, and puree *briefly* in the blender so there are still small pieces. Re-season if necessary.

♣Sauté in the same pot
2 TBS. OLIVE OIL
4 TOMATOES (about 1 lb.)
♣Stir and toss until liquid is almost evaporated, and slightly thickened.
♣Season with SESAME SALT AND PEPPER. Add potato soup back to the pot and combine.

♣In a small saucepan, sauté until fragrant
2 TBS. OIL
1 CUP FRESH CHOPPED BASIL
1/2 teasp. SESAME SALT

1 teasp. TARRAGON VINEGAR
1/4 teasp. BLACK PEPPER

♣Pureé in the blender until smooth
♣Ladle soup into bowls. Swirl a spoonful of basil pureé into each bowl and grind on a little pepper.

Nutritional analysis: per serving; 173 calories; 2gm. protein; 24gm. carbohydrate; 3gm. fiber; 8gm. fats; 7gm. cholesterol; 36mg. calcium; 1mg. iron; 32mg. magnesium; 469mg. potassium; 338mg; sodium; trace zinc.

455   VERY LOW FAT WATERCRESS SOUP

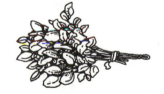

For 4 servings:

♣Sauté for 5 minutes until fragrant
1 TB. OIL
3 LEEKS, chopped
1 1/2 LBS. ZUCCHINI, chopped

♣Add 4 CUPS CHICKEN or ONION STOCK and bring to a boil. Simmer 1 minute.
♣Add 1 BUNCH WATERCRESS, stemmed.
♣Season with SALT, PEPPER and GREAT 28 MIX.

♣Blender blend until smooth. Re-season if necessary.

High Protein Soups
*Soups can be strengthening and building as well as cleansing and purifying.
The recipes in this section are a good way to get protein for healing.*

456 ITALIAN VEGETABLE WITH CHICKEN DUMPLINGS

For 6 people:

♣Making the chicken dumplings takes a little more time, but it is the authentic way for this soup. If you don't have the time, simply use 1¹/₂ CUPS COOKED DICED CHICKEN instead.

♣Make the CHICKEN DUMPLING BALLS. Combine and form into 6 balls. Chill for 1 hour.

♣Grind in a blender or food processor 1¹/₂ CUPS COOKED CHICKEN. Add and mix together
2 TBS. MINCED PARSLEY
¹/₂ CUP WHOLE GRAIN BREAD CRUMBS   1 BEATEN EGG
¹/₄ teasp. LEMON PEPPER   1 TB. ROMANO CHEESE

♣Bring 6 CUPS LIGHT CHICKEN STOCK to a simmer. Add the chicken balls, ¹/₄ teasp. OREGANO, and ¹/₄ teasp. GARLIC/LEMON SEASONING.

♣Simmer for 10 minutes. Remove balls with a slotted spoon and set aside. Keep the soup stock hot.

♣Sauté in a skillet in 1 TB. OLIVE OIL for 5 minutes
¹/₂ CUP SLICED MUSHROOMS   1 teasp. LEMON JUICE
¹/₄ CUP MINCED GREEN ONIONS   ¹/₄ teasp. OREGANO
DASHES PAPRIKA   ¹/₄ teasp. THYME

♣Add to hot stock and stir in 4-OZ. ORZO PASTA. Simmer 5 minutes. Add chicken balls to heat.

♣Beat together in a small bowl
3 EGGS
1 CUP PLAIN YOGURT
6 TBS. GRATED ROMANO CHEESE

♣Add ¹/₂ cup soup to warm the eggs and return mixture to the soup pot. Heat just briefly to warm.

♣*Do not boil.* Sprinkle with more ROMANO, PEPPER, and OREGANO. Serve hot.

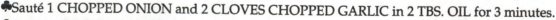

457 QUICK POTATO TOFU STEW

For 6 people:

♣Sauté 1 CHOPPED ONION and 2 CLOVES CHOPPED GARLIC in 2 TBS. OIL for 3 minutes.

♣Add 3 DICED POTATOES, ¹/₂ teasp. SEA SALT, ¹/₄ teasp. PEPPER and sauté for 5 minutes.

♣Add and bring to a bubble.
1 16 OZ. JAR TOMATO SAUCE   3 CUPS WATER
1 LB. DICED TOFU   1 CUP WHITE WINE
1 BOUILLON CUBE

♣Reduce heat and simmer for 20 minutes til potatoes are just tender but not crumbly. Remove from heat and stir in 1¹/₄ CUPS GRATED CHEDDAR. Stir until cheese is just melted.

458   CHINESE HOT & SOUR SOUP

For 8 large servings:

♣Soak 8 DRY SHIITAKE BLACK MUSHROOMS until soft. Slice into slivers, discard woody stems, and save soaking water.
♣Sauté 1 CLOVE MINCED GARLIC and 1 TB. FRESH MINCED GINGER in 1 TB. PEANUT OIL in a large soup pot until aromatic.

♣Add 1½ QTS. CHICKEN STOCK or MISO SOUP and the reserved SLIVERED MUSHROOMS.
♣Bring to a boil, and add 1 LB. FRESH CUBED TOFU. Cover and simmer for 3 minutes.
♣Add 3 TBS. BROWN RICE VINEGAR.
♣Mix 3 TBS. KUZU CHUNKS or ARROWROOT POWDER IN 1½ TBS. TAMARI until dissolved and add to soup.

♣Add
1 10 OZ. PACKAGE FRESH FROZEN PEAS   ½ teasp. CHILI OIL
4 GREEN ONIONS in thin matchstick pieces   1 teasp. BLACK PEPPER

♣Heat for 3 minutes until peas turn a bright green.
♣Remove to a serving tureen and top with CRISPY CHINESE NOODLES.

Nutritional analysis: per serving; 145 calories; 9gm. protein; 16gm. carbohydrate; 4gm. fiber; 7gm. fats; 0 cholesterol; 85mg. calcium; 4mg. iron; 81mg. magnesium; 244mg. potassium; 173mg. sodium; 1mg. zinc.

459   COOL CUCUMBER SHRIMP SOUP

For 6 servings:

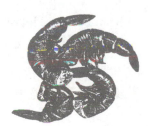

♣Peel and chop 2 LARGE CUCUMBERS. Toss with
¼ CUP WHITE WINE or BASMATI VINEGAR
1 teasp. SESAME SALT
1 TB. FRUCTOSE
♣Let stand for 30 minutes to marinate.

♣Drain and purée in the blender until smooth. Add 1 CUP PLAIN YOGURT and ½ CUP WATER and blend again. Add ¾ CUP OR 1 SMALL BUNCH FRESH DILL WEED and whirl again.
♣Chill for 1 hour.

♣Heat 2 TBS. OIL in a skillet, and toss 1 LB. TINY COOKED SHRIMP to coat. Remove and reserve.
♣Add ¼ CUP SHERRY or WHITE WINE, and PINCHES of SEA SALT and PEPPER to the pan, and boil down until flavor is concentrated, about 3 minutes.
♣Pour over shrimp and add the mixture to the soup. Chill again before serving.

Nutritional analysis: per serving; 176 calories; 19gm. protein; 9gm. carbohydrate; 1gm. fiber; 6gm. fats; 150mg. cholesterol; 126mg. calcium; 3mg. iron; 49mg. magnesium; 437mg. potassium; 342mg. sodium; 2mg. zinc.

460   ONION & WHITE WINE SOUP

Put PUFFY YOGURT CHEESE SQUARES in each bowl to pour the soup over. Or use them as dippers.
For 6 to 8 servings:

♣Make the SQUARES. Preheat oven to 350°.
♣Blend the batter in the blender

1 EGG
1 TB. WHOLE WHEAT FLOUR
1/4 CUP PLAIN LOW-FAT YOGURT
1/3 CUP GRATED MOZARELLA

1/4 teasp. SEA SALT
PINCH WHITE PEPPER
1/4 teasp. LEMON/GARLIC SEASON

♣Soak 3 to 4 trimmed WHOLE GRAIN BREAD SLICES in batter. Melt 3 to 4 TBS. BUTTER on a baking sheet. Put bread slices on the sheet, and toast until golden, turning once.
♣Cut in quarters, and put in soup bowls.

♣Make the soup.
♣Sauté in a skillet 2 LARGE SLICED YELLOW ONIONS in 2 TBS. OIL until translucent - 10 minutes.
♣Add to 6 CUPS CHICKEN or ONION STOCK in a large soup pot. Bring to a boil and simmer gently.

♣Heat 3 TBS. BUTTER and 3 TBS. OIL in the skillet and add
1/3 CUP UNBLEACHED FLOUR
2 teasp. DRY MUSTARD
1/2 teasp. SEA SALT

1/4 teasp. WHITE PEPPER
1/4 teasp. NUTMEG

♣Stir all together til bubbly and well blended, about 5 minutes.

♣Add 2 CUPS WHITE WINE and heat gently until aromatic. Add wine mixture to onion soup pot, and simmer a few minutes to blend. Add 8-OZ SWISS or MOZARELLA CHEESE CUBES.
♣Rremove from heat and let rest for a few minutes to melt cheese.

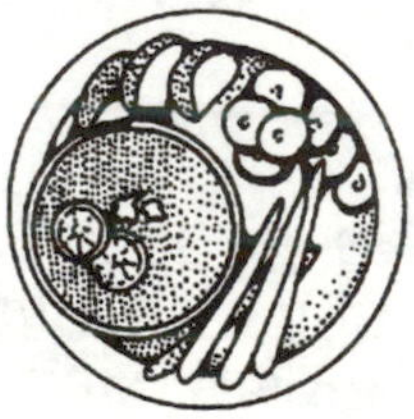

�֍

461   FRESH TOMATO CHEESE SOUP

For 4 to 6 people:

♣Sauté 1 CUP ONION chopped and 3 CLOVES GARLIC, minced in 3 TBS. OLIVE OIL for 5 minutes.
♣Pureé in the blender with 7 FRESH CHUNKED TOMATOES, 1 TB. FRESH CHOPPED BASIL, and 1 teasp. BASMATI VINEGAR.

♣Add to a large soup pot with 2 CUPS VEGETABLE STOCK (Pg. 652).

♣Heat and add
1 CUP ROSÉ WINE
2 TBS. SHERRY

1/2 teasp. SEA SALT
1/4 teasp. PEPPER

♣Simmer for 15 minutes. Remove from heat.
♣Beat 2 EGG YOLKS with 1/2 CUP PLAIN YOGURT, and 1/3 CUP PARMESAN CHEESE. Add a little soup to warm eggs and pour all back into the soup pot. Heat gently, whisking until blended. Serve.

Vegetable Soups For Complex Carbohydrates

462   GOLDEN SOUP

For 8 servings:

♣Sauté 1 CHOPPED YELLOW ONION or the white parts of 2 CHOPPED LEEKS in 2 TBS. OIL in a large soup pot for 10 minutes.
♣Add 2 TOMATOES, CHOPPED, 1 LB. (about 4) YELLOW CROOKNECK SQUASH, and 1 CUP CHOPPED CARROTS. Sauté for 5 more minutes.
♣Add 3 CUPS CHICKEN BROTH or VEGETABLE BROTH. Bring to a boil and simmer until tender, about 15 minutes. Remove from heat and cool slightly.

♣Purée in the blender in batches with
1/2 CUP LOW-FAT YOGURT   1/4 CUP WHITE WINE
1/4 CUP CHOPPED FRESH BASIL LEAVES   1/4 CUP WATER
♣Serve warm or cool with TOMATO SLICES on top.

Nutritional analysis: per serving; 84 calories; 2gm. protein; 19gm. carbohydrate; 2gm. fiber; 4gm. fats; trace cholesterol; 54mg. calcium; 1mg. iron; 25mg. magnesium; 329mg. potassium; 67mg. sodium; trace zinc.

463   HEARTY LENTIL SOUP

For 6 servings:

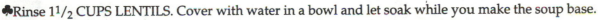

♣Rinse 1 1/2 CUPS LENTILS. Cover with water in a bowl and let soak while you make the soup base.
♣In a large soup pot, sauté in 2 TBS. BUTTER and 2 TBS. OIL for 5 minutes.
♣Add
3 CLOVES MINCED GARLIC   2 SLICED CARROTS
2 ONIONS, CHOPPED   1 RIB CHOPPED CELERY with leaves

♣Add 1/3 CUP BROWN RICE and sauté until coated and shiny, about 2 minutes. Add drained lentils.
♣Stir and add
1 1/2 QTS. WATER   1/2 teasp. BLACK PEPPER
3 TBS. SMOKED BREWER'S YEAST   1/2 teasp. DRY BASIL
1 teasp. SEA SALT   1/4 teasp. CUMIN POWDER

♣Mix 1/2 cup of the soup with 2 TBS. MISO PASTE. Add back to soup. Simmer for 20 minutes until aromatic and flavor concentrates. Remove from heat, cool slightly and purée in the blender til smooth.
♣Return to soup pot. Add 1 teasp. ZEST or other vegetable seasoning salt, and 1 TB. SOY BACON BITS.
♣Heat through and serve with thin LEMON SLICES on top.

Nutritional analysis: per serving; 255 calories; 14gm. protein; 36gm. carbohydrate; 7gm. fiber; 7gm. fats; 7mg. cholesterol; 60mg. calcium; 4mg. iron; 71mg. magnesium; 572mg. potassium; 455mg. sodium; 2mg. zinc.

464   TARRAGON TOMATO

For 6 servings:

♣Sauté 1¹/₂ CUPS SLICED ONIONS in 4 TBS. OIL and 4 TBS. BUTTER in a large soup pot until golden.
♣Add 4 CUPS FRESH CHOPPED TOMATOES and mash in with a potato masher.

♣Add ¹/₂ CUP WHITE WINE, 1 TB. FRUCTOSE, and 1 teasp. DRY TARRAGON and simmer for 20 minutes. Turn off heat and let sit for 15 minutes to let the flavors blend.

♣Pureé in the blender and return to soup pot. Simmer for 5 more minutes.
♣Re-season if necessary, (it usually is with tomatoe soups) and serve.

Nutritional analysis: per serving; 173 calories; 2gm. protein; 11gm. carbohydrate; 2gm. fiber; 13gm. fats; 15mg. cholesterol; 22mg. calcium; 1mg. iron; 21mg. magnesium; 352mg. potassium; 14mg. sodium; trace zinc.

465   RED ONION, RED WINE SOUP

New research is showing that some red wines have active anti-carcinogens, making the combination with onions a potent healing recipe.
For 12 servings:

♣Make the stock. Use as many fresh, whole ingredients as possible. Bring everything to a boil, and simmer for 25 minutes.
1 TB. FRESH THYME LEAVES (¹/₂ teasp. dry)
8 FRESH SPRIGS PARSLEY (2 teasp. dry flakes)
3 BAY LEAVES
3 PEELED CLOVES GARLIC
¹/₂ teasp. SEA SALT
1 TB. DRY LEMON GRASS LEAVES
8 CUPS WATER

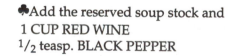

♣Strain out solids, discard and set stock aside while you prepare the soup.

♣Sauté 2 LBS. SLICED RED ONIONS and 4 MINCED CLOVES in a large soup pot in 4 TBS. OLIVE OIL til soft and aromatic, about 20 minutes.

♣Add
1 LB. TOMATOES CHOPPED
¹/₂ teasp. SEA SALT
1 CUP TOMATO JUICE

♣Add the reserved soup stock and
1 CUP RED WINE
¹/₂ teasp. BLACK PEPPER

♣Partially cover and simmer for 35 to 40 minutes.

♣While soup is simmering, toast in the oven 2 CUPS WHOLE GRAIN BREAD CUBES drizzled with 4 TBS. OLIVE OIL. Place in the serving tureen and pour hot soup over.

Nutritional analysis: per serving; 130 calories; 2gm. protein; 13gm. carbohydrate; 2gm. fiber; 7gm. fats; 0 cholesterol; 32mg. calcium; 1mg. iron; 24mg. magnesium; 291mg. potassium; 137mg. sodium; trace zinc.

466 SWEET CARROT PUREE

Definitely a soup with a difference.

For 6 people:

♣Blanch in a large soup pot with 1 CUP CHICKEN or LIGHT ONION STOCK until color changes. Add 1$\frac{1}{2}$ LBS. SLICED CARROTS, 2 STALKS CHOPPED CELERY, and 3 CUPS SLICED LEEKS (mostly white parts).

♣Cool slightly and pureé in the blender with 1 CUP PLAIN YOGURT until smooth. Return to soup pot.

♣Add

5 MORE CUPS STOCK	$\frac{1}{2}$ teasp. LEMON/GARLIC SEASON
$\frac{1}{3}$ CUP CHOPPED FRESH PARSLEY	2 PINCHES NUTMEG
3 TBS. BUTTER	$\frac{1}{4}$ teasp. WHITE PEPPER

♣Heat just gently. Do not boil.

♣Melt and cook $\frac{1}{2}$ teasp. BROWN SUGAR for 3 minutes in a saucepan til caramelized.

♣Add

$\frac{1}{2}$ CUP MINCED CARROT	$\frac{1}{2}$ teasp. SEASME SALT
$\frac{1}{4}$ CUP PLAIN YOGURT	$\frac{1}{4}$ teasp. WHITE PEPPER

♣Cook for 10 minutes until carrots are tender crisp. Add to hot soup. Season again if necessary.

♣Sprinkle with 1 TB. FRESH CHOPPED MINT LEAVES.

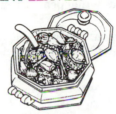

Whole Meal Stews

Hearty stews have been whole meals since time began, serving man then for the same reasons that they do today; hot nutrition that reaches the system and satisfies fuel and energy needs quickly.

467 FRENCH ONION STEW

For 6 servings:

♣Slice 4 LARGE ONIONS and sauté in 2 TBS. BUTTER or OIL until translucent.

♣Add

4 CUPS ONION BROTH	$\frac{1}{2}$ teasp. PEPPER
1$\frac{1}{2}$ CUPS SLICED BABY RED POTATOES	1 teasp. VEGETABLE SALT

♣Cover and cook until tender. Remove from heat. Cool slightly, and purée in the blender, in batches with 1 CUP PLAIN YOGURT. Return to the soup pot, and re-season.

♣Put 6 SLICES of TRIMMED WHOLE WHEAT SOURDOUGH BREAD on a baking sheet. Sprinkle with GRATED CHEDDAR CHEESE and toast until cheese melts.

♣Put a slice of toast in the bottom of each soup bowl and pour soup over.

468 VEGETABLE HERB STEW

For 6 to 8 servings:

♣Chunk 1 RED POTATO, and boil until tender in 1 CUP WATER and 3 CUPS VEGETABLE BOUILLON.

♣Sauté 1 CHOPPED ONION and 1 CLOVE CHOPPED GARLIC in 2 TBS. BUTTER and 1 TB. OIL until aromatic.

♣Add and sauté until color changes
1 CARROT, sliced   1/2 teasp. DILL WEED
1 STALK CELERY with leaves, sliced   1/2 teasp. DRY BASIL
8 OZ. SLICED MUSHROOMS   1/2 teasp. BLACK PEPPER
1/2 teasp. THYME   1/2 teasp. VEGETABLE SALT
♣Add this mixture to the potato stock, and simmer for 20 minutes.

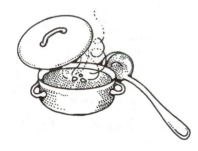

♣Add and heat gently
1 CAKE TOFU, cubed   2 TBS. SHERRY
3/4 CUP WHITE WINE   1 TB. TAMARI

♣Just before serving, add 1 CUP FROZEN PEAS.
♣Remove from heat, and let sit for 5 minutes while peas warm and turn bright green.

Nutritional analysis: per serving; 124 calories; 4gm. protein; 13gm. carbohydrate; 3gm. fiber; 6gm. fats; 8mg. cholesterol; 47mg. calcium; 2mg. iron; 37mg. magnesium; 342mg. potassium; 132mg. sodium; 1mg. zinc.

469 ITALIAN CIAMBOTTA

This is a wonderful, fragrant southern Italian stew.
For 6 people:

♣Sauté in 1/3 CUP OLIVE OIL until fragrant, about 10 minutes
3 CLOVES CHOPPED GARLIC
3 CHOPPED ONIONS
3 CHOPPED BELL PEPPERS (one of each color if possible)

♣Add 3 POTATOES in chunks and 1/2 teasp. SEA SALT, and cook for 20 minutes.

♣Add 1 LB. ROMA TYPE TOMATOES, chopped and 1 CUP TOMATO JUICE, (or ONE 28 OZ. CAN TOMATOES WITH JUICE). Simmer for 20 more minutes.

♣Add 2 ZUCCHINI, sliced and simmer for 5 minutes.

♣Serve hot and top with 6 LARGE BLACK OLIVES sliced, and 1/2 teasp. BLACK PEPPER.

Nutritional analysis: per serving; 178 calories; 3gm. protein; 23gm. carbohydrate; 4gm. fiber; 9gm. fats; 0 cholesterol; 32mg. calcium; 1mg. iron; 37mg. magnesium; 612mg. potassium; 147mg. sodium; trace zinc.

470   EVERYTHING VEGETABLE SOUP

This is one of those recipes where you can add practically anything you have in the house and it will taste good. Here are some suggestions, but feel free to add and change to your liking. It's really all in the herbs and spices.
For 4 to 6 people:

♣Cover the bottom of a large soup kettle with OIL. Saute until aromatic, about 5 to 7 minutes

1 teasp. LEMON/GARLIC SEASONING	1 RED POTATO, CUBED
1/4 CUP BROWN RICE	1 CARROT, SLICED
1/4 CUP CORN KERNALS	2 STALKS CELERY SLICED
1 ONION, CHOPPED	1 CUP SLICED MUSHROOMS
1 CLOVE GARLIC, CHOPPED	1/4 CUP CHOPPED GREEN BEANS

♣Add 2 VEGETABLE BOUILLON CUBES dissolved in 1 CUP WHITE WINE
♣Add 5 CUPS WATER and bring to a boil.
♣Add 2 TOMATOES pureed in the blender with 1/2 CUP WATER and 1 1/2 CUPS TOMATO SAUCE.
♣Add 1 SMALL SLICED ZUCCHINI and 1/4 HEAD SHREDDED GREEN CABBAGE

♣Add the herbs and spices

1 TB. FRESH CHOPPED BASIL (1/2 teasp. dry)	1/4 teasp. PAPRIKA
1/2 teasp. TARRAGON	1/4 teasp. OREGANO
1/2 teasp. VEGETABLE SALT	1/4 teasp. THYME
2 TBS. TAMARI SAUCE	1/4 teasp. PEPPER
1 teasp. BALSAMIC VINEGAR	

♣Simmer until fragrant, about 30 to 45 minutes. Just before serving, add 1/2 CUP FROZEN PEAS. Remove from heat and let sit for a few minutes until peas turn bright green.

471   BROCCOLI SOUP WITH KING CRAB

For 4 servings:

♣Sauté in 3 TBS. BUTTER and 1 TB. OIL in a soup pot until tender crisp and broccoli turns bright green.
1 CUP SLICED BROCCOLI
1/2 teasp. LEMON/GARLIC SEASONING
1 CUP SLICED LEEKS (mostly white parts)
1 CUP SLICED BUTTON MUSHROOMS or CHANTERELLES

♣Stir in and stir until bubbly and blended

4 TBS. UNBLEACHED FLOUR	1/4 teasp. PEPPER
1/4 teasp. DRY THYME	1/4 teasp. DRY CHERVIL

♣Add 3 CUPS LIGHT CHICKEN BROTH or VEGETABLE BOUILLON and 1 CUP PLAIN YOGURT. Cook until bubbly and thickened.
♣Add 6-OZ. KING CRAB LEG CHUNKS and heat through gently. Remove from heat, and add 3/4 CUP SHREDDED SWISS or JARLSBERG CHEESE.
♣Remove from heat and allow to melt for a few minutes before serving.

472 SPICY TOFU GOULASH

For 4 to 6 people:

♣Sauté in 2 TBS. OIL in a large soup pot for 5 minutes

2 SLICED CARROTS

1 RED or GREEN BELL PEPPER, chopped

1 LARGE ONION, chopped

3 RED POTATOES, cubed

♣Add 8 OZ. TOMATO SAUCE, 1/2 CUP WATER, and 1/2 CUP ROSÉ WINE and simmer for 10 minutes to blend flavors.

♣Add 2 CAKES CUBED TOFU, 1 TB. PAPRIKA, 1 teasp. VEGETABLE SALT, and 1 teasp. PEPPER.

♣Cover and simmer for 10 minutes more.

♣Remove from heat. Add 1 cup soup to the blender with 1 CUP PLAIN YOGURT.

♣Whirl until smooth and add back to the pot. Serve with more paprika, nutmeg and pepper sprinkles.

Dumpling Soup Toppers

Dumplings can make soup into dinner. Any soup is a speciality with dumpling tidbits added.
They are tender and light, very easy to make, and may be used in all kinds of soups.
Just mix ingredients. Roll into balls. Chill to set. Drop into simmering soup.
Do not open pot lid while cooking so dumplings will steam properly. They are ready when they rise to the surface.

LEMON HERB DUMPLINGS

For 25 dumplings:

1/2 CUP WATER or STOCK

2 TBS. BUTTER

6 TBS. UNBLEACHED FLOUR

1 EGG

1 TB. MINCED PARSLEY

1 TB. LEMON JUICE

1/2 teasp. HERB SALT

1/4 teasp. ground CELERY SEED

1/4 teasp. LEMON PEPPER

1 TB. MINCED CHIVES

TENDER TOFU DUMPLINGS

For about18 dumplings:

2 CAKES MASHED TOFU

2 TBS. FRESH CHOPPED PARSLEY

1/2 CUP WHOLE WHEAT FLOUR

1 EGG

2 teasp. BAKING POWDER

1 teasp. VEGETABLE SALT

BURNT ALMOND DUMPLINGS

♣Mix for 30 dumplings: Simmer 3 TBS. BUTTER to very dark in a saucepan.

1 CUP CRUSHED WH. GRAIN CRACKER CRUMBS

1/2 CUP CHOPPED ALMONDS

1 teasp. SEA SALT

1/2 CUP PLAIN YOGURT

1 EGG

2 PINCHES LEMON PEPPER

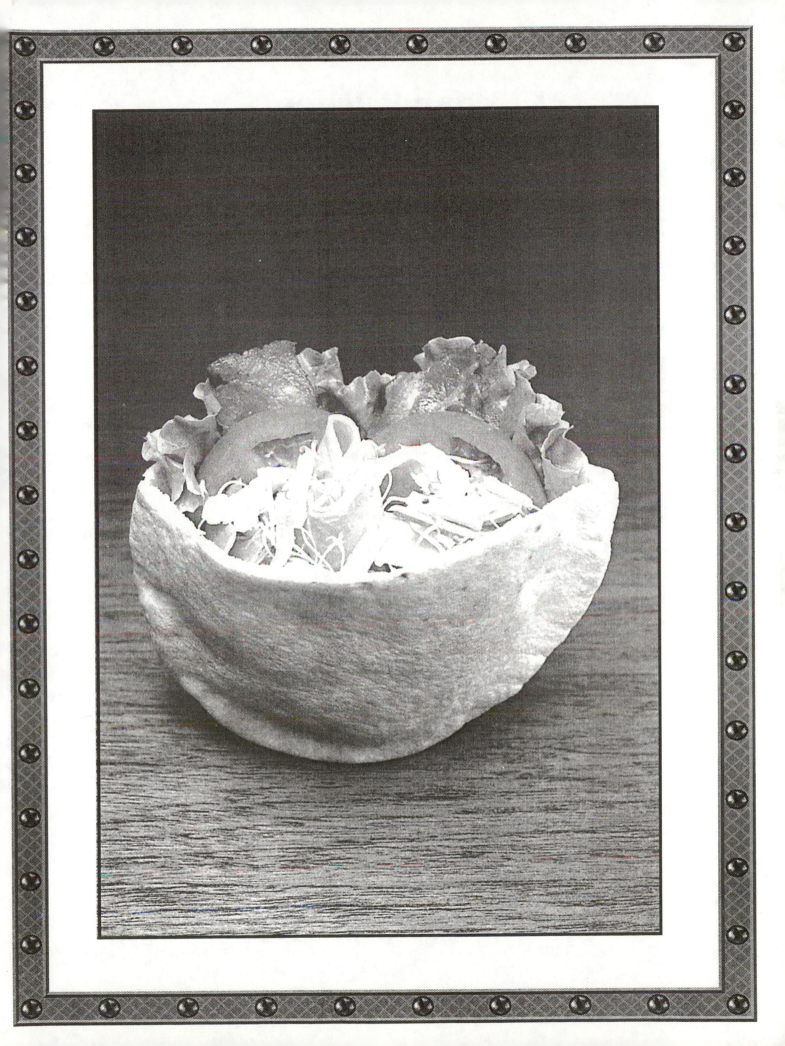

Sandwiches
Salads In Bread

Sandwiches are so easy and convenient; they are marvelously portable. Every nation has its version of a sandwich, from French *croque-monsieurs* to Italian *tostas* to Mexican *tacos* to Greek *pitas* to Lebanese *arams* and Chinese *egg rolls*. A sandwich can be a wonderful, satisfying, nutritious meal, full of good things to keep you healthy. A sandwich provides a balanced lunch or dinner that is delicious hot or cold, and uses almost anything from gourmet ingredients to leftovers.

Seafoods, poultry, vegetables, beans, tofu and seasoned grains are all sandwich ingredients that offer main substance, while whole grain breads replace rice or potatoes for complex carbohydrates. A wholesome sandwich has fresh greens and vegetables, low-fat or non-dairy dressings, cheeses, and herbal seasonings; in short, it is a *salad in bread*.

Open face, a sandwich becomes a salad on toast, with even less density. Pita breads add a new dimension to favorite fillings. They are fun to eat, low in calories, fat and cholesterol. You can stuff them in a neat self-contained pocket so that everything doesn't fall out. Sandwiches are a practical way to use good food combining principles.

Just a little rethinking can change the way you might have felt about sandwiches. Many people see them as foods that fill you up and out - heavy, meat-packed, with fatty spreads on empty calorie bread. We recommend toasting the bread for your sandwich. The density is less if you are dieting, and it tastes better.

The sandwiches in this section are tasty meals with high protein, minerals and fiber, plenty of complex carbohydrates, low fats and no sugars. The recipe categories include:
❧LOW-FAT and CALORIE SANDWICHES ❧HIGH PROTEIN SANDWICHES ❧SEAFOOD SANDWICHES ❧POCKET SANDWICHES ❧OPEN FACE SANDWICHES ❧ARAM SANDWICHES ❧

Go ahead. Create a great sandwich. It's good for you!

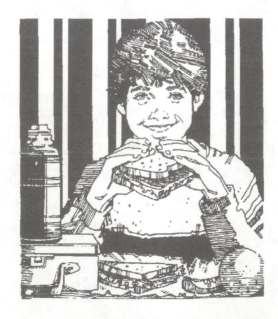

Low Fat, Low Calorie Sandwiches

473   SMALL PLANET BURGER

This is a delicious, perennial favorite for people that love hamburgers, but don't like how the meat-eating economic chain affects the environment.
For 2 large burgers:

♣Make 2 TOFU BURGERS or 2 GRAIN BURGERS according to package directions, from any good whole grain mix. We use *Fantastic Foods brand, Nature Burger Mix or Tofu Burger Mix.*
♣Toast 2 WHOLE GRAIN BURGER BUNS. Spread the 4 halves with 2 TBS. MAYONNAISE spiced with 1 teasp. SOY BACON BITS.
♣Put the burger together with SLICED TOMATO, ALFALFA SPROUTS, A SLICE of LOW-FAT or SOY CHEESE, and LETTUCE. Heat briefly in the oven to melt the cheese.

Nutritional analysis: per serving; 413 calories; 15gm. protein; 56gm. carbohydrate; 10gm. fiber; 9gm. fats; 11mg. cholesterol; 124mg. calcium; 4mg. iron; 132mg. magnesium; 387mg. potassium; 508mg. sodium; 3mg. zinc.

474   LIGHT GUACAMOLE SANDWICH

For 2 sandwiches:

♣Mix and mash until smooth

2 PEELED SEEDED AVOCADOS, sliced	2 teasp. SALSA
2 TBS. LEMON JUICE	1 TB. TAMARI
2 teasp. LEMON GARLIC SEASONING	

♣Make this sandwich with plenty of GREEN LEAF LETTUCE, and fresh THICK TOMATO SLICES on WHOLE GRAIN TOAST or a ROLLED CHAPATI.

475   LOW FAT PARTY SANDWICHES

For about 24 cocktail sandwiches:

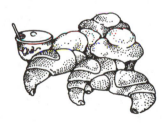

♣Mix together and chill

3 to 4 OZ. YOGURT CHEESE or KEFIR CHEESE or SOY CREAM CHEESE
16-OZ. LOW-FAT COTTAGE CHEESE
1 PEELED MINCED CUCUMBER
1/2 CUP SNIPPED WATERCRESS or PARSLEY
♣Pile on TOASTED RYE ROUNDS and serve.

Nutritional analysis: per serving; 46 calories; 4gm. protein; 6gm. carbohydrate; 1gm. fiber; trace fats; 1mg. cholesterol; 32mg. calcium; trace iron; 6mg. magnesium; 74mg. potassium; 154mg. sodium; trace zinc.

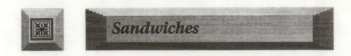

476 EGGPLANT SANDWICH WITH AVOCADO SALSA

In this sandwich, the eggplant rounds become the "bread" base for the filling.
For 4 sandwiches: Preheat oven to 450∞.

♣Peel and trim a 1 LB. EGGPLANT and slice into 8 ¹/₂" rounds. Lay slices in a single layer on a baking sheet brushed with OLIVE OIL. Brush eggplant with olive oil and bake until brown and soft - 20 to 25 minutes.

♣Top each eggplant slice with a slice of LOW-FAT MUENSTER or JACK CHEESE and return to oven until cheese melts. Transfer two rounds to each sandwich plate.

♣Sauté 8 thin slices RED ONION in 1 TB. OLIVE OIL until quite brown and fragrant.

♣Make the salsa while onion is browning.   ♣Mash together
1 LARGE PEELED SEEDED AVOCADO   1 LARGE CHOPPED TOMATO
2 TBS. LIME JUICE   1 to 2 TBS. CHILI SAUCE
♣Pile onions on eggplant slices. Top with dollops of salsa and 2 TBS. CHOPPED FRESH CILANTRO.

Nutritional analysis: per serving; 220 calories; 6gm. protein; 17gm. carbohydrate; 9gm fiber; 15gm. fats; 9mg. cholesterol; 137mg. calcium; 2mg. iron; 37mg. magnesium; 700mg. potassium; 84mg. sodium; 1mg. zinc.

477 LOW-FAT TURKEY CLUB

For 2 sandwiches:

♣Toast 4 slices of your favorite WHOLE GRAIN BREAD. Spread each slice with a low calorie RUSSIAN DRESSING.

♣Shred in a salad shooter 1 SMALL ZUCCHINI and 1 SMALL CARROT.

♣Layer 2 slices with
A THIN SLICE OF LOW-FAT SWISS CHEESE
A THIN SLICE OF COOKED TURKEY BREAST
A LARGE BOSTON LETTUCE LEAF
A LARGE SLICE OF TOMATO
SOME ALFALFA SPROUTS
THE CARROTS and ZUCCHINI
♣Top with remaining toast slices. Cut diagonally in both directions to make four triangles. Secure with toothpicks.

Nutritional analysis: per serving; 278 calories; 16gm. protein; 43gm. carbohydrate; 7gm. fiber; 7gm. fats; 21mg. cholesterol; 161mg. calcium; 3mg. iron; 83mg. magnesium; 594mg. potassium; 662mg. sodium; 2mg. zinc.

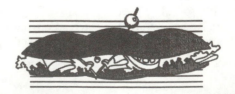

High Protein Sandwiches

478   FRENCH TOFU BURGERS

This sandwich was a great favorite from a summer spent in France during college. They were made with meat there, and served open face, (on French toast, of course) with a red wine sauce. When I stopped eating meat, this was one of the first recipes that I "changed over" to Tofu and other healthy ingredients.
Two dressing sauces are offered - the original French for an open face sandwich, and a Tamari Mustard spread for a regular burger bun.
For 6 burgers:

♣Sauté in a large skillet in 1 TB. OIL and 1 TB. BUTTER until soft
$3/4$ CUP MINCED ONIONS $1/2$ teasp. THYME
1 teasp. SEA SALT $1/4$ teasp. PEPPER
♣Remove from heat and set aside.

♣Use a packaged TOFU BURGER MIX such as *Fantastic Foods* or *Lite Chef,* and make up enough mix with TOFU, WATER and EGG to make 6 burgers.

♣Add onions and form into burgers. Dredge TOFU BURGERS in flour on a plate and set aside to rest.

♣Heat 2 teasp. oil and butter in the onion skillet and sauté burgers until brown on both sides. Remove and keep warm in a low oven while you make the sauce.

Nutritional analysis: per serving; 137 calories; 5gm. protein; 14gm. carbohydrate; 2gm. fiber; 7gm. fats; 41mg. cholesterol; 39mg. calcium; 2mg. iron; 48mg. magnesium; 130mg. potassium; 393mg. sodium; 1mg. zinc.

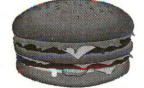

FRENCH WINE SAUCE:

For 1 cup:

♣Sauté 2 MINCED SHALLOTS in the large onion skillet with 1 teasp. butter until sizzling.
♣Add $1/2$ CUP BOUILLON and $2/3$ CUP ROSÉ WINE and bring to a boil. Cook rapidly until sauce reduces to $1/2$ cup.
♣Remove from heat, and stir in 1 teasp. ARROWROOT mixed in 1 teasp. WATER. Return to heat briefly, season with SALT and PEPPER, and snip in 2 TBS. FRESH PARSLEY.
♣Serve immediately over burgers.

TAMARI MUSTARD SAUCE:

For $1 1/2$ cups:

♣Blend well: 1 CUP LIGHT MAYONNAISE, $1/3$ CUP SWEET HOT MUSTARD, 1 teasp. HONEY, and 2 TBS. TAMARI.
♣Serve over burgers.

479   GRILLED BRIE WITH MUSHROOMS

For 4 sandwiches: Preheat griddle or broiler.

♣Sauté 4 to 6 LARGE BUTTON MUSHROOMS or CHANTERELLES in 2 TBS. OIL AND 1 TB. BUTTER until soft, about 2 to 3 minutes.

♣Add 2 CHOPPED GREEN ONIONS and sauté until bright green.

♣Remove from heat and season with LEMON PEPPER.

♣Slice 4-OZ. COLD BRIE or TELEME CHEESE into 4 SLICES. Put each slice of cheese on a slice of whole grain bread.

♣Soak 2 teasp. DRY TARRAGON in water for 10 minutes. Drain and divide over each cheese slice.

♣Divide mushroom mix on cheese. Top with another slice of bread, and grill for 4 minutes until light brown (or broil on a greased sheet until cheese melts).

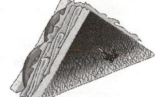

480   PEANUT BUTTER TOMATO CLUB

For 2 sandwiches:

♣Spread 2 SLICES of WHOLE GRAIN TOAST with PEANUT BUTTER. Top each with a LETTUCE LEAF. Sprinkle with 1 teasp. SOY BACON BITS and top with a TOMATO SLICE.

♣Spread 2 more slices of toast with PEANUT BUTTER & place <u>face up</u> on top of the tomatoes.

♣Cover each with a lettuce leaf and a slice OF CHEDDAR CHEESE. Top with 1 more slice of tomato if you want a really big sandwich - *or* just spread LIGHT MAYONNAISE on the last 2 pieces of toast.

♣Cover, press down to put the whole thing together, and cut diagonally into quarters.

Nutritional analysis: per serving; 564 calories; 25gm. protein; 42gm. carbo.; 10gm. fiber; 34gm. fats; 15mg. cholesterol; 181mg. calcium; 4mg. iron; 165mg. magnesium; 628mg. potassium; 448mg. sodium; 3mg. zinc.

481   CLASSIC AVO JACK

Another seventies classic. This is the Rainbow Kitchen restaurant version.
For 1 sandwich:

♣Mix $1/4$ teasp. GREAT 28 MIX (Pg. 645) with 2 TBS. LIGHT MAYONNAISE, and spread on 2 SLICES of WHOLE GRAIN TOAST. Cover each side with a LETTUCE LEAF.

♣Fill with
2 or 3 SLICES OF AVOCADO   1 SLICE JACK CHEESE
HALF A HANDFUL of ALFALFA SPROUTS   2 or 3 SLICES CUCUMBER
♣Sprinkle with TOASTED SUNFLOWER SEEDS and SOY BACON BITS.

Nutritional analysis: per serving; 677 calories; 17gm. protein; 32gm. carbohydrate; 8gm. fiber; 30gm. fats; 53mg. cholesterol; 287mg. calcium; 4mg. iron; 108mg. magnesium; 408mg. potassium; 660mg. sodium; 3mg. zinc.

Loaves & Fishes - Seafood Sandwiches

Ocean foods are finally gaining the popularity in America that they enjoy in the rest of the world.
Since Americans have a continuing love affair with sandwich meals, seafood sandwiches are also coming of age.

482 APPETIZER CRAB ROLLS

For 4 to 6 people as appetizers: Preheat oven broiler when ready to serve.

♣Whisk together
1/2 CUP LIGHT MAYONNAISE
1/4 CUP PLAIN LOW-FAT YOGURT
2 teasp. LIME JUICE
2 teasp. LEMON JUICE

♣Stir in
1 to 2 MINCED CELERY RIBS
1 MINCED GREEN ONION
1/4 teasp. TARRAGON
1/4 teasp. LEMON PEPPER

♣Fold in 1 LB. DUNGENESS CRABMEAT picked over for shells. Cover and chill.

♣Toast RYE COCKTAIL ROUNDS in the oven until crisp. Top with spoonfuls of crab mix. Broil briefly just to brown on top. Sprinkle with MINCED WATERCRESS or FRESH PARSLEY for garnish.

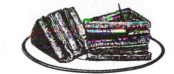

483 SALMON CLUB

This sandwich is good with either thin Lox slices or slices of salmon filet.
For 4 sandwiches: Preheat broiler.

♣Toast 8 SLICES WHOLE GRAIN BREAD in the broiler until golden. Remove and set aside.

♣Season 1 LB. SALMON FILET or LOX SLICES with LEMON PEPPER. Broil 3" from heat in an oiled pan for 2 to 3 minutes. Salmon will be pale pink and opaque when ready.

♣Spread all toast slices with FRESH MAYONNAISE or GREEN MAYONNAISE (page 648). Top 4 pieces with Salmon slices, FRESH BOSTON LETTUCE LEAVES, and thin overlapping TOMATO SLICES. Season with more lemon pepper, top with remaining 4 bread slices. Cut in half and serve.

484 AHI TUNA MELT

Thin-sliced ahi tuna steaks are perfect for a melt. They have the taste and texture of beef steaks, but hardly any fat, and all the valuable Omega oils.
For 6 sandwiches: Preheat broiler.

♣Combine filling in a bowl and spread on whole grain buns.
3/4 CUP MINCED CELERY
1/4 CUP LOW-FAT MAYONNAISE

1/2 teasp. DILLWEED
2 TBS. MINCED ONION

♣Season 6 THIN SLICED AHI TUNA STEAKS with LEMON PEPPER. Drizzle with LEMON JUICE.
♣Broil for 5 minutes. Place 1 steak slice on each of 4 filled bun halves. Top with a SLICE of LOW-FAT MOZZARELLA and broil again until cheese bubbles.
♣Top with a TOMATO SLICE, a LETTUCE LEAF and the top bun.

Terrific Tuna Sandwiches

*Tuna sandwiches are traditional favorites. We are only now realizing how healthy this oldy but goody really is -
a tasty, low fat source of protein and heart-wise Omega-3 oils.The three salad sandwiches offered here are all good
open-face on toast or in pita pockets, as well between bread slices.*

485   TUNA ITALIAN

For 2 sandwiches:

♣Mix gently together in a bowl

1/2 SIX OZ. CAN WATERPACKED TUNA

1 to 2 MINCED GREEN ONIONS

1/3 CUP MOZZARELLA CHUNKS

4 teasp. ITALIAN VINAIGRETTE DRESSING

2 TBS. RED BELL PEPPER

2 TBS. FRESH CHOPPED PARSLEY

8 SLICED BLACK OLIVES

♣Pile on WHOLE GRAIN TOAST, and top with another SLICE OF TOAST.

Nutritional analysis: per serving; 369 calories; 27gm. protein; 33gm. carbohydrate; 7gm. fiber; 15gm. fats; 38mg. cholesterol' 284mg. calcium; 4mg. iron; 84mg. magnesium; 325mg. potassium; 390mg. sodium; 2mg. zinc.

486   TUNA MEXICANO

For 2 sandwiches:

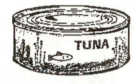

♣Mix together in a bowl

1/2 SIX OZ. CAN WATERPACKED TUNA

1/4 CUP GRATED HOT PEPPER or JALAPEÑO JACK CHEESE

2 MINCED GREEN ONIONS

1 SMALL TOMATO, chopped

1 CUP SHAVED LETTUCE

4 teasp. SALSA or BARBECUE SAUCE

♣Pile on WHOLE GRAIN TOAST. Top with another SLICE OF TOAST, or stuff into PITA POCKETS.

Nutritional analysis: per serving; 245 calories; 21gm. protein; 35gm. carbohydrate; 7gm. fiber; 3gm. fats; 23mg. cholesterol; 73mg. calcium; 4mg. iron; 88mg. magnesium; 509mg. potassium; 378mg. sodium; 2mg. zinc.

487   HOT DOG TUNA

For 2 sandwiches:

♣Mix together in a bowl .

1/2 SIX OZ. CAN WATERPACKED TUNA

1 HARD BOILED EGG, crumbled

1 teasp. YELLOW MUSTARD

1 to 2 teasp. SWEET RELISH

1 teasp. TAMARI

2 TBS. LIGHT MAYONNAISE

♣Pile on half a TOASTED BUN. Top with ALFALFA SPROUTS if desired, and top with the other half.

Pocket Sandwiches

Greek cuisine pioneered the use of pita pockets by stuffing them with falafel, a spicy garbanzo bean mixture. Today we use pitas for every kind of filling imaginable, from a stossed salad to deli stuffings, to pocket pizzas. They are light, fun to eat, and low in fat and calories. They come in all sizes from minis for appetizers to large ones the size of tortillas. They can be split at the top, or cut in half for filling, or sliced lengthwise for open-face or pizza rounds. They seem to go well with all kinds of cuisines, and are delicious broiled, toasted or cold. Use whole wheat pitas for whole grain goodness.

488   LOW-FAT POCKET FALAFELS

This section wouldn't be complete without falafels, a whole wheat, garbanzo bean and spice combination from the Middle East that became one of the foundation foods for the healthy eating movement in the sixties. This version is from The Rainbow Kitchen of the seventies, has a California touch, and has stood the test of time.
For 4 large pitas split. Enough for 8 pita pockets: Preheat oven to 350∞.

♣Have ready 4 CUPS COOKED GARBANZO BEANS. Process in the blender until smooth with

3 CLOVES PEELED GARLIC	1/2 teasp. CUMIN
1/3 CUP CHOPPED CELERY	1/4 teasp. TURMERIC
1/2 CUP CHOPPED ONION	1/4 teasp. CAYENNE
3 TBS. BREAD CRUMBS	1/4 teasp. SEA SALT
2 TBS. SESAME TAHINI	1/4 teasp. PEPPER

♣Chill in the fridge to blend flavors.

♣Form mixture into 1" balls. (makes about 48 balls.) Place on a lecithin-sprayed baking sheet and bake until golden brown, about 15 minutes.
♣Divide 1 THIN SLICED CUCUMBER, 4 THIN SLICED TOMATOES, ONE 4-OZ. TUB ALFALFA SPROUTS, and FALAFEL BALLS into 8 pita pocket halves. Top with spoonfuls of PLAIN LOW-FAT YO-GURT.

Nutritional analysis: per serving; 275 calories; 12gm. protein; 47gm. carbohydrate; 9gm. fiber; 6gm. fats; 0 cholesterol; 99mg. calcium; 4mg. iron; 81mg. magnesium; 546mg. potassium; 153mg. sodium; 2mg. zinc.

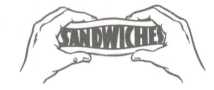

489   EASY CALIFORNIA FALAFELS

This is the quick, easy, pre-prepared version - also delicious.
For 4 large pitas split. Enough for 8 pita pockets: Preheat oven to 375∞.

♣Use a packaged Falafel or Grain Burger mix such as *Lite Chef*, or *Fantastic Foods*. Mix with 1 LB. FRESH TOFU crumbled and mashed, 1 EGG, and 1/2 CUP WATER. Form into 25 to 30 balls.
♣Flatten slightly, and bake on oiled sheets for 20 minutes until brown. Loosen about halfway through the baking with a spatula so they won't stick and crumble. Remove and cool slightly.

♣Halve and open 4 PITA BREADS. Toast for a few minutes in the oven until aromatic. Remove, cool slightly, and line bottom and sides with SHREDDED LETTUCE.

♣Divide FALAFELS, 2 CHOPPED TOMATOES, 1 PEELED, SLICED CUCUMBER, a 4-OZ. TUB of AL-FALFA SPROUTS, and an 8-OZ. JAR of MILD TACO SAUCE between the pita pockets.

490   HOT SALSA PIZZARITO

This was a popular recipe during the Rainbow Kitchen years. We used to change the filling a lot according to the fresh ingredients of the day, but nobody seemed to mind. It was always a fresh salad in a pocket.
For 4 sandwiches:

♣Mix the filling in a bowl

1/4 CUP CHOPPED ZUCCHINI	2 TBS. CHOPPED GREEN PEPPER
1/4 CUP CHOPPED TOMATO	2 TBS. GREEN ONION
2 TBS. SLICED BLACK OLIVES	2 teasp. PARMESAN
2 TBS. LOW-FAT MOZZARELLA or JACK CHEESE	

2 TBS. FALAFEL CRUMBLES (We made up falafels every day in the restaurant for regular falafel sand-wiches and salads, and then used the crumbled pieces in the pan for these sandwiches to give a spicy crunch to the filling. Falafels make up and keep beautifully from a natural packaged mix. You might want to make some up and have them around for these and lots of other recipes.)

♣If you don't have falafels, substitute ROASTED SUNFLOWER SEEDS.

♣Stuff the filling into SPLIT and HALVED PITA POCKETS .

♣Top with dollops of a quick, fresh, blender-made **HOT TOMATO SALSA.**

It is delicious on lots of things. You might want to keep some of this around, too.
Makes 1 1/2 cups sauce:

♣Whirl in the blender

1 1/4 CUPS CHOPPED TOMATOES	1/4 CUP GRATED JACK CHEESE
1 TB. SOY BACON BITS	1/2 teasp. OREGANO
2 TBS. CHOPPED GREEN CHILIES	1/2 teasp. MEXICAN SEASONING

♣Toast in the oven to melt cheese and top with 2 TBS. SPICY SPROUTS per sandwich. Serve hot.

Nutritional analysis: per serving; 120 calories; 4gm. protein; 18gm. carbohydrate; 2gm. fiber; 4gm. fats; 1mg. choles-terol; 49mg. calcium; 1mg. iron; 21mg. magnesium; 139mg. potassium; 100mg. aodium; trace zinc.

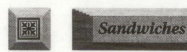

491   HAWAIIAN CHICKEN PITAS

For 6 pita pockets:

♣Sauté in a wok 3/4 LB. BONELESS, SKINLESS BITE SIZE CHICKEN BREAST PIECES until opaque. Re-move from heat.

♣Mix in a bowl

1/2 CUP PLAIN LOW-FAT YOGURT	1/4 CUP CHOPPED CELERY
1 CUP PINEAPPLE CHUNKS	1 TB. LEMON JUICE
3/4 CUP HALVED SEEDLESS GRAPES	1/2 TB. VANILLA

♣Chill to let flavors blend.

♣Add chicken to yogurt mix and fill pita pockets.

Nutritional analysis: per serving; 213 calories; 21gm. protein; 24gm. carbohydrate; 2gm. fiber; 4gm. fats; 49mg. cho-lesterol; 66mg. calcium; 1mg. iron; 34mg. magnesium; 296mg. potassium; 103mg. sodium; 1mg. zinc.

Open Face Sandwiches

492   ORIENTAL TUNA & BLACK MUSHROOM

Very exotic for a sandwich - the creme de la creme of tuna sandwiches.
For 4 sandwiches:

♣Mix 1 teasp. GREAT 28 MIX and 1 TB. MUSTARD with $1/2$ CUP MAYONNAISE. Let sit to blend.

♣Soak 4 to 6 LARGE SHIITAKE BLACK MUSHROOMS until soft. Sliver and discard woody stems.
♣Slice 1 LB. RINSED SKINNED FRESH AHI TUNA FILET into 4 slices. Brush tuna and mushrooms with OLIVE OIL, and let sit while you heat a skillet or griddle to hot. Add tuna and mushrooms to griddle and grill <u>one minute on each side.</u>

♣Spread spiced mayonnaise on 4 WHOLE GRAIN TOAST SLICES. Top each slice with 2 LARGE LETTUCE LEAVES, TUNA, and MUSHROOMS. Squeeze LEMON JUICE over.

Nutritional analysis: per serving; 438 calories; 31gm. protein; 19gm. carbohydrate; 4gm. fiber; 15gm. fats; 56mg. cholesterol; 55mg. calcium; 3mg. iron; 82mg. magnesium; 444mg. potassium; 389mg. sodium; 2mg. zinc.

493   CHICKEN MELT CROISSANTS

These can be lovely little brunch sandwiches. Form the filling to the shape of the croissant half and let chill on the baking sheet before broiling.
For 8 sandwich halves:

♣Split and toast 4 CROISSANTS until light brown on a baking sheet, 1 to 2 minutes.
♣Shred 2 CUPS COOKED CHICKEN BREAST into a bowl. Mix with MAYONNAISE to moisten.
♣Add DIJON MUSTARD to taste, and

$1/2$ teasp. DRY TARRAGON	1 TB. SWEET PICKLE RELISH
3 MINCED GREEN ONIONS	$1/4$ teasp. HOT PEPPER SAUCE

♣Spread each croissant half with chicken mix. Top with grated CHEDDAR or SWISS CHEESE.
♣Broil until cheese melts, about 30-45 seconds.

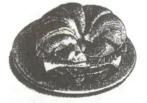

494   TERIYAKI TOFU SANDWICH

For 4 sandwiches:

♣Slice ONE 12 OZ. TUB of TOFU into thin slabs and marinate in 4 TBS. BOTTLED TERIYAKI SAUCE.
♣Split a SMALL WHOLE WHEAT FRENCH BREAD LENGTHWISE.
♣Make the sandwich spread. Mix and cover WHOLE GRAIN BREAD SLICES with 2 TBS. LIGHT MAYONNAISE and 1 teasp. HOT ORIENTAL MUSTARD.
♣Top each with slices of SWISS or FARMER CHEESE. Heat briefly under the broiler to melt cheese.
♣Top cheese with TOFU SLICES. Pour over any remaining marinade and broil until brown.

495   HOT BROWN

For 4 sandwiches:

♣Make the sauce. Melt 3 TBS. BUTTER. Add 3 TBS. FLOUR and 2 TBS. SOY BACON BITS. Roux stirring together until bubbly. Add and stir in 1 teasp. SWEET HOT MUSTARD.
♣Add 1 CUP CUBED LOW-FAT CHEDDAR and 1/2 CUP LOW-FAT JACK. Mix in and add 2 TBS. SHERRY and 2 TBS. PLAIN LOW-FAT YOGURT.
♣Toast 4 WHOLE GRAIN BREAD SLICES. Cover each with a tablespoon of sauce, and SLICES of COOKED TURKEY BREAST. Spoon rest of cheese sauce over and broil until sauce browns.
♣Top with FRESH TOMATO SLICES and serve hot.

Nutritional analysis: per serving; 311 calories; 21gm. protein; 21gm. carbohydrate; 4gm. fiber; 15gm. fats; 48mg. cholesterol; 360mg. calcium; 2mg. iron; 61mg. magnesium; 247mg. potassium; 460mg. sodium; 2mg. zinc.

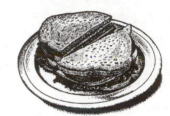

496   SPICY NEW ORLEANS EGG SALAD

For 4 sandwiches:

♣Hard boil 4 EGGS. Chop into a bowl.
♣Sauté 2 TBS. DICED RED ONION and 1 CLOVE CHOPPED GARLIC in 1 TB. OLIVE OIL until soft.
♣Remove from heat and add enough light MAYONNAISE to moisten.
♣Add

4 TBS. DICED CELERY	1 1/2 teasp. SHERRY
3 TBS. DICED PICKLES or SWEET RELISH	1 teasp. LEMON JUICE
2 teasp. PAPRIKA	1/2 teasp. DILL WEED
1/2 teasp. HOT PEPPER SAUCE	1/2 teasp. LEMON PEPPER

♣Combine gently with eggs. Serve on OPEN FACE TOAST SLICES covered with WATERCRESS LEAVES. Top with SUNFLOWER SPROUTS or SNIPS of CILANTRO LEAVES.

497   TOMATO WITH BASIL MAYONNAISE

For 2 sandwiches:

♣Mix 4 TBS. MAYONNAISE with 4 TBS. MINCED FRESH BASIL LEAVES and 1 teasp. MUSTARD.
♣Sauté 1/4 CUP CHOPPED RED ONION in 1 teasp. OIL and 1/4 teasp. GARLIC/LEMON SEASONING until aromatic and soft.
♣Toast 2 WHOLE GRAIN BREAD SLICES. Cover with BASIL MAYONNAISE.
♣Top with the ONIONS, a LIGHT CHEDDAR CHEESE SLICE, and FRESH TOMATO and CUCUMBER SLICES. Dab a spoonful of BASIL MAYONNAISE on top and serve.

Nutritional analysis: per serving; 401 calories; 12gm. protein; 21gm. carbohydrate; 4gm. fiber; 18gm. fats; 28mg. cholesterol; 247mg. calcium; 2mg. iron; 46mg. magnesium; 223mg. potassium; 465mg. sodium; 2mg. zinc.

498   ZUCCHINI BURGERS

These are delicious, low fat and surprisingly hearty.
For 6 burgers:

♣Split, toast and butter 3 ENGLISH MUFFINS. Run under the broiler to crisp and brown tops.
♣Shred 1¹/₂ LBS. ZUCCHINI into a colander. Salt and let drain for 30 minutes to remove moisture.

♣Sauté 1 LARGE CHOPPED ONION in 1 TB. OIL in a skillet until soft, about 10 minutes. Remove to a bowl, and add the zucchini, ¹/₄ CUP BREAD CRUMBS, 2 EGGS, and ¹/₄ CUP PARMESAN.
♣Season with SEA SALT and BLACK PEPPER.

♣Heat 1 TB. BUTTER, and 1 TB. SOY BACON BITS in the skillet until sizzling. Ladle 3 mounds of zucchini mix into pan and spread to make 3" cakes. Cook until bottoms are light brown, about 3 minutes. Turn and cook for 3 more minutes. Repeat for 3 more cakes.

♣Spread muffin halves with ample spoonfuls of **QUICK LIGHT CHEESE SAUCE.**
For 1 cup:

♣Stir 1 TB. BUTTER and 1 TB. WHOLE WHEAT FLOUR together until bubbly. Add ¹/₄ CUP CHOPPED ONION and sauté for 7 minutes until aromatic.
♣Add ¹/₄ CUP PLAIN LOW-FAT YOGURT and ¹/₄ CUP WHITE WINE or WATER. Reduce heat and cook slowly until thickened. Season with 2 PINCHES NUTMEG, SESAME SALT and PEPPER.

♣Turn off heat. Add ¹/₂ CUP GRATED LOW-FAT CHEESE and let melt.
♣Top burgers with TOMATO SLICES and another dollop of cheese sauce. Run under the broiler for 30 seconds to bubble, and serve hot.

Nutritional analysis: per serving; 303 calories; 12gm. protein; 25gm. carbo.; 3gm. fiber; 17gm. fats; 98mg. cholesterol; 234mg. calcium; 2mg. iron; 47mg. magnesium; 617mg. potassium; 480mg. sodium; 1mg. zinc.

499   CALIFORNIA SUNSHINE MELT

For 2 sandwiches: Preheat broiler.

♣Toast 2 SLICES MIXED GRAIN BREAD. Spread with 2 TBS. LOW-FAT MAYONNAISE.
♣Top with
¹/₂ CUP THIN SLICED RED RADISHES or TOMATOES
2 TO 4 LARGE THIN SLICED MUSHROOMS
1 SMALL CARROT, shredded
3-OZ. (¹/₂ CUP) LOW-FAT MONTEREY JACK CHEESE
♣Run under the broiler just to melt cheese.
♣Top with ALFALFA SPROUTS.

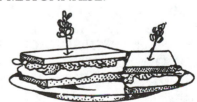

Nutritional analysis: per serving; 314 calories; 17gm. protein; 23gm. carbohydrate; 5gm. fiber; 11gm. fats; 29gm. cholesterol; 350mg. calcium; 2mg. iron; 57mg. magnesium; 426mg. potassium; 472mg. sodium; 2mg. zinc.

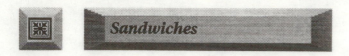
Aram Sandwiches

Aram sandwiches are the newest thing to hit the American sandwich stage since pocket pitas. They are neat roll up sandwiches of Armenian origin, and can be gourmet elegant perfect for picnics and parties or brown bag simple for lunches. The flavor and thinness of these sandwiches provides light, satisfying eating. You can make them by covering big sheets of Lebanese cracker bread for several hours with damp kitchen towels, until the crackers are soft and pliable. Or you can buy the rolling dough in big, soft, flat circles all ready to fill. The result is delicious either way.

♣**How to make an aram sandwich:**
    1) Cover entire round with cream cheese (or other cream cheese type base).
    2) Layer all filling ingredients pizza fashion an the roller, **Leave 4 inches at one end covered only with the cream cheese.**
    3) Beginning at the end covered with filling, roll the bread as tightly as possible jelly-roll fashion toward the end covered with the cream cheese only. The ingredients will move down as you roll. Just tuck them under and keep rolling. The last roll with only the cream cheese will act as a seal.
    4) Wrap in plastic wrap to chill. To serve, slice like a jelly roll into rounds. Each roll produces approximately 16 one-inch slices for about 30 calories per slice, and 3gm. fat.

♣**Tips on making aram sandwiches:**
    1) Make sure the cracker dough is soft and pliable before rolling.
    2) Begin with a base of cream cheese, Neufchatel cheese, kefir cheese or soy cream cheese. A mayonnaise base will separate, and cottage cheese is too watery to work.
    3) Make up half sheets for appetizer rolls so you can use different fillings. Just roll from the rounded edge to the straight side.
    4)Make rolls up ahead of time and chill in the fridge for several hours, to let the filling flavors blend.

✸

500   THREE DELICIOUS ARAM SANDWICHES

TURKEY & LOX

♣Mix 3 to 4 OZ. NEUFCHÂTEL CREAM CHEESE with 1 TB. LIGHT MAYONNAISE and 2 teasp. MUSTARD. Spread on entire round. Sprinkle with SALT and PEPPER.
♣Layer on <u>alternating</u> THIN-SLICED DELI TURKEY SLICES, LOX SLICES and BIG LEAF LETTUCE LEAVES - about 4 of each. Roll and chill as in directions above.

VEGETABLE & HERB

♣Mix 3 to 4-OZ. NEUFCHÂTEL CREAM CHEESE with 1 TB. MAYONNAISE. Spread on entire round. Sprinkle with SESAME SALT and PEPPER.
♣Layer on FRESH SPINACH LEAVES, THIN SLICES of TOMATO, MUSHROOMS, OLIVES and AVOCADO or MARINATED ARTICHOKES. Sprinkle with GRATED CARROT and 2 TBS. ROASTED SUNFLOWER SEEDS. Roll and chill as in directions above.

TEX-MEX BURRITO

♣Mix 3 to 4 OZ. NEUFCHÂTEL CREAM CHEESE with 2 TBS. PLAIN YOGURT and 2 teasp. HOT SALSA. Spread on entire round. Sprinkle with PINCHES of CUMIN and ONION SALT.
♣Cover with a layer of REFRIED BEANS, a layer of THIN-SLICED TOMATOES, and a layer of THIN-SLICED MONTEREY JACK CHEESE. Roll and chill as in directions above.

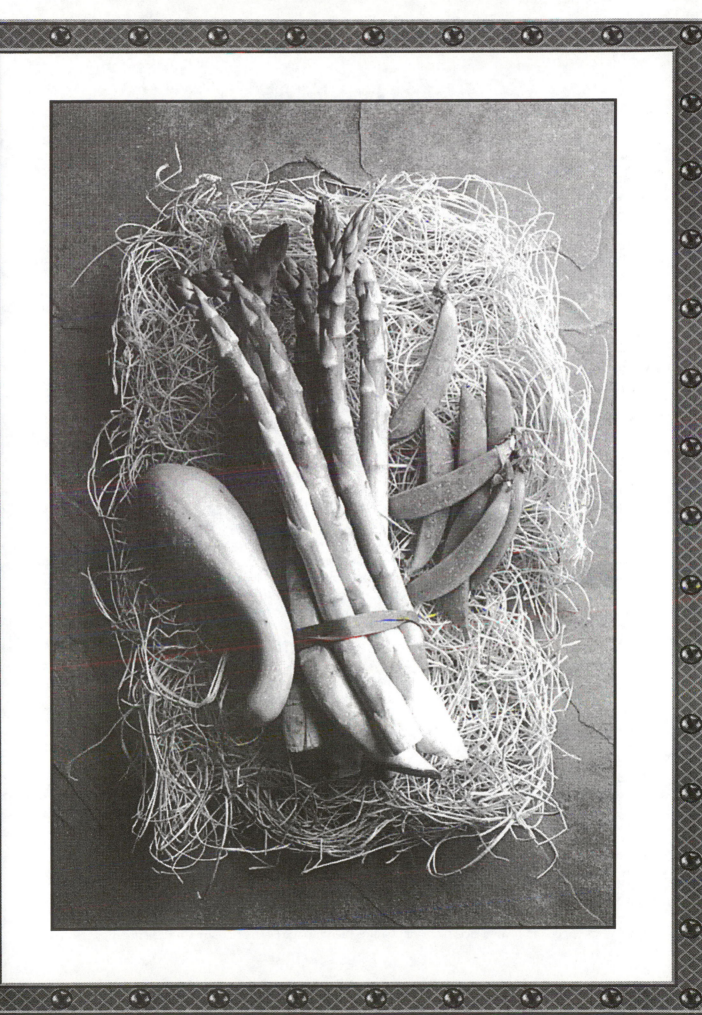

Stir-Fries
Oriental Steam Braising

Steam sautéing is a fast, tasty, cooking technique that is also very healthful. It is best done in a hot wok with a spare amount of peanut oil or broth. A cooking broth or sauce is then added, and the ingredients steam and stir for a few minutes to absorb flavors and heighten colors. Stir-frying does wonderful things to food, especially vegetables. It quickly seals in nutrients with short, intense heat, while preserving fresh vitamins and minerals and softening vegetable cellulose.

Stir-fries are wonderful for party meals. You can do all the prep work ahead of time and let the guests help with the fast cooking, right at the table if you have an electric wok or skillet. Serve everything hot and sizzling, with hot sake or cold white wine.

Although originally an Oriental system of cooking, stir frying adapts beautifully to western tastes and ingredients. We have incorporated several international applications into this section, using stir frying as a more healthful cooking technique for other cuisines.

The recipe categories in this chapter include:

❧STIR-FRIES UNLIMITED ❧HOT SALAD STIR-FRIES ❧STIR-FRIES WITH PASTA and NOODLES ❧STIR-FRIES WITH VEGETABLES ❧STIR-FRIES WITH SEAFOOD, TURKEY and CHICKEN❧STIR-FRIES FROM AROUND THE WORLD ❧STIR-FRY SAUCES ❧

Tips For Great Stir-Fries:

☛Have all ingredients prepared before you start. Many of the health benefits, and most of the taste, comes from the fast, even cooking, and keeping the food constantly moving.

☛Use a large heavy-bottomed wok or skillet, that can conduct heat evenly. It should have high sides and a handle that stays cool.

☛Cut all stir-fry ingredients as uniformly as possible. Pat all food dry before you stir-fry; otherwise it will steam and stew. Moist poultry can be dusted with flour for better browning.

☛Use just enough oil to lightly coat the bottom of the pan.

☛Heat your wok over medium high heat <u>first,</u> then add the oil or your liquid of choice; then add your choice of spices and heat until fragrant; then add the stir-fry ingredients.

☛Don't crowd the pan. Adding too many ingredients at a time means they will steam and stew, rather than brown and sear in the valuable juices and flavor.

Stir-Fries Unlimited

You can do almost anything with a steam-sauté/stir-fry. The following technique gives you choices all in one place so that you can: 1) use your fresh garden harvest; 2) use up perfectly good leftovers in a new way; 3) suit your individual tastes.

Step By Step To The Perfect Vegetable Stir-Fry:

1) Heat wok alone for 1 minute over **high heat. The key to perfection is quick, hot cooking.**

2) Add oil and seasonings or spices of your choice. Heat for 1 to 2 minutes until aromatic.

3) Add onions if you are using them, and heat for 1 to 2 minutes until fragrant.

4) Add dense vegetables first: cauliflower, broccoli, potato slices, carrots, celery, cabbage, etc. Stir and toss for about 2 minutes.

4) Add lighter vegetables next: mushrooms, daikon slices, summer squash, bell peppers, chinese cabbage, etc. Stir and toss for 1 minute.

5) Add even lighter vegetables next: water chestnuts, black mushrooms, bok choy, tofu chunks, scallions, etc. Toss for 1 more minute.

6) Add seasoning sauce and stir through for 1 minute to let bubble.

7) Add the following ingredients on top. Do not stir in. Just cover and steam for 2 minutes: spinach, bean sprouts, cooked noodles, chard leaves, toasted nuts, etc.

8) Serve over cooked brown rice, Gourmet Grains blend (page 647), or crispy Chinese noodles.

Hot Salad Stir-Fries
These are easy, uncomplicated, light, low-fat, hot salads, done with an Oriental touch.

501   HOT CHINESE GINGER SALAD

For 6 people:

♣Heat the wok briefly, then add and sizzle until aromatic
3 TBS. PEANUT OIL
1 CLOVE MINCED GARLIC
1 teasp. FRESH GRATED GINGER

♣Add and brown
2 CAKES CUBED TOFU (opt.)

♣Add the following greens, and toss just to coat with oil and turn bright green, *about 1 minute.*
8 to 10 CUPS WASHED, STEMMED, CHOPPED or TORN CHINESE GREENS MIXTURE. Use NAPPA CABBAGE, BOK CHOY, CHARD, ROMAINE, SPINACH, CELERY, etc.

♣Add 1 CAN SLICED WATER CHESTNUTS

♣Add and toss just to heat through
1/4 CUP MIRIN or SAKÉ or SHERRY
1 TB. BROWN RICE VINEGAR
2 TBS. TAMARI OR OYSTER SAUCE

1 teasp. TOASTED SESAME OIL
1 teasp. HONEY

♣Serve immediately - hot, over BROWN RICE.

Nutritional analysis: per serving with rice; 258 calories; 8gm. protein; 33gm. carbo.; 5gm. fiber; 10gm. fats; 0 cholesterol; 125mg. calcium; 4mg. iron; 116mg. magnesium; 452mg. potassium; 108mg. sodium; 1mg. zinc.

502   SPICY PEAS, MUSHROOMS & CELERY

For 4 people as a main dish:

♣Have ready
4 CUPS DIAGONALLY SLICED CELERY
1 CUP SLICED ONION, in rings
2 1/2 CUPS SLICED MUSHROOMS

1 CUP SNOW PEAS, strung
1 SMALL BELL PEPPER, slivered

♣Mix the sauce
1 TB. TAMARI
2 TBS. ARROWROOT or KUZU
1/2 teasp. HOT CHILI OIL

1 teasp. SAKÉ or SHERRY
1 teasp. FRUCTOSE

♣Heat the wok briefly, about 1 minute. Add 1 TB. PEANUT OIL and 1 teasp. TOASTED SESAME OIL.
♣Heat briefly. Add CELERY, BELL PEPPER and ONION SLICES. Steam sauté for 3 minutes.
♣Add the MUSHROOMS and 1/2 teasp. BLACK PEPPER. Add the SNOW PEAS and 1 3/4 CUPS CHICKEN STOCK or MISO BROTH Add the sauce and bring to a boil. Let bubble until thickened.
♣Serve over crispy CHINESE NOODLES.

503 SWEET & SOUR GREENS

For 4 to 6 people:

♣Heat the wok briefly, then add 3 TBS. OIL to sizzling. Add 1 HEAD BOK CHOY or RADICCHIO LETTUCE cut in 1" pieces and toss for <u>30 seconds only.</u>
♣Add and steam, covered for 1 minute
1/4 CUP BROWN RICE VINEGAR   1/4 CUP BROWN SUGAR
1 teasp. FRESH SHREDDED GINGER
♣Mix 1 TB. ARROWROOT in 1 TB. TAMARI. Add to 1/4 CUP WATER and 1/4 CUP SHERRY or MIRIN.
♣Add to greens and steam until thickened.

※

504 QUICK SKILLET SPROUTS

For 2 servings:

♣Heat 1 TB. OIL to hot. Add 1/2 CUP CHOPPED GREEN ONION and 1 CUP GRATED CARROTS.
♣Sauté until color changes.
♣Add 4 CUPS MUNG BEAN SPROUTS, 1/4 CUP LIGHT VEGETABLE STOCK, 1 teasp. SESAME SALT and 1/4 teasp. PEPPER.
♣Stir and toss over high heat for 30 seconds until sprouts are hot. Serve immediately.

Nutritional analysis: per serving; 162 calories; 8gm. protein; 20gm. carbohydrate; 8gm. fiber; 8gm. fats; 0 cholesterol; 69mg. calcium; 3mg. iron; 62mg. magnesium; 570mg. potassium; 405mg. sodium; 1mg. zinc.

※

505 ASPARAGUS, SHALLOTS & SPROUTS

For 6 servings:

♣Toast 1/2 CUP SLIVERED ALMONDS in the oven until golden brown.
♣Trim 2 LBS. FRESH ASPARAGUS IN 1" PIECES.
♣Chop 4 TBS. FRESH SHALLOTS.
♣Have ready 3 CUPS SUNFLOWER SPROUTS or BEAN SPROUTS.
♣Make the sauce. Mix ingredients to blend and then set aside.
1 TB. ARROWROOT OR KUZU   2/3 CUP VEGETABLE BROTH
1 TB. TAMARI   2 teasp. SHERRY or MIRIN
2 teasp. SHREDDED GINGER ROOT
♣Heat the wok for about 1 minute. Add 3 TBS. PEANUT OIL and heat for one more minute.
♣Add ASPARAGUS and 2 TBS. WATER, and steam/braise until water evaporates, about 2 minutes.
♣Add the SHALLOTS and cooking sauce. Bring to a boil and toss.
♣Add the SPROUTS and cook until sauce thickens and sprouts are tender.
♣Top with the TOASTED ALMONDS and serve.

506 SNOW PEAS WITH BLACK MUSHROOMS

This is a particularly good therapeutic recipe when you use reishi or shiitake mushrooms.
For 6 to 8 people:

♣Soak 15 to 20 DRIED BLACK SHIITAKE MUSHROOMS in water until soft. Sliver and discard woody stems. *Save soaking water.*

♣Mix the sauce in a small bowl

1 teasp. ARROWROOT OR KUZU
1 teasp. FRUCTOSE

1/2 teasp. SESAME SALT
1 teasp. TAMARI

♣Toss with black mushrooms to coat, and set aside.

♣Trim 8-OZ. FRESH SNOW PEAS. Chop 4 GREEN ONIONS. Shred 2 SLICES FRESH GINGER.

♣Heat wok for about 1 minute over medium heat. Add 2 TBS. PEANUT OIL and the GINGER and heat until sizzling and aromatic, about 1 minute.

♣Add the MUSHROOMS and GREEN ONIONS and toss to coat, about 1 minute.

♣Add 1 1/2 CUPS MISO BROTH and the MUSHROOM SOAKING LIQUID. Bring to a boil, cover and simmer for 5 minutes.

♣Add 2 to 3 TBS. OYSTER SAUCE and the arrowroot mixture. Stir to thicken and blend. Remove from heat to a serving platter.

♣Add 2 teasp. OIL to the wok, heat briefly and add the SNOW PEAS and 1/2 teasp. SESAME SALT

♣Toss and sauté until color changes to bright green. Spoon over the mushroom mix and serve.

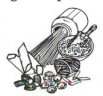

Stir-Fries With Pasta & Noodles

All kinds of pasta and noodles can be stir-fried for a hearty, quick, one-dish, healthy meal.
This chapter shows you the delicious possibilities.

507 SZECHUAN NOODLES WITH PEANUT SAUCE

For 6 servings:
♣Make the sauce first. Combine in a bowl and set aside to let flavors blend

2 TBS. PEANUT BUTTER
2 TBS. SESAME TAHINI
2 TBS. OYSTER SAUCE
1/3 CUP CHICKEN STOCK or MISO BROTH

2 teasp. BROWN RICE VINEGAR
2 teasp. HOT CHILI OIL
2 TBS. FRUCTOSE
1 CHOPPED SCALLION

♣Bring 3-qts. water to a boil. Add 8-OZ. CAPELLINI or THIN FETTUCINI and cook just to al dente, about 3 minutes. Drain and toss with 2 TBS. SESAME OIL. Pour sauce over noodles and sprinkle with DRY ROASTED PEANUTS and 1 TB. CHOPPED FRESH CILANTRO.

Nutritional analysis: per serving; 290 calories; 9gm. protein; 36gm. carbohydrate; 3gm. fiber; 13gm. fats; 0 cholesterol; 23mg. calcium; 2mg. iron; 56mg. magnesium; 180mg. potassium; 73mg. sodium; 1mg. zinc.

508   SOBA NOODLES & SAUCE

Japanese noodles are buckwheat - a good choice for those with wheat sensitivity.
For 4 servings:

♣Toast 3 TBS. SESAME SEEDS in the oven until golden.

♣Heat the wok for 1 minute. Add 2 TBS. PEANUT OIL and heat for 1 minute more until sizzling.
♣Add 1 CLOVE MINCED GARLIC and 1 SMALL SLICED ONION and sauté until aromatic.
♣Add and stir-fry til color changes

1 CHOPPED GREEN BELL PEPPER	$1/2$ CHOPPED RED BELL PEPPER
$1/3$ CUP SLIVERED DAIKON RADISH	1 SLICED CARROT

♣Add and let bubble stirring, until thickened

$2/3$ CUP WATER	1 TB. HONEY
3 TBS. TAMARI	3 TB. MINCED CILANTRO
$1^1/2$ TBS. KUZU mixed in 2 TBS. WATER	

♣While sauce is cooking, bring 2-QTS. WATER to a boil for 8-OZ. BUCKWHEAT SOBA. Add noodles and bring to a rapid boil. Add 1 cup *cold water* and bring to another boil. Add another cup *cold water* and bring to another boil. Add 1 more cup cold water, and when water reboils on high heat, pasta should be done. Drain and toss with sauce right away, so it won't stick. Top with sesame seeds.

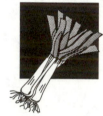

509   CANTONESE NOODLES WITH GINGER & LEEKS

For 6 people:

♣Mix the sauce ingredients and set aside to blend flavors.

$1^1/2$ TB. OYSTER SAUCE	1 teasp. TOASTED SESAME OIL
$1^1/4$ teasp. TAMARI	2 PINCHES WHITE PEPPER
3 TBS. CHICKEN STOCK	1 PINCH FRUCTOSE

♣Bring 2-QTS. WATER to a boil. Add 8-OZ. THIN CHINESE DRIED or FRESH EGG NOODLES (or FINE LINGUINE). Cook for $1^1/2$ minutes if fresh and for 10 minutes if dried. Drain in a colander. Run under cold water and drain again. Set aside in the colander while you complete the stir-fry.

♣Heat wok over medium high for 1 minute. Add 2 TBS. PEANUT OIL and heat for 1 minute. When a wisp of smoke appears, add 3 TBS. SHREDDED FRESH GINGER and 1 CLOVE MINCED GARLIC and sauté until fragrant for 30 seconds.

♣Add 1 LARGE SLICED LEEK (white parts only) and toss for 1 to 2 minutes.
♣Add noodles and toss for 1 minute. Make a well in the center, and add the sauce.
♣Cook and toss for 1 minute until just coated. Serve at once.

Nutritional analysis: per serving; 110 calories; 3gm.protein; 17gm. carbohydrate; 2gm. fiber; 4gm. fats; 11mg. cholesterol; 31mg. calcium; 2mg. iron; 24mg. magnesium; 123mg. potassium; 74mg. sodium; trace zinc.

510   WOK FRIED RICE

For 4 servings:

♣Have ready 6 CUPS COLD COOKED BROWN RICE or BASMATI RICE.

♣Soak 4 LARGE DRY SHIITAKE BLACK MUSHROOMS in water until soft. Sliver and discard woody stems. Save $1/4$ cup soaking water for sauce.
♣Chop 1 BUNCH SCALLIONS.
♣Chop 1 BUNCH BROCCOLI into FLOWERETTES with some stalks.
♣String and trim 1 CUP FRESH SNOW PEAS.
♣Coarse chop 1 HEAD BABY BOK CHOY.
♣Slice 4 LARGE BUTTON MUSHROOMS.
♣Rinse 2 CUPS BEAN SPROUTS in cold water.

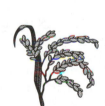

♣Heat wok over medium high heat for 1 minute. Add and heat for about 2 minutes until fragrant

2 TBS. PEANUT OIL	1 teasp. TAMARI
1 SMALL PIECE MINCED GINGER ROOT, peeled	1 teasp. TOASTED SESAME OIL
1 SMALL PIECE SNIPPED DULSE or WAKAME	1 CLOVE MINCED GARLIC

♣Remove ginger and garlic pieces.
♣Add the following and stir-fry in order for 1 minute each:
SHIITAKE MUSHROOMS, BUTTON MUSHROOMS, BROCCOLI , SNOW PEAS, BOK CHOY
♣Add mushroom soaking water,1 TB. TAMARI, 1 TB. MIRIN or SHERRY, and $1/4$ teasp. FIVE SPICE POWDER. Lower heat and add the CHOPPED SCALLIONS, RICE, BEAN SPROUTS.
♣Cover and steam for 5 minutes. Serve hot.

511   SWEET MANDARIN RICE & VEGETABLES

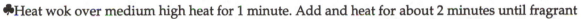

For 6 servings:

♣Have ready 4 CUPS COLD COOKED BROWN RICE or BASMATI RICE.
♣Slice 4 RIBS CELERY DIAGONALLY.
♣Slice 1 CAN WATER CHESTNUTS.
♣Slice 2 BUNCHES GREEN ONIONS DIAGONALLY.
♣Rinse 2 CUPS BEAN SPROUTS in cold water.
♣Heat wok over medium high heat for 1 minute. Add and heat 3 TBS. OIL and 1 CLOVE MINCED GAR-LIC until fragrant. Add vegetables in the order given above, and toss for 1 minute.

♣Mix together and toss for more 1 minute

$3/4$ CUP TOASTED SUNFLOWER SEEDS	$1/2$ teasp. OREGANO
2 TBS. FRESH GRATED GINGER	$1/2$ teasp. BASIL
1 TB. LEMON JUICE	$1/2$ teasp. SESAME SALT

♣Mix together $1/4$ CUP HONEY, $1/4$ CUP MIRIN or SHERRY and $1/2$ CUP TAMARI Stir in RICE and toss all together until hot, about 3 minutes. Top with 1 TB. FRESH SNIPPED CILANTRO.

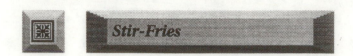

Stir-Fries With Vegetables

These can be the perfect, satisfying vegetarian meal.
All vegetables seem to be compatible, so your imagination is the only limit.

512   MUSHROOM MADNESS

You can use almost any mix of mushrooms with this recipe, and come out with a different delicious taste each time.
Try Chanterelles, Porcini, Shiitake, Enoki, Button, Straw, Golden, Oyster or Chinese Tree mushrooms. We have
used fresh, dried and canned versions of all of these with success.
For 6 servings:

♣Heat wok on high heat for 1 minute. Add 1 TB. PEANUT OIL and heat to very hot. Add and toss

1 CUP SNOW PEAS or WATER CHESTNUTS, sliced   1 TB. GINGER TAMARI SAUCE
$1/2$ CUP SLICED GREEN ONIONS $1/4$ teasp. NUTMEG

♣Stir and toss until color changes. Remove with a slotted spoon and set aside.

♣Add 2 TBS. PEANUT OIL to the wok and heat. Then add and toss

$1^1/2$ LBS. MIXED MUSHROOMS   1 TB. LEMON JUICE
1 TB. MIRIN or SHERRY   1 TB. SNIPPED PARSLEY

♣Stir fry for 1 or 2 minutes, tossing continuously to enhance delicate flavor.

♣Add vegetables back to wok and toss for 30 seconds. Turn onto a serving platter and serve hot.

Nutritional analysis: per serving; 87 calories; 3gm. protein; 9gm. carbohydrate; 3gm. fiber; 5gm. fats; 0 cholesterol;
24mg. calcium; 2mg. iron; 21mg. magnesium; 507mg. potassium; 33mg. sodium; 1mg. zinc.

513   CLASSIC VEGETABLES FOR CRISP NOODLES

For 4 servings:

♣Toast $1/2$ CUP SLIVERED ALMONDS in the oven until brown.

♣Begin the gravy before you stir-fry the vegetables. Mix in a saucepan

$1^1/2$ CUPS BOTTLED CLAM JUICE or MISO BROTH   1 TB. SHERRY
2 TBS. ARROWROOT dissolved in 4 TBS. WATER   1 TB. TAMARI

♣Reduce heat to low, and allow to bubble and thicken while you stir-fry the vegetables.

♣Heat wok over medium high heat for 1 minute. Add 3 TBS. PEANUT OIL and $1/2$ teasp. GARLIC/
LEMON SEASONING and heat until fragrant and sizzling.

♣Add in order, stir frying each ingredient til color changes, about 1 minute.

1 ONION, sliced in half moons   2 STALKS BOK CHOY, in 1" squares
2 STALKS CELERY, sliced diagonally   1 CUP LARGE MUSHROOMS, sliced
1 STALK BROCCOLI with a little stem, sliced lengthwise

♣Cover wok, and drain liquid into the saucepan. Blend liquid into the sauce.

♣Put wok back on high heat. Add the sauce, the toasted almonds, and $1^1/2$ CUPS BEAN SPROUTS.

♣Toss for 2 minutes to put a gloss on the veggies and heat through .

♣Serve over crispy Chinese noodles.

514 CLASSIC VEGETABLES WITH RICE

For 4 people:

♣Heat the wok over medium high heat for 1 minute. Add 4 TBS. PEANUT OIL and 1/4 teasp. ORIENTAL 5 SPICE POWDER and heat for 2 minutes until aromatic

♣Start the **MISO SAUCE** in a small saucepan before you add the vegetables. It can be bubbling while the vegetables are cooking, and it will all come out together.
♣Dissolve 3 TBS. ARROWROOT or KUZU CHUNKS into 1/4 CUP LOW SODIUM TAMARI.
♣Add 4 TBS. MILD CHICKPEA MISO mixed into 1 1/2 CUP WATER
♣Add a LARGE PINCH HOT CHINESE DRY MUSTARD and 2 PINCHES <u>EACH</u>: SAGE POWDER, THYME POWDER and ROSEMARY POWDER.
♣Cook until sauce begins to thicken. Reduce heat and let simmer.

♣Add the following to the hot wok in order given. Stir fry until color changes for each, about 1 minute.
2 CUPS LEEKS, sliced thin
1/2 CUP MUSHROOMS, sliced
1/2 CUP GREEN BELL PEPPER, in strips
2 CUPS CHINESE NAPPA CABBAGE in 1" square pieces
1/2 CUP GREEN CABBAGE, shaved
1 CUP BOK CHOY in 1" square pieces
1/2 CUP SWISS CHARD LEAVES in 1" square pieces
♣Cover the wok and drain excess liquid into the Miso sauce. Blend and bubble for a minute. Return wok to the heat and pour sauce over. Toss and serve over hot Basmati or Brown rice.

Nutritional analysis: per serving; 173 calories; 5gm. protein; 22gm. carbohyrate; 4gm. fiber; 8gm. fats; 0 cholesterol; 89mg. calcium; 3mg. iron; 49mg. magnesium; 375mg. potassium; 740mg. sodium; 1mg. zinc.

515 SWEET & SOUR VEGETABLES

For 4 servings:

♣Toast 1/2 CUP CASHEWS in the oven to golden. Remove and set aside.
♣Heat wok over medium hot heat for 1 minute.
♣Add 1 TB. PEANUT OIL,1 teasp. TOASTED SESAME OIL, 1 teasp. BROWN SUGAR and 1/2 teasp. NUTMEG, and heat until aromatic.
♣Add in order given and cook each ingredient for 1 minute until color changes
1 SMALL ONION in slices
1 SMALL BELL PEPPER in strips
HALF OF A RIPE PINEAPPLE in bite size chunks
♣Add and cook briefly until sauce thickens
3/4 CUP CHICKEN BROTH   4 teasp. BROWN SUGAR
2 TBS. TAMARI   2 teasp. BROWN RICE VINEGAR
2 teasp. KUZU CHUNKS mixed in 2 teasp. water
♣Top with cashews, and serve over CRISPY CHINESE NOODLES.

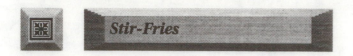

516   ZUCCHINI STIR FRY WITH TOASTED WALNUTS

This entire recipe takes about 15 minutes from cutting the veggies to pouring them out on a big serving platter. My husband and I have this frequently on busy days. He starts at one end with chopsticks and I start at the other, and that is dinner.
For 2 people:

♣Toast 1 CUP WALNUTS in the oven until brown.

♣Have ready 2 CUPS SUNFLOWER SPROUTS or BEAN SPROUTS
♣Slice 1 GREEN and 1 YELLOW ZUCCHINI in diagonal rounds
♣Sliver 1/2 GREEN PEPPER
♣Heat a wok over high heat for 1 minute.
♣Add 1 TB. OIL, 1/2 teasp. GARLIC/LEMON SEASONING and 1 LARGE SLICED ONION and heat until fragrant.
♣Add vegetables and stir fry for 3 minutes until color changes.

♣Mix the following sauce together, and add to vegetables

2 TBS. SHERRY or MIRIN   2 TBS. TAMARI
DASHES of CINNAMON and ALLSPICE   1 TB. WATER

♣Add WALNUTS and simmer for 30 seconds. Pour onto serving platter.

Nutritional analysis: per serving; 323 calories; 10gm. protein; 22gm. carbohydrate; 6gm. fiber; 23gm. fats; 0 cholesterol; 71mg. calcium; 3mg. iron; 98mg. magnesium; 662mg. potassium; 218mg. sodium; 2mg. zinc.

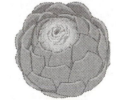

517   STIR FRY WITH ARTICHOKE HEARTS

For 4 people:

♣Slice an 11 OZ. JAR WATER-PACKED ARTICKOKE HEARTS. Sprinkle with LEMON JUICE.

♣Heat a wok over high heat for 1 minute. Add 1 TB. OIL, 1/2 teasp. GARLIC/LEMON SEASONING and 1/2 CUP SLICED ONION and heat until fragrant.
♣Add 2 CUP SLICED ZUCCHINI ROUNDS, and the artichokes and stir-fry about 5 minutes.
♣Add 1 CUP CHUNKED TOMATOES

♣Mix together and add

2 TBS. CHOPPED PARSLEY   1/2 teasp. SESAME SALT
1/2 teasp. OREGANO   1/4 teasp. PEPPER

♣Toss for 1 to 2 minutes to heat through.
♣Sprinkle with 1/4 CUP GRATED MOZZARELLA CHEESE. Turn off heat. Cover wok and let cheese melt. Serve hot.

Nutritional analysis: per serving; 115 calories; 5gm. protein; 14gm. carbohydrate; 8gm. fiber; 5gm. fats; 3mg. cholesterol; 107mg. calcium; 2mg. iron; 56mg. magnesium; 524mg potassium; 198mg. sodium; 1mg. zinc.

518 CHINESE VEGETABLES WITH TOFU

For 4 people:

♣Soak 8 DRY SHIITAKE MUSHROOMS in 1/2 CUP WATER until soft. Sliver and discard woody stems. ♣Reserve soaking water.

♣Mix the sauce ingredients in a small sauce pan and heat briefly to blend while you begin the stir-fry.

1/2 CUP CHICKEN STOCK or MISO BROTH
1 TB. ARROWROOT mixed with 1 TB. WATER

1 TB. OYSTER SAUCE
the MUSHROOM SOAKING WATER

♣Heat the wok over high heat for 1 minute. Add 3 CHOPPED SHALLOTS and 1 TB. FRESH CHOPPED GINGER and heat until aromatic.
♣Add 3 CAKES TOFU in strips and sizzle until brown. Pour sauce over and let bubble until thickened.
♣Add vegetables in order given. Stir. Cover and let steam for 5 minutes.

1 ONION in rings
1/2 BELL PEPPER in strips
2 STALKS BROCCOLI sliced lengthwise with some stem
3 LEAVES CHINESE CABBAGE in 1" squares

3 STALKS BOK CHOY in 1" squares
THE SHIITAKE MUSHROOMS
4-OZ. STRUNG SNOW PEAS

♣Lift cover and add
2 CUPS MUNG BEAN SPROUTS
1 TB. TAMARI
♣Toss for 1 minute and serve hot.

 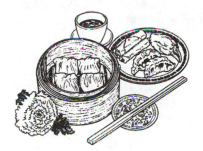

Stir-Fries With Seafood, Turkey & Chicken

519 SZECHUAN CHICKEN CHOW MEIN

This is northern Chinese cuisine at its spicy best. Use a spicy pasta, too.
For 4 people:

♣Cook 3/4 LB. SPICY FETTUCINI for 3 minutes in boiling water. Drain, and toss with oil in a bowl.

♣Heat the wok over high heat for 1 minute. Add 2 TBS. OIL, 1 CLOVE MINCED GARLIC, and 1 teasp. GROUND GINGER, and heat until aromatic.
♣Add and brown 1 1/2 LBS. BONED, SKINNED CHICKEN BREAST in 1" squares.
♣Add 2 CUPS SNOW PEAS, 1 RED BELL PEPPER in thin slices, and 2 CHOPPED GREEN ONIONS.
♣Mix the sauce in a bowl, and stir into the vegetables

3 TBS. TAMARI
1 TB. RICE VINEGAR

1 teasp. CHILI OIL
1/2 teasp. CRUSHED RED PEPPER

♣Toss everything with pasta in the bowl. Top with DRY ROASTED PEANUTS.

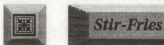

520   SWORDFISH & BLACK MUSHROOM STIR FRY

For 3 people:

♣Soak 5 or 6 BLACK SHIITAKE MUSHROOMS in water until soft.
Sliver and discard woody stems. Save soaking water for sauce.

♣Skin and cube about 12-OZ. SWORDFISH STEAKS.
♣Cut 1 SMALL CARROT into julienne.
♣Slice 1 SMALL ZUCCHINI in rounds.
♣String 4-OZ. FRESH SNOW PEAS.
♣Slice 1/2 RED BELL PEPPER in strips.

♣Heat wok over high heat for 1 minute.
♣Add 2 TBS. OIL and 1 teasp. SHREDDED FRESH GINGER and heat until aromatic, for 3 minutes.
♣Add SWORDFISH, CARROTS, MUSHROOMS and ZUCCHINI and stir-fry for 5 minutes.
♣Add SNOW PEAS, BELL PEPPER, and 1 TB. TAMARI. Stir-fry til fish is opaque.
♣Reduce heat and stir in 1 TB. ARROWROOT dissolved in 1 TB. WATER, 1 teasp. FRUCTOSE, and the MUSHROOM SOAKING WATER.
♣Return to a fast bubble and cook until sauce thickens, about 3 minutes.

♣Turn onto a large serving platter and sprinkle with SESAME SEEDS.

Nutritional analysis: per serving; 228 calories; 5 gm. protein; 5 gm. carbohydrate; 1 gm. fiber; 11 gm. fat; 75 mg. cholesterol; 28 mg. calcium; 1 mg. iron; 76mg. magnesium; 590mg. potassium; 228 mg. sodium; 1mg. zinc.

521   SPICY GREENS WITH CHICKEN & CAPERS

For 6 people:

♣Have ready 4 CUPS MIXED SPICY GREENS, such as SPINACH, ROMAINE, RED LETTUCE and ENDIVE in a serving bowl.

♣Cut 1 LB. BONED SKINNED CHICKEN BREASTS into bite size chunks.

♣Make the **CAPER SAUCE:** mix together in a saucepan and heat until reduced to 1/4 cup. Mix 3/4 CUP CHICKEN BROTH, 1 TB. LEMON JUICE, and 2 TBS. DRAINED CAPERS.
♣Heat the wok over high heat for 1 minute. Add 2 TBS. OIL and 1 ONION in 1" squares. Stir-fry for 2 minutes and remove to a bowl.
♣Add 1 TB. OIL to hot wok, and stir-fry chicken pieces until opaque. Remove to bowl with onions.
♣Add CAPER SAUCE to the wok and deglaze until fragrant and bubbly. Pour over greens and toss to coat. Top with chicken and onions and toss again.

Nutritional analysis: per serving; 244 calories; 25gm. protein; 15gm. carbohydrate; 4gm. fiber; 9gm. fats; 44mg. cholesterol; 34mg. calcium; 2mg. iron; 63mg. magnesium; 683mg. potassium; 171mg. sodium; 2mg. zinc.

522   ORIENTAL TURKEY STIR FRY

For 4 servings:

Marinate ³/₄ LB. COOKED TURKEY BREAST in bite size chunks for 30 minutes in

1 CUP CHICKEN BROTH
2 TBS. ARROWROOT dissolved in 2 TBS. TAMARI
2 TBS. OYSTER SAUCE
2 TBS. SHERRY

1 TB. TOASTED SESAME OIL
1/2 teasp. CINNAMON
1/2 teasp. GROUND ANISE

♣Heat wok on high heat for 1 minute. Add 1¹/₂ teasp. SHREDDED FRESH GINGER, 2 CLOVES MINCED GARLIC, and 3 CHOPPED RED CHILIES and heat until aromatic, about 1¹/₂ minutes.
♣Add in order given, and stir-fry until color changes for each ingredient
2 CUPS SHREDDED CHINESE CABBAGE or BOK CHOY
3 RIBS DIAGONALLY SLICED CELERY
1 CAN SLICED WATER CHESTNUTS or SLICED JICAMA
1 CUP JULIENNED GREEN ONIONS

♣Add TURKEY and MARINADE and stir until sauce bubbles and thickens. Serve over chinese noodles.

Nutritional analysis: per serving; 351 calories; 31gm. protein; 30gm. carbohydrate; 4gm. fiber; 12gm. fats; 58mg. cholesterol; 107mg. calcium; 4mg. iron; 66mg. magnesium; 724mg. potassium; 268mg. sodium; 3mg. zinc.

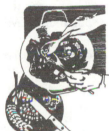

523   CHICKEN SALAD STIR FRY

For 6 people:

♣Cut 3 BONED, SKINNED CHICKEN BREASTS into bite size chunks.

♣Heat wok over medium high heat for 1 minute. Add 2 TBS. PEANUT OIL, 1 CLOVE MINCED GARLIC, 1 teasp. LEMON PEPPER, 1/2 teasp. HOT CHINESE MUSTARD POWDER and 1 teasp. SESAME SALT, and heat for 2 minutes until aromatic.

♣Add in order given and stir fry until color changes for each ingredient
1 CUP SLICED BROCCOLI FLORETS
1 CUP SLICED CAULIFLOWERETTES

2 STALKS CELERY sliced diagonally
1/2 CUP GREEN ONIONS in julienne

♣Remove veggies with a slotted spoon and set aside.
♣Add 1 TB. oil and the CHICKEN BREAST CHUNKS to the wok. Stir-fry until opaque for 4 minutes.

♣Return vegetables to the wok.
♣Add 1/2 CUP LIGHT MAYONNAISE mixed with 1/2 teasp. GREAT 28 MIX (or other vegetable seasoning) and 1 TB. TAMARI.
♣Simmer for 1 minute to heat through and serve over hot basmati rice.

Nutritional analysis: per serving; 448 calories; 31gm. protein; 33gm. carbohydrate; 2gm. fiber; 12gm. fats; 81mg. cholesterol; 55mg. calcium; 3mg. iron; 49mg. magnesium; 438mg. potassium; 300mg. sodium; 2mg. zinc.

524   PRAWNS AND VEGETABLES

For 8 people with rice:

♣Toast ¹/₂ CUP SLICED ALMONDS in a 350° oven until golden.

♣Heat wok for 1 minute over medium high heat. Add and heat until fragrant
3 TBS. PEANUT OIL	1 teasp. SESAME SALT
1 teasp. GINGER POWDER	¹/₂ teasp. LEMON PEPPER

♣Add 1 LB. PEELED SLICED PRAWNS and toss until pink. Remove with a slotted spoon and set aside.
♣Add in order and stir-fry for 1 minute each
1 SMALL ONION in slices	1 STALK CELERY sliced diagonally
1¹/₂ CUPS NAPPA CABBAGE in 1" squares	¹/₂ GREEN PEPPER in 1" squares

♣Add, cover and let steam for 5 minutes.
1¹/₂ teasp. CHICKPEA MISO	1 teasp. SHERRY
¹/₃ CUP WATER	1 teasp. FRUCTOSE
2 TBS. FRESH CHOPPED CILANTRO	

♣Lift lid and place 2 CUPS BEAN SPROUTS on top. <u>Do not stir in.</u> Place 1 CUP TRIMMED SNOW PEAS on top of sprouts. <u>Do not stir in</u>. Place Prawns on top of snow peas. <u>DO NOT STIR IN</u>. Cover and steam for 2 minutes to heat through.
♣Sprinkle ALMONDS over top. Serve with brown rice or GOURMET BLEND rice (pg. 647).

Nutritional analysis: per serving; 267 calories; 17gm. protein; 31gm. carbohydrate; 4gm. fiber; 9gm. fats; 86mg. cholesterol; 79mg. calcium; 3mg. iron; 98mg. magnesium; 349mg. potassium; 2mg. zinc.

Stir Fries From Around The World

Although we in the western world tend to think of stir-fry as an Oriental cooking method, almost every cuisine has developed this type of technique as a more healthful way fo frying.

525   ENGLISH STIR-FRY

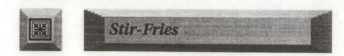

For 6 people:

♣Toast 1 CUP CASHEWS in a 350° oven until golden.

♣Heat wok for 1 minute over medium high heat. Add 1 ONION in thin rings and 1 LEMON in thin slices and toss until fragrant.
♣Add ¹/₂ LB. SLICED MUSHROOMS and stir, tossing for 5 minutes.
♣Add 1 HEAD SLICED GREEN CABBAGE and toss to coat. Season with SEA SALT, PEPPER and TAMARI SAUCE.
♣Add cashews, and toss again until blended.

526   MEXICAN SHRIMP FAJITAS STIR FRY

For 8 servings:

♣Warm 8 FLOUR TORTILLAS in the oven to crisp.

♣Mix and marinate 1¹/₂ LBS. LARGE PEELED SHRIMP for 1 hour in the following sauce
1 CLOVE MINCED GARLIC
1¹/₂ teasp. VEGETABLE SEASONING SALT
1¹/₂ teasp. CUMIN POWDER
¹/₂ teasp. HOT PEPPER SAUCE

2 TBS. OIL
2 TBS. LEMON JUICE
¹/₂ teasp. CHILI POWDER

♣Heat the wok for 1 minute over high heat. Add 3 TBS. OIL and ¹/₂ teasp. OREGANO and heat until aromatic, about 2 minutes.
♣Add in order given and stir-fry until color changes
1 SLICED RED BELL PEPPER IN STRIPS
¹/₂ CUP SLICED ONION RINGS
¹/₂ CUP GREEN ONIONS in julienne slices
♣Remove with a slotted spoon and keep warm.

♣Add shrimp and the marinade, and stir fry for 4 minutes until opaque and tender
♣Add back vegetables and toss to heat.
♣Spoon over tortillas. Top with AVOCADO SLICES and drops of MILD SALSA.

Nutritional analysis: per serving; 307 calories; 21gm. protein; 25gm. carbohydrate; 4gm. fiber; 15gm. fats; 129mg. cholesterol; 83mg. calcium; 3mg. iron; 58mg. magnesium; 400mg. potassium; 288mg. sodium; 1mg. zinc.

527   ITALIAN STYLE STIR-FRY

For 4 servings:

♣Bring 3-qts. water to a boil. Add 8-OZ. SMALL PASTA SHELLS and cook just to al dente, about 3 minutes. Drain. Toss with 2 TBS. OLIVE OIL and put in a serving bowl while you stir-fry the rest.

♣Slice 1 LARGE RED ONION in rings.
♣Grate 4 CARROTS in a salad shooter or food processor.
♣Chop 1 HEAD BROCCOLI into bite size pieces.

♣Heat the wok for 1 minute over high heat. Add 4 TBS. OIL, ¹/₄ teasp. BASIL and ¹/₄ teasp OREGANO, and toss until fragrant.

♣Add vegetables and stir and toss for 5 minutes over medium high heat.
♣Add and toss with pasta in the serving bowl. Top with GRATED MOZARRELLA and serve hot.

Nutritional analysis: per serving; 356 calories; 13gm. protein; 54gm. carbohydrate; 5gm. fiber; 10gm. fats; 7mg. cholesterol; 151mg. calcium; 3mg. iron; 50mg. magnesium; 423mg. potassium; 106mg. sodium; 1mg. zinc.

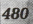

528   CHICKEN CARBONARA STIR FRY

For 4 people:

♣Pan roast 4 TBS. SOY BACON BITS and 1/2 CUP PINE NUTS for 5 minutes and set aside.

♣Cook 8-OZ. DRY LINGUINI in boiling water for 8 minutes. Drain, toss with 1 teasp. oil and set aside.
♣Heat wok over high heat for 1 minute. Add 3 CLOVES MINCED GARLIC, 2 TBS. OLIVE OIL and 2 teasp. DRY BASIL and heat until aromatic.

♣Add 1 1/2 CUPS CHICKEN BREASTS IN BITE SIZE CHUNKS and stir-fry until opaque and tender.
♣Reduce heat to medium. Add and toss for 1 minute
1/2 CUP PARMESAN CHEESE
1/4 CUP CHOPPED FRESH PARSLEY
THE HOT LINGUINI

♣Add 4 EGGS BEATEN with 1/3 CUP PLAIN YOGURT and 2 TBS. WATER. Stir and cook until just set and shiny. Turn onto a serving platter and top with the pine nuts and bacon bits.

Nutritional analysis: per serving; 481 calories; 36gm. protein; 46gm. carbo.; 3gm. fiber; 15gm. fats; 200mg. cholesterol; 257mg. calcium; 5mg. iron; 75mg. magnesium; 408mg. potassium; 305mg. sodium; 3mg. zinc.

529   INDIAN CURRY STIR-FRY

For 8 people:

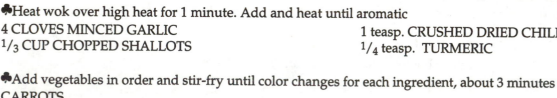

♣Toast 1 CUP CASHEWS in the oven until golden. Season with SESAME SALT.
♣Have ready
4 CARROTS julienned
1 CUCUMBER in matchsticks
1 CAULIFLOWER in halved flowerettes
1 RED BELL PEPPER in strips

♣Heat wok over high heat for 1 minute. Add and heat until aromatic
4 CLOVES MINCED GARLIC   1 teasp. CRUSHED DRIED CHILIS
1/3 CUP CHOPPED SHALLOTS   1/4 teasp. TURMERIC

♣Add vegetables in order and stir-fry until color changes for each ingredient, about 3 minutes
CARROTS
CAULIFLOWER
BELL PEPPER
CUCUMBER

♣Add 1/2 CUP BROWN RICE VINEGAR, 1/2 CUP WHITE WINE, and 2 TBS. FRUCTOSE.
♣Turn to high heat and stir-fry until liquid boils and veggies are tender crisp about 3 minutes.
♣Stir in cashews and serve in shallow soup plates.

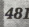

530   THAI NOODLE STIR FRY

For 6 servings:

♣Bring 4 qts. water to a boil. Add 1 LB. DRY LINGUINE and cook just to al dente, about 3 minutes.
♣Drain. Toss with 1 TB. OLIVE OIL and set aside in a serving bowl while you stir-fry the rest.

♣Heat wok over high heat for 1 minute. Add and stir-fry for 1 minute until fragrant
2 CLOVES MINCED GARLIC   1 teasp. BROWN SUGAR
3 SCALLIONS sliced diagonally   4 TBS. TAMARI
3 TBS. FRESH LIME JUICE   1/4 teasp. HOT PEPPER SAUCE
♣Turn off heat and add 2 CUPS BEAN SPROUTS. Toss and pour over noodles. Serve hot.

Nutritional analysis: per serving; 326 calories; 12gm. protein; 62gm. carbohydrate; 4gm. fiber; 4gm. fats; 0 cholesterol; 29mg. calcium; 4mg. iron; 50mg. magnesium; 228mg. potassium; 127mg. sodium; 1mg. zinc.

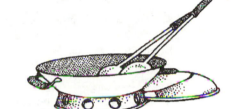

531   INDONESIAN STIRRED VEGGIES

For 8 servings:

♣Hot spicy rice is a must for this dish. Have it ready on a serving platter.

♣Cook 2 SLICED RED POTATOES in boiling water until tender. Drain, and spoon over rice.
♣Make the sauce in a small saucepan. Sauté 1 CLOVE MINCED GARLIC, 2 TBS. OIL, and 1 SMALL
CHOPPED ONION for a few minutes until fragrant. Add, stir until smooth and set aside
1 CUP CRUNCHY PEANUT BUTTER
1 CUP PIÑA COLADA YOGURT
1/2 teasp. SAMBAL OELEK or HOT PEPPER SAUCE
2 TBS. or more WATER for consistency

♣Heat wok for 1 minute. Add 2 TBS. OIL, and 1/4 teasp. TURMERIC and heat until fragrant.
♣Add 1 LB. PEELED PRAWNS or SHRIMP and stir-fry just until pink. Remove with a slotted spoon and
arrange on top of rice and potatos.

♣Add and steam/sauté until tender crisp, about 8 minutes
1/2 PACKAGE FROZEN FRENCH CUT GREEN BEANS
1 SMALL HEAD CAULIFLOWER in halved flowerettes
1/2 SMALL GREEN CABBAGE shaved in strips
♣Add 8 OZ. BEAN SPROUTS and steam covered for 2 minutes.
♣Remove veggies to a serving platter, and arrange attractively around prawns and rice.

♣Add 1 TB. OIL and 1 ONION sliced in rings to the hot wok and stir-fry until *very brown*.
♣Add 1 CUP PINEAPPLE CHUNKS and toss to coat.
♣Remove with a slotted spoon to the serving dish. Pour remaining liquid into peanut butter sauce, stir to
blend and pour over. Crumble a HARD BOILED EGG on top for a Dutch touch.

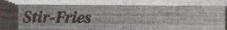

Sauces For Stir-Fries

There is delightful variety in sauces for stir fries. Each country, region and cuisine seems to have its own unique taste combination. Making your own individual specialty sauce is easy. Here are a few for inspiration.

MISO SAUCE

For ³/₄ cup:

♣Sauté 1 TB. OLIVE OIL, 1 CLOVE MINCED GARLIC, ¹/₂ CUP SLICED SHALLOTS, and 1 teasp. GRATED FRESH GINGER in a saucepan until very fragrant.
♣Add and bring to a gentle boil, 2 TBS. TAMARI, 1 teasp. HONEY, 2 TBS. CHICKPEA MISO dissolved in 2 TBS. WATER, and 1¹/₂ TBS. KUZU CHUNKS OR ARROWROOT dissolved in 2 TBS. WATER. Stir one minute and remove from heat.

SWEET & SOUR SAUCE

For 1 cup:

♣Sauté 2 teasp. SESAME OIL, 2 TBS. FRUCTOSE, 1 CLOVE MINCED GARLIC, and 1 TB. FRESH GRATED GINGER ROOT in a saucepan until fragrant.
♣Add ¹/₄ CUP TAMARI, ¹/₂ CUP PINEAPPLE JUICE, and 2 TBS. ARROWROOT mixed with 2 TBS. SHERRY. Stir until just beginning to thicken and add to stir-fry.

SPICY OYSTER SAUCE

For ³/₄ cup:

♣Dry roast ¹/₂ teasp. grated GINGER, ¹/₄ teasp. 5 SPICE POWDER, 2 PINCHES CHILI POWDER, and ¹/₂ teasp. SESAME SALT in a small pan until aromatic.

♣Add 2 TBS. SHERRY, 2 TBS. OYSTER SAUCE, 1 teasp. FRUCTOSE, DASHES of HOT PEPPER SAUCE, and 2 teasp. ARROWROOT dissolved in ¹/₂ CUP CHICKEN BROTH.
♣Let simmer to blend flavors and stir to thicken.

HOT MUSTARD SAUCE

For ¹/₂ cup:

♣Combine in a small sauce pan:
4 TBS. TAMARI, 4 teasp. BROWN RICE VINEGAR, 1 teasp. GINGER POWDER, 1 TB. FRUCTOSE, 2 teasp. PEANUT OIL, 2 teasp. TOASTED SESAME OIL, 1 TB. SHERRY and 1 teasp. HOT CHINESE DRY MUSTARD.

♣Heat until fragrant and pour over stir-fry.

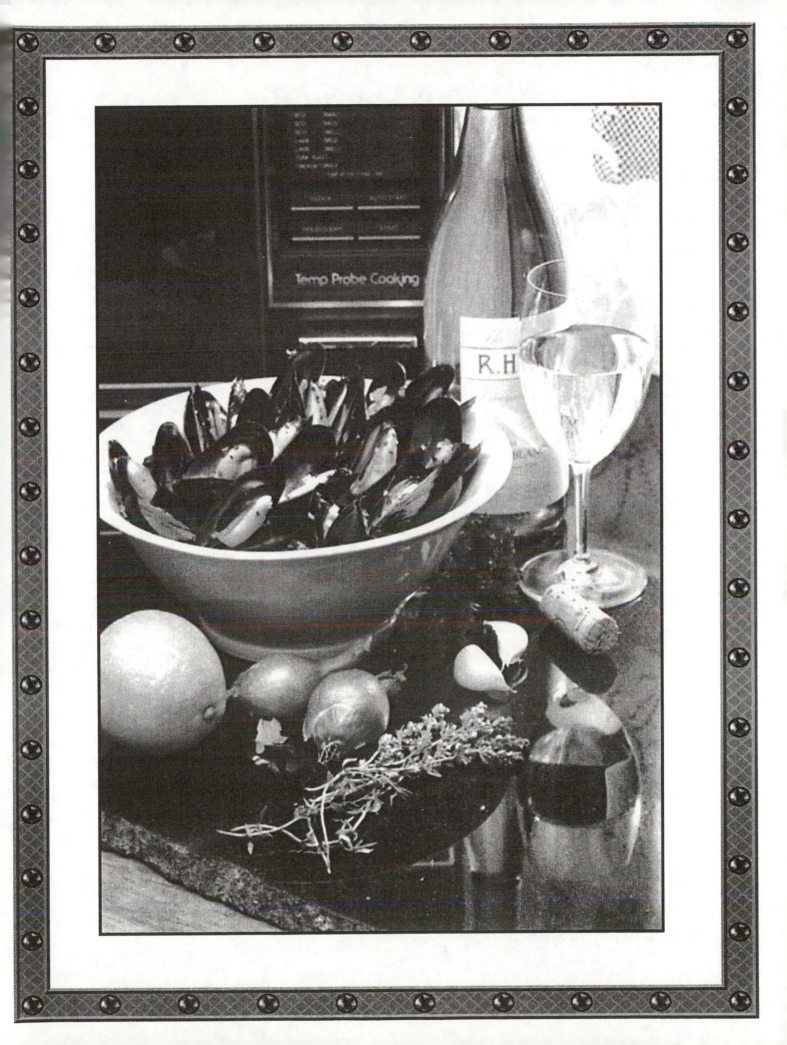

Fish & Seafoods

Over the past few years, a great deal of research has been concentrated on complex Omega 3 fatty acids for the prevention and healing of heart and circulatory disease. These oils not only help deter harmful clogs, clots, and platelet aggregation, but also seem to neutralize the bad effects of saturated fats already in the bloodstream.

Including cold water fish and seafood in your diet is a delicious way to put these oils into your system. In fact, with no other change in diet, both cholesterol and triglyceride fat levels have shown substantial drops with the addition of omega-3 oils and fatty acids from ocean fish. Even a small quantity of the oil from cold water fish can have a beneficial effect on blood viscosity (thickness) and the blood's propensity to clot - factors that have a great deal to do with heart attacks. Salmon heads the list, but tuna (especially fresh tuna), mackerel, shad, cod, shark, bass, halibut, trout, red snapper and swordfish are all beneficial, and so are many of the Hawaiian and Alaskan fish now arriving into west coats markets from these unpolluted waters. There are lots of choices for your healing diet. Both fish and shellfish are quick and easy to prepare, and low in saturated fat, cholesterol and calories. We know now that shellfish **is also not high in cholesterol.** Initial tests and studies were measured with faulty and incomplete information regarding cholesterol types. Even shellfish with moderate cholesterol counts are heart healthy, because of their low saturated fats and omega-3 oils.

I was raised on the Southern Atlantic coast, where fresh-caught crab is a favorite food, and my mother had lots of delicious ways to fix it. As kids, we would take chicken necks tied on a string, go sit in an old abandoned row boat that had washed up in an inlet behind our house, and go crabbing for supper. The crabs always seemed to know when we had that chicken neck. We would just barely let the string down in the water before two or three of them grabbed it. Sometimes they would even swim up close to the surface and watch us *tie on* the chicken necks. Anyway, we would pull them up, pick them off the string, throw them in a bucket, and take them home to eat. I can still see my father sitting at our newspaper-covered kitchen table, cracking crab claws.
Now the coastal waters are too polluted, of course, but those were the days of really fresh seafood.

The secrets to moist, tender, delicious fish are freshness and timing. Whether you broil, poach, bake, sauté or grill it, the moment the fish turns from its natural translucent white or pink, to opaque white (like egg whites), it is done. Remove it from the heat *immediately*. Even brief overcooking toughens and dries out the meat. I have learned this the hard way many times by not paying attention, or not gauging the thickness of the fish correctly, or not testing it for doneness. When you put the fish on to cook, the rest of the meal should either already be together, or done later, because fish needs almost undivided attention for the few minutes it takes to come to that lovely perfect tenderness.

☞Use the professional 10 minute rule for best results: cook 10 minutes for each inch of thickness.

☞If you are baking or barbecuing fish in foil or parchment, or simmering it in a sauce, then 15 minutes per inch of thickness is about right.

☞Do not fry fish! Poach, bake, steam, broil or grill it for the best health benefits.

☞To test for doneness, cut into the thickest part of the fish with a knife and fork. If it is just opaque, it is just right. If it flakes easily, it is probably overcooked. Many older recipes recommend flaking as the proper doneness point, but we have found again and again that the best flavor and texture have already gone by then. Newer thinking for the most healthful way to eat fish is to cook it less, and leave the meat firmer and fresher.

This chapter offers recipes in categories where fish and seafood are particularly ideal.
❧APPETIZERS and HORS D'OEUVRES FROM THE SEA ❧SEAFOOD SALADS ❧SEAFOOD and PASTA ❧HEALTHY FISH and SEAFOOD STEWS ❧PASTA DISHES ❧MAIN MEAL STARS FROM THE SEA ❧DELECTABLE SAUCES FOR FISH and SEAFOOD ❧

☛*See "GREAT OUTDOOR EATING" for seafood on the grill.*

Appetizers & Hors D'oeuvres From The Sea

532   NORFOLK CRAB

This traditional Eastern Seaboard recipe demands absolutely fresh crabmeat. When it's available, there's nothing like it for crab lovers.
Enough for 2:

♣Use about ¹/₂ LB. FRESH CRAB MEAT - pick over for cartilege, rinse in a colander, and let drain.
♣Melt 4 TBS. BUTTER and sizzle 1 TB. MINCED FRESH SHALLOTS until transparent. Remove from heat. Add ¹/₂ teasp. DILL WEED, and 1 TB. CHOPPED FRESH WATERCRESS or PARSLEY.
♣Toss with crab just to coat and serve on toast with a squeeze of FRESH LEMON.

Nutritional analysis: per serving; 375 calories; 24gm protein; 15gm. carbo.e; 3gm. fiber; 26gm. fats; (15gm. sat., 8gm. mono., 3gm. poly.); 134mg. cholesterol; 33IU beta carotene; 506mg. potassium; 521mg. sodium; 5mg. zinc.

533   CRAB PUFFS

For 6 puffs: Preheat oven to 350°.

♣Pick over 1 LB. washed, drained, LUMP CRAB MEAT.
♣Melt 2 TBS. BUTTER in a skillet Add 2 TBS. UNBLEACHED FLOUR and roux, stirring until bubbly.
♣Add ¹/₂ teasp. SEA SALT and TWO PINCHES WHITE PEPPER
♣Add ¹/₂ CUP YOGURT mixed with 4 TBS. WATER and 4 TBS. WHITE WINE to roux gradually.
♣Stir until a smooth thick sauce is formed. Remove from heat.

♣Beat 2 EGG YOLKS until frothy. Add a little of the hot sauce to the yolks to warm them, then add them back to the sauce and stir in well.
♣Add ¹/₄ teasp. PAPRIKA, 1 CUP KEFIR CHEESE or YOGURT CHEESE and the CRAB. Mix well.

♣Beat 2 EGG WHITES to stiff with A PINCH of CREAM OF TARTER so they will hold up better, and fold into crab mixture. Place in individual greased ramekins. Place the ramekins in a pan of hot water, and bake for 40 to 45 minutes til puffs are high and firm.
♣These are good just as they are, or with a very easy-to-make **HOMEMADE TARTAR SAUCE.**

DELUXE HOMEMADE TARTAR SAUCE

For about 1¹/₂ cups:
♣Blend together in a bowl

¹/₂ CUP PLAIN or LEMON YOGURT	2 TBS. SWEET PICKLE RELISH
¹/₄ CUP LIGHT MAYONNAISE	2 TBS. CHOPPED GREEN ONIONS
1 HARD BOILED EGG, crumbled	2 TBS. WHITE WINE

♣Chill and serve.

Nutritional analysis: per serving; 107 calories; 3gm. protein; 5gm. carbo.; trace fiber; 3gm. fats; (trace sat., 1gm. mono., 1gm. poly.); 49mg. cholesterol; 3IU beta carotene; 100mg. potassium; 86mg. sodium; trace zinc.

534 MARYLAND CRAB CAKES

This recipe is from an old, well-known restaurant located right on the Chesapeake Bay. The simplicity makes it healthy; the fresh-caught Chesapeake crab makes it delectable.
For 6 servings:

♣Mix the crab cakes in a large bowl
$3/4$ LB. FRESH LUMP CRAB MEAT, picked over and rinsed

$1/4$ CUP PLAIN YOGURT OR KEFIR CHEESE
$1/4$ CUP WHOLE GRAIN BREAD CRUMBS
2 TBS. FRESH CHOPPED PARSLEY
1 teasp. LEMON/GARLIC SEASONING

$3/4$ CUP GRATED PARMESAN
1 EGG
2 GREEN ONIONS, minced
$1/2$ teasp. DRY OREGANO

♣Add 2 teasp. OIL to a *hot* skillet. Spoon in 3 to 4 TBS. crab cake mix in mounds and flatten into cakes.
♣Cook 2 minutes until lightly browned. Turn once with a spatula and cook another minute. Remove and keep warm. Repeat until all are done.
♣Peel and slice a LARGE RIPE AVOCADO. Arrange Bibb or Boston lettuce on salad plates. Arrange avocado slices and crab cakes on top.

Nutritional analysis: per serving; 232 calories; 19gm. protein; 8 carbo.; 5gm. fiber; 14gm. fats; (3gm. sat., 7gm. mono., 4gm. poly.); 101mg. cholesterol; 45IU beta carotene; 551mg. potassium; 417mg. sodium; 3mg. zinc.

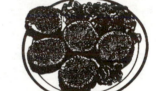

535 CRAB STUFFED MUSHROOMS

For 24 appetizers: Preheat oven to 400°.

♣Clean, stem, and scoop out ribs from 24 LARGE WHITE MUSHROOMS to make a filling bowl.

♣Mix the filling in the blender
$1/2$ LB. FRESH DUNGENESS CRABMEAT
2 teasp. LEMON JUICE.
$1/4$ CUP NEUFCHATEL or SOY CREAM CHEESE

$1/4$ teasp. GARLIC POWDER
$1/4$ teasp. ONION POWDER
$1/4$ teasp. BASIL

♣Turn into a bowl and mix in $1/3$ CUP CHOPPED BLACK OLIVES AND 2 TBS. FRESH CHOPPED PARSLEY. Fill mushroom caps.

♣Rinse a baking sheet with water. Shake off excess and place filled caps on the sheet. Cover with foil and bake 12 to 15 minutes. Remove foil and bake for 5 more minutes until tops are golden. Serve hot.

536 SWEET CALAMARI SLICES

For 6 delectable pieces:

♣Pound about 1 LB. FRESH CALAMARI, ABALONE STYLE, until thin. Add to a quart of <u>cold water</u>.
♣Bring to a boil. Lower heat, and simmer 10 minutes. Add 3 TBS. SAKE, 2 TBS. FRUCTOSE , and 1 TB. TAMARI. Simmer for 5 - 8 minutes. Cool and cut into slices.

537 JAPANESE FISH ROLL

They cook these rolls right at the table in authentic Japanese restaurants, in a <u>square</u> skillet. I have made them successfully in a regular heavy square 8" baking pan on medium low heat, or a regular round skillet. Just trim the rounded edges to square before you arrange them on a serving plate.
For 12 slices:

♣Grind together in a food processor until fine
1/2 LB. FRESH WHITE FISH FILLETS
3 TBS. FRUCTOSE
1/2 teasp. SESAME SALT
 3 TBS. SAKE or SHERRY

♣Beat together in a bowl
6 EGGS
4 TBS. WATER
2 TBS. TAMARI

♣Combine the two mixtures together.

♣Heat 2 teasp. OIL in a skillet. When hot, pour in half the fish/egg mixture. Cook until set on the top and brown on the bottom. Turn the egg sheet over very carefully. Brown the other side. Turn out onto a piece of waxed paper and roll up like a jelly roll. Fasten ends with toothpicks to hold the shape. Repeat with other half of fish mixture and another 2 teasp. OIL. Let rolls sit for 15 minutes to fully set while you make a **RUMAKI DIPPING SAUCE.** Then cut into 12 slices .

Nutritional analysis: for 2 slices; 175 calories; 15gm. protein; 8gm. carbo.; trace fiber; 8gm. fats; (2gm. sat., 4gm. mono.; 2gm. poly.); 220mg. cholesterol; trace beta carotene; 248mg. potassium; 199mg. sodium; 1mg. zinc.

RUMAKI DIPPING SAUCE

For about 1 1/4 cups:
♣Sauté 1 TB. FRESH GRATED GINGER, 1/2 teasp. GARLIC POWDER, and 2 TBS. MINCED GREEN ONIONS in 1 teasp. oil until aromatic. Add 1 cup TAMARI SAUCE, 1 TB. FRUCTOSE, and 1/2 teasp. CINNAMON. Remove from heat and serve in a dipping bowl at room temperature.

538 HOT CLAM BALLS

For about 24 balls: Preheat oven to 325°.

♣Drain 2 CANS of CHOPPED CLAMS into a bowl. (Save the clam juice for your pets if you don't have other uses for it. They love it.) Blend clams in the blender so there are still chewy pieces.
♣Add to the blender. Blend until just right for balls.
1/2 CUP CRUSHED WHOLE GRAIN CRACKERS
1 SMALL CHOPPED ONION
1/4 CUP CHOPPED BELL PEPPER
1 TB. WHITE WORCESTERSHIRE SAUCE
1 teasp. LEMON/GARLIC SEASONING

1 TB. FRESH SNIPPED PARSLEY
1 teasp. PAPRIKA
1/2 teasp. HOT PEPPER SAUCE
1/2 teasp. SESAME SALT
1/4 teasp. PEPPER

♣Mix everything with the clams. Form into balls.
♣Add a little WHEAT GERM if necessary to hold them together. Roll in WHEAT GERM for crustiness. Set on lecithin-sprayed baking sheets and chill, covered for 1 hour to set.
♣Bake for 15 to 20 minutes until aromatic. Serve hot with toothpicks.

Nutritional analysis: per serving; 78 calories; 9gm. protein; 7gm. carbo.; 1gm. fiber; 2gm. fats; (less than 1gm. sat., mono., and poly.); 19mg. cholesterol; 249mg. potassium; 121mg. sodium; 1mg. zinc.

539 SCALLOP MOLD WITH GREEN MAYONNAISE

This is a San Francisco version of a traditional French terrine; but much lighter, using Bay scallops.
For 8 slices: Preheat oven to 350°.

♣Combine in a blender until smooth
15 CHOPPED GREEN ONIONS **WHITE PARTS ONLY** (save green parts for the green mayonnaise)
1/2 LB. FRESH WHITE FISH FILLETS, rinsed
1/2 LB. FRESH BAY SCALLOPS, rinsed   1 EGG
1/3 CUP PLAIN YOGURT or COTTAGE CHEESE   1/4 teasp. WHITE PEPPER
1/2 teasp. DRY TARRAGON   1/2 teasp. SEA SALT
♣Scrape out into a buttered loaf pan.
♣Scatter on 2 TBS. DRAINED CAPERS.
♣<u>Cover</u> and place the pan in a larger pan. Fill halfway up the sides with water and bake until set in the center, 40 to 50 minutes. Uncover, and let cool. Re-cover again and chill until firm, overnight.
♣Cut into 1/2" slices and serve on a large lettuce leaf with a thin lemon wedge.
♣Top each with a **GREEN MAYONNAISE** dollop and some green onion top snips.

GREEN MAYONNAISE
♣Add rest of the reserved green onion tops to the blender. Add 1/2 CUP LOW-FAT MAYONNAISE and 1 TB. LEMON JUICE. Blend until smooth. Scrape into a serving bowl and sprinkle with 1 TB. CAPERS.

540 SHRIMP WITH SPICY GREEN SAUCE

For 6 people as an appetizer:

♣Boil 1 LB. SHELLED SHRIMP in SEAFOOD BOIL for 3 minutes until opaque. Drain, mound on a platter and make the sauce.
♣Dry roast 1/4 CUP SLIVERED ALMONDS in a skillet until golden. Blend in the blender with
2 CUPS CHOPPED FRESH PARSLEY   3 TBS. WHITE WINE VINEGAR
1/3 CUP OLIVE OIL   1 TB. DRAINED CAPERS
1 JALAPEÑO or GREEN CHILI, seeded and chopped   1/2 teasp. LEMON PEPPER
♣Spoon sauce on the shrimp and serve with toothpicks.

541 LEMON PRAWNS CEVICHE

For 8 people as an appetizer:

♣Simmer 1 LB. SHELLED PRAWNS in 3/4 CUP CIDER VINEGAR and 3/4 CUP LEMON JUICE with 1 teasp. DIJON MUSTARD until opaque. Remove with a slotted spoon and put in a bowl. Boil liquid over high heat until reduced to 1 cup - about 4 minutes. Pour over prawns and chill overnight.
♣Mix together 4 THIN SLICED GREEN ONIONS, 2 DICED TOMATOES, SEA SALT and PEPPER..
♣Place drained prawns on lettuce leaves. Top with green onion mix; garnish with LEMON WEDGES.

Seafood Salads

Definitely not your ho hum "shrimp and sauce" salads. These recipes have all the health benefits, but none of the boredom. These are sea foods and greens with a difference.

542   LIGHT CRAB LOUIS

For 2 to 3 people: (Use about half the LOUIS DRESSING recipe for 2 to 3 people.)

♣This salad looks the best when you serve it in a big "cup" of stiff overlapping cabbage leaves. Make up each "cup" on individual salad plates and fill about halfway up with SHAVED HEAD LETTUCE.
♣Top the shaved lettuce with 1/2 LB. CHUNKED KING CRAB LEGS or FRESH LUMP DUNGENESS CRABMEAT and 2 MINCED CELERY STALKS with leaves.

♣Make the **LOUIS DRESSING** in the blender. Whirl until smooth

1/2 CUP LIGHT MAYONNAISE	2 TBS. CHILI SAUCE
1/2 CUP PLAIN YOGURT	1 TB. CHIVES
1/2 teasp. LEMON PEPPER	1 teasp. LEMON JUICE

♣Spoon dressing over crab, and top with 2 CHOPPED HARD BOILED EGGS and 2 TBS. CRUMBLED FETA CHEESE (optional).

Nutritional analysis: per serving; 260 calories; 22gm. protein; 6gm. carbo.; 2gm. fiber; 9gm. fats; (2gm. sat., 3gm. mono., 4gm. poly.) 228mg. cholesterol; 75IU beta carotene; 584mg. potassium; 330mg. sodium; 4mg. zinc.

543   HAWAIIAN CRAB SALAD

Because of its enzyme-producing action, papaya works with both fruit and vegetable "food-combining" categories.
For 4 salads:

♣Peel, seed and chop 3 RIPE PAPAYAS.   ♣Mix in a bowl with
1 LB. FRESH LUMP or KING CRAB MEAT, in chunks   1/3 CUP LEMON/LIME YOGURT
3/4 CUP CHOPPED SCALLIONS   1 teasp. CURRY POWDER
♣Cover and chill.
♣Pour 2 CUPS BOILING WATER over 1 CUP BULGUR or KASHA. Let sit 1 hour until water is absorbed. Drain off excess water. Fluff and add to crab mixture, tossing gently. Serve in large lettuce cups.

544   SIMPLE JAPANESE CRAB SALAD

For 4 salads:

♣Mix and chill for 1 hour to marinate
6 OZ. FRESH LUMP CRABMEAT   1 TB. FRESH MINCED GINGER
1 TB. TAMARI   1 TB. CHOPPED GREEN ONION
1 TB. SAKE or MIRIN
♣Halve and scoop out flesh from 2 LARGE CUCUMBERS to make shells. Fill with crab mixture. Slice in rounds and serve.

545   AVOCADO CRAB SALAD

Very southern California - this salad. It's from a small restaurant overlooking the water in Santa Barbara.
For 3 or 4 salads:

♣Sauté 1/2 LB. LUMP CRAB or KING CRAB LEG MEAT CHUNKS IN 2 teasp. OIL until just opaque.

♣Combine marinade ingredients; pour over crab and marinate for 1 hour.

1 CUP THIN SLICED CELERY
1 TB. LEMON JUICE
1/2 teasp. GRATED LEMON ZEST
2 MINCED GREEN ONIONS

1/2 teasp. SESAME SALT
2 PINCHES PAPRIKA
1/4 CUP WHITE WINE

♣Peel a LARGE AVOCADO and cut in small cubes. Mix with 1/3 CUP LIGHT MAYONNAISE, and then toss with the crab and marinade dressing. Serve on SHAVED LETTUCE.

※

546   ELEGANT LOBSTER ARTICHOKE SALAD

The key to this salad is the fresh mustard mayonnaise. Make it right before serving.
For 6 salads:

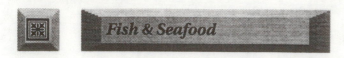

♣Purchase an 11-OZ. JAR WATER-PACKED ARTICHOKE HEARTS and cut in bite size pieces.

♣Boil 1 1/2 LBS. (3 large tails) LOBSTER MEAT in seafood boil for 5 minutes until opaque. Cut in 1" pieces. Line salad plates with watercress.

♣Divide lobster and artichokes between the plates and chill while you make the mayonnaise.

♣Blend in the blender

1 EGG
1/3 CUP TARRAGON VINEGAR

1 1/2 TBS. DIJON MUSTARD
1/2 teasp. SEA SALT

♣With the blender running, pour in 1/2 CUP OIL in a thin steady stream until mayonnaise thickens. Remove from blender to a bowl and stir in

1 MINCED SHALLOT
3 TBS. FRESH MINCED PASRLEY

3 TBS. FRESH MINCED CHIVES
1/2 teasp. CRACKED PEPPER

♣Serve in generous dollops over the lobster and artichokes.

※

547   QUICK BROWN RICE & TUNA SALAD

For 4 servings:

♣Combine the following ingredients with 2 1/2 CUPS COOKED BROWN RICE or MIXED GRAINS.

1 SMALL CAN WATER-PACKED TUNA
1 CRUMBLED HARD BOILED EGG
2 RIBS CELERY, chopped
1/2 CUP LIGHT MAYONNAISE

2 GREEN ONIONS chopped
1 TB. LEMON JUICE
1/2 teasp. SWEET HOT MUSTARD

Nutritional analysis: per serving; 377 calories; 17gm. protein; 31gm. carbo.; 3gm. fiber; 8gm. fats; (2gm. sat., 3gm. mono., 4gm. poly.); 90mg. cholesterol; 5IU beta carotene; 289mg. potassium; 259mg. sodium; 2mg. zinc.

※

548 PRAWNS & ASPARAGUS SALAD

For 6 salads:

♣Snap 1 LB. ASPARAGUS in 1" pieces, discarding parts. Parboil in boiling salted water until bright green and just tender. Drain and rinse in cold water to set color and stop the cooking.
♣Cook 1 LB. LARGE PRAWNS in seafood boil for 3 minutes until opaque. Drain and chill both asparagus and prawns.

♣When ready to serve, arrange on lettuce-lined salad plates, and top with dollops of **LIGHT MUSTARD LEMON CREAM.**

For 1 cup:
♣Mix in a pan, and stir over low heat until the dressing coats a spoon.

1 EGG YOLK	1 TB. LEMON JUICE
1/4 CUP DIJON MUSTARD	1 TB. BUTTER
1 TB. WHITE WINE	1/2 TB. FRUCTOSE

♣Set in ice water and stir until cool. Add 1 small carton PLAIN YOGURT and chill.

Nutritional analysis: per serving; 155 calories; 21gm. protein; 7gm. carbohydrate; 1gm. fiber; 5gm. fats; (2gm. sat., 2mono., 1 poly.); 190mg. cholesterol; 64IU beta carotene; 453mg. potassium; 235mg. sodium; 2mg. zinc.

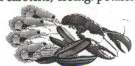

549 SEAFOOD SALAD DELUXE WITH TARRAGON DRESSING
This is a real company salad.
For 8 servings:

♣Bring 4-qts. salted water to a boil. Drop in 1 LB. PEELED SHRIMP; *then* drop in 1 LB. SCALLOPS, *then* drop in 1/2 LB. LOBSTER MEAT CHUNKS. *Just before* water returns to a boil, *drain,* and cool seafood.
♣Bring fresh salted water to a boil. Add 1 CUP FROZEN PEAS. Drain and cool as soon as color changes to bright green. Add to the seafood, and pop it all into the fridge while you make the dressing.

TARRAGON DRESSING

♣Measure and mix in the blender

1 EGG	1/4 CUP BALSAMIC VINEGAR
2 EGG YOLKS	1 teasp. DRY TARRAGON
1/3 CUP DIJON MUSTARD	1/4 teasp. BLACK PEPPER

♣Whirl briefly in the blender, then while blender is running, add 1/2 CUP SALAD OIL and 1/2 CUP OLIVE OIL in a thin steady stream until mixture thickens.

♣To serve, shred 4 CUPS mixed SPINACH and ROMAINE LEAVES and place in a ring around the edge of a serving plate. Spoon seafood in the middle, and spoon Tarragon Mayonnaise over top.

Nutritional analysis: per serving; 424 calories; 31gm. protein; 6gm. carbos; 2gm. fiber; 31gm. fats; (4gm. sat., 14gm. mono., 13gm. poly.); 230mg. cholesterol; 168IU beta carotene 544 potassium; 470mg. sodium; 3mg. zinc.

550 LOBSTER SALAD WITH GINGER DRESSING

For 4 servings:

♣Trim, string and blanch ¹/₂ LB. FRESH PEA PODS in boiling water until color changes to bright green. Remove with a slotted spoon and rinse in ice water to set color.

♣Return water to a boil, and add 2 LOBSTER TAILS (6 to 8-OZ. each). Simmer covered until meat turns opaque in the center, about 7 minutes.
♣Drain, clip fins and shell, and lift out meat. Slice meat into thin chunks and chill.

♣Tear 3-QTS. CRISP LETTUCE PIECES in a large salad bowl. Arrange 2 SLICED FRESH KIWI in a ring over top. Fill the middle of the ring with fresh sliced STRAWBERRIES.
♣Top with lobster and pea pods. Chill again while you make the **GINGER DRESSING.**

GINGER DRESSING
♣Mix 1 teasp. GRATED ORANGE ZEST, ³/₄ CUP ORANGE JUICE, 2 TBS. RED WINE VINEGAR and 2 TBS. MINCED CRYSTALLIZED GINGER. Pour over salad, and serve.

551 MIXED SEAFOOD SALAD WITH GOURMET GRAINS
This salad is excellent hot or cold. We have tried it with several different sea food blends. All were good; so you have lots of choice with this recipe.
If you are serving the salad hot, don't precook the frozen peas; add them right from the freezer, and just heat them briefly with the whole salad until the cheese melts.
For 4 main meal servings:

♣Have ready 2 CUPS COOKED GOURMET GRAINS. (See page 647).

♣Sauté ¹/₂ LB. PEELED HALVED SHRIMP and ¹/₂ LB. BAY SCALLOPS in 1 teasp. CHILI OIL briefly, until just opaque and tender. Remove from skillet and toss with the COOKED GOURMET GRAINS.
♣Add 1 teasp. PLAIN OIL to the skillet and sauté ¹/₂ CUP RED or GREEN BELL PEPPER julienne cut, about 3 minutes until aromatic.
♣Add 1 cup FROZEN PEAS and toss together another 2 minutes until color changes to bright green.
♣Mix with seafood and grains.

♣Add and toss and mix together gently
¹/₄ CUP TOASTED SUNFLOWER SEEDS
¹/₄ CUP RAISINS
1 CUP SWISS CHEESE, julienne cut

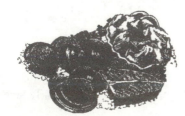

♣Make the **LEMON YOGURT DRESSING.** Mix
1 CUP PLAIN YOGURT
¹/₄ CUP CHOPPED CHIVES
¹/₄ CUP CHOPPED CUCUMBER

3 TBS. LEMON JUICE
¹/₂ teasp. LEMON PEPPER
2 TBS. GINGER/TAMARI SAUCE

♣Pour over salad. Mix gently and serve in lettuce cups.

Seafood & Pasta

Sea foods and light vegetable or whole grain pastas complement each other beautifully for a light meal, offering good high protein and complex carbohydrates with low fats. We present just a few favorites here, but this is an area you will probably want to expand yourself for a successful healing diet.

552   SMOKED SALMON WITH PASTA PRIMAVERA

For 4 to 6 servings:

♣Purchase a 6-OZ. PACKAGE of SMOKED SALMON or 6-OZ. LOX and cut in slivers. Set aside.
♣Bring 2-QTS. WATER to a boil. Blanch 2 CARROTS cut in matchsticks, and 8-OZ. FRENCH CUT GREEN BEANS just until color changes. Remove with a slotted spoon and set aside.

♣Make the PARMESAN SAUCE in a small bowl and set aside

3 TBS. WHITE WINE VINEGAR	2 TBS. PARMESAN
1/3 CUP OLIVE OIL	1/2 teasp. CRUSHED CHILIES
1 teasp. GARLIC/LEMON SEASONING	1/2 CUP FROZEN PEAS
1/2 CUP GREEN ONIONS sliced lengthwise	

♣Bring water to boil again. Add 8-OZ. SMALL SHAPED PASTA and cook to al dente. Drain and toss with sauce.
♣Set up LETTUCE CUPS on salad plates. Fill with pasta salad. Top with salmon or lox slivers. Sprinkle with CHOPPED TOMATOES. Season with SEA SALT and CRACKED PEPPER.

Nutritional analysis: per serving; 325 calories; 13gm. protein; 37gm. carbo.; 4gm. fiber; 14gm. fats; (2gm. sat., 10gm. mono., 2gm. poly.); 9mg. cholesterol; 9IU beta carotene; 374mg. potassium; 302mg. sodium; 1mg. zinc.

553   PASTA & HOME-SMOKED SALMON

We have used this home-smoking technique for several years to give a hickory flavor to both chicken and salmon. It's so easy, and lends a delectable outdoor aroma to your food and kitchen.
For 4 people:

♣Remove the skin from a 3/4 LB. SALMON FILET. Cut in 1/2" strips.
♣Pour about 3 TBS. LIQUID SMOKE into a steaming pan. Set the steaming rack on top, put the salmon on the rack, cover tightly, and steam for 10-12 minutes. Remove and let stand to absorb flavors.

♣Make the sauce in a small saucepan. Boil 2 TBS. BALSAMIC or WHITE WINE VINEGAR and 1/2 CUP CHOPPED RED ONION until liquid evaporates. Add 1 CUP HALF & HALF or 1 cup plain yogurt, 3/4 CUP WHITE WINE, and 1 TB. DIJON MUSTARD. Cook until liquid is reduced to 1 3/4 cups.

♣Bring 2-QTS. of WATER to a boil. Cook 12-OZ. DRY LINGUINI for 10 minutes to *al dente*. Drain and toss with the sauce. Divide pasta onto individual serving plates. Top each with smoked salmon slices, snips of FRESH PARSLEY, sprinkles of PARMESAN CHEESE and CRACKED BLACK PEPPER.

Nutritional analysis: per serving; 364 calories; 22gm. protein; 47gm. carbo.; 3gm. fiber; 8gm. fats; (2gm. sat., 3gm. mono., 3gm. poly.); 41mg. cholesterol; 8IU beta carotene; 452mg. potassium; 110mg. sodium; 1mg. zinc.

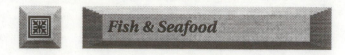

554 FETTUCINI & FRESH AHI

Delicious ahi tuna is now available everywhere. It has the taste and texture of steak, but is heart healthy.
For 6 servings:

♣Sauté 1 LARGE CHOPPED ONION in 4 TBS. OLIVE OIL until fragrant.

♣Add one 14-OZ. CAN ROMA TYPE TOMATOES with juice, 1 TB. FRESH CHOPPED BASIL, SEA SALT and PEPPER. Heat until juices thicken, about 5 minutes. Remove from heat and set aside.

♣Cube 1 LB. FRESH AHI TUNA and season with GARLIC SALT, PEPPER, CHOPPED MINT LEAVES and 1 teasp. LEMON JUICE. Heat 2 TBS. OLIVE OIL in another skillet, and sauté ahi until just barely opaque, about 2 minutes.

♣Bring 3-QTS. WATER to a boil and cook 16-OZ. FETTUCINI to al dente, about 9 minutes. Drain and toss with tomato sauce. Top with the ahi cubes and serve hot.

❈

555 EASY TUNA MAC

For 4 servings: Preheat oven to 350°.

♣Saute 1 CHOPPED GREEN ONION, 1/4 CUP CHOPPED BELL PEPPER, and 1/4 STALK CHOPPED CELERY in 1 TB. OIL until color changes to bright green. Add 2 TBS. WHOLE WHEAT FLOUR and stir for a few minutes until bubbly.

♣Add 1 CUP PLAIN YOGURT **or** 1 CUP LOW-FAT COTTAGE CHEESE and 1/2 CUP WATER. Stir and cook til thickened. Add a small can of WATER PACKED TUNA, drained. Remove from heat.

♣Bring 3-QTS. WATER to a boil, and add about 1 1/2 CUPS VEGETABLE ELBOW MACARONI. Cook for 7 minutes until almost tender. Drain and mix with tuna.

♣Pour everything into a lecithin-sprayed casserole and bake <u>covered</u> for 15 minutes until hot through.

Nutritional analysis: per serving; 280 calories; 21gm. protein; 37gm. carbo.; 2gm. fiber; 5gm. fats; (1gm. sat., 1gm. mono., 3gm. poly.); 26mg. cholesterol; 7IU beta carotene; 369mg. potassium; 173mg. sodium; 1mg. zinc.

❈

556 TRADE WINDS TUNA

For 4 people: Preheat oven to 350°.

♣Sauté 1/2 CUP CHOPPED ONION in 1 TB. OIL until translucent.

♣Remove from heat and add an 8-OZ. CAN SLICED WATER CHESTNUTS.

♣Add 1 CAN CREAM of CELERY SOUP, <u>or</u> make a MUSHROOM SAUCE from a natural mix, such as MAYACAMAS MUSHROOM SOUP MIX, and add about 10 to 12-OZ. (This is delicious both ways)

♣Add
ONE 7-OZ. CAN WATER PACKED TUNA <u>with the water</u>

1/2 teasp. CURRY POWDER   1/4 CUP LOW-FAT PLAIN YOGURT
2 CUPS CRISPY CHOW MEIN NOODLES   2 TBS. FRESH MINCED PARSLEY

♣Pour everything into a lecithin-sprayed 1-qt. casserole dish.

♣Top with more CHOW MEIN NOODLES to cover and bake for 35 to 40 minutes until light brown.

❈

Healthy Fish & Seafood Stews

So What's The Catch? You can use almost any fish or seafood in these wonderful stews. It seems every cuisine has discovered them - calling them bouillabaisse, paella, yosenabe, or cioppino. They all represent delicious ways to get healthy food from the sea. Serve them in big shallow soup bowls for best effect.

557   BIARRITZ BOUILLABAISSE

For 8 servings: Preheat oven to 375°.

♣Sauté 1½ CUPS SLICED LEEKS (white parts with a little green) in 2 TBS. OLIVE OIL until aromatic.
♣Add 2 DICED GREEN BELL PEPPERS and sauté until color changes.

♣Add and stir for 10 minutes
1/4 teasp. DRY THYME
2 teasp. GROUND FENNEL
1 teasp. SEA SALT
2 CLOVES MINCED GARLIC
3 ROMA TOMATOES, CHOPPED
2 teasp. DRY BASIL (or 2 TBS. fresh)
ONE 8-OZ. CAN TOMATOES with juice, chopped

♣Add and simmer for 15 minutes
1 TB. grated LEMON ZEST
1 CUP VEGETABLE or FISH STOCK
1 teasp. DRY TARRAGON
JUICE OF 1 LEMON
2 TBS. CHOPPED FRESH PARSLEY
PINCH SAFFRON
PINCH OF PAPRIKA

♣Place 3 LBS. MIXED or WHITE FISH FILETS about 1" thick, or 3 LBS. MIXED SEA FOODS (shrimp, scallops, clams, prawns, etc.) in a shallow oiled baking dish. Pour bouillabaisse Sauce over, and bake <u>covered</u> for 20 minutes until fish or seafood is opaque.
♣Snip on parsley or cilantro and serve in shallow soup bowls.

558   LIGHT ITALIAN CIOPPINO

For 12 bowls:

♣In a large heavy soup pot, heat 1/2 CUP OLIVE OIL, and sauté 2 CUPS CHOPPED ONIONS and 2 CLOVES MINCED GARLIC for 5 minutes.
♣Add 1 CHOPPED GREEN BELL PEPPER and 1/2 CUP SLICED MUSHROOMS and sauté for 5 minutes until aromatic.
♣Add

3 TBS. FRESH CHOPPED PARSLEY
1½ CUPS CHOPPED ROMA TOMATOES
1½ CUPS ROSÉ WINE

2 teasp. ITALIAN SEASONING
1 teasp. HERB SALT
PINCH CAYENNE or PAPRIKA

♣Cover and cook over low heat for 1 hour.
♣Uncover, and add

3 LBS. FRESH CHUNKED THICK FISH FILETS
1 LOBSTER TAIL IN CHUNKS (or 6 shucked oysters)

2 CUPS SCALLOPS or CLAMS whole
1 CUP PEELED PRAWNS

♣Simmer for 15 minutes until all the sea foods are just tender and opaque.
♣Serve in big shallow soup plates with crusty sour dough bread.

559   QUICK BOUILLABAISSE

For 8 servings:

♣Sauté 2 CHOPPED ONIONS and 3 CLOVES CHOPPED GARLIC in 3 TBS. OLIVE OIL until transparent and fragrant.
♣Add ONE 28-OZ. CAN PLUM TOMATOES with their juice, 2 PINCHES CAYENNE, 1 PINCH SAFFRON and a 7-OZ. BOTTLE of CLAM JUICE.
♣Add 2 LBS. mixed SEAFOOD - CRAB MEAT, SCALLOPS, OYSTERS, LEFT-OVER FISH PIECES, etc. and heat through. Serve in large shallow soup bowls.

Nutritional analysis: per serving; 202 calories; 21gm. protein; 13gm. carbo.; 2gm. fiber; 7gm. fats; (1gm. sat., 4gm. mono., 2gm. poly.); 62mg. cholesterol; 67mg. beta carotene; 671mg. potassium; 430mg. sodium; 7mg. zinc.

560   GINGER CRAB IN WINE BROTH

For 6 to 8 servings:

♣Melt 4 TBS. BUTTER in a large soup pot. Add 4 CUPS CHICKEN BROTH, 2 CUPS REISLING WINE, 1/4 CUP CHOPPED GREEN ONIONS, 6 SLICES FRESH PEELED GINGER, 1 TB. TAMARI and 1 TB. LEMON JUICE. Simmer for 10 minutes until fragrant -10 to 15 minutes.
♣Add the meat of 3 COOKED, CLEANED DUNGENESS CRABS. Heat and ladle into soup bowls.

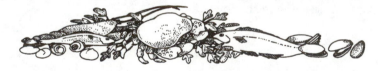

Main Meal Stars From The Sea

Fish and seafood are so versatile, with tastes ranging from delicate to hearty, and the familiar to the exotic. The main dishes in this section offer something for everybody.

561   DELUXE CRAB QUICHE

For 6 people: Preheat oven to 300°.

♣Use an unbaked <u>whole grain</u> quiche shell <u>or</u> individual shallow casseroles, oiled and lined with chapatis or flour tortillas.
♣Sauté 2 TBS. CHOPPED SHALLOTS in 1 teasp. BUTTER until translucent.
♣Make the sauce in the blender. Add and whirl until frothy, 1 CUP SOUR CREAM or a blend of 3/4 CUP YOGURT and 1/4 CUP LIGHT MAYONNAISE. Plus
THE SAUTÉED ONIONS   3 EGGS
1 teasp. TAMARI   1 teasp. SESAME SALT
♣Distribute 1 1/2 CUPS LUMP CRAB MEAT KING CRAB LEG CHUNKS over the quiche shell.
♣Top with 1 CUP GRATED LOW-FAT SWISS or CHUNKS of BRIE CHEESE.
♣Pour sauce over and bake for 55 minutes until set. Let rest for 10 minutes before cutting.

562 SEAFOOD & MIXED MUSHROOMS

This is an ordinary title for a pretty gourmet dish. Very aromatic. You can taste it with your nose.
For 6 servings:

♣Dry roast 1 CUP GOURMET GRAIN BLEND (pg. 647) or BASMATI RICE for 5 minutes in a pan.
♣Add 2 CUPS WATER. Bring to a boil, cover, reduce heat and steam for 25 minutes until water is absorbed. Fluff and set aside.

♣Soak 4 or 5 BLACK SHIITAKE MUSHROOMS in water until soft. Sliver mushrooms and discard woody stems. Save soaking water.

♣Sauté 2 MINCED SHALLOTS in a large skillet in 3 TBS. OIL til aromatic. Add 1 CUP SLICED BUTTON MUSHROOMS, the soaked SHIITAKE MUSHROOMS, 4 or 5 SLIVERED CHANTERELLES or OYSTER MUSHROOMS. Sauté until light brown and liquid is almost evaporated, about 8 minutes.

♣Add and sauté until just opaque and firm, about 3 minutes
1/2 LB. RINSED SCALLOPS   1/4 CUP WHITE WINE
1/2 LB. PEELED PRAWNS or LARGE SHRIMP   1/2 teasp. PAPRIKA
♣Add 2 MINCED SCALLIONS and 1 TB. FRESH SNIPPED PARSLEY. Heat 1 minute, and serve over rice.

Nutritional analysis: per serving: 180 calories; 12gm. protein; 30gm. carbo.; 3gm. fiber; 1gm. fats; (less than 1gm. for any type of fat.); 73mg. cholesterol; 15IU beta carotene; 313mg. potassium; 94mg. sodium; 2mg. zinc.

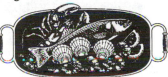

563 PESCADO CANCUN

This recipe is a speciality of Cancun's lovely resort area. It is beautifully spiced, and very light.
For 8 people: Preheat oven to 350°.

♣Rinse and skin 2 LBS. THICK FRESH FISH FILETS (shark and swordfish are both good). Sprinkle with LEMON JUICE.

♣Sauté in 3 TBS. OLIVE OIL til aromatic
1 CUP CHOPPED ONION   1/4 teasp. GROUND CLOVES
1 CLOVE CHOPPED GARLIC   1/4 teasp. GROUND CUMIN
1 TB. DRY CHILI FLAKES   1/4 teasp. GROUND CORIANDER

♣Add and simmer 15 minutes until bubbly and blended
3 CUPS CHOPPED TOMATOES   3 TBS. LEMON JUICE
1 TB. HONEY   1 teasp. SEA SALT
1 CUP CHOPPED BLACK OLIVES   1/2 teasp. BLACK PEPPER
♣Pour over fish. Snip a generous amount of PARSLEY over top and bake for 20 minutes until tender and fish is white all the way through.

Nutritional analysis: per serving; 203 calories; 25gm. protein; 9gm. carbo.; 2gm. fiber; 7gm. fats; (1gm. sat., 4gm. mono., 2gm. poly.); 36mg. cholesterol; 77IU beta carotene; 737mg. potassium; 242mg. sodium; 1mg. zinc.

564 FISH IN FRESH BASIL SAUCE

This is a wonderful, light summer recipe.
For 6 people: Preheat oven to 350°.

♣Whirl 1/2 LEMON peeled and seeded, and 1/2 CUP OLIVE OIL in the blender until emulsified.
♣Pour into a <u>hot</u> skillet and let sizzle for a minute.

♣Add 2 MINCED SHALLOTS, and 3 to 4 TBS. FRESH MINCED BASIL LEAVES. Sauté until aromatic.
♣Add 2 CUPS WHOLE GRAIN BREAD CRUMBS and stir until dry.
♣Remove from heat and add 2/3 CUP PARMESAN CHEESE and 1/4 teasp. BLACK PEPPER.

♣Oil a shallow baking dish and place 2 LBS. RINSED THICK FISH FILETS in a single layer. Cover with the sauce and bake for 15 to 20 minutes, until fish whitens to opaque and sauce bubbles.

Nutritional analysis: per serving: 413 calories; 35gm. protein; 6gm. carbo.; 1gm. fiber; 27gm. fats; (6gm. sat., 17gm. mono., 4gm. poly.); 65mg. cholesterol; 3IU beta carotene; 505mg. potassium; 330mg. sodium; 2mg. zinc.

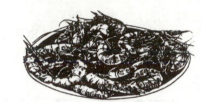

565 CREOLE SHRIMP ETOUFEÉ

Right from the Louisiana bayous to you.
For 8 people:

♣Cook about 1 1/2 LBS. FRESH PEELED SHRIMPS in seafood boil until just pink, about 3 minutes.

♣Melt 4 TBS. BUTTER and 2 TBS. OLIVE OIL in a skillet. Sprinkle on 1/4 CUP UNBLEACHED FLOUR and stir until bubbly and light gold.

♣Add and stir and toss for 15 minutes

1 CUP SCALLIONS, chopped	1/2 CUP CELERY, chopped
1 CUP YELLOW ONIONS, chopped	2 CLOVES GARLIC, minced
1/2 CUP GREEN BELL PEPPER, chopped	1 BAY LEAF
1 TB. FRESH BASIL chopped (or 1 teasp. dry)	1/4 teasp. DRY THYME

♣Add and bring to a boil

8 OZ. TOMATO SAUCE, canned or fresh	1/2 CUP WATER
1 CUP WHITE WINE	1/2 teasp. BLACK PEPPER
ONE 7 OZ. BOTTLE of CLAM JUICE	1/2 teasp. HOT PEPPER SAUCE
1 TB. WHITE WORCESTERSHIRE SAUCE	

♣Lower heat and simmer until thickened, and sauce is reduced to about 4 1/2 cups, about 45 minutes.

♣Remove from heat. Stir in 1 TB. grated LEMON ZEST, 1 TB. LEMON JUICE, and 1/4 CUP CHOPPED FRESH PARSLEY. Serve immediately over BROWN OR BASMATI RICE.

Nutritional analysis: per serving: 309 calories; 22gm. protein; 30gm. carbohydrate; 3gm. fiber; 11gm. fats; (4gm. sat., 5gm. mono., 2gm. poly.); 181mg. cholesterol; 78IU beta carotene; 510mg. potass.; 337mg. sodium; 2mg. zinc.

566   SALMON SOUFFLÉ

This is very light-textured for such a meaty fish. I have made many fish soufflés over the years, but those made with white fish never seem to have the flavor that salmon has; and salmon and eggs go so well together.
For 6 people: Preheat oven to 325°.

♣Make a light white sauce with 2 TBS. MELTED BUTTER or OIL and 2 TBS. UNBLEACHED FLOUR. Stir together until bubbly, blended and golden.
♣Add 1/2 CUP PLAIN YOGURT mixed with 1/4 CUP WATER and 1/4 CUP WHITE WINE. Whisk until thick and smooth.

♣Separate 2 EGGS. Beat a little of the yogurt sauce into the yolks to warm them, then add back to the sauce. Season with
1/2 teasp. SEASONING or HERB SALT
1/4 teasp. PEPPER
1/4 teasp. NUTMEG
♣Open and add a 16-OZ. CAN of RED SALMON with skin and bones removed.
♣Beat EGG WHITES TO STIFF and fold into salmon mix.
♣Put into lecithin-sprayed individual casseroles and bake for 45 minutes until puffy and golden brown.

♣While the soufflés are cooking, make the **EGG SAUCE.** It adds a little more fat and calories, but you only need about 2 to 3 TBS. per individual soufflé, and it does make a taste difference. This sauce is also very good on nut or grain loaves, and on steamed cauliflower.

EGG SAUCE: Use about 2 to 3 TBS. per person on soufflé servings. Makes about 1 1/2 cups:

♣Hard boil 2 EGGS. Chop them into a med. hot skillet with 2 TBS. BUTTER and 2 TBS. UNBLEACHED FLOUR. Stir until bubbly and blended. Add 1 CUP PLAIN YOGURT and 1/2 CUP WATER. Whisk until sauce thickens and comes to a boil. Reduce heat and simmer for 3 minutes.
♣Stir in 1 TB. LEMON JUICE, 1/2 teasp. SEA SALT and 1/4 teasp. WHITE PEPPER

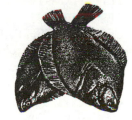

567   SOLE OR FLOUNDER ROLLATINI

Try this for a quick, easy week-night dinner.
For 4 to 6 people: Preheat oven to 375°.

♣Mix the filling

1/2 CUP GRATED PARMESAN or SOY PARMESAN	1 TB. CHOPPED FRESH BASIL
1/2 CUP CHOPPED <u>TOASTED</u> ALMONDS	1/2 CUP CHOPPED FRESH PARSLEY

♣Place 2 LBS. SOLE or FLOUNDER FILETS flat and spoon a little filling on one end. Roll up. PLace seam side down in a shallow oiled baking dish. Pour over 3 TBS. LEMON JUICE and 3 TBS. MELTED BUTTER.
♣Spread on remaining filling.
♣Cover with foil and bake for 30 minutes until fish is opaque and white all through. Serve with asparagus and brown rice.

568 SALMON CAKES PIQUANTE

Serves 4 people: Preheat oven to 350°.

♣Mix together in a bowl

3 SLICES WHOLE GRAIN BREAD, crumbled
$^1/_4$ CUP MINCED ONION
1 EGG lightly beaten
1 TBS. LEMON JUICE

$^1/_2$ teasp. THYME
PINCH PAPRIKA
2 TBS. WHEAT GERM
1 teasp. DIJON MUSTARD

♣Mix in one 16-OZ. CAN of RED SALMON with skin and bones removed. Form into patties.

♣Crush cracker crumbs into a dish. Roll patties in the crumbs. Put on a plate and chill.

♣Oil a shallow baking dish and bake patties for 30 minutes until golden.

♣Serve with a spicy **PIQUANTE SAUCE.** Mix everything and chill to blend flavors.

$^1/_4$ CUP PLAIN YOGURT
2 TBS. LIGHT MAYONNAISE
1 MINCED GREEN ONION
$^1/_4$ CUP FRESH MINCED PARSLEY

1 teasp. DIJON MUSTARD
1 TB. NATURAL LOW SALT CATSUP
1 TB. SWEET PICKLE RELISH

Nutritional analysis: per serving; 308 calories; 28gm. protein; 17gm. carbo.; 3gm. fiber; 11gm. fats; (3gm. sat., 4gm. mono., 4gm. poly.); 120mg. cholesterol; 30IU beta carotene; 569mg. potassium; 505mg. sodium; 2mg. zinc.

569   CREOLE RED SNAPPER WITH MUSHROOMS

An authentic choice for a little company dinner, easy and light, with lots of gourmet flair.
For 4 servings: Preheat oven to 350°.

♣Bring 1-qt. water to a boil. Simmer a few minutes until aromatic.

1 SLICED CARROT
1 SLICED ONION
A HANDFUL FRESH PARSLEY LEAVES
A TABLESPOON OF LEMON JUICE

♣Add
A FEW WHOLE CLOVES
A FEW PEPPERCORNS
A PINCH OF SALT

♣Simmer five minutes until aromatic. Add a 1 LB. FILET RED SNAPPER, rinsed, cleaned and *wrapped in cheesecloth to maintain its shape.* Poach for 3 minutes only. Remove and cut into 4 serving pieces.

♣Reserve $^1/_2$ CUP of the POACHING STOCK to make the sauce. Melt 2 TBS. BUTTER, and stir with 2 TBS. UNBLEACHED FLOUR and $^1/_4$ teasp. SEA SALT until bubbly and golden. Season with WHITE PEPPER and ONE PINCH CHERVIL. Add $^1/_3$ CUP PLAIN YOGURT and 2 TBS. WHITE WINE.

♣Bring to a boil. Add reserved poaching stock and bubble for 1 minute until thickened. Remove from heat and let sit while you sauté $^3/_4$ LB. (about 12) PEELED, RINSED SHRIMP until opaque in 1 TB. BUTTER. Remove from the pan with a slotted spoon. Add 1 TB. more BUTTER and 8 SLICED MUSHROOMS. Sauté until just coated and beginning to brown. Add mushrooms to the sauce.

♣Make up the baking packets. Cut out four 8 x 12" rectangles of foil or baking parchment. Put about 3 TBS. sauce on the bottom half of each rectangle. Lay on a piece of fish, and top with 3 to 4 shrimp. Spoon on a little more sauce. Fold other half of rectangle over, close and seal all edges. Put in a shallow baking dish, and bake for 15 to 20 minutes until fish is tender and firm. Put one packet on each plate, and let each person open his own to enjoy and savor the aroma.

Delectable Sauces For Fish & Seafood

Fish and seafood is often so light and mild that the sauce or marinade can sometimes literally "make the dish."
You can mix and match these with almost any fish you buy.

HONEY MUSTARD SAUCE
This is good with salmon, shrimp or a substantial fish like shark.

♣Mix together and chill: $1/4$ CUP DIJON MUSTARD, $3/4$ CUP HONEY, $1/4$ CUP LIGHT MAYONNAISE, 2 TBS. TAMARI, $1/4$ CUP PLAIN YOGURT, $1/2$ teasp. sea salt, and $1/4$ teasp. PEPPER.

ORIENTAL GREEN PEPPERCORNS MARINADE & SAUCE
This is good with swordfish, ahi tuna and halibut.

♣Whisk all together: $1/4$ CUP TAMARI, $1/4$ CUP MIRIN or SHERRY, $1/4$ CUP SAKE, $1/4$ CUP + 1 TB. BROWN RICE VINEGAR, 2 TBS. DRAINED CRUSHED CAPERS, 1 TB. MINCED FRESH GINGER, 1 CLOVE MINCED GARLIC, and $1/2$ CUP + 2 TBS. LIGHT OIL.

MUSTARD MAYONNAISE
This is good with salmon, scallops and thick fish steaks.

♣Blend in the blender. Cover and chill. For $2 1/4$ cups: $3/4$ CUP GRAINY MUSTARD, 2 TBS. DRY MUSTARD, $1/3$ CUP DARK BROWN SUGAR, 1 CUP LIGHT MAYONNAISE, and $1/2$ CUP FRESH CHOPPED DILL WEED.

DILL TOPPING
Dill is a perfect accompaniment to salmon, and also good with delicate white fish.

♣Mix together and chill: $1/4$ CUP PLAIN YOGURT, $1/4$ CUP LIGHT MAYONNAISE, and $1/4$ teasp. DILLWEED.

MUSTARD DIP FOR SEAFOOD COCKTAIL
A welcome change from regular old cocktail sauce.

♣Mix together and chill: 2 TBS. LIGHT MAYONNAISE, 2 teasp. DIJON MUSTARD, $1/2$ teasp. DRY THYME, 2 PINCHES LEMON PEPPER.

CRUMB SPRINKLE FOR BAKED FISH
An excellent enhancement for light, white fish.

♣Mix together in a bowl and sprinkle over fish before baking: 3 TBS. MELTED BUTTER, $1/2$ CUP WHOLE GRAIN BREAD CRUMBS, 1 TB. GRATED PARMESAN, $3/4$ teasp. THYME, and $1/4$ teasp. LEMON PEPPER.

The hardest thing in life
is learning
which bridge to cross
and which bridge to burn.

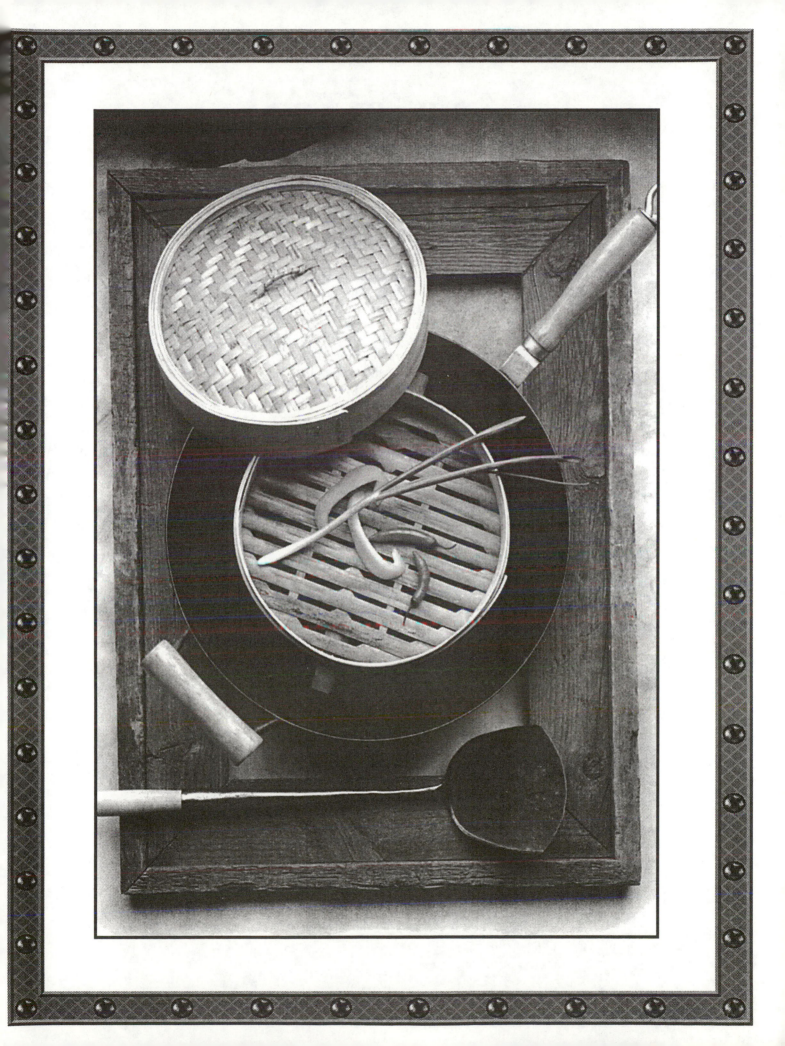

Tofu For You
Cooking With Soy Foods

Tofu is definitely a winner at our house. The more I work with, eat and enjoy tofu, the more I believe it can contribute much to health.

Tofu is a convenient, nutritious meat replacement, and can take on any flavor perfectly, from savory to sweet. When combined with whole grain foods, tofu yields a complete protein that is much less expensive than protein from animal sources. It provides dairy and egg richness without the fat or cholesterol, but with all the calcium and iron. Tofu can be elegant or homey. You can blend it into drinks, make it into frozen desserts, or use it as "pasta." You can toast it or bake it or crunchy-sauté it, or braise it or broil it or freeze it - and it's all tasty. You can use it in soups and salads, dips, sauces and dressings, pancakes and muffins, and even desserts. Have I left anything out? If we don't have tofu every 2 or 3 days in <u>something,</u> we feel deprived. I wonder how we ate before tofu?

It is the most versatile, stress-free, success-guaranteed food I have ever come across. In addition to its culinary talents, tofu is a nutritionally balanced healing food. Tofu is cholesterol free. You can readily substitute it for many cholesterol loaded meats or dairy products. It is a delicious, non-mucous-forming way to add richness and creamy texture to your recipes, easy on the digestive system, and full of soluble fiber.

☞Tofu is low in calories. 8-oz. supplies only 164 calories.

☞Tofu is rich in organic calcium. 8 oz. supplies the same amount of calcium as 8 oz. of milk, but with far more absorbability.

☞Tofu is high in Iron. 8-oz. supplies the same amount of iron as 2-oz. of beef liver or 4 eggs.

☞Tofu has high quality protein. 8-oz. supplies the same amount of protein as $3^1/_4$ oz. of beef steak, or $5^1/_2$ oz. of hamburger, or $1^2/_3$ cups of milk, or 2-oz. of regular cheese, or 2 eggs; but it is lower in fat than any of these.

☞Tofu is an adequate source of complex carbohydrates, minerals and vitamins.

What more could you ask of a food? Shouldn't tofu be for you, too?

Tofu is not the same old yucky but healthy, food any more. As its popularity has risen in America, so has the variety of ways you can buy, prepare and eat it. Tofu now comes firm-pressed into cubes, in a soft delicate form, or silken, with a sweeter custard-like texture. It comes smoked and pre-cooked in seasonings to give it a cheese-like flavor and firmness. It comes freeze-dried so that it can be stored at room temperature and reconstituted; especially suited for camping and traveling. It comes in deep-fried pouches as age (pronounced "ah-gay") that are hollow inside for filling.

The recipes in this chapter cover areas where tofu particularly shines; and some new areas, where even if you are already a tofu fan, you might not have thought to use it.
❧TOFU BASICS, MARINADES and SAUCES ❧TOFU DIPS and APPETIZERS ❧TOFU SALADS ❧TOFU BURGERS and SANDWICHES ❧TOFU and PASTA ❧TOFU WITH RICE and GRAINS ❧WHOLE MEAL DISHES WITH TOFU ❧TOFU DESSERTS ❧
In addition to these recipes, check the index for others throughout this book.

Tofu consists of soybeans water and a curdling agent such as Nigari, a mineral-rich seawater precipitate. For those of you with sensitivity to beans and legumes, tofu may be simmered in water-to-cover for 15 minutes before using. This will normally precook the soybeans enough so that they won't bother your tummy.

For babies, tofu can be blended in the blender or ground in the baby food grinder with a flavoring, fruit or vegetable of your choice.

Tofu Equivalent Source; "Tofu Goes West" Free Press; Ca.

Tofu Basics

Fresh tofu has a light delicate flavor of its own that becomes a wonderful addition or foundation for almost any type of recipe or cuisine. Marinating tofu in a sauce or dressing is the essence of successful cooking with this food. Cut tofu into strips or cubes before marinating for best results. Chill while marinating for best blending of flavors.

570   GINGER MISO MARINADE

For about 2$\frac{1}{2}$ cups:

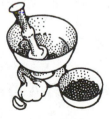

♣Blend in the blender

3 to 4 TBS. LIGHT CHICKPEA MISO
2 teasp. FRESH GRATED GINGER
1/4 CUP BROWN RICE VINEGAR

1/2 CUP WATER
1/4 CUP WHITE WINE
2 TBS. TOASTED SESAME OIL

♣Whirl briefly just to mix and add 3/4 CUP OIL very slowly while blending, to form an emulsion.

Nutritional analysis: for 1 cake Tofu; 30 gm.; 115 calories; trace protein; 1gm. carbohydrate; trace fiber; 13gm. fats; 0 cholesterol; 3mg. calcium; trace iron; 2mg. magnesium; 14mg. potssium; 118mg. sodium; trace zinc.

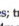

571   FRENCH COOKING MARINADE

This is the basic flavoring sauce used for meats in many French haute cuisine recipes. We have found that it also works beautifully with tofu.
For 2 cups:

♣Blend in the blender

1/4 CUP RED WINE VINEGAR
1 EGG
1 CLOVE CHOPPED GARLIC
1/4 CUP OLIVE OIL

1/4 teasp. WHITE PEPPER
1/2 teasp. DRY MUSTARD
1/2 teasp. SEA SALT

♣Whirl briefly and add 1 CUP LIGHT OIL in a slow steady stream until a thick emulsion forms.
♣Scrape into a bowl, and add 1 CHOPPED HARD BOILED EGG, 1/2 BUNCH CHOPPED WATERCRESS LEAVES, and 2 MINCED GREEN ONIONS with tops.

572   SESAME MARINADE

For about 1/2 cup:

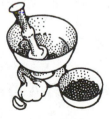

♣Shake in a jar to blend
2 TBS. TAMARI
2 TBS. TOASTED SESAME OIL
2 TBS. TOASTED SESAME SEEDS
1/2 teasp. SESAME SALT

1 TB. BROWN RICE VINEGAR
1/2 teasp. BLACK PEPPER
1/4 teasp. HOT PEPPER SAUCE

573 TOMATO CAESAR MARINADE

For 1¹/₂ cups:

♣Blend in the blender

¹/₄ CUP LEMON JUICE	2 TBS. WATER
¹/₄ CUP BALSAMIC VINEGAR	2 TBS. WHITE WINE
¹/₂ teasp. LEMON GARLIC SEASONING	3 TBS. ROMANO CHEESE
¹/₄ teasp. BLACK PEPPER	1 TB. TOMATO PASTE
1 teasp. FRUCTOSE or HONEY	

♣Whirl briefly and add ³/₄ CUP OLIVE OIL slowly in a steady stream while blending until thickened.

♣Chill to blend flavors while marinating.

574 BASIC VINAIGRETTE MARINADE

For 2 cakes of tofu :

♣Shake all ingredients in a jar and pour over

¹/₄ CUP LIGHT OIL	PINCH FRUCTOSE
1 TB. WHITE WINE VINEGAR	PINCH BLACK PEPPER
1 TB. LEMON JUICE	PINCH DRY MUSTARD
¹/₄ teasp. SESAME SALT	PINCH PAPRIKA

Nutritional analysis: per 1-oz. serving; 165 calories; 1gm. protein; 1gm. carbohydrate; 1gm. fiber; 18gm. fats; 0 cholesterol; 2mg. calcium; trace iron; 1mg. magnesium; 15mg. potassium; 63mg. sodium; trace zinc.

575 POPPYSEED MARINADE

This is good for tofu salads with fruit and nuts. Pour marinade over as a dressing when you make the salad.
For about 1¹/₂ cups:

♣Combine in a jar, and shake vigorously to blend

¹/₃ CUP HONEY	2 TBS. POPPY SEEDS
²/₃ CUP CANOLA OIL	1 teasp. TAMARI
1¹/₂ teasp. SWEET HOT MUSTARD	2 TBS. RASPBERRY VINEGAR
2 TBS. LEMON or LIME JUICE	

576 HOT HONEY AND SPICE TOFU SAUCE

♣Sauté briefly to concentrate flavors, and pour over tofu and steamed veggies.

3 TBS. TAMARI	¹/₂ teasp. SWEET HOT MUSTARD
3 TBS. HONEY	3 TBS. LEMON JUICE
3 TBS. CASHEWS	¹/₄ teasp. BLACK PEPPER
3 TBS. SESAME or other mild oil	¹/₂ teasp. WORCESTERSHIRE SAUCE

577 FOREVER MARINADE
This is a continuing favorite, one I have been making "forever."
For about ¹/₂ cup:

♣Mix in a small bowl, and pour over tofu

2 teasp. TAMARI	1 teasp. ITALIAN HERBS
¹/₂ teasp. DRY MUSTARD	¹/₂ teasp. BLACK PEPPER
2 teasp. SOY BACON BITS	2 teasp. BALSAMIC VINEGAR

♣Whisk with a fork to blend and add *either* ¹/₄ CUP LIGHT MAYONNAISE *or* ¹/₄ CUP LIGHT OIL.

♣Chill for about 30 minutes. This is a good combination when baking tofu, as well as for cold salads.

Nutritional analysis: per 1 oz. serving; 197 calories; 1gm. protein; 1gm. carbohydrate; 1gm. fiber; 16gm. fats; 0mg. cholesterol; 3mg. calcium; 1mg. iron; 2mg. magnesium; 17mg. potassium; 63mg. sodium; 1mg. zinc.

☙YOU CAN ALSO: Marinate tofu in **bottled Italian dressing**; or **Bragg's Liquid Aminos** or **Vegex Yeast Broth**; or a good **bottled hickory, mesquite** or **barbecue sauce**; or **natural liquid smoke with a little water and wine** for an outdoor flavor.

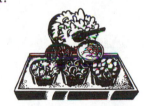

Tofu Salads

578 HOT SPANISH RICE & TOFU SALAD

For 6 salads:

♣Sauté 2 TBS. OIL, 2 CLOVES MINCED GARLIC and ¹/₂ CHOPPED RED ONION until aromatic.
♣Add ¹/₂ GREEN BELL PEPPER in julienne strips and sauté until color changes.
♣Mix in 1 LB. DICED TOFU.

♣Drain, and turn into a large mixing bowl, and add

2¹/₂ CUPS COOKED BROWN RICE or GOURMET GRAINS	
¹/₂ CUP GRATED CHEDDAR or JACK CHEESE	2 teasp. SPANISH SEASONING
¹/₂ HEAD SHAVED ICEBERG LETTUCE	2 DICED TOMATOES

♣Turn into a large shallow serving bowl.

♣Mix the topping ingredients in a bowl and scatter over: 1 DICED AVOCADO, ¹/₄ CUP PLAIN YOGURT or SOUR CREAM, and MILD SALSA to taste.
♣Finish the salad by sticking taco or pinta chips points down around the salad, or surround the salad with chips.

Nutritional analysis: per serving; 297 calories; 13gm. protein; 28gm. carbohydrate; 6gm. fiber; 16gm. fats; 6mg. cholesterol; 196mg. calcium; 5mg. iron; 139mg. magnesium; 590mg. potassium; 116mg. sodium; 2mg. zinc.

579 RAINBOW TOFU SALAD

This was the Rainbow Kitchen restaurant's basic salad. It was varied daily with the fresh ingredients available. It is easy, inexpensive, and highly nutritious.

For 2 large salads:

♣Whisk the dressing in a bowl, and add 3 to 4 CAKES of TOFU to marinate

1 TB. HONEY
1 TB. OLIVE OIL   1/4 CUP SWEET RELISH
1 1/2 teasp. SWEET HOT MUSTARD   1 TB. SMOKED YEAST POWDER

♣Toss in a salad bowl lined with large overlapping lettuce leaves

2 CHOPPED SCALLIONS   1 SMALL CHOPPED TOMATO
1 STALK SLICED CELERY   1 CHOPPED CARROT
2 TBS. TOASTED SLIVERED ALMONDS   1/2 CUP SHAVED RED CABBAGE
3 TBS. TOASTED SUNFLOWER SEEDS   1/2 PEELED CHOPPED CUCUMBER

580 CLASSIC TOFU "EGG" SALAD

Versions of this quick, easy recipe have been around since the popularity of tofu began, and it is still a favorite. It is good in lettuce cups, as a sandwich filling, or on top of a mixed sprout bed.

For 4 salads:

♣Mash together in a bowl
1 LB. TOFU   1/2 teasp. SESAME SALT
3 CHOPPED SCALLIONS   1/2 teasp. BLACK PEPPER
1 STALK CELERY, diced   1/2 teasp. TAMARI
1/2 MINCED GREEN BELL PEPPER   2 teasp. DIJON MUSTARD
1/2 teasp. GREAT 28 MIX (or other herb seasoning)   1 TB. LEMON JUICE
1/3 CUP LIGHT MAYONNAISE PINCH TURMERIC for color

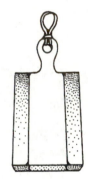

581 TOFU MAYONNAISE

This dressing and sauce can see lots of service in a healing diet. It is a low-fat, no cholesterol, dairy-free mayonnaise. It may be used as a creme fraiche, sour cream, or a base for cream sauces, with the advantages of a dairy product without the problems.

♣Blend in the blender to mayonnaise consistency
1/2 LB. TOFU   1/2 teasp. SESAME SALT
1 1/2 TBS. LEMON JUICE   2 TBS. OIL
1/2 teasp. DIJON MUSTARD (OR 1 1/2 teasp. LIGHT MISO)
♣Add 4 TBS. PLAIN YOGURT and 1/2 teasp. TARRAGON VINEGAR to use as a substitute for creme fraiche or sour cream.

Tofu Burgers & Sandwiches

No section on tofu would be complete without these - the recipes that put tofu into the American mainstream, great low-fat burgers without the beef.

582   TOFU BURGER SUPREME

These burgers use frozen, thawed tofu. Freezing tofu gives it a chewy meaty taste that is perfect for "hamburger" type recipes. Squeezing out the liquid leaves more facets on the tofu crumbles to soak up the seasonings.
For 6 to 8 burgers: Preheat oven to 375°.

♣Freeze $1^1/_2$ LBS. TOFU. Thaw, squeeze out water and crumble in a bowl. Mix in 2 EGGS and $^3/_4$ CUP ALMOND or PEANUT BUTTER.

♣Sauté 1 CHOPPED ONION, 1 TB. MUSTARD and $^1/_2$ teasp. ZEST SEASONING SALT in 2 TBS. BUTTER or OIL until fragrant. Add to TOFU in the bowl and stir.

♣Mix in and form into patties

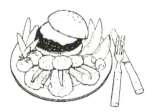

$^1/_2$ CUP GRANOLA $^1/_2$ CUP KETCHUP
$^3/_4$ CUP BEAN SPROUTS or CHOPPED CARROTS $^1/_2$ teasp. LEMON PEPPER

♣Roll in TOASTED WHEAT GERM or CRUSHED GRANOLA.
♣Bake on greased sheets until brown on the outside and moist on the inside, about 25 minutes.

Nutritional analysis: per serving; 330 calories; 14gm. protein; 18gm. carbohydrate; 5gm. fiber; 24gm. fats; 61mg. cholesterol; 176mg. calcium; 6mg. iron; 183mg. magnesium; 478mg. potassium; 245mg. sodium; 2mg. zinc.

583   OPEN FACE TOFU A LA KING

For 4 sandwiches:

♣Squeeze out and crumble 1 LB. TOFU, previously frozen, thawed. Sauté with 1 CHOPPED ONION in 2 TBS. BUTTER or OIL for 10 minutes.

♣Add $^1/_4$ CUP MINCED CELERY, and 2 CUPS SLICED MUSHROOMS.
♣Sprinkle with 4 TBS. UNBLEACHED FLOUR and stir until bubbly.

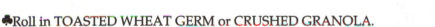

♣Blender blend the sauce
1 CUP PLAIN YOGURT   4 TBS. WHITE WINE
8 OZ. KEFIR CHEESE $^1/_2$ teasp. SESAME SALT
$^1/_2$ CUP LIGHT MAYONNAISE $^1/_4$ teasp. PEPPER
2 VEGETABLE or CHICKEN BOUILLON CUBES
♣Pour into skillet and bring to a boil. Simmer stirring constantly until thickened, and sauce is reduced by about $^1/_4$ to concentrate flavors.
♣Place hand-cut slices of whole grain toast on a baking sheet. Top with sauce, and bake or broil until bubbly and browned.

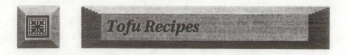
584 TOFU SLOPPY JOES

The ultimate outdoor food.
For 6 open face sandwiches:

♣Sauté in 2 TBS. OIL in a large skillet until brown
1/2 LARGE ONION, chopped
1/2 GREEN BELL PEPPER, diced
1/4 teasp. GARLIC POWDER
1 teasp. ITALIAN HERBS
2 CAKES CRUMBLED TOFU

♣Add 1 CUP ITALIAN TOMATO SAUCE (canned if you like), and simmer until aromatic, and moisture is reduced by one quarter.

♣Toast ENGLISH MUFFIN HALVES on a baking sheet and cover each with some Sloppy Joe mix. Top with CHUNKS of MOZARRELLA CHEESE and a little PARMESAN. Serve hot.

Nutritional analysis: per serving; 199 calories; 10gm. protein; 19gm. carbohydrate; 2gm. fiber; 9gm. fats; 7gm. cholesterol; 201mg. calcium; 3mg. iron; 58mg. magnesium; 413mg. potassium; 296mg. sodium; 1mg. zinc.

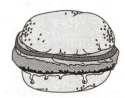

585 EASY TOFU BURGERS WITH GREAT SAUCE

For 6 burgers:

♣Combine all burger ingredients in a bowl
2 EGGS
1 LB. TOFU mashed
ONE 14-OZ. PACKAGE TOFU BURGER MIX such as FEARN or FANTASTIC FOODS
2 teasp. BOTTLED BARBECUE or HICKORY SAUCE.
1/2 teasp. THYME
♣Shape into thick patties and broil for 3 minutes on each side.
♣Serve on whole grain burger buns with lettuce, tomato and the GREAT 28 SAUCE below.

GREAT 28 SAUCE

♣Blend in the blender
1/2 CUP SESAME TAHINI   1 TBS. LEMON JUICE
1/2 CUP KEFIR CHEESE   1 teasp. GREAT 28 MIX
1/4 CUP SWEET PICKLE RELISH
♣Add 2 TBS. WATER if needed for consistency.

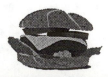

Tofu Dips, Appetizers & Hors D'oeuvres

586   TOFU PASTIES WITH MUSHROOM FILLING

Tofu makes this dough very light and tender. The filling is like your favorite egg rolls without deep fat frying.
For about 30 pasties:

♣Mix the dough in the blender until smooth
1 CUP SOFT BUTTER
1 LB. VERY FRESH TOFU
1 teasp. SEA SALT
♣Scrape in to a bowl and add $2^1/_4$ CUPS UNBLEACHED FLOUR. Mix to form a smooth soft dough. Cover bowl and chill.

♣Make the filling. Soak 2 LARGE BLACK SHIITAKE DRIED MUSHROOMS in water until soft. Sliver, chop, and discard woody stems.

♣Mix together in a big bowl

THE BLACK MUSHROOMS	2 teasp. FRESH GRATED GINGER
4-OZ. CHOPPED BUTTON MUSHROOMS	1 TB. TAMARI
6 to 8 CHOPPED WATER CHESTNUTS	1 TB. SHERRY
$1/_4$ CUP DICED CELERY	3 SHALLOTS, chopped
1 SMALL DICED CARROT	3 GREEN ONIONS, chopped
1 CUP CHOPPED SPINACH or BOK CHOY GREENS	
1 HANDFUL SUNFLOWER or BEAN SPROUTS	

♣Sauté all in a skillet in 2 TBS. OIL for 3 minutes just to soften and blend.

♣When ready to fill, roll dough out on a floured surface, and cut into 3" squares. Fill each square with 1 teaspoon of filling and fold over to form a triangle. Seal edges with fork tines. Put filled pasties on oiled baking sheets and bake for 30 minutes at 350°.

Nutritional analysis: per pasty; 116 calories; 3gm. protein; 9gm. carbohydrate; trace fiber; 8gm. fats; 16mg. cholesterol; 25mg. calcium; 1mg. iron; 22mg. magnesium; 90mg. potassium; 83mg. sodium; trace zinc.

※

♣Dip the pasties in **MOCK SOUR CREAM** if desired.

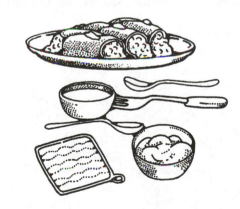

MOCK SOUR CREAM

For six 2 oz. servings:

♣Blend in the blender and process until creamy
1 CUP LOW-FAT COTTAGE CHEESE
2 TBS. LEMON JUICE
2 TBS. LIGHT MAYONNAISE
$1/_4$ CUP PLAIN YOGURT
ZEST of $1/_2$ LEMON

Nutritional analysis: per serving; 6 calories; 5gm. protein; 2gm. carbohydrate; trace fiber; 1gm. fats; 4mg. cholesterol; 43mg. calcium; 1mg. iron; 64mg. potassium; 160mg. sodium; trace zinc.

※

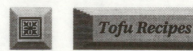

587 TOFU TORTILLAS

These are very versatile. We have used them as chapati dippers, as flour tortillas for wrapping burritos, as crepes for rolling fillings, as light crusts for pizzas and quiches and tortillas, as pasties and as eggroll wrappers. They are light, low fat, tender, and elastic. The dough freezes well, and the recipe can be cut down easily if you don't want to use it all at once. One could hardly ask for more than all that!
Enough for 16 crusts:

♣Mix in the blender
1 LB. VERY FRESH TOFU   1^1/$_2$ teasp. SEA SALT
^{1}/$_2$ CUP BUTTER   2 TBS. BAKING POWDER
♣Turn into a mixing bowl. Add 3 CUPS UNBLEACHED FLOUR. Mix until smooth and elastic. Chill.

♣Divide into 16 parts and form into balls. Roll out each one into an 8" circle. Bake on a preheated <u>ungreased</u> skillet or griddle over medium high heat, until done but not brown. Stack with waxed paper between each layer for storage and freezing.

Nutritional analysis: per serving; 142 calories; 6gm. protein; 13gm. carbohydrate; 2gm. fiber; 8gm. fats; 15mg. cholesterol; 123mg. calcium; 2mg. iron; 56mg. magnesium; 538mg. potassium; 204mg. sodium; 1mg. zinc.

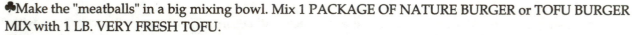

Try the crust above as the base for this TOFU MEATBALL PIZZA.

588 TOFU "MEATBALL" PIZZA

The tofu "meatballs" also freeze very well if you have too many.
For 35 to 40 small balls: Preheat oven to 400∞.

♣Make the "meatballs" in a big mixing bowl. Mix 1 PACKAGE OF NATURE BURGER or TOFU BURGER MIX with 1 LB. VERY FRESH TOFU.
♣Add
1 EGG   2 TBS. OLIVE OIL
^{1}/$_4$ CUP GRATED PARMESAN   1 TB. RED WINE VINEGAR
^{1}/$_4$ CUP FRESH CHOPPED PARSLEY
♣Roll into balls and place on an oiled baking sheet. Bake for 18 to 20 minutes until brown and crusty.

♣Make the sauce. Sauté in a skillet til aromatic, about 5 minutes
3 TBS. OLIVE OIL
1 CUP CHOPPED ONION
1 CUP CHOPPED GREEN PEPPER
^{1}/$_2$ teasp. ANISE SEED or FENNEL SEED
♣Add one 15-OZ. JAR of ALL NATURAL ITALIAN PIZZA SAUCE and stir until bubbly. Reduce heat and let simmer for about 20 minutes.

♣Assemble the pizza. Fit the TOFU TORTILLA CRUST above onto a round pizza pan, or put 2 on a 15 x 11" baking sheet. Spoon on sauce to cover. Top with chunks of MOZARRELLA CHEESE, and arrange tofu meatballs around the pizza. Bake for 30 minutes <u>on the bottom rack</u> of the oven.

Nutritional analysis: per 4oz. serving; 168 calories; 9gm. protein; 14gm. carbohydrate; 3gm. fiber; 10gm. fats; 20mg. cholesterol; 134mg. calcium; 3mg. iron; 62mg. magnesium; 351mg. potassium; 297mg. sodium; 1mg. zinc.

589   ELEGANT BAKED TOFU KABOBS

If you have skewers with fancy handles, now is the time to use them.
Marinate large TOFU CUBES for 1 hour in your favorite marinade. (See first part of this chapter for some suggestions.)

♣Marinate cubes of PEELED EGGPLANT, GREEN PEPPER, LARGE WHOLE MUSHROOMS, and RED ONION CHUNKS for 1 hour in
1 TB. FRUCTOSE
2 TBS. TAMARI
3 TBS. ROSÉ WINE
4 TBS. ITALIAN DRESSING

♣Alternate Tofu cubes with each of the veggie cubes on the skewers, and bake on oiled sheets, or on the outside grill, until tender. If you use the oven, run them under the broiler for 30 seconds to "charcoal" the kabobs.

590   TOFU DIPPING STICKS

These are best as dunkers for light sauces or creamy dips.
For about 30 sticks: Preheat oven to 375°.

♣Blend in the blender
1 LB. FRESH TOFU
3/4 CUP SOFT BUTTER
1 teasp. SEA SALT
2 1/2 teasp. BAKING POWDER
♣Beat until very elastic and smooth.

♣Pour into a mixing bowl and beat with
2 1/4 CUPS UNBLEACHED FLOUR
1/2 CUP POPPY SEEDS
   or PARMESAN CHEESE

♣Divide into 30 parts and roll between your palms into 4" to 5" sticks. Place on oiled sheets and bake for 35 minutes. Serve warm if possible, with **FRENCH ONION TOFU DIP** if desired.

Nutritional analysis: per stick; 92 calories; 3gm. protein; 6gm. carbohydrate; 1gm. fiber; 6gm. fats; 12mg. cholesterol; 74mg. calcium; 1mg. iron; 34mg. magnesium; 178mg. potassium; 74mg. sodium; trace zinc.

FRENCH ONION TOFU DIP

♣Sauté 1/2 SMALL ONION, chopped, and 1 CLOVE GARLIC, minced in 2 TBS. OLIVE OIL until aromatic and browning.

♣Add 1/2 SMALL CARROT, grated, and PINCHES of CHILI POWDER and PAPRIKA, and sauté for 3 minutes.

♣Put in a blender and blend until smooth with
2 TBS. CIDER VINEGAR
1 TB. TAMARI
2 CAKES SOFT TOFU

1/4 teasp. PEPPER
2 TBS. CHOPPED CHIVES

591 BASIL BITES WITH TOMATO OLIVE SAUCE

For about 18 bites:

♣Make the sauce first. Sauté for 10 minutes until fragrant

3 TBS. OLIVE OIL — $1/2$ teasp. OREGANO
1 ONION, chopped — $1/2$ teasp. THYME
1 teasp. LEMON GARLIC SEASONING — $1/2$ teasp. HOT PEPPER SAUCE
1 TB. FRESH CHOPPED BASIL

♣Add 1 LARGE CAN ITALIAN TOMATOES and simmer uncovered until sauce is reduced to 3 cups, about 45 minutes. Let cool slightly, pureé in the blender, and add back to the pot.
♣Stir in $1/3$ CUP CHOPPED CILANTRO and 12 CHOPPED BLACK OLIVES.
♣Make the tofu bites. Preheat oven to 325°.
♣Make up $1/2$ PACKAGE TOFU BURGER MIX with 2 CAKES FRESH TOFU as directed.
♣Add 2 TBS. PARMESAN CHEESE and 2 TBS. FRESH CHOPPED BASIL. Roll into 2" balls and place on oiled sheets. Bake turning for 15 minutes until golden.

Nutritional analysis: per bite; 66 calories; 3gm. protein; 6gm. carbohydrate; 2gm. fiber; 4gm. fats; 0 cholesterol; 35mg. calcium; 1mg. iron; 26mg. magnesium; 163mg. potassium; 55mg. sodium; trace zinc.

592 TOFU FALAFEL BITES

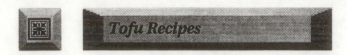

For 36 homemade falafel bites:

♣Mix in a bowl and form into 1" balls

3 CAKES MASHED TOFU — 3 TBS. TAMARI
1 CUP DICED ONIONS — 3 TBS. OIL
1 CUP BREAD WHOLE GRAIN CRUMBS — $1/4$ teasp. BLACK PEPPER
4 TBS. SESAME TAHINI — 4 TBS. LEMON JUICE
$1/4$ CUP CHOPPED PARSLEY — $1 1/2$ TBS. TOASTED SESAME OIL
1 teasp. GROUND CUMIN SEED — 2 teasp. GROUND TURMERIC

♣Roll in $1/2$ CUP SESAME SEEDS. Place on oiled baking sheets as you make them. Chill for an hour before baking until crusty. Serve with **GINGER TAHINI DIP**.

Nutritional analysis: per serving; 51 calories; 2gm. protein; 2gm. carbohydrate; trace fiber; 4gm. fats; 0 cholesterol; 37mg. calcium; 1mg. iron; 25mg. magnesium; 52mg. potassium; 23mg. sodium; trace zinc.

GINGER TAHINI DIP

For about 1 cup:

♣Blend in the blender

2 CAKES CRUMBLRED TOFU — 1 teasp. HONEY
2 teasp. LIGHT MISO — 2 TBS. SESAME TAHINI
$1/2$ teasp. GRATED FRESH GINGER — PINCH CURRY POWDER

♣Add 2 TBS. YOGURT CHEESE or LIGHT MAYONNAISE for creaminess if desired.

Tofu & Pasta

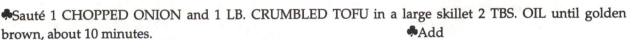

593   TOFU TETRAZZINI

Enough for 4 people: Preheat oven to 350°.

♣Bring 2 qts. salted water to a boil for the noodles.

♣Sauté 1 CHOPPED ONION and 1 LB. CRUMBLED TOFU in a large skillet 2 TBS. OIL until golden brown, about 10 minutes.   ♣Add
1 LB. FRESH DICED TOMATOES $1/_2$ teasp. SESAME SALT
$1/_2$ teasp. DRY THYME $1/_2$ teasp. LEMON PEPPER

♣Remove from heat and add 1 CUP COTTAGE CHEESE, $1/_2$ CUP CHOPPED PARSLEY, and $1/_4$ CUP GRATED JACK CHEESE.
♣Cook about 6-OZ. EGG or SESAME NOODLES to *al dente*. Pour into a lecithin-sprayed casserole and toss with tofu mixture. Sprinkle with more JACK CHEESE, and bake for 30 minutes until bubbling.

❀

594   TOFU TEMPEH STROGANOFF
Tempeh is a fermented soy food with a meaty, dense texture. It lends itself well in sandwiches or to dishes like this where the chewiness enhances the traditional stroganoff recipe richness.
Enough for 6 people:

♣Cube 2 CAKES of TOFU and 8-OZ. TEMPEH. Sprinkle well with LEMON PEPPER and CUMIN POWDER, and marinate in a shallow pan with $1/_3$ CUP TAMARI and 3 TBS. SHERRY for 1 hour.

♣Meanwhile sauté 1 CHOPPED ONION and 4 CUPS SLICED MUSHROOMS in 4 TBS. BUTTER or OIL in a large pan for 5 minutes. Drain off tofu/tempeh liquid and add them to the onion mix.

♣Toss and stir briefly to heat and add
$1/_2$ teasp. SESAME SALT $1/_2$ teasp. DRY BASIL
$1/_4$ teasp. PEPPER   2 PINCHES NUTMEG
♣Reduce heat to low and cook partially covered for 15 minutes. Stir occasionally and add 1 to 2 teasp. of the marinade if mixture is getting too dry.

♣Add $1/_4$ CUP WHITE WINE and 1 CUP PLAIN YOGURT. Taste for seasoning and add a little more of the marinade if seasoning is bland.

♣While stroganoff is cooking, bring salted water to a boil for the noodles. Use 6 to 8-OZ. WHOLE EGG or SESAME NOODLES and cook to *al dente*. Toss with 1 teasp. OIL to keep separated. Pour onto a serving platter and spoon stroganoff sauce over the top. Snip on FRESH PARSLEY.

Nutritional analysis: per serving; 286 calories; 13gm. protein; 24gm. carbohydrate; 4gm. fiber; 15gm. fats; 20mg. cholesterol; 173mg. calcium; 6mg. iron; 110mg. magnesium; 458mg. potassium; 222mg. sodium; 2mg. zinc.

❀

595   LOW FAT TOFU LASAGNA WITH FRESH HERBS

Enough for 12 servings: Preheat oven to 350°.

♣Use about 1 LB. FROZEN TOFU for the "lasagna noodles" in this recipe. Thaw, squeeze out water, and slice into very thin slabs.
♣Make the LASAGNA SAUCE. For about 3 cups, sauté 1 LARGE CHOPPED ONION and 2 CLOVES MINCED GARLIC in 4 TBS. OIL until aromatic.
♣Add 1 CHOPPED GREEN BELL PEPPER and sauté until color changes to bright green.
♣Add and simmer for 5 minutes

2 LBS. CHOPPED PLUM TOMATOES	$1/4$ teasp. ZEST SEASONING SALT
2 TBS. SNIPPED PARSLEY	$1/4$ teasp. PEPPER
$1/2$ teasp. FRESH OREGANO ($1/4$ teasp. DRY)	$1/4$ teasp. NUTMEG
$1/2$ teasp. FRESH THYME ($1/4$ teasp. DRY)	2 teasp. TAMARI
$1/2$ teasp. FRESH ROSEMARY ($1/4$ teasp. DRY)	$1/2$ teasp. GRATED LEMON ZEST

♣Add 1 CUP SLICED MUSHROOMS, $1/2$ CUP ROSÉ WINE, and $1/2$ CUP VEGETABLE BROTH and simmer on low heat for 15-20 minutes.
♣Remove from heat, and mix in 2 LBS. LOW-FAT RICOTTA or COTTAGE CHEESE and 1 EGG.
♣Slice 4 LARGE TOMATOES.

♣Assemble the lasagna. Layer half the tofu slices on the bottom of a greased lasagna pan to cover.
♣Spread with half the ricotta mix. Top with half the tomato slices and cover with lasagna sauce.
♣Mix $1/2$ CUP CHOPPED FRESH BASIL with $1/2$ CUP FETA CHEESE and sprinkle over sauce.
♣Repeat layers, topping the whole thing with tomato slices. Bake covered with foil until bubbling, about 20 to 25 minutes. Sprinkle with more feta cheese. Let rest 10 minutes before cutting to serve.

Nutritional analysis: per serving; 198 calories; 16gm. protein; 11gm. carbohydrate; 3gm. fiber; 10gm. fats; 29mg. cholesterol; 150mg. calcium; 3mg. iron; 63mg. magnesium; 459mg. potassium; 460mg. sodium; 1mg. zinc.

596   PASTA, VEGETABLES & TOFU

Enough for 4 people: Preheat oven to 350°.

♣Bring 2 qts. salted water to boil for the pasta. Add 2 CUPS SPINACH or ARTICHOKE PASTA SHAPES while you are doing the sauté, and cook rapidly to *al dente*. Drain and toss with 1 TB. oil.
♣Sauté 1 CHOPPED ONION and 1 LB. CUBED TOFU in a large pot in 2 TBS. OIL until brown.
♣Add and sauté until color changes 4 SMALL SLICED CARROTS, 1 STALK CELERY, SLICED, and 8-OZ. SLICED MUSHROOMS.
♣Mix and toss vegetables with the hot pasta. Pour half the mixture into a lecithin-sprayed casserole.
♣Top with GRATED CHEDDAR. Repeat layers.
♣Make the sauce in the sauté pan. Melt 3 TBS. BUTTER and add 4 TBS. WHOLE WHEAT FLOUR. Stir until brown and bubbly.
♣Add 1 TB. TAMARI, 1 CUP WHITE WINE or VEGETABLE STOCK, $1/2$ CUP PLAIN YOGURT, and $1/2$ CUP WATER. Cook and stir until thick and bubbly. Pour over tofu and veggies and top with crunchy Chinese noodles. Bake until bubbly.

Tofu With Rice & Grains

This special section acknowledges the outstanding protein complementarity of tofu and grains. Both foods are high in proteins, and when eaten together, assimilation is even greater - a case of one and one making three.

597   HAPPY PANCAKES

These are like baby Egg Foo Yung patties. You can stack them with a little sauce in between, or fold them over, and dip them in the sauce with your fingers.
For about 20 small pancakes: Preheat a griddle to hot.

♣Whisk together 1³/₄ CUPS RICE FLOUR and 2 CUPS COLD WATER until smooth.
♣Add ³/₄ CUP OIL and ¹/₄ teasp. TURMERIC. Whisk and set aside.

♣Sauté in 3 TBS. OIL until aromatic
1 SMALL ONION, chopped	1 teasp. SESAME SALT
1 LB. TOFU, in small dice	1 teasp. BLACK PEPPER
10 MUSHROOMS, chopped	

♣Add 1 LB. TINY COOKED SHRIMP and 2¹/₂ CUPS BEAN SPROUTS. Toss and sizzle for 1 minute.

♣Make the pancakes on the hot oiled griddle. Dab spoonfuls of the shrimp mixture around the griddle, and pour ¹/₃ CUP WHOLE GRAIN PANCAKE MIX <u>over top of each</u>. Smooth out and cook until edges turn a deep brown and curl up, about 5 minutes. Drain on towels.
♣Fold in half for dipping, and turn out onto a serving plate. Serve with the following **SWEET & SOUR DIPPING SAUCE.**

Nutritional analysis: per serving; 147 calories; 8gm. protein; 8gm. carbohydrate; 1gm. fiber; 10gm. fats; 34mg. cholesterol; 42mg. calcium; 2mg. iron; 46mg. magnesium; 127mg. potassium; 72mg. sodium; 1mg. zinc.

SWEET & SOUR BARBECUE DIPPING SAUCE

For 2 cups:

♣Sauté 1 CHOPPED ONION and 2 CLOVES GARLIC in 2 TBS. OIL in a saucepan until very brown.
♣Add, reduce heat, and simmmer for 15 minutes until thick
1 CUP CATSUP	³/₄ CUP PINEAPPLE JUICE
1 TB. SWEET/HOT MUSTARD	¹/₄ CUP PINEAPPLE CHUNKS
3 TBS. MOLASSES	
2 teasp. GREAT 28 MIX (page 645) or other broth/seasoning mix.	

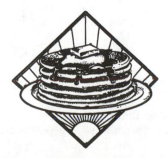

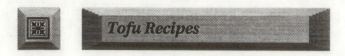

598 TOFU MILLET MIX

For 6 to 8 servings: Preheat oven to 350°.

♣Marinate 1 LB. CUBED TOFU for 30 minutes in 1/2 CUP TAMARI, 1 TB. BROWN RICE VINEGAR, and 2 teasp. LEMON GARLIC SEASONING.

♣Bring 4 CUPS SALTED WATER to a boil. Sauté and stir 1 1/3 CUPS MILLET in 1 TB. OIL in a large pot until fragrant and color changes. Pour boiling water over millet, reduce heat and simmer partially covered for 20 to 25 minutes until water is absorbed. Fluff and set aside.

♣Sauté in a medium skillet until aromatic

3 TBS. OIL	1/2 teasp. PAPRIKA
1 teasp. GROUND ROSEMARY	1 teasp. THYME
1 teasp. GROUND SAGE	1 SLICED ONION

♣Add and sauté 1 CHOPPED RED or GREEN BELL PEPPER and 2 CUPS SLICED MUSHROOMS.
♣Drain tofu and add to mushroom mix. Toss/stir for 10 minutes. Add millet, and toss to combine.
♣Add

1/2 LB. GRATED LOW-FAT CHEDDAR CHEESE	1/4 CUP PLAIN YOGURT
1/2 CUP CHOPPED FRESH PARSLEY	1/4 CUP LIGHT MAYONNAISE

♣Turn into an oiled 9 x 13" baking pan and bake for 30 minutes to heat through.

Nutritional analysis: per serving; 366 calories; 18gm. protein; 33gm. carbohydrate; 3gm. fiber; 15gm. fats; 18mg. cholesterol; 306mg. calcium; 5mg. iron; 359mg. potassium; 128mg. magnesium; 3mg. zinc.

599 GOLDEN TOFU CURRY OVER KASHI

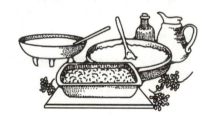

For 6 servings:

♣Have ready 2 to 3 CUPS COOKED KASHI or BROWN RICE.
♣Steam 2 POTATOES and 2 CUPS of DICED, PEELED EGGPLANT.

♣Sauté 1 SLICED ONION, 1 CLOVE MINCED GARLIC, and 1 teasp. GROUND GINGER in 2 TBS. OIL for 2 minutes until aromatic.
♣Add 1 LB. CUBED TOFU, sprinkle with 1 TB. MILD CURRY and sauté for 10 more minutes.
♣Add potatoes and eggplant and toss briefly to heat.
♣Remove from heat and add

1/4 CUP RAISINS	1 teasp. SESAME SALT
1/4 CUP CHOPPED NUTS	2 TBS. CHOPPED CILANTRO
THE VEGETABLES and TOFU	1 CUP PLAIN YOGURT

♣Serve over the cooked rice or Kashi, and have a good homemade chutney on the side.

Nutritional analysis: per serving; 258 calories; 12gm. protein; 33gm. carbohydrate; 5gm. fiber; 10gm. fats; 2mg. cholesterol; 201mg. calcium; 6mg. iron; 144mg. magnesium; 476mg. potassium; 145mg. sodium; 2mg. zinc.

600   TOFU RICE MOLD WITH MUSTARD GLAZE

Enough for 8 servings: Preheat oven to 350°.

♣Have ready 1/2 CUP COOKED BROWN RICE.

♣Sauté 1 LARGE CHOPPED ONION, 1 DICED BELL PEPPER, 1 DICED STALK CELERY and 1 teasp. THYME in a large skillet until color changes.

♣Add 2 LBS. FROZEN TOFU thawed, squeezed out and crumbled.
♣Add 1/4 CUP WHEAT GERM, 1/3 CUP NATURAL KETCHUP, 2 EGGS, 1 teasp. FRESH PEPPER.
♣Mix all well and pack into a large bowl. Turn out onto a shallow oiled baking dish, and pat into a smooth rounded mold.
♣Press 2 TBS. SOY BACON BITS into the top. Drizzle with 2 TBS. SHERRY. Bake for 1 hour until cooked through but still moist. Let stand for 10 minutes while you make the **HONEY MUSTARD GLAZE**.

HONEY MUSTARD GLAZE

♣Bring to boil in a small pan

1/2 CUP HONEY   1/4 CUP SWEET HOT MUSTARD
1/4 CUP FRUCTOSE   1/3 CUP ROSÉ WINE
1/3 CUP BALSAMIC VINEGAR

♣Reduce heat and simmer for 20 minutes until thickened. Let cool and spoon glaze over mold.

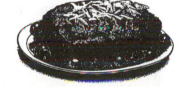

601   TOFU BULGUR LOAF

For 8 servings: Preheat oven to 400°.

♣Dry roast 1 CUP BULGUR in a pan until aromatic. Add water to cover and soak for 15 minutes. Drain, press out water and set aside.
♣Add 1 LB. FROZEN TOFU thawed, squeezed of liquid and crumbled to bulgur.

♣Mix 6 TBS. WHOLE WHEAT FLOUR, 3 EGGS and a 6-OZ. CAN TOMATO PASTE dissolved in 1 CUP WATER in a large mixing bowl.

♣Sauté in 4 TBS. OIL in a skillet until very fragrant

2 CHOPPED RED ONIONS   1/4 teasp. HOT PEPPER SAUCE
1 teasp. LEMON GARLIC SEASONING   1/2 teasp. CUMIN POWDER
2 TBS. CHOPPED GREEN ONIONS   1/2 teasp. LEMON PEPPER
1 teasp. FRESH GRATED GINGER   1 teasp. OREGANO

♣Add to mixing bowl and combine. Add bulgur and tofu and combine all together well.
♣Turn into a large greased loaf pan and drizzle with OLIVE OIL. Sprinkle with 1 teasp. PAPRIKA, and bake for 1 1/4 hours until very brown and crusty on top.

Whole Meal Dishes With Tofu

602 GIANT TOFU & VEGETABLE BALL

For 6 servings: Preheat oven to 350°.

♣Sauté in a skillet in 3 TBS. OIL until fragrant, about 15 minutes
1 SMALL CHOPPED ONION
2 CLOVES CHOPPED GARLIC

2 teasp. ITALIAN SEASONING
$1/_4$ teasp. HOT PEPPER SAUCE

♣Wash and chop 1 BUNCH FRESH SPINACH or ROMAINE. Add to skillet and let wilt for a few minutes. Remove pan from heat and cool slightly.

♣Turn into a large mixing bowl and add
TWO 12-OZ. TUBS TOFU, frozen, thawed, squeezed out and crumbled
$1/_2$ CUP WHOLE GRAIN BREAD CRUMBS or CORN BREAD CRUMBS
2 EGGS
1 teasp. SESAME SALT
$1/_4$ CUP PARMESAN CHEESE
♣Turn mixture onto a lecithin-sprayed shallow baking dish and form into a big rounded smooth hemisphere. Bake for $1^1/_2$ hours until well browned. Let stand for 10 minutes to set.

♣Serve in wedges with a FRESH TOMATO SAUCE. (See index for choices.)

Nutritional analysis: per serving; 212 calories; 14gm. protein; 12gm. carbohydrate; 3gm. fiber; 13gm. fats; 74mg. cholesterol; 213mg. calcium; 7mg. iron; 139mg. magnesium; 369mg. potassium; 331mg. sodium; 1mg. zinc.

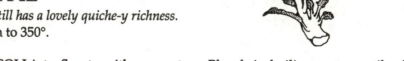

603 TOFU BROCCOLI PIE

This has no eggs, cream or milk, but still has a lovely quiche-y richness.
Enough for 6 people: Preheat oven to 350°.

♣Chop 1 LARGE HEAD BROCCOLI into florets with some stem. Blanch in boiling water until color changes to bright green. Drain. Rinse in cool water and set aside.
♣Sauté 1 SMALL CHOPPED ONION in 4 TBS. BUTTER and 2 TBS. OIL for 5 minutes. Add 2 TB. WHOLE GRAIN FLOUR and 1 TB. LIGHT MISO PASTE and stir til bubbly and browning.

♣Add 1 CUP CHICKEN or VEGETABLE STOCK and cook until thickened.
♣Add 2 CAKES MASHED TOFU or 2 READY-MADE TOFU BURGERS, crumbled.
♣Add $1/_2$ CUP GRATED LOW-FAT CHEDDAR (or soy cheddar) and $1/_2$ CUP CRISPY CHINESE NOODLES or TOASTED SLICED ALMONDS.

♣Pour into a lecithin-sprayed quiche dish. Sprinkle with PARMESAN CHEESE, TOASTED WHEAT GERM, and MORE TOASTED ALMONDS or NOODLES. Bake for 30 minutes until set and bubbly.

604   SAVORY ONIONS, MUSHROOMS & TOFU

For 8 servings: Preheat oven to 325°.

♣Oven fry 1 LB. SLICED TOFU STRIPS in a large flat baking/serving dish with a little VINAIGRETTE DRESSING until just tender and aromatic, about 15 minutes.
♣Sauté in 4 TBS. OIL until very fragrant, about 5 minutes

6 SLICED ONIONS	1 teasp. PAPRIKA
1 CLOVE MINCED GARLIC	3 TBS. TAMARI

♣Add and sauté for 5 more minutes

4 CUPS SLICED MUSHROOMS	1/4 teasp. SAGE POWDER
3 TBS. SOVEX SMOKED YEAST	1/4 teasp. THYME
1/2 teasp. VEGETABLE SALT	1/2 teasp. PAPRIKA

♣Reduce heat and simmer, covered for 5 to 7 minutes until tender. Add 2 TBS. WHITE WINE if mixture gets too dry. Remove tofu from the oven and spoon onion/mushroom mixture over to smother. Serve right away.

605   TOFU ENCHILADAS

For 6 big enchiladas: Preheat oven to 350°.

♣Soak 1 SMALL RED ONION in 1/4 CUP WINE VINEGAR while you make the sauce.

♣Sauté 1 SMALL CHOPPED ONION, 2 CLOVES MINCED GARLIC, and 1 CHOPPED RED BELL PEPPER until transparent in 2 TBS. OLIVE OIL.
♣Add

11/2 CUPS TOMATO SAUCE	1 teasp. CUMIN
1 VEGETABLE BOUILLON CUBE	1/2 teasp. CHILI POWDER
PINCHES of OREGANO and BASIL	

♣Bring to a boil. Reduce heat and simmer covered for 30 minutes.
♣Mix the filling in a bowl; 1 LB. FROZEN TOFU, thawed, squeezed out and crumbled, the soaked RED ONION, ONE 4 OZ. CAN CHOPPED BLACK OLIVES, and 2 CHOPPED GREEN ONIONS.

♣Assemble the enchiladas.
♣Heat a fresh WHOLE WHEAT FLOUR TORTILLA. Dip into the sauce and spoon on about 1/2 cup of filling. Top filling with some SHREDDED LETTUCE or ROMAINE, GRATED JACK CHEESE, and CRUMBLED HARD BOILED EGG. Roll up, and place seam side down in a large shallow baking dish.
♣Repeat until filling is used and enchiladas are side by side in a single layer in the dish.
♣Top with rest of sauce and scatter on A LITTLE MORE CHEESE and some CRUSHED TORTILLA CHIPS. Bake covered for 30 minutes to heat through.

Nutritional analysis: per serving; 318 calories; 15gm. protein; 32gm. carbohydrate; 5gm. fiber; 16gm. fats; 43mg. cholesterol; 255mg. calcium; 7mg. iron; 116mg. magnesium; 518mg. potassium; 13mg. sodium; 2mg. zinc.

606   TOFU SHEPHERD'S PIE
This is a hearty winter meal specialty.
For 10 servings: Preheat oven to 375°.

♣Make the topping.
♣Bake 6 POTATOES in the oven until soft. Mash them in a large bowl and beat until fluffy with

1/2 CUP PLAIN YOGURT	1/2 teasp. BLACK PEPPER
1/2 CUP COTTAGE CHEESE	3 TBS. BUTTER
1/2 teasp. SOVEX SMOKED YEAST	1 TB. TAMARI

♣Set aside.

♣Make the filling. Sauté 1 LARGE SLICED YELLOW ONION and TWO 12 OZ. TUBS FROZEN TOFU thawed, squeezed out and crumbled, in 2 TBS. OIL for 15 minutes until brown.
♣Add and sauté for 5 more minutes
5 or 6 SLICED MUSHROOMS
1/2 teasp. DRY BASIL
1/2 teasp. DRY THYME
2 teasp. ZEST SEASONING SALT or other vegetable salt
♣Place in the bottom of a greased 9 x 13 pan.

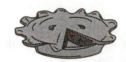

♣Spoon over 2 CUPS MAYACAMAS MUSHROOM SOUP MIX made up as a SAUCE. (See directions on the package. It's easy). You can also use 2 cups of any favorite mushroom sauce or gravy.
♣Scatter over 1 CUP FROZEN GREEN PEAS right from the freezer. Cover with the mashed poatato mix.
♣Spread evenly. Bake for 35 minutes to heat through and brown potato crust.

Nutritional anlysis:per serving; 275 calories; 11gm. protein; 38gm. carbohydrate; 5gm. fiber; 10gm. fats; 10mg. cholesterol; 122mg. calcium; 6mg. iron; 110mg. magnesium; 720mg. potassium; 210mg. sodium; 1mg. zinc.

607   ZUCCHINI TOFU PUFF

For 4 people: Preheat oven to 350°.

♣Steam 2 to 3 SMALL ZUCCHINI until just barely tender. Drain and set aside.

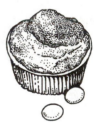

♣Mix in a bowl

1 CUP GRATED LOW-FAT CHEDDAR CHEESE	3/4 teasp. DILL WEED
3 CAKES FRESH MASHED TOFU	3 EGGS
1 teasp. ZEST SEASONING SALT or other vegetable salt	
1/2 CUP SEASONED STUFFING CUBES	

Add ZUCCHINI and mix well. Turn into a shallow lecithin-sprayed baking dish, and top with crunchy Chinese noodles or crushed corn chips. Bake for 30 minutes to blend flavors.

Nutritional analysis: per serving; 293 calories; 22gm. protein; 24gm. carbo.; 3gm. fiber; 13gm. fats; 170mg. cholesterol; 311mg. calcium; 7mg. iron; 124mg. magnesium; 428mg. potassium; 380mg. sodium; 2mg. zinc.

608   TOFU GREEN BEAN STROGANOFF

For 6 servings:

♣Bring 2-qts. salted water to a boil for 8-OZ. EGG NOODLES, and cook until just barely tender. Drain and toss with 1 teasp. OIL to separate. Place in a serving bowl.

♣Marinate 1 LB. CUBED TOFU for 30 minutes in 1/4 CUP LIGHT MISO dissolved in 2 TBS. SHERRY and 2 TBS. WATER.

♣Sauté 2 SLICED ONIONS in 3 TBS. OIL until brown.
♣Add 1 SMALL PACKAGE FRENCH CUT GREEN BEANS and sauté until tender and color changes to bright green. Add to the NOODLES and set aside.

♣Add marinade and tofu to the hot skillet. Sprinkle with 1/2 teasp. OREGANO, 1 teasp. DRY BASIL, and 1 TB. ARROWROOT dissolved in 1 TB. TAMARI. Toss to coat and add 1 CUP PLAIN YOGURT.
♣Simmer to heat through and serve over the green beans and noodles.

Nutritional analysis: per serving; 310 calories; 14gm. protein; 35gm. carbohydrate; 5gm. fiber; 13gm. fats; 26mg. cholesterol; 201mg. calcium; 7mg. iron; 122mg. magnesium; 418mg. potassium; 476mg. sodium; 2mg. zinc.

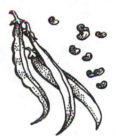

609   TOFU WITH SWEET & SOUR VEGETABLES
A nice summer meal. You can serve it in individual bowls or over a bed of thin oriental noodles.
For 4 servings:

♣Cut 1 LB. FIRM TOFU in 1/2" thick slices. Pat dry and cut into 1" squares.
♣Combine 3 TBS. TAMARI and 2 TBS. WATER in a large baking pan. Add tofu pieces and turn to coat. Let marinate for 15 minutes. Transfer to a plate and reserve marinade.

♣Sauté tofu in 1 TB. OIL until both sides are golden, about 8 minutes. Remove and keep warm.

♣Add 1 MORE TB. OIL to the skillet and sauté 1 CLOVE MINCED GARLIC and 4 THIN SLICES FRESH GINGER until aromatic.
♣Add 1/4 CUP BROWN RICE VINEGAR, 1/4 CUP RICE SYRUP, (or 2 TBS. HONEY and 3 TBS. RESERVED MARINADE) and bring to a simmer.
♣Remove ginger and stir in 1 TB. + 1 teasp. ARROWROOT POWDER mixed in 1/3 CUP WATER.
♣Cook until sauce simmers and thickens, about 2 minutes.

♣Blanch 2 JULIENNED CARROTS and 1 BUNCH BROCCOLI in florets in boiling, salted water until color changes, and they are tender crisp, about 5 minutes. Drain and set aside.
♣Combine tofu and vegetables. Pour sauce over them.
♣Toss gently and serve.

Nutritional analysis: per serving; 244 calories; 12gm. protein; 26gm. carbohydrate; 4gm. fiber; 12gm. fats; 0 cholesterol; 182mg. calcium; 7gmg. iron; 147mg. magnesium; 530mg. potassium; 170mg. sodium; 1mg. zinc.

Tofu Desserts
Tofu can take the heaviness out of dessserts
It is a smooth, non-dairy, low fat substitute for cream cheese, or ricotta cheese, or just to lighten texture.

610   TOFU LEMON RICE PUDDING

For 8 servings: This is a good kid bid. Preheat oven to 350°.

♣Toast 1 CUP SHREDDED COCONUT until light gold.

♣Mix in the blender until very light

1 LB. VERY FRESH TOFU
3 EGGS
1/2 CUP HONEY
1/4 CUP LEMON YOGURT
2 TBS. LEMON JUICE
1 1/2 teasp. VANILLA

2 TBS. MAPLE SYRUP
2 TBS. FRUCTOSE
1/2 teasp. LEMON PEEL
1/2 teasp. CINNAMON
1/2 teasp. NUTMEG

♣Turn out into a large bowl and mix with 1 CUP COOKED BROWN RICE, THE TOASTED COCONUT and 3/4 CUP RAISINS or CURRANTS.

♣Put in an oiled casserole and bake for 1 hour until fragrant and set.

Nutritional analysis: per serving; 297 calories; 9gm. protein; 44gm. carbohydrate; 4gm. fiber; 11gm. fats; 80mg. cholesterol; 109mg. calcium; 4mg. iron; 89mg. magnesium; 319mg. potassium; 37mg. sodium; 1mg. zinc.

611   CREAMY TOFU CHEESECAKE

This dessert is a custard cheesecake. Scatter sweet chopped fruits over the top before serving for a fresh touch.

For 6 slices. Use a crumb crust, or no crust at all. Preheat oven to 350°.

♣Mix the cake in the blender
2 EGGS
1 LB. VERY FRESH TOFU
2/3 CUP HONEY
2 TBS. MAPLE SYRUP
2 TBS. FRUCTOSE
8-OZ. KEFIR CHEESE or PLAIN YOGURT
3 TBS. LEMON JUICE
1 1/2 teasp. VANILLA

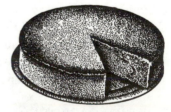

♣Turn into crust or oiled 8 x 8" square pan. Bake for 1 hour. Remove, dust with a little NUTMEG, cool and chill.

Nutritional analysis: per serving w/o crust; 253 calories; 10gm. protein; 44gm. carbo. 1gm. fiber; 6gm. fats; 73mg. cholesterol; 167mg. calcium; 5mg. iron; 89mg. magnesium; 241mg. potassium; 41mg. sodium; 1mg. zinc.

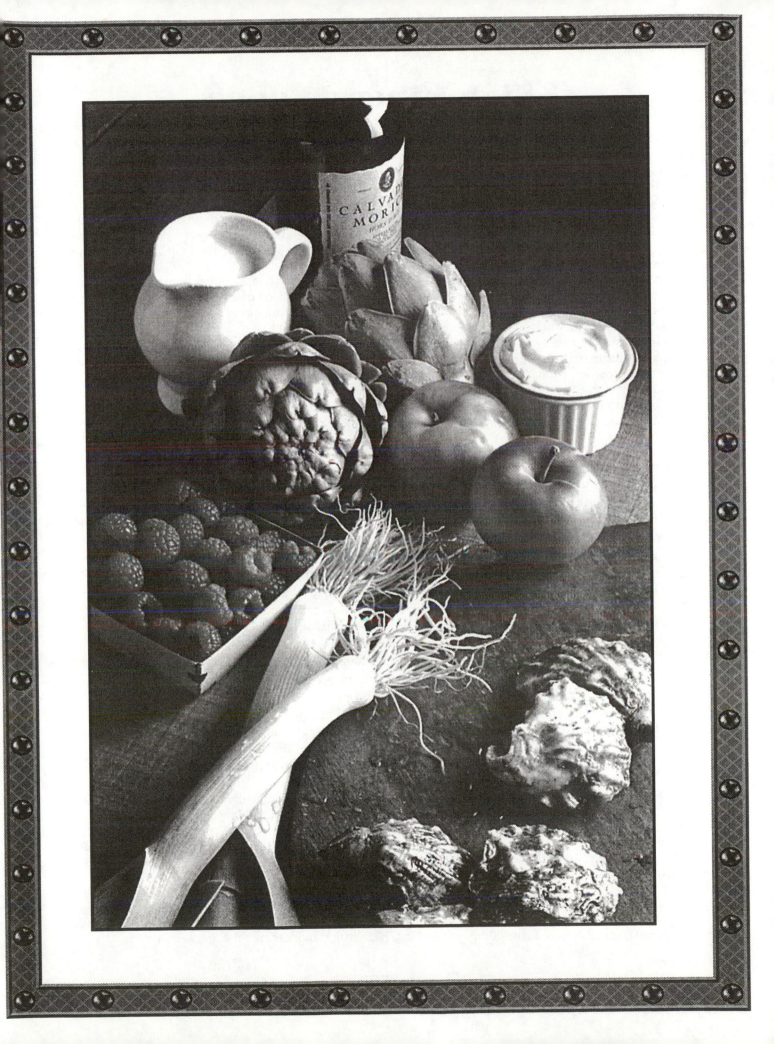

High Mineral Foods

MINERALS - the building blocks of life. Absolutely necessary for athletes and sporty people, because you must have minerals to run. Needed by everybody for good health and an active life.

Hardly any of us get enough.

Minerals are the most basic of nutrients. They are the bonding agents between you and your food. Without them, the body cannot absorb its nutrition.

Minerals are essential to bone formation, and to the digestion of food. They regulate the body's acid/alkaline balance, the osmosis of cellular fluids, electrical activity in the nervous system, and most metabolic actions. They transport oxygen through the system, balance heart activity, help you sleep, give you strength, and are keys to mental and spiritual balance.

Even small deficiencies can cause severe depression, paranoia, P.M.S. and other menstrual disorders, hyperactivity in children, sugar imbalances such as hypoglycemia or diabetes, nerve and emotional problems, heart disease, high blood pressure, osteoporosis, premature aging of skin and hair, memory loss, and the inability to heal quickly.

Minerals cannot be synthesized by the body, but must be obtained through food, drink or mineral baths. Unfortunately, many minerals and trace minerals are no longer present in the foods we eat. They have been leached from the soil by the chemicals, sprays and other current practices of commercial farming. Even many foods that still show measurable amounts of mineral composition have less quality and quantity than we are led to believe. Most testing was done decades ago, when sprays, pesticides, fertilizers and chemicals were not as prolific as they are now.

To help you incorporate high mineral foods in your diet, the listing below includes the most important mineral rich foods. The recipes in this section will concentrate on the use of these foods.

❦**Foods rich in calcium:** sesame seeds, salmon, sea veggies, tofu, cheese, oysters, leafy greens, most nuts and legumes, olives, broccoli, brown rice, wheat germ, figs, dates, raisins, onions, leeks and chives.

❦**Foods rich in potassium:** sea vegetables, brown rice, tofu and other soy foods, beans, nuts and seeds, most dried fruits, raisins, dates, bananas, broccoli, garlic, mushrooms, potatoes and yams.

❦**Foods rich in iron:** amaranth, wheat and wheat germ, millet, fish, molasses, chard, spinach and other dark greens, pumpkin and sunflower seeds, turkey, black beans, raisins, prunes and peaches.

❦**Foods rich in chromium:** potatoes, bananas, turkey and chicken, green peppers, leafy greens, brewer's yeast, organ meats, mushrooms, corn, carrots, wheat germ and fish.

❦**Foods rich in magnesium:** poultry, organ meats, mushrooms, cheese, brewer's yeast, lettuce, celery, water chestnuts, tofu, soy foods, nuts, seeds, sea plants and sea foods, whole grains and legumes.

❦**Foods rich in zinc:** nuts and seeds, oysters, liver and organ meats, eggs, raw milk, brewer's yeast, beans, peas and leafy greens, whole grains, mushrooms, maple syrup, onions and leeks.

❦**Foods rich in chlorine:** tomatoes, celery, lettuce, kelp and sea vegetables, dark leafy greens, cabbage, radishes, eggplant, cucumber, potatoes and yams, carrots, cauliflower, leeks and onions.

❦**Foods rich in copper:** oysters, liver and organ meats, nuts, peas and beans, mushrooms, avocados, leafy greens, whole grains, sea vegetables, blueberries, raisins, and fish.

❦**Foods rich in phosphorus:** yogurt, poultry, fish, nuts, brewer's yeast, cereals, peas and beans.

Mineral content is higher and more absorbable in fresh foods. Organically grown, unsprayed fruits, vegetables and herbs are the best sources of both vitamins and minerals. This section includes:
❧HIGH MINERAL SOUPS & SALADS ❧HIGH MINERAL SEAFOODS ❧MINERAL PACKED ONION FAMILY FOODS FOR HEALING ❧QUICHES & VEGETABLE PIES - FULL OF MINERALS ❧TURKEY & CHICKEN - HIGH MINERAL MEATS ❧SAVORY BAKING FOR MINERALS ❧MINERAL RICH DESSERTS ❧

Minerals help keep the body pH balanced - alkaline instead of acid. For our purposes in these diets, high calcium recipes include more than 200mg., and high magnesium more than 100mg. per serving. High potassium is more than 400mg. per serving. High iron is more than 2 mg. per serving.

High Mineral Soups & Salads

These recipes are particularly beneficial to the bone, muscle and tissue re-building part of a healing diet.

612   BLACK BEAN SOUP

This soup has outstanding nutrition. It is purifying, strengthening, and alkalizing, with protein for healing.
Enough for 10 servings:

♣Use a very large soup pot. This recipe makes enough for 10 servings or several days. It also freezes well for use later.

♣Soak $2^1/_2$ CUPS DRIED BLACK BEANS in 10 CUPS WATER overnight.

♣Sauté 2 CLOVES MINCED GARLIC and 1 CHOPPED ONION in 2 TBS. OIL until very brown.

♣Add and bring to a boil
THE SOAKED BEANS   1 CUP WATER
2 TBS. VEGEX YEAST PASTE or DARK MISO PASTE   1 CUP ROSÉ WINE
9 CUPS VEGETABLE STOCK or BOUILLON

♣Reduce heat. Simmer uncovered for $1^1/_2$ to 2 hours stirring occasionally. Keep beans covered with liquid. Remove from heat to cool slightly. Purée soup in the blender in batches and return to the pot.

♣Add $1/_4$ CUP MADIERA or MARSALA WINE, 1 teasp. BLACK PEPPER, and 1 teasp. SEA SALT.
♣Heat through and ladle into shallow bowls. Top with crumbled hard boiled egg and lemon slices.

Nutritional analysis: per serving; 177 calories; 9gm. protein; 26gm. carbohydrate; 9gm. fiber; 3gm. fats; 21mg. cholesterol; 56mg. calcium; 83mg. magnesium; 2mg. iron; 416mg. potassium; 480mg. sodium; 2mg. zinc.

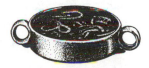

613   REAL FRENCH ONION SOUP

The secret to the real thing is the fresh herbs. A small herb garden can be a wonderful culinary goldmine.
For 4 to 6 servings:

♣Make a *bouquet garni* in a muslin bag or piece of cheesecloth with a twisty: Use 1 fresh sprig of <u>each</u>: BAY LEAF, PARSLEY, THYME, GARLIC CLOVE, ROSEMARY, MARJORAM, and DILL WEED.

♣Sauté 4 to 6 CUPS THIN SLICED ONIONS in 2 TBS. OLIVE OIL with a PINCH of SEA SALT for about 5 minutes until aromatic. Partially cover and sauté for 45 minutes more, until onions are $1/_3$ of their original volume and are sweet and golden brown.

♣Add 6 CUPS WATER or LIGHT STOCK and bouquet garni, with SEA SALT, and TAMARI or LIGHT MISO to taste. Simmer for 30 minutes. Remove *bouquet garni*, re-season if necessary.

♣Serve over buttered toast rounds. Snip on GREEN ONIONS and PARSLEY for garnish.

Nutritional analysis: per serving w/ toast; 104 calories; 3gm. protein; 18gm. carbohydrate; 3gm. fiber; 3gm. fats; 0 cholesterol; 46mg. calcium; 29mg. magnesium; 278mg. potassium; 1mg. iron; 200mg. sodium; 1mg. zinc.

614   PAELLA POLLO

This is a low-fat version of the usual Spanish stew; but still very fragrant with tomatos and peppers.
For 8 servings: Preheat oven to 350°.

♣Peel ¹/₂ LB. FRESH SHRIMP and sprinkle with 1 TB. LEMON JUICE in a bowl.

♣Open and drain ONE JAR FIRE ROASTED BELL PEPPERS.

♣Chop 2 LARGE TOMATOES.

♣Skin and bone 3 WHOLE CHICKEN BREASTS. Cut in long strips. Season with SEA SALT and LEMON PEPPER.

♣Sauté 2 CLOVES MINCED GARLIC in 4 TBS. OLIVE OIL in a paella pan or very large ovenproof skillet until aromatic. Add chicken pieces and sauté until opaque and tender, about 7 to 8 minutes. Remove with a slotted spoon and reserve.

♣Add SHRIMP and toss until just pink, about 2 minutes. Remove with a slotted spoon and reserve.

♣Add 1 MORE TB. OLIVE OIL and sauté 1 SLICED ONION until transparent, about 3 minutes. Add 2 SLICED TURKEY WEINERS, THE TOMATOES and ROASTED PEPPERS and sauté for 2 minutes.

♣Add 2 CUPS BROWN RICE and toss til grains are opaque amd coated with oil.

♣Add

3¹/₂ CUPS CHICKEN STOCK   PINCH SAFFRON

¹/₂ CUP DRY VERMOUTH or WHITE WINE   ¹/₂ teasp. PEPPER

2 TBS. CHOPPED CHIVES   ¹/₂ teasp. HERBS DE PROVENCE

♣Add 1 cup FROZEN PEAS and cook uncovered just until color changes to bright green. Most of the liquid should now be absorbed. Re-season if necessary.

♣Lay chicken and shrimp over rice, burying shrimp and pushing chicken halfway under.

♣Place pan in oven and bake for 15 minutes. Remove from oven. Cover loosely with foil and let rest to steam for 5 minutes. Sprinkle with CHOPPED CILANTRO.

Nutritional analysis: per serving; 430 calories; 25gm. protein; 46gm. carbohydrate; 4gm. fiber; 15gm. fats; 95mg. cholesterol; 88mg. calcium; 4mg. iron; 107mg. magnesium; 536mg. potassium; 380mg. sodium; 3mg. zinc.

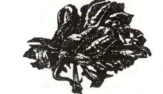

615   FLORENTINE SPINACH SOUP

For 4 one cup servings:

♣Sauté ¹/₂ CUP SLICED GREEN ONIONS, ¹/₂ CUP SLICED CELERY, and 2 teasp. ANISE SEED in 1 TB. OLIVE OIL for 8 minutes until fragrant.

♣Add 1 BUNCH RINSED, DRAINED, CHOPPED SPINACH LEAVES, ¹/₄ teasp. PEPPER, and 3 CUPS CHICKEN BROTH. Bring to a boil, reduce heat and simmer for 10 minutes.

♣Pour into serving bowls and top with THIN LEMON SLICES and PARMESAN CHEESE.

Nutritional analysis: per serving; 72 calories; 3gm. protein; 6gm. carbohydrate; 3gm. fiber; 4gm. fats; 2mg. cholesterol; 110mg. calcium; 2mg. iron; 47mg. magnesium; 474mg. potassium; 200mg. sodium; 1mg. zinc.

616   ITALIAN SPINACH SALAD

For 6 people: Preheat oven to 400°.

♣Toss together 1¹/₂ CUPS WHOLE WHEAT BREAD CUBES, 1 TB. SOY BACON BITS, 2 TBS. ITALIAN DRESSING and 2 TBS. PARMESAN CHEESE. Bake for 10 minutes until light brown. Set aside.

♣Wash and tear 1 BUNCH SPINACH LEAVES. Mix in a large salad bowl with 2 CUPS SHREDDED RED CABBAGE, 1 CUP TOFU CUBES and 1 CUP SLICED WATER-PACKED ARTICHOKE HEARTS. Pour over ¹/₂ CUP MORE ITALIAN DRESSING and marinate for 30 minutes.

♣Toss all together with the toasted crouton blend and serve.

Nutritional analysis: per serving; 142 calories; 8gm. protein; 17gm. carbohydrate; 6gm. fiber; 6gm. fats; 3mg. cholesterol; 134mg. calcium; 4mg. iron; 100mg. magnesium; 373mg. potassium; 400mg. sodium; 1mg. zinc.

617   FRESH BROCCOLI SALAD

For 4 to 6 people:

♣Blanch 2 BUNCHES CHOPPED BROCCOLI FLORETS and STEMS in a large pot of boiling salted water until bright green. Rinse under cold water to set color. Drain and set aside in a serving dish.

♣Mix and toss the sauce
JUICE OF 2 LEMONS
¹/₂ CUP LIGHT MAYONNAISE
¹/₂ CUP PLAIN YOGURT
4 TBS. CHOPPED CHIVES

¹/₂ teasp. DIJON MUSTARD
¹/₂ teasp. TARRAGON
¹/₂ teasp. BLACK PEPPER

♣Chill to blend flavors, spoon over broccoli and grate LOW-FAT CHEDDAR CHEESE over the top.

618   HOT POTATO GREEN BEAN SALAD

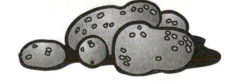

For 4 to 6 people:

♣Steam 1 LB. SMALL THIN SLICED RED POTATOES, and 8-OZ. FRENCH CUT FROZEN GREEN BEANS for 10 minutes until just tender.

♣Heat 2 TBS. OIL in a skillet and sauté 2 TBS. SESAME SEEDS until golden.
♣Add ¹/₂ CUP THIN SLICED SCALLIONS, 1 TB. LEMON JUICE, ¹/₄ teasp. SEA SALT, and ¹/₄ teasp. PEPPER and sauté until fragrant.
♣Toss with potatoes and beans and serve hot.

Nutritional analysis: per serving; 204 calories; 5gm. protein; 34mg. carbohydrate; 5gm. fiber; 6gm. fats; 0 cholesterol; 59mg. calcium; 3mg. iron; 65mg. magnesium; 653mg. potassium; 149mg. sodium; 1mg. zinc.

619   HOT PASTA SALAD WITH BROCCOLI & CASHEWS

For 6 to 8 servings:

♣Bring 4-qts. salted pasta water to a boil while you are making the salad. Add 1 LB. PASTA SHELLS and cook until *al dente*. Drain and toss with 1 teasp. OIL.
♣Toast 1 CUP CASHEWS in the oven til golden.
♣Sauté 6 CUPS BROCCOLI FLORETS and STEMS, 2 CUPS SLICED MUSHROOMS and 2 CUPS CHOPPED SCALLIONS in 4 TBS. OIL until color changes.
♣Sprinkle with 1¹/₂ CUPS FRESH CHOPPED PARSLEY and remove from heat.

♣Mix a quick dressing
¹/₃ CUP LIGHT MAYONNAISE
¹/₂ CUP PLAIN YOGURT
1 teasp. DIJON MUSTARD
♣Toss pasta, vegetables and dressing together, and serve in large shallow salad/soup bowls. Top with DICED TOMATOES and THE TOASTED CASHEWS.

620   TUNA TOMATO SALAD

This is like a fresh tuna casserole.
For 2 people:

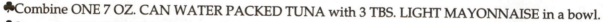

♣Combine ONE 7 OZ. CAN WATER PACKED TUNA with 3 TBS. LIGHT MAYONNAISE in a bowl.
♣Steam 1 CUP FROZEN PEAS until bright green and drain. Add to tuna. Add 2 CHOPPED TOMA-TOES, and 3 CHOPPED GREEN ONIONS. Season with GREAT 28 MIX or other vegetable salt, and 1 teasp. TAMARI. Serve in lettuce cups. Sprinkle CRUNCHY CHINESE NOODLES over top.

Nutritional analysis: per serving; 336 calories; 31gm. protein; 20gm. carbohydrate; 6gm. fiber; 6gm. fats; 56mg. cholesterol; 57mg. calcium; 3mg. iron; 66mg. magnesium; 742mg. potassium; 530mg. sodium; 2mg. zinc.

621   LOW-FAT SWEET & SOUR COLESLAW

For 4 salads:

♣Shred 2 CUPS GREEN CABBAGE in a food processor.
♣Mix the dressing in a bowl and toss with cabbage.

2 TBS. PLAIN YOGURT
2 TBS. LIGHT MAYONNAISE
¹/₂ teasp. DIJON MUSTARD
¹/₂ teasp. MIXED SALAD HERBS (pg. 645)
1¹/₂ TBS. LEMON JUICE

1 teasp. FRUCTOSE
¹/₄ teasp. VEGETABLE SALT
¹/₄ teasp. SESAME SALT
¹/₄ teasp. PEPPER

♣Chill for 1 hour before serving to blend flavors.

High Mineral Seafoods

Ocean foods of all kinds are a primary source of nutritional minerals.
Here are some delicious ways to add them to your diet.

622 BAKED SALMON LOAF WITH FRESH BASIL SAUCE

For 4 servings: Preheat oven to 375°.

♣Mix all ingredients together and press into a greased loaf pan

1/2 CUP GRANOLA
1/2 CUP WHITE WINE
2 TBS. LIGHT MAYONNAISE
2 BEATEN EGGS
One 16 OZ. CAN or 1 LB. FRESH SKINNED SALMON

2 TBS. CHOPPED PARSLEY
2 TBS. MINCED SHALLOTS
1 teasp. HERB SALT
1/2 teasp. PEPPER

♣Bake for 50 to 60 minutes until set. Let rest for 10 minutes while you make the FRESH BASIL SAUCE.

♣Make the sauce in the blender

1/3 CUP PACKED FRESH BASIL LEAVES
1/2 teasp. GARLIC/LEMON SEASONING

2 TBS. PARMESAN CHEESE
6 TBS. OLIVE OIL

♣Pour over loaf before cutting, and sprinkle with 2 TBS. CHOPPED WALNUTS.

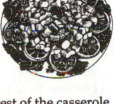

623 SALMON NOODLE CASSEROLE

For 4 people: Preheat oven to 425°.

♣Bring 2-qts. salted water to boil in a large pot for the pasta while you make the rest of the casserole.

♣Sauté 1/4 CUP CHOPPED ONION and 1/4 LB. SLICED MUSHROOMS in 2 TBS. OIL until aromatic.
♣Sprinkle with 2 TBS. WHOLE WHEAT FLOUR and stir until bubbly. Add 3/4 CUP PLAIN YOGURT and 1/4 CUP WATER and cook stirring until mixture is the consistency of heavy cream.
♣Season with

1/2 teasp. ZEST or SPIKE SEASONING SALT
1/2 teasp. SALAD HERBS (page 645)
1/4 teasp. WHITE PEPPER

♣Add 1 CUP FROZEN GREEEN PEAS and 1 SMALL 7 OZ. CAN SALMON with LIQUID.

♣Cook 4-OZ. SPINACH NOODLES in the boiling water to *al dente.* Drain and toss with the salmon mixture.
♣Turn all into a buttered casserole and sprinkle with crushed whole grain cracker crumbs *or* seasoned bread crumbs.
♣Bake for 20 minutes until golden brown and heated through.

Nutritional analysis: per serving; 300 calories; 19gm. protein; 36gm. carbohydrate; 4gm. fiber; 9gm. fats; 38mg. cholesterol; 110mg. calcium; 58mg. magnesium; 3mg. iron; 589mg. potassium; 119mg. sodium; 2mg. zinc.

624   ARTICHOKE & SALMON PASTA SALAD

This recipe can be really fancy if you cook four fresh artichokes; remove the the hearts, and fill the artichoke cup with the salad.

For 4 entree size salads:

♣Rinse and slice FRESH COOKED ARTICHOKE HEARTS, or ONE 11 OZ. JAR WATER-PACKED ARTI-CHOKE HEARTS. Set aside.

♣Cook 8 OZ. ORZO (rice style pasta) in boiling salted water, until just tender but still separate grains.

♣Mix in a bowl

1/2 CUP LIGHT MAYONNAISE   4 teasp. DIJON MUSTARD
1/2 CUP PLAIN YOGURT   4 teasp. DRY DILL WEED
4-OZ. COOKED or CANNED FLAKED SALMON   1/4 teasp. LEMON PEPPER
1 GREEN ONION, CHOPPED   1/4 teasp. SEA SALT

♣Toss with artichoke hearts and orzo and serve in artichoke leaf or lettuce cups.

Nutritional analysis: per serving; 365 calories; 19gm. protein; 55gm. carbohydrate; 9gm. fiber; 8gm. fats; 28mg. cholesterol; 126mg. calcium; 83mg. magnesium; 4mg. iron; 569mg. potassium; 530mg. sodium; 2mg. zinc.

625   SCALLOPS WITH SWEET ONIONS

For 2 entree salads:

♣Tear, rinse and pat dry 2 CUPS TART GREENS, such as RADICCHIO, ARUGULA, ENDIVE or RO-MAINE. Set aside to chill.

♣Slice and sauté 3/4 CUP THIN-SLICED SWEET ONIONS and 4-OZ. SLICED SCALLOPS in 1 TB. OLIVE OIL and 1 TB. BALSAMIC VINEGAR until scallops are just opaque and onions are translucent.

♣Mix onions and scallops together with

2 TBS. OLIVE OIL   1/4 teasp. SEA SALT
2 teasp. LEMON JUICE   1/4 teasp. WHITE PEPPER

♣Divide greens on salad plates and spoon on scallops.

Nutritional analysis: per serving; 204 calories; 11gm. protein; 9gm. carbohydrate; 2gm. fiber; 14gm. fats; 18mg. cholesterol; 55mg. calcium; 1mg. iron; 44mg. magnesium; 457mg. potassium; 361mg. sodium; 1mg. zinc.

626   HALIBUT IN HERB DRESSING

For 4 servings:

♣Have ready 4 TRIMMED HALIBUT STEAKS. Bring to a boil and boil rapidly for 5 minutes

4 CUPS WATER   1 CHOPPED CARROT
2 CUPS WHITE WINE   8 to 10 PEPPERCORNS
1 CHOPPED ONION   1 BOUQUET GARNI

♣Reduce to a simmer and poach halibut until almost opaque, about 5 minutes. Remove and transfer to a serving plate while you make the **HERB SAUCE.**

♣Whisk together
1 teasp. DIJON MUSTARD
2 TBS. SHERRY
2 TBS. BALSAMIC VINEGAR
1/4 CUP OLIVE OI
1/4 CUP SALAD OIL
1 teasp. DRY CHERVIL
2 TBS. MINCED SHALLOTS

1 teasp. SESAME SALT
1/2 teasp. WHITE PEPPER
1 TB. MINCED CHIVES
1 teasp. DRY TARRAGON

Mineral Packed Onion Family Foods For Healing

Onions, garlic, scallions, shallots, leeks and chives have long been known for their anti-biotic,
anti-viral and anti-carcinogenic qualities. And they are so delicious, too.
This recipe section concentrates on ways to add the onion family to your nutritional healing program.

627   LEEK AND PASTA TERRINE

Definitely a company recipe. Show off your gourmet talents and give them mineral riches at the same time.
For 8 people: Preheat oven to 350°.

♣Soak 4 BLACK SHIITAKE MUSHROOMS in water until soft. Sliver and discard woody stems. Save soaking water.
♣Heat 3 TBS. OLIVE OIL and sauté 3 CLOVES MINCED GARLIC, 1 SLICED YELLOW ONION, 4 DICED CARROTS and 8-OZ. SLICED MUSHROOMS for 8 to 10 minutes until aromatic.
♣Reduce heat to medium and add

2 CUPS CHOPPED ROMA TOMATOES
THE SLIVERED BLACK MUSHROOMS
1/2 CUP ROSÉ WINE

2 teasp. DRY THYME
2 teasp. ITALIAN SEASONING

♣Partially cover and let bubble for 30 minutes. Turn off heat and set aside.

♣Meanwhile, trim and slice 12 LEEKS (mostly white parts).
♣Bring 4 CUPS SALTED WATER and the MUSHROOM SOAKING WATER to a boil, and simmer LEEKS for 15 minutes until tender. Drain and rinse in cool water to stop cooking. Set aside.
♣Melt 4 TBS. BUTTER in a saucepan. Add 6 TBS. WHOLE WHEAT FLOUR and stir until bubbly for 1 minute. Add 1 CUP PLAIN YOGURT and 1 CUP CHICKEN BROTH. Whisk until thick and smooth.
♣Stir in 1 CARTON KEFIR CHEESE and 1/2 SMALL CARTON COTTAGE CHEESE. Re-season with Italian herbs if necessary. Remove from heat and set aside.

♣Assemble the terrine in a large buttered mold. Line mold with waxed paper, and spray paper with lecithin spray. Distribute LEEK SLICES over bottom of dish. Spoon on 1 CUP TOMATO/VEGETABLE mix.
♣Top with another layer of Leeks. Cover with YOGURT/CHEESE sauce. Repeat layers until dish is filled, ending with the cheese sauce. Bake til bubbly and set for 45 minutes. Let sit for 30 minutes to an hour. ♣Unmold onto a serving platter. Remove waxed paper and slice.

Nutritional analysis: per serving; 277 calories; 10gm. protein; 35gm. carbohydrate; 7gm. fiber; 11gm. fats; 20mg. cholesterol; 189mg. calcium; 4mg. iron; 70mg. magnesium; 757mg. potassium; 222mg. sodium; 1mg. zinc.

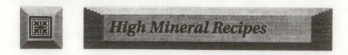
628   ROAST YORKSHIRE PUDDING

The ultimate onion popover; it's really a savory dinner side dish.

For 8 servings: Preheat oven to 500°.

♣Roast 4 LARGE QUARTERED YELLOW ONIONS in 1/4 CUP BALSAMIC VINEGAR and 2 TBS. OLIVE OIL in a shallow baking pan until brown and sweetly aromatic, about 40 minutes. Baste with the marinade avery 10 minutes to keep moist and flavorful.
♣Remove from the oven and let cool in the pan. Keep quarters intact. Dot with butter.
♣Reduce oven to 375°. Heat onions until sizzly - about 5 minutes.
♣Whirl 1 CUP WHOLE WHEAT FLOUR, 1/2 CUP PLAIN YOGURT, 1/2 CUP WATER and 2 EGGS in the blender until smooth. Pour *around* onions, (not on top) and bake until well browned and puffy, about 35 to 40 minutes. Serve hot with butter.

629   GLAZED PEARL ONIONS & BABY CARROTS

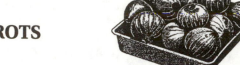

For 4 servings:

♣Braise one 10-OZ. PACKAGE of PEARL ONIONS in a little water or broth in a skillet for 10 minutes until tender. Set aside.
♣Add a little more water or broth and braise 1 LB. SLICED BABY CARROTS for 7 minutes. Drain and set aside.
♣Add 2 TBS. BUTTER, 2 TBS. LEMON JUICE, 1 TB. HONEY, 1 TB. COCOA or CAROB POWDER and 1 teasp. FRESH GRATED GINGER. Stir til fragrant.
♣Add vegetables and raise heat. Stir til sauce thickens and coats vegetables, about 2 to 3 minutes.
♣Serve hot in a bowl with SNIPPED PARSLEY.

Nutritional analysis: per serving; 158 calories; 2gm. protein; 25gm. carbohydrate; 6gm. fiber; 6gm. fats; 15mg. cholesterol; 68mg. calcium; 1mg. iron; 31mg. magnesium; 568mg. potassium; 46mg. sodium; 1mg. zinc

630   ROAST SHALLOTS

Shallots are such sweet little morsels. I wish they weren't so expensive so that we could have them more often. These are excellent with grilled fish.
For 6 servings: Preheat oven to 350°.

♣Peel 24 LARGE SHALLOTS but leave the root end on. Toss them *on a cast iron skillet* with

3/4 teasp. SESAME SALT
2 BAY LEAVES or 2 MINT SPRIGS
3 THYME SPRIGS or 1/2 teasp. DRY

1/4 teasp. WHITE PEPPER
2 TBS. OLIVE OIL
PINCH FRUCTOSE

♣Cover skillet with foil, and roast in the oven for 30 minutes. Uncover and roast for 30 minutes more until tender. Increase heat to 450° and roast for 10 minutes to caramelize.

631   SAVORY ONION TORTE

For 6 servings: Preheat oven to 350°.

♣Make a simple, quick crust by crushing 35 WHOLE GRAIN CRACKERS, mixing them with 6 TBS. MELTED BUTTER and pressing into a 9" pie plate. Bake for 5 minutes to brown. Remove from oven and set aside.

♣Sauté 5 SLICED YELLOW ONIONS in 3 TBS. BUTTER until aromatic. Spread over the crust.

♣Make the filling in the blender.
4 EGGS
1 LB. SOFT FRESH TOFU
1 TB. CHOPPED PARSLEY
1 teasp. DRY BASIL

♣Add
1 teasp. DRY THYME
1 teasp. SEA SALT
1/4 teasp. PEPPER
1/4 teasp. NUTMEG

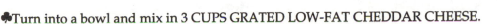

♣Turn into a bowl and mix in 3 CUPS GRATED LOW-FAT CHEDDAR CHEESE.
♣Spread over onions. Dust with PAPRIKA. Bake for 1 hour until set.

Nutritional analysis: per serving; 475 calories; 27gm. protein; 27gm. carbo.; 5gm. fiber; 28gm. fats; 180mg. cholesterol; 493mg. calcium; 6mg. iron; 128mg. magnesium; 497mg. potassium; 598mg. sodium; 3mg. zinc.

632   ROMAN ONIONS

As you can probably tell by now, we love Italian and Mediterranean cooking, for its simplicity and of- the -earth quality. One always feels like the garden is right around the corner, and the sun is smiling on it. It's the reason eating al fresco is such a pleasure.
For 6 servings: Preheat oven to 350°.

♣Sauté 4 SLICED YELLOW ONIONS in 2 TBS. OIL and 2 TBS. BUTTER until golden.
♣Add 4 SLICED HARD BOILED EGGS and toss to combine. Put in a lecithin-sprayed baking dish.

♣Make a **WHITE WINE SAUCE** in the sauté pan.
♣Melt 2 TBS. BUTTER and add 2 TBS. UNBLEACHED FLOUR. Stir until bubbly and golden.
♣Add
1/2 CUP PLAIN YOGURT
1/2 CUP WHITE WINE
1/2 teasp. DRY MUSTARD
♣Stir and cook til thickened and smooth.

♣Pour over onions. Top with 1 CUP GRATED CHEDDAR CHEESE and 2 TBS. CHOPPED PARSLEY.
♣Sprinkle with 1/2 CUP WHOLE WHEAT BREAD CRUMBS or TOASTED WHEAT GERM, and bake for 25 to 30 minutes. Let rest for a few minutes before serving.

Nutritional analysis: per serving; 230 calories; 15gm. protein; 11gm. carbos; 1gm. fiber; 14gm. fats; 169mg. cholesterol; 255mg. calcium; 1mg. iron; 23mg. magnesium; 148mg. potassium; 370mg. sodium; 1mg. zinc.

Quiches & Vegetable Pies; Full Of Minerals

Quiches and vegetable pies are a delicious way to get vegetables and other ingredients that are rich in minerals. They are easy to make, one-dish meals that just about everybody likes. They are light, yet full of nutrition. You can eat just a small amount and feel satisfied. Each quiche is enough for 8 to 10 servings.

A quiche is good place to use your imagination, starting with the crust. Use vegetable crusts, crumb crusts, light dough crusts, chip crusts, or no crust at all. See page 226 for suggestions. A lovely one is included below.

633   QUICHE CRUST PERFECTION

Preheat oven to 450°.

♣Mix until foamy
1/3 cup PLAIN YOGURT
1/3 CUP WATER
1 teasp. BAKING SODA
2 teasp. CREAM OF TARTAR

♣Add and mix in
1/2 CUP OIL
4 TBS. MELTED BUTTER
1/4 CUP HONEY
1/2 teasp. SEA SALT

♣Mix together
1 3/4 CUP UNBLEACHED FLOUR
1/4 CUP OAT OR RYE FLOUR

1/2 CUP BRAN FLAKES
2 TBS. TOASTED SESAME SEEDS

♣Combine the 2 mixtures. Knead briefly on a floured surface, and roll or pat into a greased quiche pan. Prick bottom and bake for 5 minutes. Remove and cool for filling.

634   DEEP GREENS QUICHE

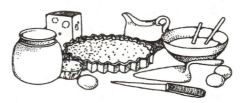

Preheat oven to 400°.

♣Prepare a quiche crust. See our suggestions or use your own.

♣Make the filling. Sauté 1 CUP SLICED MUSHROOMS in a skillet in 3 TBS. BUTTER til aromatic.
♣Sprinkle on 1 TB. WHOLE WHEAT FLOUR and stir for 1 minute. Spoon onto the quiche crust.
♣Add a little more butter in the skillet if it is dry and sauté 2 TBS. CHOPPED SHALLOTS and 1/2 teasp. HERBS DE PROVENCE until fragrant. Add 2 CUPS CHOPPED MIXED GREENS (such as SPINACH, CHARD, or ROMAINE), and simmer just until wilted, about 1 minute. Puree in the blender until smooth. Pour greens over mushrooms. Sprinkle with 1 CUP GRATED LOW-FAT SWISS CHEESE.

♣Make the sauce in the blender
4 EGGS
1 CUP PLAIN YOGURT
1/4 CUP WHITE WINE
1/4 CUP WATER
1/2 teasp. SESAME SALT

1/4 teasp. PEPPER
1/4 teasp. NUTMEG
1/2 teasp. FRUCTOSE
DASHES HOT PEPPER SAUCE

♣Pour over quiche and bake on the bottom oven rack for 15 minutes. Reduce heat to 325° and bake for 30 minutes more, until puffy, brown and set. Cool slightly and serve.

635   BROCCOLI CHEESE QUICHE

For 8 slices: Preheat oven to 400°.

♣This is a good quiche to use with a seasoned bread crumb crust. Just mix 2 1/2 CUPS CRUMBS with 1 EGG and 2 to 3 TBS. WATER and bake for 15 minutes until crisp and golden. Reduce heat to 325°.

♣Cover crust with 1 CUP GRATED CHEDDAR (or ONE 8-OZ. CARTON SOY CREAM CHEESE).

♣Blanch 1 BUNCH *SLICED* BROCCOLI FLORETS in boiling water until color changes to bright green.
♣Drain and layer on top of cheese. Top with 1 CUP GRATED LOW FAT SWISS CHEESE.

♣Make the sauce in the blender
1 CUP PLAIN YOGURT	2 TBS. CHOPPED SCALLIONS
1/4 CUP WHITE WINE	1 teasp. SALAD HERB MIX
1/4 CUP WATER	1/2 teasp. PAPRIKA
4 EGGS	1/4 teasp. WHITE PEPPER

♣Pour over quiche and bake for 1 hour until puffy and brown, and a knife inserted in the center comes out clean. Let set 5 minutes before slicing.

Nutritional analysis: per serving; 270 calories; 16gm. protein; 28gm. carbo.; 2gm. fiber; 10gm. fats; 152mg. cholesterol; 304mg. calcium; 2mg. iron; 33mg. magnesium; 280mg. potassium; 370mg. sodium; 2mg. zinc.

636   PARTY ARTICHOKE QUICHE

Preheat oven to 325°.

♣The best crust for this quiche is a simple one. Mix 1 1/4 CUPS UNBLEACHED FLOUR with 4 TBS. BUTTER, and 1 EGG until crumbly. Press into a quiche pan and bake at 350∞ for 5 to 8 minutes. Remove and cool for filling.

♣Grate your choice of CHEESES or SOY CHEESES ONTO THE CRUST to a 1" thickness.
♣Slice 1 LARGE (11 OZ.) JAR of water packed ARTICHOKES and arrange on top of the cheeses.

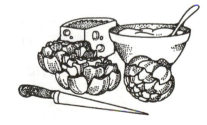

♣Sauté in 2 TBS. BUTTER until aromatic
1 teasp. DIJON MUSTARD
1/2 CUP SLICED MUSHROOMS
1/4 CUP SLICED GREEN ONIONS
♣Layer on top of artichokes.

♣Make the sauce in the blender
3 EGGS	2 TBS. SHERRY
1/2 CUP PLAIN YOGURT	1/2 teasp. 5 SPICE POWDER
1/4 CUP WATER	

♣Pour over quiche . Lightly sprinkle with nutmeg and bake until firm.

637   SHRIMP & SCALLION QUICHE

For 8 slices: Preheat oven to 375°.
♣Have ready a prepared quiche shell or crust.

♣Slice 1 BUNCH SCALLIONS CROSSWISE. Separate green and white parts. Sauté WHITE PARTS in 4 TBS. Butter and 4 TBS. OIL with 1 TB. CHOPPED FRESH GINGER until fragrant.
♣Stir in 8-OZ. TINY COOKED SHRIMP. Heat briefly and turn into quiche shell.
♣Add seasonings to the skillet and stir until fragrant

1 teasp. TAMARI	3 TBS. SHERRY
3 TBS. WHOLE GRAIN FLOUR	1 teasp. FRUCTOSE

♣Combine custard ingredients in the blender

4 EGGS	1/2 teasp. SEA SALT
1 CUP PLAIN YOGURT	1/4 teasp. PEPPER
1/2 CUP WATER	PINCH NUTMEG
1/2 CUP KEFIR CHEESE	3 TBS. SHERRY

♣Pour over quiche and bake for 45 minutes until set when shaken. Let set for 10 minutes. Serve hot.

Nutritional analysis: per serving with crust; 453 calories; 18gm. protein; 35gm. carbos; 4gm. fiber; 24gm. fats; 172mg. cholesterol; 157mg. calcium; 3mg. iron; 90mg. magnesium; 566mg. potass.; 446mg. sodium; 2mg. zinc.

638   SEVEN VEGGIE CHEESE PIE

This quiche is good with or without a crust. If you use a crust, pre-bake it, and make it very simple, like the one at the beginning of this section, or just use some toasted crumbs scattered on the bottom of the quiche plate.

Preheat oven to 350°.

♣Sauté in a large skillet, until aromatic
2 TBS. OIL
1 teasp. GARLIC LEMON SEASONING
1 teasp. GINGER TAMARI SAUCE
1 ONION, in rings or half moons

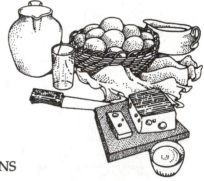

♣Add and sauté until color changes
1 STALK BROCCOLI FLOWERETTES, sliced lengthwise
1 CUP CAULIFLOWERETTES, sliced lengthwise
1 CUP SLICED ZUCCHINI or FROZEN FRENCH-CUT GREEN BEANS
1/2 CUP SLICED CARROTS
1/2 CUP MUSHROOMS

♣Scatter a few SOY BACON BITS over the shell or bottom of quiche dish. Cover with the veggies.
♣Top with LARGE TOMATO IN WEDGES
♣Sprinkle with 1 1/2 CUPS GRATED LOW FAT MIXED CHEESES of your choice.
♣Bake for 30 minutes until cheese melts and crust browns.

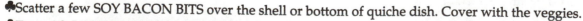

639   DEEP DISH ITALIAN PIE

This is like a mushroom pizza without the crust. It makes up very fast and easy, and is very light.
For one 9 x 13" shallow pan: Preheat oven to 375°.

♣Have ready ONE 15-OZ. JAR of PIZZA SAUCE.
♣Peel and slice 1 SMALL EGG PLANT or 2 ZUCCHINI in rounds.
Set aside.
♣Grate 1 1/2 CUPS LOW-FAT MOZZARELLA CHEESE.

♣Sauté in 2 TBS. OLIVE OIL for about 5 minutes
1 SLICED ONION   1 SLICED GREEN BELL PEPPER
1/2 teasp. GROUND ANISE SEED   1 teasp. PIZZA SEASONING

♣Add 1 LB. SLICED MUSHROOMS and toss until coated and hot.
♣Add 1 LB. FRESH TOMATOES and toss to coat.

♣Spread a little pizza sauce on the bottom of the pan, and cover with the eggplant or zucchini slices.
♣Cover with a scattering of the mozzarrella. Top with the tomato/mushroom mixture.

♣Pour on the rest of the jar of PIZZA SAUCE. Sprinkle on 1/4 CUP ROSÉ WINE.
♣Scatter on 2 TBS. PARMESAN to lightly cover the top.

♣Bake <u>COVERED</u> for 20 minutes. Remove cover and bake for 20 more minutes. Let rest for a few minutes and cut in big squares to serve.

Nutritional analysis: per serving; 169 calories; 9gm. protein; 15gm. carbohydrate; 3gm. fiber; 9gm. fats; 10mg. cholesterol; 175mg. calcium; 2mg. iron; 36mg. magnesium; 695mg. potassium; 358mg. sodium; 1mg. zinc.

640   FRESH TOMATO BASIL CHEESE TART

This quiche has the light fresh flavor of Northern Italy at harvest time. It works well with the crust given at the beginning of this section.

♣Preheat oven to 325°. Have ready a pre-baked quiche shell.

♣Sauté 1 CHOPPED RED ONION, 1 TB. SOY BACON BITS, and 1 teasp. DRY OREGANO in 2 TBS. OIL until aromatic, about 7 to 8 minutes.

♣Add and sauté briefly
4 FRESH CHOPPED TOMATOES   1 teasp. MIXED SALAD HERBS
1/4 CUP FRESH CHOPPED BASIL   1/2 teasp. PEPPER

♣Mix in 2 TBS. PARMESAN CHEESE. Spoon into the pre baked shell.
♣Cover with 2 CUPS DICED MOZZARRELLA CHEESE. Bake for 45 minutes until bubbly.

Nutritional analysis: per serving with the crust; 394 calories; 16gm. protein; 35gm. carbohydrate; 5gm. fiber; 22gm. fats; 32mg. cholesterol; 282mg. calcium; 3mg. iron; 86mg. magmesium; 543mg. potassium; 399mg. sodium; 2mg. zinc.

641   SWEET POTATO SUPPER PIE

For 6 - 8 servings: Preheat oven to 350°.

♣Toast 1¹/₄ CUPS CHOPPED PECANS in the oven for 5 to 7 minutes.
♣Make the **WHOLE GRAIN & NUT CRUST**. Mix

¹/₂ CUP FINE CHOPPED TOASTED PECANS	4 TBS. BUTTER
1¹/₄ CUP WHOLE WHEAT PASTRY FLOUR	2 to 5 TBS. COLD WATER

♣Pat into a lecithin-sprayed quiche pan or 10" pie pan. Chill.

♣Make the filling. Soak 4 to 6 DRIED APRICOTS in water until soft. Slice thin. Reserve soaking water.
♣Bake 2 LBS. YAMS or SWEET POTATOES until soft. Peel and mash with

1 TB. BUTTER	¹/₂ teasp. CINNAMON
³/₄ CUP CHOPPED TOASTED PECANS	¹/₂ teasp. SEA SALT
THE SLICED APRICOTS with 2 TBS. reserved water	1 TB. HONEY
¹/₂ CUP PLAIN YOGURT	¹/₄ teasp. NUTMEG

♣Spread onto chilled crust. Sprinkle with ¹/₃ CUP TOASTED WHEAT GERM and ¹/₂ CUP GRATED LOW-FAT CHEDDAR. Bake for 40 yo 50 minutes until browned and bubbly.

Nutritional analysis: per serving; 434 calories; 11gm. protein; 54gm. carbohydrate; 7gm. fiber; 21gm. fats; 20mg. cholesterol; 141mg. calcium; 2mg. iron; 92mg. magnesium; 822mg. potassium; 122mg. sodium; 3mg. zinc.

642   CLASSIC SWISS & SALMON QUICHE

For 6 servings: Preheat oven to 350°.

♣Have ready 1 pre-baked 9" quiche shell.

♣Drain ONE 15-OZ. CAN SALMON and trim of excess skin and bones. Mix in a bowl with 1 CUP SHREDDED SWISS CHEESE, ¹/₂ CUP THIN SLICED SCALLIONS, and ¹/₂ teasp. PEPPER. Spread on quiche shell.
♣Mix the custard in the blender

3 EGGS	6 TBS. SHERRY
¹/₂ CUP PLAIN YOGURT	1 teasp. DRY DILL WEED
¹/₄ CUP WATER	¹/₄ teasp. NUTMEG

♣Pour over salmon. Bake until firm, about 55 minutes. Cool for 10 minutes to set before slicing.

♣Serve with a chilled **FRESH SPINACH BASIL SAUCE** if desired. Mix all ingredients in the blender.

3 to 4 TOMATOES	³/₄ CUP GRATED PARMESAN
1 SMALL BUNCH FRESH WASHED SPINACH	12 FRESH BASIL LEAVES
¹/₂ CUP FRESH CHOPPED PARSLEY	¹/₂ CUP OLIVE OIL

♣Pour into a saucepan and simmer briefly just until fragrant.
♣Serve over cut quiche slices.

Chicken & Turkey; High Mineral Meats

There is such a nutrition difference in poultry that is raised out of doors naturally, chemical- free. When the birds scratch and eat in a free-run environment, the meat is lower in fat and cholesterol, higher in absorbable minerals, vitamins and proteins, without the need for hormones or growth stimulants. The quality difference is definitely reflected in the full-flavored taste and juiciness. Free-run poultry nutrients can be an excellent healing tool for people who need more concentrated protein for body building, bone and tissue formation.

Roasting is one of the most wholesome ways to fix poultry, in the traditional oven method, and also in the French clay roasters now becoming popular in America. (See page 357 for a full section on cooking in clay.) Clay pots roast in the ancient earth-oven manner and allow liquid-free, fat-free cooking, while still keeping all the flavor and nutrition intact. The new boneless turkey roasts from natural growers are perfect for cooking in this way. Just follow the directions given with the clay roaster, or roast for 25 minutes per pound at 325° when using the traditional oven method.

To enhance the flavor of roast poultry, we usually brush with a glaze. Here are two favorites.

HONEY GLAZE FOR TURKEY

♣Blend in a cup and brush on before and during roasting.

2 TBS. HONEY
2 TBS. ORANGE JUICE

1 TB. TERIYAKI SAUCE
PINCH TURMERIC

DARK BROWN GLAZE

♣Blend in a small cup and brush on poultry before and during roasting.

2 TBS. TAMARI
2 TBS. MOLASSES

1 TB. HONEY
1/4 teasp. NUTMEG

Nutritional analysis for roast turkey with glaze: to serve 8; 21 calories; trace protein; 5gm. carbo.; trace fiber; trace fats; 0 cholest.; 35mg. calcium; 1mg. iron; 14mg. magnesium; 156mg. potassium; 47mg. sodium; trace zinc.

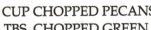

643   BAKED TURKEY SUPREME

For 8 servings: Preheat oven to 425°.

♣Use 4 CUPS COOKED DICED TURKEY
♣Make up 1 PACKAGE MAYACAMAS MUSHROOM SOUP or CREAM OF CHICKEN SOUP MIX for the <u>sauce</u> directions. You will have about 2 CUPS of sauce.

♣Mix turkey and sauce with

1 1/2 CUPS SLICED CELERY
1 CAN SLICED WATER CHESTNUTS
1 CUP GRATED LOW-FAT CHEDDAR

1 CUP CHOPPED PECANS
4 TBS. CHOPPED GREEN ONIONS
4 TBS. LEMON JUICE

♣Turn into a casserole and cover with CRUNCHY CHINESE NOODLES and a scattering of TOASTED CHOPPED PECANS. Bake for about 15 minutes, just to heat through.

Nutritional analysis: per serving; 308 calories; 26gm. protein; 11gm. carbohydrate; 2gm. fiber; 18gm. fats; 53mg. cholesterol; 119mg. calcium; 2mg. iron; 55mg. magnesium; 455mg. potassium; 236mg. sodium; 3mg. zinc.

 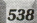

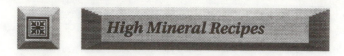

644 APPLE 'LASSES TURKEY LOAF

This is a lovely wintertime, energy source recipe.
Enough for 8 servings: Preheat oven to 350°.

♣Mix all ingredients together in a large bowl

2 LBS. GROUND TURKEY	$1/4$ CUP DARK MOLASSES
1 CUP CORN BREAD CRUMBS	$1/4$ CUP YOGURT
1 EGG	2 TBS. SHERRY
1 CHOPPED APPLE	$1^1/2$ teasp. SEA SALT
$1/2$ CHOPPED ONION	$1/4$ teasp. PEPPER

♣Place in a lecithin-sprayed loaf pan. Bake for 1 hour until crusty on top.
♣Make a **MOLASSES GLAZE** with 2 TBS. MOLASSES and 2 TBS. KETCHUP. Brush top and bake 20 more minutes to brown.

Nutritional analysis: per serving; 310 calories; 36gm. protein; 23gm. carbohydrate; 1gm. fiber; 7gm. fats; 114mg. cholesterol; 169mg. calcium; 7mg. iron; 79mg. magnesium; 879mg. potassium; 500mg. sodium; 4mg. zinc.

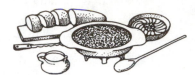

645 LIGHT TURKEY MOUSSAKA

This is a big family dinner, in the traditional Greek style, but with much healthier, lighter ingredients.

For 8 to 10 servings with leftovers: Preheat oven to 450°.

♣Cut 2 LARGE EGGPLANT in $1/2$" slices. Lay in a single layer in 2 large baking pans brushed with OLIVE OIL. Brush eggplant slices with olive oil. Bake for 20 minutes. Turn slices and bake for 10 more minutes until very soft. Lay slices from <u>one pan</u> in a single layer in a 9 x 13" shallow casserole. Set the other eggplant baking pan aside.

♣Add 2 LARGE SLICED ONIONS to the empty pan. Scatter on 2 CLOVES MINCED GARLIC. Drizzle with 2 teasp. OLIVE OIL, and add $1/2$ CUP WATER. Bake for 35 minutes, until moisture evaporates and onions are dark brown and aromatic. Stir often to keep from burning. Remove from oven. Add $1/2$ CUP WHITE WINE to deglaze, and scrape up browned bits. Distribute $1^1/2$ LBS. GROUND TURKEY over the onions, and bake until turkey is white, about 6 minutes. Remove from oven.

♣Blend in a heating saucepan with 2 TBS. WATER

$1/4$ teasp. FENNEL SEED	$1/4$ teasp. CARDAMOM POWDER
$1/4$ teasp. CINNAMON	4 teasp. ARROWROOT POWDER
$1/4$ teasp. CUMIN POWDER	1 teasp. SEA SALT

♣Add $1^1/2$ CUPS CHICKEN BROTH. Heat to boiling, and pour over turkey and onions. Sprinkle generously with CRACKED PEPPER. Pour entire mixture over the eggplant slices in the casserole and smooth top.
♣Cover with RESERVED EGGPLANT SLICES.
♣Rinse saucepan, and make a smooth paste with 2 TBS. ARROWROOT and 2 TBS. WATER. Add $1/2$ CARTON LIGHT CREME FRAICHE and $1^1/2$ CUPS CHICKEN BROTH. Bring to a rapid boil, stirring.
♣Spoon over eggplant. Cover and chill.
♣To serve, sprinkle with 2 TBS. GRATED PARMESAN and bake at 350° until hot and bubbly.

646   LOW-FAT MU SHU CHICKEN

For 8 servings:

♣Skin, bone and slice 2 CHICKEN BREASTS into strips. Marinate for 1 hour in

2 TBS. TAMARI	1 teasp. FRUCTOSE
1 MINCED SHALLOT	1/2 teasp. GINGER POWDER
1/2 CUP SHERRY	2 TBS. OIL

♣Wrap 8 FLOUR TORTILLAS IN FOIL, and warm in a 250° oven for 15 minutes until soft for wrapping.

♣Sauté in a skillet until fragrant

2 TBS. PEANUT OIL	1 SLICED ONION
2 teasp. TOASTED SESAME OIL	6 LARGE SLICED MUSHROOMS

♣Pour off marinade from chicken pieces and add to skillet. Set chicken aside.

♣Boil down to 2/3 cup liquid, about 2 minutes.

♣Add chicken pieces and 2 CUPS SHAVED HEAD LETTUCE to mushroom mix.

♣Add 2 EGGS and stir until eggs are just set.

♣Spoon some of the mixture over each tortilla. Top each with

1 teasp. HOISIN SAUCE
1 TBS. MINCED GREEN ONION
1 teasp. CHOPPED CILANTRO LEAVES
Roll up and serve hot.

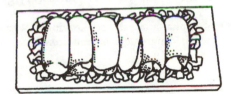

Nutritional analysis: per serving; 248 calories; 16gm. protein; 24gm. carbohydrate; 2gm. fiber; 10gm. fats; 83mg. cholesterol; 63mg. calcium; 2mg. iron; 35mg. magnesium; 365mg. potassium; 223mg. sodium; 2mg. zinc.

647   FIVE MINUTE EASY CHICKEN, PEAS & BROWN RICE

Use leftover baked or broiled chicken for this. This casserole makes it even better the second time around..

For 6 servings: Preheat oven to 325°.

♣Layer 3 CUPS DICED COOKED CHICKEN in an oiled 9 X 13" BAKING PAN.

♣Sprinkle with a layer of 2 CUPS COOKED BASMATI RICE.

♣Dot with BUTTER.

♣Top with a layer of FROZEN PEAS. Use a whole 10 OZ. BOX.

♣Sprinkle on a 4-OZ. CAN SLICED MUSHROOMS with juice.

♣Whisk together 2 CUPS WATER, 1 CHICKEN BOUILLON CUBE, 1 CUP PLAIN YOGURT, 4 EGGS, 1/2 teasp. SEA SALT, and 2 TBS. CHOPPED FRESH PARSLEY. Pour over casserole.

♣Sprinkle with 3 TBS. ROMANO CHEESE and bake 45 minutes until set.

Nutritional analysis: per serving; 336 calories; 33gm. protein; 26gm. carbo.; 4gm. fiber; 10gm. fats; 200mg. cholesterol; 156mg. calcium; 3mg. iron; 74mg. magnesium; 455mg. potassium; 351mg. sodium; 3mg. zinc.

648   ONE POT CHICKEN & VEGETABLES

This is almost a perfect whole meal dish; delicious and fragrant with herbs, high in complex carbohydrates, protein and minerals, low in fat.

Enough for 8 people: Preheat oven to 350°.

♣Bring 2 CUPS CHICKEN STOCK to a boil. Stir in 1½ CUPS BULGUR GRAINS. Reduce heat. Cover and simmer for 10 minutes. Fluff and turn into a large greased casserole.

♣Skin, bone and slice 4 CHICKEN BREASTS into strips. Brown in 1 TB. BUTTER and 1 TB. OIL until opaque, firm and tender. Arrange on top of bulgur in the casserole.

♣Add 2 TBS. OIL to the skillet and sauté for 5 minutes.
1 CHOPPED RED ONION
1 CHOPPED SHALLOT
1 SLICED RED BELL PEPPER
½ teasp. DRY BASIL

♣Add and sauté for 5 minutes more
3 LARGE DICED TOMATOES
1 teasp. CUMIN
½ teasp. OREGANO
½ teasp. PEPPER

♣Arrange vegetables over the chicken. Cover and bake for 30 minutes to heat through.

♣Uncover, and stir in 2 CUPS FRESH TRIMMED PEA PODS. Cover again, turn off oven, and let peas steam in the hot mixture until very green, about 10 minutes.

Nutritional analysis: per serving; 304 calories; 32gm. protein; 28gm. carbohydrate; 8gm. fiber; 8gm. fats; 75mg. cholesterol; 54mg. calcium; 3mg. iron; 86mg. magmnesium; 562mg. potassium; 104mg. sodium; 2mg. zinc.

649   CHICKEN IN SESAME TAHINI SAUCE

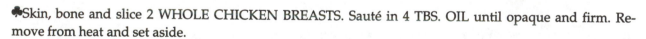

For 6 servings:

♣Skin, bone and slice 2 WHOLE CHICKEN BREASTS. Sauté in 4 TBS. OIL until opaque and firm. Remove from heat and set aside.

♣Add 2 TBS. OIL to the skillet and sauté until aromatic
2 CHOPPED ONIONS
1 teasp. GARLIC/LEMON SEASONING
4 TBS. CHOPPED FRESH CILANTRO
1 SMALL CHOPPED SEEDED CHILI PEPPER

♣Add and bring to a boil
2 CUPS LIGHT STOCK
6 TBS. SESAME TAHINI
1 TB. MIXED SALAD HERBS

½ teasp. SESAME SALT
¼ teasp. PEPPER

♣Add chicken strips. Cover and simmer over low heat for 30 minutes.
♣Serve on a platter with COOKED BASMATI RICE.

Nutritional analysis: per serving; 401 calories; 29gm. protein; 24gm. carbohydrate; 4gm. fiber; 22gm. fats; 63mg. cholesterol; 59mg. calcium; 2mg. iron; 110mg. magnesium; 405mg. potassium; 280mg. sodium; 3mg. zinc.

650 CHICKEN PESTO KIEV

For all of you who love Chicken Kiev, here it is - California style.
For 6 people: Preheat oven to 350°.

♣Split, bone, skin and pound flat 3 WHOLE CHICKEN BREASTS. Chill while you make the pesto.

♣Make the pesto in the blender

1 CUP PACKED FRESH BASIL LEAVES   3/4 CUP PARMESAN
1/2 teasp. LEMON GARLIC SEASONING   1/4 CUP OLIVE OIL

♣Spoon some pesto over each chicken breast piece. Roll up and secure with a toothpick.

♣Melt 6 TBS. BUTTER in a shallow baking dish.

♣Dip each roll in SEASONED UNBLEACHED FLOUR, and place seam side down in a single layer in the dish. Bake for 40 minutes until chicken is opaque, steaming and fragrant.

♣Serve with **RAISIN ALMOND SAUCE.** Make the sauce in a small saucepan.

♣Sauté until aromatic   ♣Add and simmer until fragrant
2 TBS. BUTTER   1/2 CUP CHOPPED ALMONDS
2 CHOPPED SHALLOTS   1/4 CUP RAISINS
1/2 teasp. LEMON/GARLIC SEASONING   1/4 teasp. PEPPER
1 TB. SOY BACON BITS

♣Pour over kiev rolls and serve immediately.

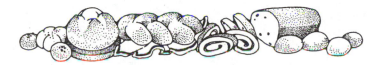

Savory Baking For Minerals

Whole grain baking is an excellent, satisfying source of balanced mineral building blocks.

651 QUICK MOLASSES BREAD

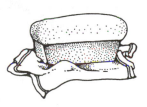

For 1 loaf, 12 slices: Preheat oven to 325°.

♣Mix all ingredients together just to blend

2 CUPS GRAHAM FLOUR or GOURMET FLOUR BLEND (page 647)
1 CUP UNBLEACHED FLOUR
1 CUP MOLASSES   1 teasp. BAKING SODA
1/2 CUP LOW-FAT COTTAGE CHEESE   1/2 CUP WATER
1/2 CUP PLAIN YOGURT   1/2 teasp. SEA SALT

♣Turn into an oiled loaf pan. Bake until bread pulls away from the sides of the pan, and a toothpick inserted in the center comes out clean, about 60 to 70 minutes.

♣Cool on a rack. Cut in very thin slices, and spread with kefir cheese to serve.

Nutritional analysis: per slice; 164 calories; 6gm. protein; 34gm. carbohydrate; 2gm. fiber; trace fats; 1mg. cholesterol; 219mg. calcium; 8mg. iron; 99mg. magnesium; 970mg. potassium; 191mg. sodium; 1mg. zinc.

652 TENDER MOLASSES GINGERBREAD
This is good eating just plain. It doesn't need a thing. Great for kids snacks.
For a 9 x 9" square pan; 6 pieces: Preheat oven to 350°.

♣Mix the dry ingredients Mix the wet ingredients
1 1/4 CUPS WHOLE WHEAT PASTRY FLOUR
3/4 teasp. BAKING SODA
1/2 teasp. CINNAMON
1/4 teasp. NUTMEG
1/2 teasp. GROUND GINGER
1/4 teasp. GROUND ALLSPICE

1 EGG
1/4 CUP OIL
3/4 CUP UNSULPHURED MOLASSES
1/2 CUP HOT WATER
2 TBS. HONEY
1/4 teasp. SEA SALT

♣Combine the two mixtures, and beat smooth. Pour into a square baking pan and bake for 20 minutes until a knife inserted in the center comes out clean.

Nutritional analysis: per piece; 134 calories; 5gm. protein; 27gm. carbohydrate; 2gm. fiber; 2gm. fats; 35mg. cholesterol; 98mg. calcium; 4mg. iron; 59mg. magnesium; 501mg. potassium; 162mg. sodium; 1mg. zinc.

653 CRUMB TOP PUMPKIN BREAD
This recipe is also delicious with golden cooked squash instead of pumpkin.
For one 8 x 12" baking pan: Preheat oven to 350°.

♣Mix the dry ingredients together until crumbly
3 CUPS WHOLE WHEAT PASTRY FLOUR
1/2 CUP FRUCTOSE
1/2 CUP DATE SUGAR
1 STICK UNSALTED BUTTER
1/4 CUP OIL

2 teasp. GROUND GINGER
1 teasp. CINNAMON
1/2 teasp. NUTMEG
1/4 teasp. CARDAMOM POWDER

♣Set aside 2/3 CUP of the mixture for topping.

♣Mix the wet ingredients
1 CAN COOKED PUMPKIN or 1 LB. COOKED GOLDEN SQUASH
1/2 CUP MOLASSES
2 EGGS
2 TBS. PLAIN YOGURT
2 TBS. WATER
1 1/2 teasp. BAKING SODA
♣Mix the two ingredients together just to moisten, and pour into an oiled 8 x 12" baking pan.
♣Sprinkle crumble mix on top. Bake until top is firm, about 50 minutes. Cool slightly. Serve warm with a
CRUNCHY ALMOND TOPPING.

♣Toast 1/2 CUP SLIVERED ALMONDS in the oven until brown, about 10 minutes.
♣Bring 1/2 CUP MAPLE SYRUP to a boil. Stir in almonds. Bring to another boil. Pour onto oiled sheets. Let set for 10 minutes, and then break up into pieces. Sprinkle over pumpkin bread.

654   DONA'S IRON SKILLET CORN BREAD

For 1 9 x 9" pan or cast iron skillet; 9 pieces: Preheat oven to 425°.

♣Combine the dry ingredients
1 CUP UNBLEACHED FLOUR
2 TBS. WHEAT GERM
1½ CUPS YELLOW CORNMEAL
½ teasp. SESAME SALT
4 teasp. BAKING POWDER
3 TBS. FRUCTOSE

♣Blender blend the wet ingredients
2 EGGS
1 CUP PLAIN YOGURT
½ CUP WATER
¼ CUP OIL
2 teasp. MAPLE SYRUP

♣Combine the two together just to moisten. Pour into cast iron skillet, or an oiled 9 x 9" pan and bake for 15 to 20 minutes until springy and golden.

Nutritional analysis: per serving; 227 calories; 7gm. protein; 31gm. carbohydrate; 3gm. fiber; 9gm. fats; 47mg. cholesterol; 156mg. calcium; 1mg. iron; 52mg. magnesium; 642mg. potassium; 70mg. sodium; 1mg. zinc.

655   POLENTA WITH FRESH TOMATOES & BASIL

This is another rare treat we found in northern Italy. Polenta looks and acts like a cornmeal, and it is; but the flavor is definitely different than the American grain.
For 8 pieces: Preheat oven to 350°.

♣Combine 1 CUP WATER and 1½ CUPS LOW-FAT MILK in a large pot and bring to a boil. Add 8-OZ. POLENTA and cook for 20 minutes until thick and smooth.

♣Stir in
1 CUP PARMESAN CHEESE
½ teasp. SEA SALT

½ teasp. NUTMEG
¼ teasp. PEPPER

♣Spread mixture on a moist flat surface, like a cutting board or wax paper covered counter to cool.

♣Make the sauce in a saucepan. Sauté 1 CUP CHOPPED ONION in 2 TBS. BUTTER and 2 TBS. OLIVE OIL for 5 minutes.

♣Add and let simmer til thick and fragrant
3 STALKS CELERY, chopped
3 LARGE TOMATOES, chopped
2 TBS. FRESH BASIL, chopped

1 teasp. OREGANO
1 teasp. SESAME SALT
¼ teasp. PEPPER

♣Turn off heat, but leave pan to slowly cool while you bake the polenta.
♣Cut cooled polenta into slabs. Dip each slab in a bowl of BEATEN EGG, then into a dish of WHOLE WHEAT BREAD CRUMBS. Place slabs on a baking sheet brushed with OLIVE OIL and bake until dark golden brown, about 30 minutes.
♣Put on small plates and serve with spoonfuls of the sauce.

Nutritional analysis: per serving; 237 calsoies; 10gm. protein; 32gm. carbohydrate; 5gm. fiber; 9gm. fats; 44mg. cholesterol; 226mg. calcium; 2mg. iron; 51mg. magnesium; 388mg. potassium; 352mg. sodium; 1mg. zinc.

656   SWEET POTATO MUFFINS

For 12 muffins: Preheat oven to 350°.

♣Bake until soft and peel 2 MEDIUM SWEET POTATOES or 1 LARGE YAM.

♣Combine dry ingredients in a bowl.

$1^1/_3$ CUPS GOURMET FLOUR MIX (page 647)   2 teasp. BAKING POWDER
$1/_3$ CUP FRUCTOSE $1/_2$ CUP DATE SUGAR
$1^1/_2$ teasp. SWEET TOOTH BAKING MIX (page 645) $1/_2$ teasp. SEA SALT

♣Combine the wet ingredients

3 TBS. MAPLE SYRUP   1 EGG
$1/_4$ CUP PLAIN YOGURT   4 TBS. MELTED BUTTER
$1/_4$ CUP WATER   2 TBS. OIL

♣Combine the two ingredient mixtures together just to moisten and stir in $1/_4$ CUP CHOPPED WAL-NUTS and $1/_4$ CUP RAISINS. Spoon into paper-lined cups. Mix 1 teasp. FRUCTOSE with $3/_4$ teasp. CIN-NAMON and sprinkle a pinch on each muffin.
♣Bake for 25 minutes until muffins spring back when touched.

Nutritional analysis: per serving; 204 calories; 4gm. protein; 32gm. carbohydrate; 3gm. fiber; 7gm. fats; 28mg. cholesterol; 79mg. calcium; 1mg. iron; 31mg. magnesium; 414mg. potassium; 102mg. sodium; 1mg. zinc.

657   VEGETABLE CHEESE BREAD

This quick bread is perfect for lunch or savory spreads.
For 1 loaf pan; 12 slices: Preheat oven to 350°.

♣Combine the dry ingredients   ♣Combine the wet ingredients
3 CUPS WHOLE WHEAT FLOUR $1/_2$ CUP PLAIN YOGURT
$1/_4$ CUP PARMESAN CHEESE $1/_2$ CUP WATER
1 TB. + 2 teasp. BAKING POWDER $1/_4$ CUP HONEY
$1/_2$ teasp. BAKING SODA   6 TBS. OIL
$1^1/_2$ teasp. SEA SALT   2 EGGS

♣Add the wet to the dry ingredients and mix slowly and gently adding the vegetables gradually
1 CUP GRATED ZUCCHINI
1 CUP GRATED CARROT
$2/_3$ CUP MINCED CELERY
$1/_4$ CUP MINCED ONION
♣Spread smoothly into a lecithin-sprayed 9 x 9" square pan and sprinkle with SESAME SEEDS. Bake for 50 to 60 minutes until golden.

Nutritional analysis: per slice; 212 calories; 8gm. protein; 25gm. carbohydrate; 3gm. fiber; 9gm. fats; 37mg. cholesterol; 158mgg. calcium; 1mg. iron; 47mg. magnesium; 717mg. potassium; 340mg. sodium; 1mg. zinc.

High Mineral Desserts

Desserts aren't a place one would ordinarily expect to find high mineral foods, but it is a very good place to find them. And desserts are a good way to get minerals into your kids, who hardly ever get enough.

658   MAPLE RAISIN NUT PUDDING

This is very easy. You can put it together in about 5 minutes.
For 10 servings: Preheat the oven to 350°.

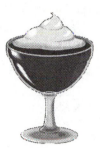

♣Make the pudding in the blender

1 LB. VERY FRESH TOFU	2 EGGS
1 STICK MELTED BUTTER	1/2 teasp. BAKING SODA
1 CUP MAPLE SYRUP	1/2 CUP RICE FLOUR
1 CUP HONEY	

♣Turn into an oiled baking dish. Stir in 1 CUP CHOPPED WALNUTS and 1 CUP RAISINS. Bake for 45 minutes until set and firm.

Nutritional analysis: per serving; 450 calories; 8gm. protein; 68gm. carbohydrate; 3gm. fiber; 20gm. fats; 66mg. cholesterol; 112mg. calcium; 4mg. iron; 89mg. magnesium; 452mg. potassium; 45mg. sodium; 1mg. zinc.

659   OLD FASHIONED MOLASSES PIE

For one 8" pie or 6 tarts: Preheat oven to 375°. Have an unbaked pie shell ready.

♣Make the filling in the blender

4 TBS. WHOLE WHEAT PASTRY FLOUR	3 EGGS
1/4 CUP HONEY	2 TBS. BUTTER
1/2 CUP APPLE JUICE	2 teasp. VANILLA
1/3 CUP MOLASSES	1/2 teasp. SEA SALT

♣Pour into prepared shell, and bake until almost firm, but still slightly wobbly in the center when shaken. ♣Remove and cool before serving.

Nutritional analysis: per serving; 176 calories; 4gm. protein; 27gm. carbohydrate; 1gm. fiber; 6gm. fats; 117mg. cholesterol; 141mg. calcium; 5mg. iron; 56mg. magnesium; 616mg. potassium; 227mg. sodium; trace zinc.

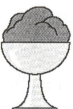

660   AVOCADO CREAM

It sounds weird, but is rich, creamy, good and nutritious. Don't miss it.
For 4 servings:

♣Combine in the blender, 1 PINT VANILLA RICE DREAM FROZEN DESSERT, 1 PEELED, CHUNKED AVOCADO, 2 TBS. ORANGE JUICE CONCENTRATE. Whirl until smooth. Spoon into dessert glasses. Top with a mint leaf and freeze. Remove 5 minutes before you want to serve.

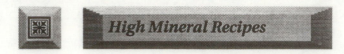

661   ANY WINTER SQUASH PIE

This recipe works with just about any squash-type vegetable. Try ACORN SQUASH, BANANA SQUASH, TURBAN SQUASH, PUMPKINS, DELICATAS, or YAMS - even CARROTS.
For one 10" pie; 8 servings: Preheat oven to 350°.

♣Bake your squash choice until soft. Scoop out and puree enough for 2 CUPS in the blender.

♣Mix the crumb crust together
1 CUP DRY WHOLE GRAIN BREAD CRUMBS
4 TBS. FRUCTOSE
4 TBS. MELTED BUTTER
2 teasp. SWEET TOOTH BAKING SPICE

♣Make the filling in the blender
2 CUPS SQUASH PURÉE
1 CUP PLAIN YOGURT
1/2 CUP HONEY
3 EGGS
1 teasp. CINNAMON
1/4 CUP MAPLE SYRUP

♣Pat into pie pan, and chill.
♣Pour filling into crust. Sprinkle on 1/2 CUP RAISINS, and bake for 45 minutes.

Nutritional analysis: per serving; 328 calories; 7gm. protein; 59gm. carbohydrate; 3gm. fiber; 8gm. fats; 96mg. cholesterol; 134mg. calcium; 2mg. iron; 45mg. magnesium; 500mg. potassium; 132mg. sodium; 1mg. zinc.

662   HAWAIIAN PUNCH DESSERT

For 4 servings:

♣Toss all ingredients together in a bowl
1 RIPE PINEAPPLE in 1" cubes
1 RIPE MANGO in 1" cubes
1/2 teasp. LIME ZEST
1/4 CUP LIME JUICE
1/4 CUP HONEY
3 TBS. CHOPPED FRESH MINT
♣Serve in dessert glasses with 4 MINT SPRIGS for garnish.

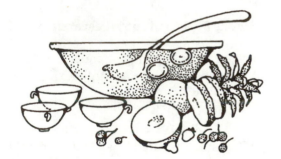

663   SMOOTHY POPS

For 8 pops:

♣Blend 2 CUPS CHILLED CUT UP FRESH FRUITS in the blender until smooth.
♣Add and blend
11/2 CUPS LOW-FAT MILK
1 CUP PLAIN YOGURT
1/3 CUP HONEY or MAPLE SYRUP

1 teasp. VANILLA
1/2 teasp. NUTMEG
1/2 teasp. CINNAMON
♣Pour into 8 paper-lined muffin cups and freeze for 1 hour. Insert a popsicle stick and freeze to firm.

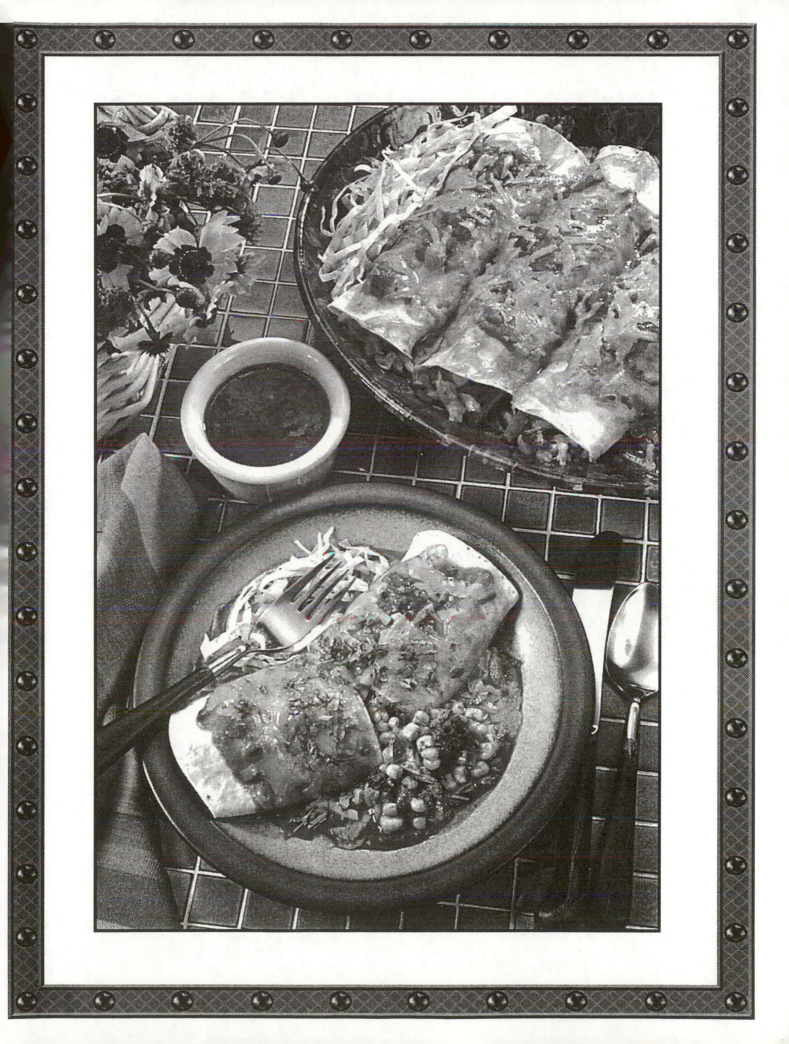

High Protein Cooking Without Meat

We all know that we need protein for daily energy, body growth and general health. After water, protein is the most plentiful substance in the body. Proteins are the major constituents of every living cell and body fluid except for bile and urine. Protein regulates acid/alkaline and body fluid balance. It helps to form enzymes and some hormones. **We also need protein to heal from injury or illness, and to maintain immune resistance.** When the body suffers a wound or surgery trauma, it loses protein, especially in skeletal muscle. For stabilization and recuperation, extra high quality protein is needed. **However, except in this restore and repair condition, or for accelerated athletic performance, the human body doesn't seem to need large amounts of protein to thrive.**

Most of us have been taught that we need much more protein than we actually do. Americans, for instance, eat 2 to 4 times more protein than is needed for good nutrition or health. In developed countries, *too much protein* is a bigger health threat than too little. Even athletes, for whom "high protein" was once the only watchword, do not need an overabundance of protein. Muscle strength, power and endurance grow from complex carbohydrates and unsaturated fats as well as from protein. (See **the Training, Competitive, and High Performance Diets** in the diet section of this book.)

Most Americans are accustomed to think in terms of meat and animal products for protein. But animal protein often comes loaded with saturated fat calories and cholesterol. Overeating on these foods adds unwanted weight because excess protein turns into fat. Too much protein impairs good kidney function, increases calcium **loss** in the bones, and poses a clear health risk to the heart and circulatory system. In addition, the latest knowledge about human needs for protein include man as a part of the ecological system of the planet, putting the question much more into perspective about eating meat. (See the section about red meats in this book).

All experts agree that plant protein sources should furnish at least half, if not all of our protein intake. Naturally occurring vegetable protein is rich in fiber and complex carbohydrates, and high in vitamins and minerals with little fat content. Vegetarian diets, even without dairy products can easily meet the RDA for protein. If you eat enough calories to maintain a reasonable weight, you will get more than enough protein. Vegetarians have lower cholesterol, denser bones and stronger teeth. Eating less total protein, with the majority of it from plant sources, can significantly increase healing capability, and reduce proneness to cancer and other diseases.

Good plant proteins come from soy foods, dried beans, nuts and seeds, potatoes, whole grains and pasta, brown rice, corn, bee pollen, bananas, brewer's yeast, and sprouts. Complete vegetable protein, such as that from tofu, tempeh, quinoa, and brewer's yeast supplies all the necessary amino acids found in animal foods without the fat and cholesterol. Even those that are not "complete" in terms of amino acids, complement other vegetable protein foods (an activity called protein complementarity), effectively enhancing the quality and absorption of both. Examples of this include rice with beans or tofu, and peas with potatoes or rice.

Today we know much more about enzyme activity in relation to different foods. You don't have to carefully mix and match beans and grains, or dairy and nuts for protein complementarity any more.

In addition, of course, good high grade, non-meat protein may be obtained from eggs, low-fat cheeses, yogurt, kefir, and other cultured foods. For healing purposes, high protein is defined in this book as 13 grams or more per serving. The recipes in this section emphasize protein from the following areas:

❧PROTEIN FROM EGGS - FRITTATAS, SOUFFLÉS and SCRAMBLES ❧PROTEIN FROM LOW-FAT CHEESES ❧PROTEIN FROM SOY FOODS - TOFU and TEMPEH ❧PROTEIN FROM MUSHROOMS ❧PROTEIN FROM BEANS and LEGUMES - MEXICAN FAVORITES ❧PROTEIN FROM WHOLE GRAINS ❧HIGH PROTEIN SALADS ❧

✤The following short list includes high quality vegetable protein sources for use in your meal and diet planning.

- ✿**Soy Foods:** Tofu, Tempeh, Miso, and Soy Cheeses.
- ✿**Nuts:** Pine Nuts, Walnuts, Almonds, Cashews, Brazils and Filberts.
- ✿**Seeds:** Pumpkin Seeds, Sesame Seeds, Sunflower Seeds and Peas.
- ✿**Beans & Legumes:** Peanuts, Lentils, Pintos, Limas, Black Beans, White And Red Beans, Mung Beans, Turtle Beans and Sprouts.
- ✿**Whole Grains:** Wheat and Wheat Germ, Brown, Basmati and Wild Rice, Millet, Barley, Bulgur, Buckwheat, Amaranth, Rye, Quinoa, and Amazake Rice Drink.
- ✿**Sea Vegetables:** Kelp, Dulse, Wakame, Sea Palm and Kombu.
- ✿**Vegetables:** Sprouts, Mushrooms.
- ✿**Fruits:** Avocados, Coconuts, Prunes, Raisins, Apples, Figs and Dates.
- ✿**Othesr: Bee Pollen;** contains all the essential Amino Acids in one natural source.

Brewer's Yeast; 2 TBS. contains as much protein as $1/4$ cup wheat germ, as much calcium as $1/2$ cup orange juice, as much phosphous as $1/4$ lb. haddock, as much iron as 1 cup spinach, as much thiamine as 1 cup wheat germ, as much niacin as $1/2$ cup brown rice, as much riboflavin as 4 eggs.

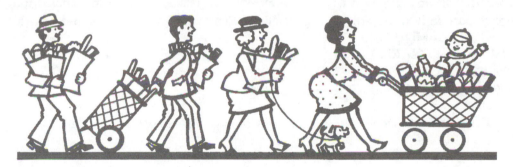

A word about Amino Acids in foods:

The body doesn't directly use the large protein molecules found in food for its protein needs. Proteins are made of amino acids that are coupled together into chains called peptides. These chains are the protein building blocks that must be provided together in the diet for the body to be able to use the protein energy that it takes in. Twenty-three amino acids have been identified. Essential amino acids must be supplied from food; the remainder can be synthesized by the body. An adult man, for example, can produce about 300gms. of new protein daily. Nine amino acids are essential to infants, and eight are essential to adults. Amino acids help detoxify sediment crystals in the system, nourish the vital organs and blood composition, release and wash out acid/ash residues, and clear the body of metabolic sludge and excess mucous. There are 22 amino acids, 8 essential, that are not synthesized by the body, and which we must get from foods.

Your protein needs can be determined by your age and ideal body weight. An adult over 20 years of age should eat about 0.36 grams of protein per pound of body weight. For example: if you are a 40 year old woman, who weighs or should weigh, 120 pounds, you would multiply 120 x 0.36 giving you 43 grams of protein a day. Exceptions to this include pregnant and nursing women, and people recuperating from illness, injury or surgery.

As we noted above, athletes also have greater protein needs. The body's ability to produce protein is decreased both during and after a workout. Protein needs for endurance athletes is often 50% higher than for the general population, and 3 to 6 times more for power lifters and strength athletes. Several studies have shown that the higher the amount of lean body mass the more protein an individual needs for maintenance.

Protein From Eggs
Frittatas, Soufflés & Scrambles

Eggs most closely approximate human protein needs. They offer complete protein with all essential amino acids, and are the standard for quality protein comparison. Regardless of current one-sided publicity concerning eggs and cholesterol, they are in fact, well-balanced nourishment, with lecithin to counterbalance cholesterol content. We know now that there are different types of cholesterol, that it is necessary to many body functions, and that it behaves differently when taken in as a whole food, rather than as an analyzed laboratory substance.

695 PIZZA FRITTATA
I have been making this recipe for at least 15 years. At one point in my life, I lived with a single mom and four children; this was a command favorite of theirs.
Enough for 4 hearty eaters:

♣Beat 8 EGGS in a bowl with $1/2$ CUP LOW-FAT COTTAGE CHEESE, $1/2$ teasp. SESAME SALT, $1/4$ teasp. PEPPER, and DASHES OF TAMARI.
♣Melt 2 TBS. BUTTER in a large **ovenproof skillet**. When it sizzles, add eggs and cook, lifting the edges to let uncooked portion flow underneath til just soft set. Remove from heat, and sprinkle with
$1/2$ CUP GRATED PARMESAN
$3/4$ CUP CHUNKY MOZZARELLA   4 SLICED MUSHROOMS
$1/4$ CUP CHOPPED SCALLIONS   4 THIN SLICES TOMATO
♣Sprinkle with 1 teasp. PIZZA SEASONING or OREGANO

Run under the broiler for 45 seconds to melt cheese. Cut in wedges to serve.

696 VEGETABLE FRITTATA

For 4 servings:

♣Make the vegetable mix. Sauté $1/2$ CUP RED ONION, CHOPPED until transparent in 2 TBS. OIL.

♣Add and toss until color changes
$1/2$ CUP GREEN PEPPER, CHOPPED
$1/2$ CUP SLICED MUSHROOMS
$1/2$ CUP DICED ZUCCHINI
♣Reduce heat and set aside.

♣Melt 2 TBS. BUTTER to medium hot in an **ovenproof skillet**. Add 6 BEATEN EGGS, and let cook, lifting edges to allow uncooked portion to flow underneath.
♣Remove the pan from heat when eggs are still moist, but not totally scrambled.
♣Spoon over and cover eggs with the sautéed veggies. Cover with 8-OZ. TOMATO SAUCE. Sprinkle with chunks of MOZZARELLA CHEESE, snipped FRESH BASIL and 1 teasp. DRY OREGANO.
♣Slide the skillet under the broiler until everything bubbles, about 3 minutes.
♣Snip FRESH PARSLEY over and serve.

697 SPANISH TORTILLA FRITTATA

Serves 4 to 6:

♣Sauté 1 SMALL CHOPPED ONION and 2 CLOVES GARLIC in 3 TBS OLIVE OIL in a large skillet until just limp, about 5 minutes.

♣Add 2 DICED POTATOES tossing until golden and tender.
♣Add 1 DRAINED 7-OZ. CAN CHOPPED OLIVES and 1 DRAINED 7-OZ. JAR ROASTED PEPPERS CHOPPED. Toss until fragrant.

♣Reduce heat to low, and add 8 BEATEN EGGS. Cover pan and cook until eggs are set around the edges but still liquid in the center. Lift edges to let uncooked egg flow underneath. Cook 5 minutes more until egg is set on top but still moist. Ease a spatula down the sides to make sure egg isn't stuck to the pan. Place a large plate over the skillet. Invert eggs onto the plate. Slide them back into pan cooked side up. Cook for 1 minute uncovered until set on the bottom. Slide out onto a serving plate. Serve hot with a light **TOMATO SAUCE** or **BLACK MUSHROOM WINE SAUCE** like the one below.

BLACK MUSHROOM WINE SAUCE: Soak 4 BLACK DRIED SHIITAKE MUSHROOMS in $1/2$ CUP ROSÉ WINE until soft. Sliver and discard woody stems. Reserve wine for the sauce.
♣Pureé 4 PLUM TOMATOES in the blender. You should have about 1 CUP purée.

♣Sauté 4 TBS. CHOPPED ONION, 1 teasp. GARLIC/LEMON SEASONING, and PINCHES of SALT and PEPPER in 1 TB. OLIVE OIL until aromatic.
♣Add
1 teasp. BASIL
1 teasp. OREGANO
1 teasp. TAMARI
♣Add TOMATO PUREÉ, $1/2$ CUP VEGETABLE BROTH, and the mushroom soaking wine. Simmer until sauce is reduced by half, about 20 minutes. Spoon over frittata.

698 ZUCCHINI FRITTATA

The first frittata I ever had was in a little omelet shop in Mill Valley, California. It was simple, delicious, and very similar to this.
For 4 people:

♣Sauté 2 TBS. CHOPPED SCALLIONS and 2 CUPS SLICED ZUCCHINI in 2 TBS. OIL for 5 minutes in an **ovenproof skillet**.
♣Mix in a bowl
6 EGGS
3 TBS. FRESH CHOPPED PARSLEY $1/2$ teasp. TAMARI
1 teasp. THYME $1/4$ teasp. PEPPER
1 teasp. CRUSHED ROSEMARY $1/4$ CUP PARMESAN
♣Pour over sizzling zucchini, and cook until almost set, shaking the pan occasionally.
♣Sprinkle with a little more PARMESAN or chunks of MOZARRELLA CHEESE, and run under the broiler for 30 seconds or so until light brown. Cut in wedges to serve.

699 BRUNCH GREENS FRITTATA

For 4 people: Preheat oven to 350°.

♣Make the sauce. Melt 1¹/₂ TBS. BUTTER. Add 1¹/₂ TBS. FLOUR and stir til bubbly. Add 2 TBS. SHER-RY and cook blending. Add ¹/₂ CUP PLAIN YOGURT, ¹/₄ CUP WATER, 2 teasp. DIJON MUSTARD and PINCHES of SALT and PEPPER. Cook stirring until just thickened and set aside.

♣Wash, chop and dry 4 CUPS MIXED GREENS, such as SPINACH, ROMAINE, and CHARD.

♣Sauté ³/₄ CUP CHOPPED ONION until transparent in 2 TBS. OIL. Add and sauté 4 OZ. SLICED MUSHROOMS for 5 minutes. Add the greens. Stir and cover the pan to wilt for 30 seconds.
♣Add 4 TBS. BUTTER and 4 EGGS to the skillet. Stir and toss until everything is coated. Turn into a straight side casserole, and pour sauce over in one layer. Do not stir.
♣Grate swiss or farmer cheese over the top to barely cover. Sprinkle with nutmeg and paprika and bake for 20 minutes.
♣Let stand before serving, while you prepare a **LIGHT MUSHROOM SAUCE** to spoon over top.

VERY LIGHT MUSHROOM SAUCE: For 1¹/₂ cups:

♣Sauté ¹/₂ CUP SLICED MUSHROOMS in 1 TB. BUTTER in a small saucepan until brown.
♣Sprinkle with 1¹/₂ TBS. WHOLE WHEAT FLOUR and blend until bubbly.

♣Add and simmer stirring until thickened

³/₄ CUP VEGETABLE STOCK or MISO BROTH   1 teasp. LEMON JUICE
¹/₄ CUP WHITE WINE   ¹/₄ teasp. PEPPER
¹/₂ teasp. SESAME SALT   PINCH NUTMEG
♣Remove from heat and add 1 TB. SHERRY if desired.

Nutritional analysis: per serving with sauce; 195 calories; 8gm. protein; 6gm. carboh.; 2gm. fiber; 10gm. fats; 100mg. choleserol; 136mg. calcium; 2mg. iron; 35mg. magnesium; 307mg. potassium; 177mg. sodium; 1mg. zinc.

700   SOUTH OF FRANCE FRITTATA

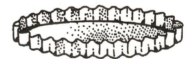

For 6 people:

♣Peel, cube and slice 1 EGGPLANT. Sauté with 2 CLOVES MINCED GARLIC for 10 minutes in 6 TBS. OLIVE OIL.
♣Add and sauté until tender
1 RED ONION, sliced   ¹/₂ RED BELL PEPPER, chopped
3 SMALL ZUCCHINI, sliced   4 TOMATOES, chopped
♣Remove from heat and stir in ¹/₄ CUP CHOPPED FRESH BASIL.
♣Add 6 BEATEN EGGS. Return to heat and cook until just set, lifting to let uncooked egg flow under-neath.
♣Sprinkle on 1 CUP ROMANO CHEESE to cover. Cook, covered for 2 minutes more just to melt cheese.

701   FOUR RING CIRCUS FRITTATA

For 6 servings: Preheat oven to 350°.

♣Slice 3 BELL PEPPERS, 1 RED, 1 YELLOW, 1 GREEN and 1 SMALL ONION into rings. Sauté in 2 TBS. OLIVE OIL until color changes and vegetables are crunchy tender. Season with SEA SALT, PEPPER, and DASHES of HOT PEPPER SAUCE. Place in a shallow baking dish.

♣Beat together

4 EGGS	2 TBS. PLAIN YOGURT
1 TBS. CHOPPED PARSLEY	2 TBS. WATER
3 TBS. GRATED PARMESAN	1/4 teasp. PAPRIKA
1/2 teasp. GARLIC SALT	1/2 teasp. DRY BASIL

♣Spoon over peppers and onions and bake for 20 minutes until set. Let rest before cutting.

Nutritional analysis: per serving; 103 calories; 8gm. protein; 5gm. carbohydrate; 1gm. fiber; 6gm. fats; 140mg. cholesterol; 73mg. calcium; 1mg. iron; 12mg. magnesium; 171mg. potassium; 136mg. sodium; 1mg. zinc.

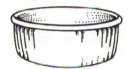

702   LOW FAT THREE VEGETABLE SOUFFLÉ

This very unusual recipe comes from The Café Chauveron in New York. It was a speciality of Monsieur Chauveron, and the recipe was a closely guarded secret. When he died, the restaurant closed and the recipe died with him. I used to order it every time I visited there. This recipe is a close approximation.
For 12 servings: Preheat oven to 400°.

♣Make the SPINACH PURÉE. Steam 1 LARGE BUNCH FRESH SPINACH until just wilted. Remove and drain in a colander. Squeeze liquid into a bowl. Purée spinach in the blender with 3 TBS. RESERVED LIQUID, 2 EGGS, 1/4 CUP WHOLE GRAIN FLOUR, 1 teasp. LEMON PEEL, 1/2 teasp. GARLIC/LEMON SEASONING and 1/4 teasp. SEA SALT. Scrape out into a bowl and set aside.

♣Make the MUSHROOM PURÉE. Sauté 2 CUPS SLICED MUSHROOMS with 1 SMALL CHOPPED ONION until fragrant. Purée in the blender with 2 EGGS, 1/4 CUP WHOLE GRAIN FLOUR, and 1/4 teasp. SEA SALT. Scrape out into a bowl and set aside.

♣Make the CARROT PURÉE. Bring 1 CUP SALTED WATER to a boil. Add 3 CHOPPED CARROTS, 1 TB. FRESH THYME LEAVES and 1 CHOPPED SMALL ONION. Cook until tender, about 15 minutes. Purée in the blender with 2 EGGS, and 1/4 CUP WHOLE GRAIN FLOUR. Scrape out into a bowl and set aside.

♣Oil a 9" springform pan. Spread with the SPINACH PURÉE. Then spread with the MUSHROOM PURÉE. Then top with the CARROT PURÉE. Bake until top feels firm when pressed, about 45 minutes.
♣Remove and sprinkle with GRATED PARMESAN CHEESE and MINCED PARSLEY.

♣Serve hot with a **LOW-FAT LEMON PEPPER SAUCE:**
♣Whisk together 1 teasp. DIJON MUSTARD, 2 teasp. GARLIC/LEMON SEASONING, 2 TBS. LEMON JUICE, 2 TBS. TOMATO JUICE, 1 teasp. TAMARI, and 1/2 teasp. CRACKED PEPPER.

703　BROCCOLI CHEESE SOUFFLÉ

For 4 servings: Preheat oven to 325°.

♣Spray a straight-sided soufflé dish with lecithin spray and cover with GRATED ROMANO CHEESE.
♣Steam 2 CUPS CHOPPED BROCCOLI FLORETS and STEMS until color changes to bright green.
♣Mix together 1 TB. MELTED BUTTER and 3 TBS. ARROWROOT POWDER and set aside.

♣Heat in a skillet 1/2 teasp. DRY BASIL, with BIG PINCHES of SEA SALT, PEPPER, and PAPRIKA.
♣Add 1/2 CUP WATER and 1/2 CUP PLAIN YOGURT. Stir until thick. Remove from heat and add 3 TBS. ROMANO CHEESE, 1 TB. LEMON JUICE and 1 EGG.
♣Bake 50 minutes until puffy and golden. Do not open oven door until baking time is up. Serve at once.

Nutritional analysis: per serving; 118 calories; 8gm. protein; 9gm. carbohydrate; 2gm. fiber; 6gm. fats; 69mg. cholesterol; 164mg. calcium; 1mg. iron; 22mg. magnesium; 246mg. potassium; 1mg. zinc; 180mg. sodium.

704　QUICK SCRAMBLED EGGS WITH SHRIMP

For 4 servings:

♣Mix 6 EGGS, 2 CHOPPED GREEN ONIONS, SEA SALT and PEPPER in a bowl.
♣Heat 2 TBS. OIL and 1/4 CUP CHOPPED ONION to sizzling. Add egg mixture and cook undisturbed until half set. Add 5-OZ. COOKED BABY SHRIMP. Scramble in and cook until set.

Nutritional analysis: per serving; 285 calories; 22gm. protein; 4gm. carbohydrate; 1gm. fiber; 19gm. fats; 218mg. cholesterol; 77mg. calcium; 3mg. iron; 30mg. magnesium; 254mg. potassium; 2mg. zinc.

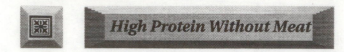

705　EGG & TOMATO RAMEKINS FOR TWO

For 2 servings: Prheat oven to 325°.

♣Sauté 1/2 CUP SLICED SCALLIONS and 1/4 CUP SLICED MUSHROOMS in 2 TBS. OIL until liquid evaporates. Sprinkle with 1 TB.WHOLE GRAIN FLOUR and stir until bubbly.

♣Add 1 LARGE CHOPPED TOMATO, 1/4 teasp. DRY BASIL, 1/4 teasp. GARLIC/LEMON SEASONING, and DASHES of SEA SALT and PEPPER.
♣Cook stirring until sauce bubbles. Blend in 3 TBS. PARMESAN CHEESE.

♣Divide between 2 ramekins. Break 1 EGG on top of each and bake for 20 minutes. Sprinkle with CHOPPED PARSLEY and serve hot.

Nutritional analysis: per serving; 200 calories; 11gm. protein; 9gm. carbohydrate; 2gm. fiber; 13gm. fats; 210mg. cholesterol; 118mg. calcium; 2mg. iron; 27mg. magnesium; 327mg. potassium; 1mg. zinc; 280mg. sodium.

Protein From Low Fat Cheeses

Cheese can be a good source of protein. The problem is always the fat that goes along with it. The recipes in this book use low fat cheeses when possible. This section in particular features cheese protein from low-fat sources.

706   ZUCCHINI, BULGUR & CHEESE

This recipe is full of good complex carbohydrates, and high minerals as well as protein.
For 8 servings: Preheat oven to 350∞.

♣Measure ³/₄ CUP BULGUR GRAINS into a bowl. Cover with ³/₄ CUP BOILING WATER and set aside to absorb.

♣Sauté 2 CUPS CHOPPED ONION and 2 CLOVES MINCED GARLIC in 3 TBS. OIL for 10 minutes.

♣Add 6 CUPS SLICED ZUCCHINI, 1¹/₂ teasp. ITALIAN HERBS and ¹/₄ teasp. PEPPER, and sauté until color changes.

♣Beat together in a bowl

1 CUP CRUMBLED FETA CHEESE (about 5-oz.)	2 EGGS
1 CUP LOW FAT COTTAGE CHEESE	¹/₄ CUP CHOPPED GREEN ONIONS
2 TBS. TOMATO PASTE	³/₄ CUP CHOPPED PARSLEY

♣Add to bulgur and mix well. Assemble casserole in a 9 x 9" baking dish. Layer bulgur mix on the bottom. Cover with zucchini mix. Top with cheese mix.

♣Layer on 2 SLICED TOMATOES and sprinkle with ONE CUP GRATED CHEDDAR. Top with 1¹/₂ TBS. SESAME SEED, and bake covered for 45 minutes. Uncover and bake for 15 minutes more. Remove and let set for 10 minutes before serving.

Nutritional analysis: per serving; 226 calories; 13gm. protein; 20gm. carbohydrate; 6gm. fiber; 11gm. fats; 67mg. cholesterol; 177mg. calcium; 2mg. iron; 69mg. magnesium; 571mg. potassium; 230mg. sodium; 2mg. zinc.

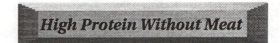

707   CHEESE & TOMATO NUT ROAST

For 4 people: Preheat oven to 350°.

♣Sauté 1 CHOPPED ONION, 1 teasp. ZEST or other HERB SALT, and ¹/₄ teasp. HOT PEPPER SAUCE in 2 TBS. OIL until aromatic.

♣Mix 2 teasp. VEGEX YEAST PASTE BROTH with 1 CUP WATER and add to onions. Heat until bubbly, and remove pan from heat.

♣Add 1¹/₂ CUPS CHOPPED NUTS ground in the blender with 4 SLICES WHOLE GRAIN BREAD.
♣Mix until well blended.

♣Turn HALF into a greased loaf pan and press in. Top with 2 SLICED TOMATOES. Top tomatoes with a covering of GRATED LOW-FAT CHEDDAR. Top with REST of nut mix and smooth top. Bake for 30 minutes. Top with a covering of PARMESAN CHEESE during the last few minutes of baking.

708 CHEESE CUTLETS WITH SHRIMP & EGG SAUCE

For 6 servings: Preheat oven to 325°.

♣Toast 1/4 CUP SESAME SEEDS in the oven until golden.

♣Mix in a large bowl

2 CUPS LOW FAT COTTAGE CHEESE	1/3 CUP FINE CHOPPED WALNUTS
2 MINCED GREEN ONIONS	1 BEATEN EGG
1 TB. WHOLE WHEAT FLOUR	1/2 teasp. PAPRIKA
2 TBS. FRESH CHOPPED PARSLEY	1/2 teasp. SESAME SALT
1 1/2 CUPS WHOLE GRAIN BREAD CRUMBS	1/4 teasp. NUTMEG

♣Mix well with hands and shape into 4 round patties. Pat on more DRY BREAD CRUMBS, and place on oiled baking sheets. Sprinkle with the sesame seeds and bake for 15 to 20 minutes until golden.

♣Make **SHRIMP & EGG SAUCE** while cutlets are baking.

♣Remove them from the oven and let set slightly before saucing and servimg.

♣Have 2 HARD BOILED EGGS ready.

♣Melt 2 TBS. BUTTER. Add 2 TBS. WHOLE WHEAT FLOUR. Stir until hot and bubbly.

♣Add

1/2 CUP PLAIN YOGURT	2 teasp. SALAD HERBS
1/3 CUP WATER	2 TBS. WHITE WINE
4 TBS. FRESH CHOPPED PARSLEY	1/4 teasp. SEA SALT
1/4 teasp. DRY MUSTARD	1/4 teasp. WHITE PEPPER

♣Cook and stir until thickened, about 7 minutes. Remove from heat and add 8 0Z. TINY COOKED SHRIMP and the CRUMBLED HARD BOILED EGGS. Spoon over cutlets and serve.

Nutritional analysis: per serving with sauce; 158 gm.; 387 calories; 33gm. carbo.; 29gm. protein; 3gm. fiber; 15gm. fats; 170 mg. cholest.; 186mg. calc.; 4 mg. iron; 77mg. mag.; 380 mg. potass.; 3mg. zinc; 435mg. sodium.

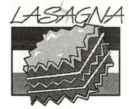

709 TOMATO CHEESE STRATA

Enough for 6: Preheat oven to 350°.

♣Bring a large pot of salted water to boil for 12 to 16 SPINACH or SESAME LASAGNA NOODLES.

♣Add 1 teasp. OIL to the pot so noodles won't stick. Cook just to *al dente*, about 10 minutes. Drain.

♣Make the sauce while lasagna is cooking. Mix together

5 EGGS	1/2 CUP ROSÉ WINE
2 CUPS PLAIN YOGURT or YOGURT CHEESE	1/2 teasp. BLACK PEPPER
1/2 teasp. LEMON/GARLIC SEASONING	

♣Assemble the strata. Line bottom of an oiled 8 x 11" baking pan with a layer of noodles. Sprinkle with 1 CUP LOW-FAT JACK CHEESE. Scatter on SLIVERED OIL-PACKED DRIED TOMATOES, or FRESH TO-MATO SLICES to cover. Cover tomatoes with a scattering of CHOPPED BLACK OLIVES.

♣Cover olives with another layer of noodles, and **repeat**.

♣Pour sauce over and scatter on CHOPPED WALNUTS to cover. Bake uncovered until edges are light brown and center is firm, about 45 minutes. Cool slightly to set and then cut in squares.

710   OVEN FETA BAKLAVA

Perfect brunch and entertaining food - looks great, low-fat, appeals to lots of tastes, with decided gourmet flair.
For 8 to 10 squares: Preheat oven to 400°.

♣Use $^1/_2$ PKG. WHOLE WHEAT FILO SHEETS, thawed, unwrapped and covered as per directions.

♣Melt together $^1/_2$ STICK BUTTER and $^1/_4$ CUP OIL

♣Make the filling. Sauté 2 CUPS CHOPPED LEEKS (mostly white parts), 2 MINCED SHALLOTS, and 1 TB. HERBS DE PROVENCE in 2 TBS. OIL for 15 minutes until fragrant.

♣Remove from heat and add
8 OZ. CRUMBLED FETA CHEESE   2 EGGS
8 OZ. KEFIR CHEESE or YOGURT CHEESE   3 TBS. WHITE WINE
$^1/_4$ CUP SLICED BLACK OLIVES $^1/_4$ teasp. NUTMEG

♣Oil an 8 X 12" baking pan. Lay one half sheet of filo on the bottom and brush with butter/oil blend.
♣Repeat until half of the filo is used ($^1/_4$ of the box). Spread with the filling.
♣Repeat with rest of the butter/oil brushed layers. Cut through pastry to make 8 to 10 serving squares.
♣Cover and chill. Bake uncovered for 40 to 50 minutes until golden. Serve hot or warm.

Nutritional analysis: per serving; 300 calories; 12gm. protein; 19gm. carbohydrate; 3gm. fiber; 20gm. fats; 93mg. cholesterol 232mg. calcium; 2mg. iron; 43mg. magnesium; 237mg. potassium; 361mg. sodium; 2mg. zinc.

711   DRIED TOMATO CHEESE CAKE

For 70 appetizer pieces: Preheat oven to 350°.

♣Make a quick press-in pastry for the cheesecake base.
♣Mix 6 TBS. OIL and $1^1/_4$ CUPS WHOLE WHEAT FLOUR until crumbly.
♣Add 1 EGG and mix until dough holds together. Press into a 10 x 15" oiled baking pan. Bake until light brown, about 10 minutes. Remove and cool before filling.

♣Make the filling.
Purée in the blender $^1/_2$ CUP OIL-PACKED DRIED TOMATOES, drained until smooth.
♣Add 1 TB. oil from the jar, 1 teasp. DRY OREGANO, 6 CLOVES MINCED GARLIC, and 3 EGGS.
♣Purée briefly and add 16 OZ. NEUFCHATEL CHEESE and 1 CARTON LOW FAT CREME FRAICHE. Blend again until smooth.

♣Turn into a bowl and stir in $^1/_2$ CUP CHOPPED GREEN ONIONS, SEA SALT and PEPPER.

♣Spread onto pastry, and bake until puffy and brown, about 25 minutes. Cool, cover and chill for several hours. Cut in 2" squares and then cut diagonally into triangles.

Nutritional analysis: per 4 pieces; 199 calories; 7gm. protein; 8gm. carbohydrate; 2gm. fiber; 16gm. fats; 81mg. cholesterol; 43mg. calcium; 1mg. iron; 17mg. magnesium; 106mg. potassium; 152mg. sodium; 1mg. zinc.

High Protein Nachos

The next three recipes are great snacks for protein hungry teenagers - and they can make them themselves.

712   FANCY CHEESE NACHOS

Enough for a trayful:

♣Toast a baking trayful (about 1 LB.) of PINTA, TACO or NACHO CHIPS until crisp.
♣Simmer in a saucepan over very low heat until cheese is smooth and melted

1/3 CUP SPARKLING WATER	4-OZ. KEFIR CHEESE
8-OZ. JALAPEÑO JACK CHEESE	1/4 CUP SALSA
8-OZ. LOW FAT CHEDDAR CHEESE	1/2 CUP CHPD. SPINACH or CHARD

♣Spoon over toasted chips, and run under the broiler to brown briefly; *or* just dunk the toasted chips in the cheese sauce right from the pan.

Nutritional analysis: per serving; 341 calories; 23gm. protein; 42gm. carbohydrate; 3gm. fiber; 12gm. fats; 31mg. cholesterol; 613mg. calcium; 3mg. iron; 66mg. magnesium; 183mg. potassium; 452mg. sodium; 3mg. zinc.

713   MINI PIZZAS ON RICE CAKES

Enough for 12 large or 24 small rice cakes:

♣Toast rice cakes on a baking sheet in the oven until crisp. Sauté until aromatic

1 SLICED RED ONION	2 TBS. OLIVE OIL
1 CLOVE MINCED GARLIC	1 teasp. OREGANO

♣Add 1 CUP TOFU BURGER made up according to package directions. Sauté in 1 TB. OIl until crumbly and brown. Divide mixture between the rice cakes. Top with 1 TOMATO SLICE, LOW-FAT MOZZARELLA CHEESE CHUNKS, and PARMESAN SPRINKLES. Run under broiler to melt the cheese.

714   JALAPEÑO CHEESE BREAD

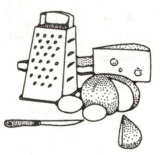

For one 9 x 9" square pan: Preheat oven to 400°.

♣Preheat empty lecithin-sprayed pan in the oven while you make the bread.
♣Mix in the blender

2 EGGS	1/4 CUP OLIVE OIL
1/2 CUP PLAIN YOGURT	1/2 CUP WATER

4 OZ JALAPEÑO or SOY JALAPEÑO JACK CHEESE, chunked
♣Mix the dry ingredients in a bowl

1 1/2 CUPS YELLOW CORNMEAL	2 TBS. HONEY
1/3 CUP UNBLEACHED FLOUR	2 TBS. FRUCTOSE
2 teasp. BAKING POWDER	1 teasp. SEA SALT

♣Combine the two mixtures together just to moisten for the batter. Pour into hot pan, and bake for 20 to 30 minutes until a toothpick comes out clean when inserted in the center. Cool and cut in squares.

Protein From Soy Foods
Tofu & Tempeh

Soy foods offer a complete, vegetarian source of protein. They also lend themselves to almost endless variations of taste and texture. The recipes in this section are only examples of the diversity of soy. See the chapter on TOFU FOR YOU and other recipes throughout this book for more delicious ways to use these foods.

715   SOY PROTEIN POWER SHAKE

For 1 shake:

♣Mix all ingredients in the blender until smooth
1 CUP HONEY-VANILLA SOY MILK
2 TBS. PROTEIN POWDER 1
2 TBS. BREWER'S YEAST
1 TB. WHEAT GERM

1 TB. LECITHIN
1/2 TB. CAROB POWDER
1 FROZEN BANANA
1/2 teasp. CINNAMON

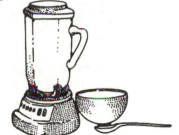

716   TOFU CLAM DIP

For 3 cups:

♣Process in the blender to smooth
1 LB. SOFT TOFU, drained
1 TB. LEMON JUICE

1 teasp. WINE VINEGAR
2 teasp. TAMARI

♣Turn into a bowl and stir in 1/2 teasp. GARLIC/LEMON SEASONING, 2 MINCED GREEN ONIONS, and ONE 6-OZ. CAN MINCED CLAMS. Sprinkle with PAPRIKA. Chill and serve.

717   TOFU SPANISH PILAF

For 6 servings: Preheat oven to 350°.

♣Sauté 1/4 CUP CHOPPED ONION in 2 TBS. OIL for 5 minutes. Turn into a 2 qt. casserole and add
2 CUPS COOKED BROWN RICE
1 CUP CHOPPED CELERY
1 CUP DICED ZUCCHINI
1/2 CHOPPED GREEN PEPPER

1 teasp. VEGETABLE SALT
1/4 teasp. PEPPER
1/4 teasp. OREGANO
PINCH CUMIN

♣Stir in ONE 16-OZ. CAN TOMATOES.
♣Drain 1 LB. TOFU. Squeeze out moisture, dice and add to casserole.
♣Sprinkle with 1/2 CUP GRATED PARMESAN.
♣Bake for 25 to 30 minutes until aromatic.

Nutritional analysis: per serving; 208 calories; 13gm. protein; 22gm. carbohydrate; 4gm. fiber; 8gm. fats; 5mg. cholesterol; 216mg. calcium; 5mg. iron; 128mg. magnesium; 431mg. potassium; 279mg. sodium; 1mg. zinc.

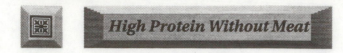

718   TOFU, CHEESE & VEGETABLES

For 6 servings: Preheat oven to 350°. Use a large covered casserole.

♣Make the tofu marinade with 2 TBS. TAMARI and, $1/2$ teasp. GARLIC/LEMON SEASONING and $1/2$ CUP WATER. Slice $3/4$ LB. FIRM TOFU into a flat dish, and pour on marinade. Let sit for 10 minutes, turning to coat all sides.

♣Make a simple, fresh herb seasoning in a small bowl. Use $1/4$ teasp. SEA SALT, $1/2$ teasp. OREGANO, $1/2$ teasp. ROSEMARY, $1/2$ teasp. SAGE and $1/2$ teasp. THYME.

♣Make the casserole layers in order as follows: Sprinkle a pinch of the herb salt over each layer.
$1^1/2$ THIN-SLICED ONIONS
THE DRAINED MARINATED TOFU
$1^1/2$ THIN-SLICED TOMATOES
4-OZ. GRATED LOW-FAT CHEDDAR
$3/4$ LB. MIXED ZUCCHINI, YELLOW SQUASH or GREEN BELL PEPPER SLICES
$1/2$ SMALL CARTON LOW-FAT COTTAGE CHEESE

♣Pour tofu marinade over all. Cover and bake for 45 minutes until aromatic and tender.

Nutritional analysis: per serving; 157 calories; 16gm. protein; 10gm. carbohydrate; 2gm. fiber; 6gm. fats; 12mg. cholesterol; 248mg. calcium; 4mg. iron; 88mg. magnesium; 404mg. potassium; 498mg. sodium; 2mg. zinc.

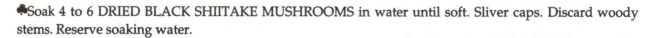

719   HAWAIIAN TOFU LAYERS

For 6 servings: Preheat oven to 350°. Use a large covered casserole.

♣Soak 4 to 6 DRIED BLACK SHIITAKE MUSHROOMS in water until soft. Sliver caps. Discard woody stems. Reserve soaking water.

♣Brown briefly in 2 TBS. OIL
12-OZ. CUBED TOFU $1/2$ ONION, chopped
$1/2$ CUP SLIVERED BAMBOO SHOOTS   THE SLIVERED MUSHROOMS
$1/2$ CAN CHOPPED WATER CHESTNUTS   1 CUP FRESH TRIMMED PEA PODS

♣Add and toss to coat
4 TBS. TAMARI
2 TB. FRUCTOSE
2 TBS. SHERRY or MIRIN

♣Turn into the casserole and top with 4 beaten eggs. Cover and bake for 30 to 40 minutes.

Nutritional analysis: per serving; 180 calories; 12gm. protein; 15gm. carbohydrate; 3gm. fiber; 8gm. fats; 142mg. cholesterol; 98mg. calcium; 5mg. iron; 79mg. magnesium; 344mg. potassium; 166mg. sodium; 2mg. zinc.

Protein From Mushrooms

Mushrooms provide a tasty source of protein for vegetarians. Current research is also showing beneficial therapeutic qulaities for many mushroom species. They are an excellent addition to a healing, body building diet.

719A   TRIPLE MUSHROOM QUICHE

This is a very delicate dish with subtle taste. It may be used with a light crust, or as a custard, with no crust at all. Just enjoy the taste of the mushrooms.
For 6 to 8 servings: Preheat oven to 350°.

♣Have ready an oiled baking dish or a pastry shell.

♣Soak 1 CUP BLACK SHIITAKE MUSHROOMS in water until soft. Sliver and discard woody stems. Reserve soaking water.

♣Melt 2 TBS. BUTTER and 2 TBS. OIL in a skillet over medium high heat. Sauté 1 SMALL CHOPPED ONION for 5 minutes. Add 4 CUPS SLICED BUTTON MUSHROOMS and the SHIITAKE MUSHROOMS for 5 more minutes. Pile into pastry shell or buttered dish.
♣Cut tough ends from a package of ENOKI MUSHROOMS and arrange over the quiche in clusters, with caps pointing toward the rim.

♣Whisk the sauce together in a bowl.

1 EGG	1/4 CUP KEFIR CHEESE
THE MUSHROOM SOAKING WATER	3 TBS. SHERRY
1/3 CUP PARMESAN CHEESE	

♣Pour over mushrooms and bake for 20 minutes until set when gently shaken. Serve hot.

Nutritional analysis: per serving; 290 calories; 21gm. protein; 10gm. carbohydrate; 3gm. fiber; 19gm. fats; 82mg. cholesterol; 589mg. calcium; 1mg. iron; 37mg. magnesium; 414mg. potassium; 274mg. sodium; 2mg. zinc.

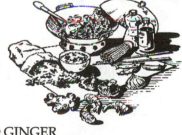

720   GINGER MUSHROOM STIR FRY

For 4 servings:

♣Combine in a bowl

3 TBS. LEMON JUICE	1 TB. GRATED GINGER
3 TBS. TAMARI	2 CLOVES MINCED GARLIC

♣Add 2 TOFU BLOCKS, cut into strips. Toss to coat.

♣Dissolve 2 teasp. ARROWROOT POWDER in 1/3 CUP CHICKEN BROTH and set aside.

♣Heat 2 TBS. OIL in a wok to sizzling. Add 2 CUPS SLICED MUSHROOM CAPS and the drained chicken strips (save liquid) and toss until chicken turns white.
♣Add 1 1/2 CUPS ASPARAGUS PIECES and 3 SLICED GREEN ONIONS and toss until color changes to bright green. Stir in arrowroot mixture and cook stirring until thickened.
♣Sprinkle with TOASTED SESAME SEEDS. Serve hot over RICE. Garnish with LEMON SLICES.

721   MUSHROOMS PARMESAN

For 6 servings:

♣Combine the marinade in a large bowl

1 CLOVE MINCED GARLIC
1 DICED ONION
2 TBS. CHOPPED PARSLEY
$1/3$ CUP OIL

2 TBS. RED WINE VINEGAR
1 teasp. SEA SALT
2 PINCHES DRY BASIL
$1/4$ teasp. BLACK PEPPER

♣Add $1^1/2$ LBS. SLICED BUTTON MUSHROOMS and marinate for several hours. Drain, reserving liquid. Sauté mushrooms in 4 TBS. marinade over high heat for 1 minutes until aromatic.
♣Reduce heat and simmer for 5 minutes, stirring frequently.
♣Turn mushrooms into a lecithin-sprayed baking dish and sprinkle with $1/2$ CUP WHOLE GRAIN BREAD CRUMBS. Drain with BUTTER, and run under broiler until brown.

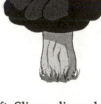

722   CHILE-CHEESE MUSHROOMS

For 4 appetizer servings:

♣Toss together to mix

1 CUP SHREDDED LOW-FAT CHEDDAR
3 TBS. CANNED DICED GREEN CHILES
2 TBS. LOW-FAT MAYONNAISE

3 TBS. SLICED GREEN ONIONS
2 TBS. PLAIN YOGURT
3 TBS. CHOPPED CILANTRO

♣Warm 4 TBS. BUTTER and 1 teasp. GARLIC/LEMON SEASONING. Brush mushroom caps. Fill each with 1 TB. cheese mixture. Sprinkle with PARMESAN and run under the broiler til bubbly.

723   WILD MUSHROOMS IN TOMATO SAUCE

For 2 cups:

♣Soak 12 to 14 DRY BLACK SHIITAKE MUSHROOMS in water to cover until soft. Sliver, discard woody stems, and reserve soaking water.
♣Sauté 2 CLOVES MINCED GARLIC in 1 teasp. OLIVE OIL and $1/3$ CUP RED WINE. Add 1 CUP MINCED ONION and sauté over high heat until aromatic, about 5 minutes.
♣Add $1/2$ CUP SLIVERED PORCINI or CHANTERELLES, and the drained shiitake mushrooms, and stir and toss for 15 minutes.
♣Add 2 CUPS CHOPPED FRESH TOMATOES. Toss to coat. Add 2 TBS. TOMATO PASTE and $1/2$ teasp. DRY BASIL. Reduce heat and simmer for 20 minutes until thickened and fragrant.

Nutritional analysis: per 2oz. serving; 58 calories; 3gm. protein; 9gm. carbohydrate; 3gm. fiber; 2gm. fats; 0 cholesterol; 13mg. calcium; 1mg. iron; 18mg. magnesium; 275mg. potassium; 9mg. sodium; 1mg. zinc.

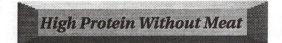

Protein From Beans & Legumes

Beans and legumes are outstanding protein sources, yielding over 20% protein, and under 20% fat.
They include black, kidney, lima and navy beans, split peas, soybeans, wheat germ, black-eyed peas, and lentils.

Mexican Favorites

Mexican food is can be healthy food. While foods in Mexican restaurants are over-fried, refried, gloppy, gooey, and full of fat, home-cooked Mexican food easily provides sound nutrition with its earthy fare. It is a perfect cuisine to provide protein from beans, rice and legumes. The Mexican kitchen is alive with a great assortment of spices, herbs, vegetables and fruits. When you are developing a healthy healing diet, it's important to keep meals tempting and flavorful. Mexican food is without a doubt, fiesta food, a feast for the eyes and taste buds. Mexican food can also be great fast food; and a busy life means that quick, easy menus are imperative. Obviously, for healing diet purposes, Mexican seasonings should be mild, and saturated fat from fried or animal foods should be kept to a minimum.

724   BLACK BEAN SOUP

For 6 to 8 servings:

♣Soak 1 LB. BLACK TURTLE BEANS overnight in a pot.

♣Drain, rinse, and just cover with cold water. Bring to a boil, and cook until soft.

♣When beans have begun to cook, sauté in 2 TBS. OIL until aromatic

2 CLOVES CHOPPED GARLIC   1 ONION, CHOPPED
2 STACK CHOPPED CELERY   2 CHOPPED CARROTS

♣Add to cooking beans and cover. Cook until tender along with the beans. Remove from heat to slightly cool. Purée in the blender briefly. Return to the pot, and add

3 CUPS CHICKEN or VEGETABLE STOCK   1 teasp. SEA SALT
1/4 CUP LEMON JUICE   1/2 teasp. PEPPER
1/2 CUP SHERRY   1/2 teasp. NUTMEG OR ALLSPICE

♣Pour into soup bowls and float a thin Lemon slice on top of each bowl.

Nutritional analysis: per serving; 208 calories; 12gm. protein; 33gm. carbohydrate; 11gm. fiber; 2gm. fats; 0 cholesterol; 55mg. calcium; 3mg. iron; 91mg. magnesium; 566mg. potassium; 331mg. sodium; 1mg. zinc.

725   DELUXE CHILI CHEESE TOSTADAS

For 6 tostadas: Preheat oven to 450°.

♣Bake 6 WHOLE WHEAT FLOUR TORTILLAS on oiled sheets for 7 minutes until golden. Set aside.

♣Sauté in 1 TB. OIL for 15 minutes   ♣Add and sauté briefly
1 CHOPPED ONION   1 CUP CHOPPED BELL PEPPER
1 teasp. DRY OREGANO   4-OZ. TINY COOKED SHRIMP
ONE 1 4-OZ. CAN CHOPPED GREEN CHILIS

♣Assemble the tostadas. Leave a small circle in the center of each tostada for the egg. Spread the vegetable mixture over the rest. Sprinkle with SHREDDED LOW FAT JACK and SHREDDED LOW-FAT CHEDDAR to cover. Bake for about 3 minutes until cheese melts. Remove and top with TOMATO SLIVERS on each tostada. Break an EGG in the center of each and bake until eggs are set.

726   THE DEVIL'S CHILI

For 6 to 8 servings:

♣Use our GOURMET BEAN MIX or your own favorites for this chili. Soak about 1 LB. beans overnight. Rinse. Cover with 2-QTS. cold water and bring to a boil. Add

2 TBS. MISO PASTE	1 teasp. TURMERIC
1 TB. PAPRIKA	1 teasp. BASIL
1 TB. CHILI POWDER	

♣Simmer for 1½ hours until tender. Set aside.

♣Sauté until aromatic

♣Add and sauté

2 TBS. OIL	4 CHOPPED GREEN ONIONS
2 TBS. MINCED GARLIC	1 CHOPPED BELL PEPPER
1½ CUPS CHOPPED ONION	16-OZ. TOMATO SAUCE

♣Add 3 LARGE CHOPPED TOMATOES and simmer until fork tender for 1 hour. Mix onions with beans. ♣Divide between individual bowls. Sprinkle with LOW-FAT CHEDDAR CHEESE and serve.

Nutritional analysis: per serving; 250 calories; 16gm. protein; 40gm. carbohydrate; 15gm. fiber; 5gm. fats; 5mg. cholesterol; 156mg. calcium; 4mg. iron; 102mg. magnesium; 934mg. potassium; 241mg. sodium; 2mg. zinc.

727   BEST BURRITOS

For 4 to 6 burritos: Preheat oven to 400°.

♣Have ready 4 to 6 WHOLE WHEAT FLOUR TORTILLAS.
♣Have ready 5 CUPS COOKED PINTO BEANS. Reserve enough of their cooking liquid to mash beans to the consistency of mashed potatoes.

♣Sauté 4 CLOVES CHOPPED GARLIC and 4 CUPS CHOPPED ONION in 4 TBS. OIL until aromatic.
♣Add and sauté until color changes
1 CHOPPED RED BELL PEPPER
1 CHOPPED GREEN BELL PEPPER
1½ TBS. CUMIN POWDER
1 TBS. GROUND CORIANDER
1 teasp. OREGANO
♣Cover, remove from heat and set aside.

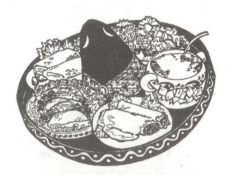

♣Add filling ingredients to the mashed beans
1 CUP CORN KERNALS
½ CUP CHOPPED OLIVES
1⅓ CUP GRATED LOW-FAT CHEDDAR

♣Oil a baking sheet. Spoon equal amounts of filling onto tortillas. Roll up from the bottom, pressing filling to distribute. Place seam side down on the oiled pan. Brush with a little olive oil. Cover with foil and bake for 20 minutes. Uncover and sprinkle with MORE CHEESE. Broil for 1 or 2 minutes to melt cheese. Sprinkle with a little MILD SALSA.

728   TEX-MEX SANDWICH

For 4 sandwiches: Have ready 4 SLICES WHOLE WHEAT TOAST

♣For the filling: Sauté 2 CAKES of CUBED TOFU, 1 SMALL CHOPPED RED ONION and $1/2$ CHOPPED BELL PEPPER in 1 TB. OIL until soft.
♣Mix with

1 CHOPPED TOMATO	$1/2$ teasp. CHILI POWDER
$3/4$ CUP CRUSHED TORTILLA CHIPS	$1/4$ teasp. PAPRIKA
$3/4$ CUP SHREDDED LOW-FAT CHEDDAR	$1/4$ teasp. SEA SALT
4 to 5 TBS. LIGHT MAYONNAISE	$1/2$ teasp. DRY OREGANO
$1/2$ JUICED LEMON	$1/2$ teasp. CUMIN

♣Pile on toast. Top with ALFALFA SPROUTS.

729   MILD MIXED VEGETABLE CHILI

For 8 to 10 servings, or have some left-overs for another delicious meal.

♣Combine all ingredients in a large pot. Bring to a simmer and cook til tender, about $1 1/4$ hours.

2 CUPS <u>COOKED</u> BLACK BEANS	2 TBS. CHILI POWDER
1 EGGPLANT in CUBES	2 TBS. DRY OREGANO
2 ZUCCHINI in CUBES	2 TBS. DRY BASIL
32-OZ. CANNED TOMATOES	1 TB. DILL WEED
2 DICED ONIONS	$1 1/2$ TB. CUMIN
$1 1/2$ CUPS CORN KERNELS	1 CUP CHICKEN BROTH
2 teasp. GARLIC/LEMON SEASONING	1 CHOPPED BELL PEPPER
$1/3$ CUP FRESH CHOPPED PARSLEY	

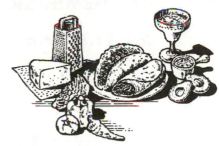

730   TOFU TAMALE NO CRUST PIE

Serves 6 to 8: Preheat oven to 350°.

♣Sauté in 3 TBS. OIL, 2 CLOVES CHOPPED GARLIC, 1 CHOPPED
ONION, 1 LB. CRUMBLED TOFU and 1 CHOPPED BELL PEPPER in a large pot until brown.
♣Remove from heat and stir in

1 CUP COOKED BROWN RICE	$1/4$ CUP ROSÉ WINE
6 to 8 CHOPPED TOMATOES	1 CUP CORNMEAL
ONE 4-OZ. CAN CHOPPED GREEN OLIVES	$1/2$ teasp. CUMIN POWDER
1 CUPS CORN KERNALS	$1/2$ teasp. PEPPER
2 BOUILLON CUBES dissolved in $1/2$ CUP WATER	2 TBS. CHILI POWDER

♣Bake for 45 minutes. Remove from oven and sprinkle on GRATED JACK CHEESE to completely cover top. Bake for 15 more minutes until bubbly.

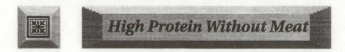

731   CHEESE & RICE ENCHILADAS

For 8 enchiladas: Preheat oven to 350°.

♣Have 8 CORN TORTILLAS ready for filling. Oil a 9 x 13" baking dish.

♣Mix 1 CUP COOKED BROWN RICE with
1 CUP GRATED CHEDDAR   2 TBS. TOASTED SUN SEEDS
1/4 CUP CHOPPED ALMONDS or PECANS   1/2 CUP CHOPPED BLACK OLIVES
DASHES of HOT PEPPER SAUCE
♣Make the sauce. Sauté 2 CLOVES MINCED GARLIC, 1 CHOPPED ONION and 2 CHOPPED JA-LAPEÑO CHILIES in 3 TBS. OIL until aromatic.
♣Add 4 CUPS CHOPPED TOMATOES and 1/2 teasp. CHILI POWDER, SPANISH SEASONING or MEX-ICAN MIX, and sauté for 20 minutes more.
♣Assemble the enchiladas. Dip a tortilla into the hot sauce until soft. Lay flat and line 1/8 of the filling down the center. Roll up and lay seam side down in the baking dish. Fill all and lay side by side.
♣Top with GRATED CHEDDAR CHEESE and CRUSHED TORTILLA CHIPS. Bake for 10 -15 minutes until cheese bubbles, and chips are toasty.

Nutritional analysis: per serving; 298 calories; 14gm. protein; 37gm. carbohydrate; 6gm. fiber; 12gm. fats; 11mg. cho-lesterol; 272mg. calcium; 2mg. iron; 78mg. magnesium; 408mg. potassium; 190mg. sodium; 2mg. zinc.

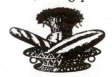

Protein From Whole Grains

732   GOURMET GRAINS & NUT LOAF

For 4 servings: Preheat oven to 350°.

♣Have ready about 1 1/2 CUPS COOKED MIXED GRAINS.

♣Mix grains together with
1 CUP TOASTED WHEAT GERM **or** GRAPENUTS   3 EGGS
3/4 CUP CHOPPED ONION   1 teasp. VEGETABLE SALT
1 CUP WALNUT PIECES   1/2 teasp. PEPPER
1 LB. LOW-FAT COTTAGE CHEESE
♣Pack into a lecithin-sprayed loaf pan, and bake for 50 minutes until brown on the top. Cool. Spoon a **YOGURT SAUCE** on top when serving.

♣For 1 1/4 cups:
♣Toast 1 CUP SESAME SEEDS in the oven until golden. Sauté 1 CHOPPED ONION in 1 TB. OIL and 1/2 teasp. GARLIC/LEMON SEASONING until fragrant.
♣Blend in the blender with SESAME SALT and PEPPER, and serve at room temperature over loaf.

❈

733   SPICY GRAINS, BEANS & MUSHROOMS

For 8 servings:

♣Have ready 2 CUPS COOKED MIXED BEANS.

♣Place $1/2$ CUP BULGUR in a bowl. Bring $2 1/2$ CUPS TOMATO JUICE to a boil and pour over bulgur. Let stand for 3 minutes. Drain and reserve juice. Set aside.
♣Sauté 2 CHOPPED ONIONS in 4 TBS. OIL in a large pot for 4 minutes.
♣Add 1 CHOPPED GREEN PEPPER and 1 CLOVE MINCED GARLIC and sauté for 2 minutes.
♣Add 2 STALKS CELERY and 1 CHOPPED CARROT and sauté for 2 minutes.
♣Add 1 LB. CHOPPED MUSHROOMS and sauté for 1 minute.
♣Add

THE RESERVED TOMATO JUICE	1 TB. TOMATO PASTE
$1 1/2$ CUPS WATER	3 TBS. CHILI POWDER
$1/2$ CUP VERMOUTH	2 teasp. CUMIN

♣Bring to a boil and simmer uncovered for 20 minutes until liquid is reduced. Add beans and simmer, partially covered for 15 minutes.

734   MOROCCAN COUSCOUS

For 4 servings:

♣Combine 1 CUP COUSCOUS, 2 CUPS BOILING WATER and $1/2$ teasp. SEA SALT in a large bowl.
♣Let stand for 15 minutes until grains swell. Pour off any excess water and rub out lumps. Add 2 TBS. OLIVE OIL and toss. Add 1 SLIVERED HOT PEPPER and $1/2$ teasp. CINNAMON.
♣Steam in a large wok or steamer

2 CUPS COOKED GARBANZOS	4 CUPS CHUNKED ZUCCHINI
1 LARGE SLICED ONION	3 CUPS CAULIFLOWER CHUNKS
2 CARROTS in matchsticks	or CHUNKED POTATOES

♣Make the sauce. Cook 4 CUPS DICED TOMATOES with $1/2$ teasp. SEA SALT in a saucepan until fragrant. Put grains on a serving platter. Surround with vegetables and top with tomato sauce.

735   AUTHENTIC YELLOW RICE

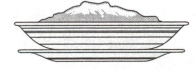

For 4 to 6 servings:

♣Sauté 1 CHOPPED ONION in 2 TBS. oil in a large pot until soft.
♣Add 1 CUP BASMATI RICE and $1/4$ teasp. TURMERIC. Stir until rice is opaque, about 5 minutes.
♣Add $1 3/4$ CUPS WATER. Bring to a boil and cook uncovered until water is below surface of the rice. Cover and cook on low til rice is tender, about 10 minutes.

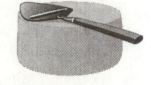

736   BROWN RICE WITH CHEESE

For 6 servings: Preheat oven to 350°.

♣Have ready 3 CUPS COOKED BROWN BASMATI RICE.
♣Blanch 2 CUP BROCCOLI FLORETS until color changes to bright green.

♣Mix rice and broccoli together with

1 CUP SHREDDED SWISS CHEESE	1/4 CUP MINCED PARSLEY
3/4 CUP CHICKEN BROTH	2 TBS. DIJON MUSTARD
1/3 CUP PLAIN YOGURT	1/4 teasp. PEPPER
1/2 CUP CHOPPED GREEN ONIONS	3 TBS. LIGHT MAYONNAISE

♣Turn into a lecithin-sprayed casserole, and sprinkle with 1/4 CUP WHOLE GRAIN BREAD CRUMBS mixed with 2 TBS. MELTED BUTTER. Bake for 15 to 20 minutes until hot and brown.

Nutritional analysis: per serving; 258 calories; 10gm. protein; 29gm. carbohydrate; 3gm. fiber; 9gm. fats; 22mg. cholesterol; 172mg. calcium; 1mg. iron; 66mg. magnesium; 242mg. potassium; 221mg. sodium; 2mg. zinc.

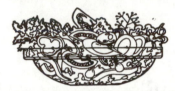

High Protein Salads

Believe it or not, a salad can be full of satisfying protein, and still light and low in fat. It is an excellent way to use complementary proteins from nuts, seeds and dark green vegetables.

737   SPINACH & MUSHROOMS SUPREME

This salad is especially good with Champagne Vinegar Dressing. Every time we go to the wine country of California, we stock up on Champagne vinegar from one of the winerys. It makes wonderful light salad dressings.
For 8 salads:

♣Toast 1/2 CUP SESAME SEEDS in the oven until golden.
♣Trim and wash 2 BUNCHES OF SPINACH or 1 BUNCH OF SPINACH and SOME ROMAINE and CHARD LEAVES. Tear into bite size pieces, and put in a big mixing bowl. Slice 1 RED ONION, 4-OZ. FRESH MUSHROOMS and 2 HARD BOILED EGGS into the bowl in thin slices.

CHAMPAGNE VINEGAR DRESSING

♣Combine in a saucepan to simmer	♣Whisk in
2 TBS. FRUCTOSE	1 EGG
1 1/2 TBS. UNBLEACHED FLOUR	3 TBS. CREAM
1 teasp. DIJON MUSTARD	1/2 teasp. SESAME SALT
1 CUP CHAMPAGNE VINEGAR	1/2 teasp. PEPPER

♣Whisk in 2 TBS. OIL in a steady stream until blended. Remove from heat and pour over salad.

♣Top with FRESH ENOKI MUSHROOMS and toss with the dressing until everything is coated.

738   TOFU POTATO SALAD

For 8 salads:

♣STEAM 1$\frac{1}{2}$ LB. SLICED RED POTATOES til tender. Set aside.

♣Have ready ONE 8-OZ. PACKAGE CALIFORNIA BURGER, NATURE BURGER, or FALAFEL MIX.

♣Mix with
1 LB. CRUMBLED TOFU
$\frac{1}{2}$ CUP WATER
$\frac{1}{4}$ CUP FRESH CHOPPED PARSLEY

1 TB. TARRAGON VINEGAR
$\frac{1}{4}$ CUP GRATED PARMESAN

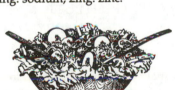

♣Sauté in a skillet until aromatic
$\frac{1}{2}$ CUP CHOPPED ONION
2 TBS. PIMENTOS
$\frac{1}{2}$ CUP CHOPPED CELERY
♣Add burger mix and simmer for 15 minutes until browned. Add potatoes, toss and chill.

♣Blend the dressing while salad is chilling. Mix in a small bowl
$\frac{1}{3}$ CUP CIDER VINEGAR
1 TB. TAMARI

$\frac{1}{3}$ CUP OIL
$\frac{1}{4}$ CUP KETCHUP
♣Pour over and serve. Sprinkle with CHOPPED FRESH PARSLEY.

Nutritional analysis: per serving; 298 calories; 9gm. protein; 41gm. carbohydrate; 7gm. fiber; 12gm. fats; 0 cholesterol; 67mg. calcium; 7mg. iron; 89mg. magnesium; 577mg. potassium; 139mg. sodium; 2mg. zinc.

739   CALIFORNIA FALAFEL SALAD

For 6 salads:

♣Boil 1 LB. CUBED TOFU in 1 CUP BOILING WATER for 5 minutes. Drain. Toss with 6 to 8-OZ. FALAFEL MIX or SESAME BURGER MIX and set aside.

♣Sauté $\frac{1}{2}$ CUP CHOPPED GREEN ONION in 1 TB. OIL until color changes.
♣Add $\frac{1}{2}$ CUP WATER and let bubble. Remove from heat. Add tofu and falafel mix. Toss to coat and set aside to absorb water.
♣Slice 2 HARD BOILED EGGS and 1 CUP CELERY into mixture.
♣Add 1 TB. SWEET HOT MUSTARD, $\frac{1}{2}$ CUP LIGHT MAYONNAISE and $\frac{1}{2}$ CUP SWEET PICKLE RELISH.

♣Stir just lightly to moisten. Chill for 1 hour and serve over SHREDDED LETTUCE on toast.

Nutritional analysis: per serving on toast; 420 calories; 18gm. protein; 44gm. carbos; 10gm. fiber; 13gm. fats; 79mg. cholesterol; 165mg. calcium; 8mg. iron; 158mg. magnesium; 567mg. potass.; 245mg. sodium; 3mg. zinc.

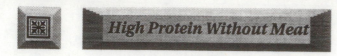

740   HIGH ENERGY SALAD

For 3 salads:

♣Mix in a large bowl just to moisten
1/2 CUP "ORIENTAL PARTY MIX" (You can buy this in most Health Food stores. Or use your own favorite crunchy snack mix.)
2 TBS. TOASTED SESAME SEEDS   1 CARROT JULIENNED
2 TBS. SUNFLOWER SEEDS   2 TBS. GRANOLA
3 TBS. CHOPPED FRESH PARSLEY   1/4 teasp. PEPPER
8-OZ. CARTON OF LEMON/LIME YOGURT
♣Mound onto big lettuce cups and top with HARD BOILED EGG SLICES, GRATED CHEESE SPRINKLES and A HANDFUL of ALFALFA SPROUTS.

Nutritional analysis: per serving; 379 calories; 20gm. protein; 24gm. carbo.; 5gm. fiber; 24gm. fats; 107mg. cholesterol; 281mg. calcium; 3mg. iron; 127mg. magnesium; 615mg. potassium; 238mg. sodium; 3mg. zinc.

❊

741   MIXED SPROUT & MUSHROOM SALAD

For 4 salads:

♣Rinse, drain and toss to aerate 11/2 CUPS ALFALFA SPROUTS, 1 CUP BEAN SPROUTS and 1 CUP SUNFLOWER SPROUTS. Place in a salad bowl.
♣Thin slice 8 OZ. FRESH BUTTON MUSHROOMS and add to bowl.
♣Mix together 1/3 CUP SHERRY, 1/4 CUP SOY SAUCE, and 1 teasp. HONEY. Pour over salad and toss to coat.

Nutritional analysis: per serving; 116 calories;10gm. protein; 20mg. carbohydrate; 4gm. fiber; trace fats; 0 cholesterol; 22mg. calcium; 2mg. iron; 44mg. magnesiium; 349mg. potassium; 180mg. sodium; 1mg. zinc.

❊

742   TAMARI ALMOND RICE SALAD

For 4 salads:

♣This is delicious tossed with **ORIENTAL ORANGE DRESSING (see index)**

♣Toss all ingredients with 2 CUPS COOKED BROWN RICE or COOKED GOURMET GRAINS.

1/2 CUP CHOPPED RED BELL PEPPER   1/2 CUP SLICED CELERY
1/2 CUP STRUNG SLICED SNOW PEAS   2 CHOPPED SCALLIONS
1/2 CUP *TOASTED* SLIVERED ALMONDS   1/2 CUP CURRANTS
♣Toss with a dressing choice. Serve in lettuce cups.

❊

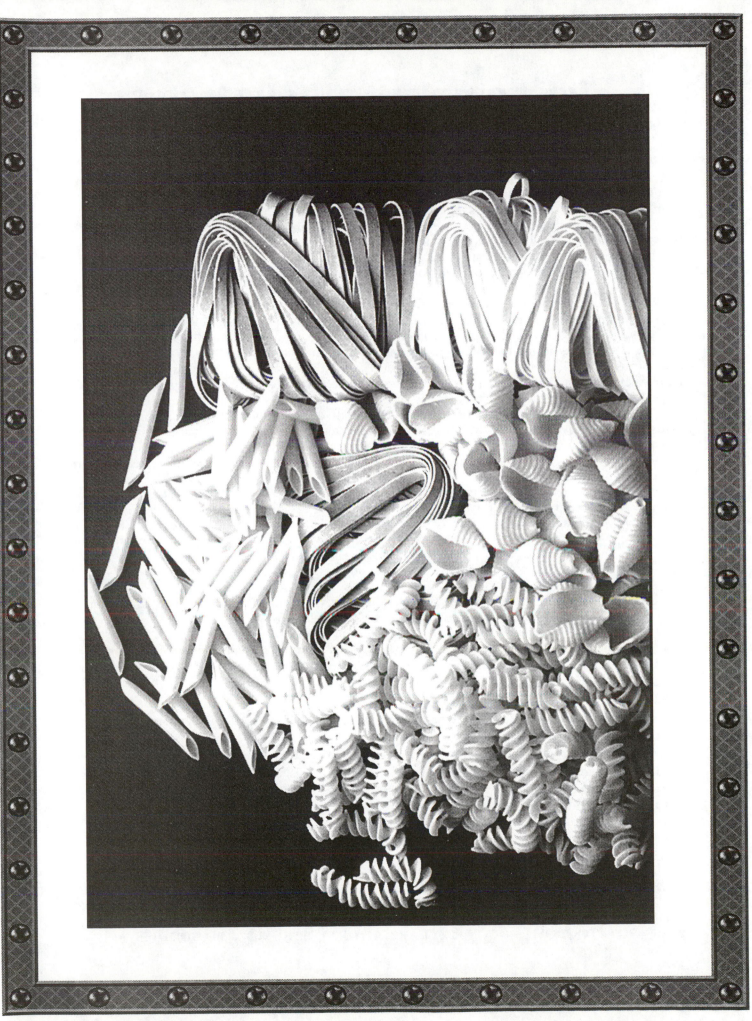

High Complex Carbohydrates For Energy

Complex carbohydrates supply energy and fuel for activity, regulate blood sugar levels, and transport nutrients through the system. The main function of <u>all</u> carbohydrates is the production of energy. *Simple carbohydrates* such as sugars, enter the blood stream quickly, supply a quick "rush" and subsequent drop. *Simple carbohydrates* from sugars or refined foods are digested quickly and encourage the body to use fats as <u>**stored**</u> fuel instead of metabolizing it for energy. *Complex carbohydrates* such as whole grains and high fiber vegetables are digested gradually, enter the bloodstream more slowly, provide a steadier source of fuel, and help stabilize blood sugar after simple carbohydrate intake.

Advanced research on weight control indicates that complex carbohydrates are one of the best ways to keep weight down and the body trim. The soluble fiber in these foods fills hunger needs rapidly, actually reducing total calorie absorption. You don't eat as much, and **almost one-third** of the fiber is excreted unabsorbed as it provides bulk to the bowel elimination process. Even a moderately high fiber intake means 100 to 150 *fewer* calories that are turned into fat *every day*. In fact, if you still ate the same number of calories, but built them around complex carbohydrates such as whole grains, nuts, seeds, vegetables, beans, legumes and fruit, instead of simple carbohydrates such as milk, meats, sweets and refined foods, you would lose about 5 to 8 pounds a month on a continuing basis. High complex carbohydrate foods are even better for weight loss than most commercial diet foods, because they contain less fat calories and take more energy to digest. In a weird twist of body mechanics, we know that obese people actually tend to eat **fewer** calories; but those calories are fat calories, that the system converts into body fat.
Twenty-three calories of energy are needed to turn 100 calories of complex carbohydrates into body fat, so only 77 calories remain to gird your hips. In contrast, only 3 calories of energy are needed to turn 100 calories of dietary fat into body fat; ninety-seven calories are left to be turned into stored body fat.

Athletes and body builders can also improve performance with a complex carbohydrate rich diet, because these foods promote storage of muscle fuel and enhance recovery after exertion.

Heart disease, hypoglycemia and diabetic conditions respond to a complex carbohydrate diet, as weight, high blood pressure, and sugar imbalances are reduced.

To help you add more complex carbohydrates to your diet, a short list of the best sources is included:
 ☛**Whole grains:** wheat, rye, amaranth, buckwheat, triticale, brown rice, wild rice, oats, barley, corn, bulgur, and millet.
 ☛**Pasta:** whole grain and vegetable pasta.
 ☛**Vegetables:** potatoes, squashes, spinach, celery, yams, asparagus, chard, bell peppers, broccoli, carrots and cauliflower.
 ☛**Fruits:** apples, prunes, raisins, cranberries, peaches, pears, papaya, pineapple, figs and bananas.
 ☛**Nuts & Seeds:** cashews, almonds, brazils, coconuts, chestnuts, pine nuts, pistachios, walnuts, sesame seeds, sunflower seeds, pumpkin seeds, and water chestnuts.
 ☛**Beans & Legumes:** peas, split peas, peanuts, soy bean products, black beans, lentils, garbanzos, limas, aduki and mung beans.

❋

The recipes in this section emphasize:
☙COMPLEX CARBOHYDRATES FROM RICE & WHOLE GRAINS ☙COMPLEX CARBOHYDRATES FROM BEANS and LEGUMES ☙ITALIAN LESSONS: COMPLEX CARBOHYDRATES FROM WHOLE GRAIN PASTA ☙COMPLEX CARBOHYDRATES FROM VEGETABLES ☙POTATO PROFITS ☙COMPLEX CARBOHYDRATES FROM BAKED GOODIES ☙

Complex Carbohydrates From Rice & Whole Grains

743   WHEAT GERM & WALNUT LOAF

This recipe is both a father and son favorite; and excellent for a man's system balance and growth.
For 6 servings: Preheat oven to 350°.

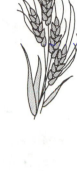

♣Toast 1 CUP CHOPPED WALNUTS and 1 CUP WHEAT GERM on a tray until brown.

♣Sauté 1 LARGE ONION CHOPPED, 1 teasp. THYME and 1/4 teasp. MARJORAM in 2 TBS. BUTTER until transparent.
♣Turn into a large bowl and mix with walnuts and wheat germ.

♣Add and mix in

1 teasp. SESAME SALT

1/2 teasp. PEPPER

1 CUP GRATED CHEDDAR

3 EGGS

3/4 CUP TOMATO JUICE

♣Pack into a greased loaf pan and bake for 45 minutes until moist but firm. Let rest before slicing. Serve with a **FRESH TOMATO SAUCE**.

For 2 cups:

♣Brown 1/2 CHOPPED ONION and 2 CLOVES MINCED GARLIC in 2 TBS. OIL until aromatic.
♣Add 1 GRATED CARROT, 2 TBS. CHOPPED GREEN PEPPER, 4 CUPS TOMATOES, 1 teasp. OREGANO, 1/2 teasp. THYME, 1/2 teasp. BASIL, 1 teasp. SEA SALT, 1/4 teasp. FRUCTOSE, and 1/4 teasp. PEPPER.
♣Simmer for 30 minutes to reduce liquid and spoon over loaf.

744   GREEN RICE

For 6 servings: Preheat oven to 350°.

♣Toast 1/2 CUP CHOPPED WALNUTS in the oven. Remove and sprinkle with melted butter. Leave oven on.
♣Have ready 3 CUPS COOKED BROWN RICE in a large mixing bowl.
♣Add and mix to blend

1/3 CUP PLAIN LOW-FAT YOGURT

3/4 CUP FRESH MINCED PARSLEY

1/2 CUP MINCED GREEN BELL PEPPER

1/2 teasp. GARLIC/LEMON SEASONING

2 CUPS GRATED CHEDDAR

2 TBS. WATER

2 TBS. MELTED BUTTER

♣Turn into a greased casserole. Sprinkle with the BUTTERED WALNUTS. Bake for 45 minutes.

Nutritional analysis: per serving; 290 calories; 12gm. protein; 27gm. carbohydrate; 3gm. fiber; 15gm. fats; 25mg. cholesterol; 262mg. calcium; 74mg. magnesium; 2mg. iron; 206mg. potassium; 172mg. sodium; 2mg. zinc.

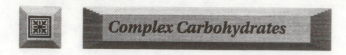
745   WHOLE GRAIN STUFFING BAKE

For 6 servings: Preheat oven to 350°.

♣Toast 4 CUPS WHOLE GRAIN BREAD CUBES until dry and crisp. Remove and leave oven on.

♣Sauté 1 CUP CHOPPED ONION, 1/2 teasp. SESAME SALT and 1/2 teasp. PEPPER in 2 TBS. BUTTER until transparent.

♣Add and sauté for 10 minutes
2 STALKS CELERY   1 TB. DIJON MUSTARD
1 teasp. HERB POULTRY SEASONING   2 CUPS SLICED MUSHROOMS

♣Add 2 TBS. FLOUR and stir for 5 minutes until flour is blended in. Add 4 TBS. SHERRY, and cook for 5 minutes more.

♣Mix and toss with bread cubes, and spread into a shallow buttered baking casserole. Sprinkle with 1 CUP CHOPPED WALNUTS or PECANS. Sprinkle with 1/2 CUP GRATED CHEDDAR.

♣Beat 4 EGGS with 1/3 CUP PLAIN LOW-FAT YOGURT and 2 TBS. WATER. Pour over casserole.
♣Dust with NUTMEG and PAPRIKA and bake for 45 minutes until firm and brown.

Nutritional analysis: per serving; 356 calories; 14gm. protein; 26gm. carbos; 3gm. fiber; 22gm. fats; 151mg. cholesterol; 168mg. calcium; 3mg. iron; 61mg. magnesium; 406mg. potassium; 257mg. sodium; 2mg. zinc.

746   WHOLE GRAINS QUICHE

This can be made with the crust given here, or with no crust at all.
It becomes a totally different dish with no crust, but is very good.
For 8 pieces: Preheat oven to 400°.

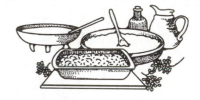

♣Make the crust if desired. Mix
3/4 CUP UNBLEACHED FLOUR   6 TBS. STICK BUTTER
1/2 CUP WHOLE WHEAT PASTRY FLOUR   1/4 CUP PARMESAN

♣Add 4 TBS. ICE WATER. Mix to form a dough ball. Wrap and chill for 30 minutes or more.
♣Fit into a greased quiche pan, and bake for 18 minutes. Remove from oven, and reduce heat to 375°.
♣Make the filling in the blender
1 CUP LOW-FAT RICOTTA CHEESE (or fresh TOFU)   2 TBS. BUTTER
2 EGGS   PINCH NUTMEG
2 TBS. WATER   PINCH PEPPER
1/3 CUP PLAIN YOGURT

♣Mix with 1 1/2 CUPS COOKED GOURMET GRAINS or BROWN RICE and 3/4 CUP PARMESAN.
♣Turn into the baked shell or into a greased casserole and bake for 30 minutes.

747 BROCCOLI & GOURMET GRAINS

For 6 servings:

♣Blanch 4 CUPS BROCCOLI FLORETS in a large pot of boiling salted water until color changes to bright green. Drain and rinse immediately with cold water. Set aside.

♣Heat 4 TBS. BUTTER, $1/4$ teasp. NUTMEG and dashes HOT PEPPER SAUCE in a skillet until sizzling.

♣Add $2^1/2$ CUPS COOKED GOURMET WHOLE GRAIN BLEND (pg. 647), or BROWN RICE and $1/2$ CUP TOASTED SUNFLOWER SEED and toss until coated.

♣Remove from heat and add 5-OZ. KEFIR CHEESE or DICED SWISS CHEESE, $1/2$ CUP PLAIN YO-GURT and $1/4$ CUP LIGHT MAYONNAISE.
♣Add BROCCOLI and toss until coated. Return to heat; stir and toss until cheese melts. Serve right away.

Nutritional analysis: per serving; 365 calories; 14gm. protein; 27gm. carbos; 4gm. fiber; 20gm. fats; 38mg. cholesterol; 265mg. calcium; 2mg. iron; 102mg. magnesium; 381mg. potassium; 171mg. sodium; 2mg. zinc.

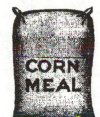

748 POLENTA MILANESE

For 10 people: Preheat oven to 350°.

♣Bring 6 CUPS WATER to a boil and add 2 CUPS POLENTA in a thin stream, stirring.
♣Add 4 TBS. BUTTER, 1 teasp. SEA SALT and $1/2$ teasp. PEPPER and simmer for 20 minute. Stir occasionally to prevent sticking. When thickened, remove from heat and stir in $3/4$ CUP PARMESAN.
♣Pour mixture into a large buttered casserole. Cool and then chill.

♣Sauté 2 GARLIC CLOVES, CHOPPED and 4 CUPS CHOPPED ONION in 3 TBS. OIL until transparent.

♣Add and sauté until color changes
3 STALKS CELERY
3 TBS. DRY BASIL
2 teasp. DRY OREGANO
1 teasp. SESAME SALT
$1/4$ teasp. PEPPER

♣Add and sauté til color changes
1 LG. PEELED EGGPLANT in cubes
1 GREEN BELL PEPPER in squares
$1^1/2$ CUPS SLICED ZUCCHINI

♣Add and simmer until blended
$1^1/2$ CUPS ROSÉ WINE
3 TBS. TOMATO PASTE
$1^1/2$ CUPS CHOPPED FRESH TOMATOES

♣Remove from heat and stir in
$1/2$ CUP GRATED PARMESAN

♣Pour vegetable mix on top of polenta. Top with 3 CUPS CUBED MOZZARELLA, and bake for 45 minutes until cheese browns and bubbles.

Nutritional analysis: per serving;411 calories; 20gm. protein; 34gm. carbohydrates; 6gm. fiber; 20gm. fats; 44mg. cholesterol; 550mg. calcium; 3mg. iron; 81mg. magnesium; 593mg. potass.; 450mg. sodium; 3mg. zinc.

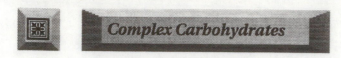

749 CREOLE RED RICE

This recipe is authentic and came with me when I moved to California from Atlanta. I have only changed the real bacon to soy bacon bits and cut down on the oil.
For 4 people:

♣Sauté 1 CUP CHOPPED RED ONION and $1/2$ CUP CHOPPED RED BELL PEPPER in 4 TBS. OLIVE OIL til aromatic, about 5 minutes.

♣Add $1/2$ CUP WHITE BASMATI RICE and stir til coated. Add and stir in

2 CHOPPED TOMATOES	$1/8$ teasp. TABASCO SAUCE
$11/2$ CUPS COLD WATER	1 teasp. PAPRIKA
$3/4$ teasp. SEA SALT	1 teasp. FRUCTOSE

♣Reduce heat, cover, and simmer for 20 minutes til water is absorbed and rice is tender. Remove from heat and set aside, covered for 10 minutes. Serve in a large bowl sprinkled with SOY BACON BITS.

Nutritional analysis: per serving; 215 calories; 3gm. protein; 26gm. carbohydrate; 3gm. fiber; 11gm. fats; 0 cholesterol; 28mg. calcium; 1mg. iron; 52mg. magmesium; 292mg. potassium; 344mg. sodium; 1mg. zinc.

750 DIXIE DRY RICE

The Old South recipe for perfect rice.
For 4 people:

♣Wash 1 CUP BASMATI RICE in a colander until water runs clear.
♣Bring $11/2$ CUPS COLD WATER, 2 TBS. BUTTER, 1 teasp. LEMON JUICE and 1 teasp. SEA SALT to a rapid boil in a pot. Pour in rice, stir and reduce heat to low. Cover and simmer for 20 minutes until tender, and water is all absorbed. Remove from heat and let steam, covered for 10 minutes. Serve with a sauce or gravy for authentic style.

751 HERBED WILD RICE & BREAD STUFFING

The savory goodness of this dish is both delicious and nutritious with baked squash recipes.
For 6 people, about 5 cups:

♣Have ready 3 CUPS COOKED WILD RICE.
♣Heat 2 teasp. OLIVE OIL with $1/4$ CUP WHITE WINE or VEGETABLE STOCK.
♣Add $1/3$ CUP MINCED ONION and stir to coat. Sauté for 5 minutes until fragrant.
♣Add $1/3$ CUP MINCED CELERY and toss for 3 minutes until color changes to bright green.

♣Turn off heat and stir in just to heat through

THE WILD RICE	2 TBS. DRIED CHIVES
2 to 3 SLICES WHOLE WHEAT BREAD crumbled	$1/2$ teasp. DRY SAGE
$1/2$ CUP FRESH MINCED PARSLEY	$1/2$ teasp. DRY THYME
$1/2$ CUP CURRANTS	$1/2$ teasp. SESAME SALT

Complex Carbohydrates From Beans & Legumes

Beans and legumes are good sources of complex carbohydrates as well as quality protein.

752   LENTIL NUT ROAST

Enough for 8 people: Preheat oven to 350°.

♣Have ready 4 CUPS COOKED LENTILS.

♣Sauté 3 CLOVES MINCED GARLIC, 2 CHOPPED ONIONS and SEVERAL SMALL STALKS CHOPPED CELERY WITH LEAVES in 3 TBS. OIL for 5 minutes until fragrant.

♣Add 1¹/₂ CUPS WHOLE GRAIN BREAD CRUMBS, 2 teasp. THYME and 2 teasp. SAGE and toss to coat. Remove from heat and mix in the COOKED LENTILS, ¹/₄ CUPS FRESH CHOPPED PARSLEY, and 1 CUP CHOPPED WALNUTS.

♣Press into a 9 x 13" baking dish. Sprinkle with ¹/₂ CUP MORE BREAD CRUMBS. Cover and bake for 40 minutes. Uncover and bake for 5 more minutes to brown and crisp. Let rest for 10 minutes to set before slicing. Serve with a spicy tomato sauce, or the following **LEMON CHEESE SAUCE.**

LEMON CHEESE SAUCE

♣For 1¹/₂ cups: Make the sauce in the blender. 1 CUP LOW-FAT COTTAGE CHEESE

2 TBS. LEMON JUICE   ¹/₂ teasp. SEA SALT
4 TBS. LIGHT MAYONNAISE   ¹/₂ teasp. PEPPER
¹/₄ CUP PLAIN YOGURT   ¹/₄ teasp. TARRAGON
2 TBS. SNIPPED CHIVES

♣Serve in dollops on NUT ROAST slices.

Nutritional analysis: per serving w. sauce; 412 calories; 19gm. protein; 47gm. carbos; 8gm. fiber; 16gm. fats; 5mg. cholesterol; 125mg. calcium; 6mg. iron; 80mg. magnesium; 651mg. potassium; 360mg. sodium; 2mg. zinc.

753   EASY, SLOW SIMMER LENTIL SOUP

For 6 servings:

♣Sauté 1 CLOVE MINCED GARLIC and 1 CHOPPED ONION in 2 TBS. OIL until fragrant.

♣Add and bring to a boil

4 CUPS WATER   1 CUP LENTILS, rinsed and drained
ONE 14¹/₂ OZ. CANNED TOMATOES with liquid   2 TBS. TAMARI

♣Reduce heat and simmer 1¹/₂ hours until lentils are tender.

♣Add 1 CUP THIN SLICE CARROTS and 2 TBS. LEMON JUICE during last 15 minutes of cooking.

♣Garnish with SNIPPED PARSLEY or cilantro and serve hot.

Nutritional analysis: per serving; 165 calories; 10gm. protein; 26gm. carbohydrates; 6gm. fiber; 3gm. fats; 0 cholesterol; 36mg. calcium; 4mg. iron; 52mg. magnesium; 564mg. potassium; 79mg. sodium; 1mg. zinc.

754   DRESSED UP BEANS

For 6 servings:

♣Cook 1 LARGE PACKAGE FROZEN FRENCH CUT GREEN BEANS in boiling water until just tender and bright green. Drain.

♣Make up 1 PACKAGE MAYACAMAS MUSHROOM SOUP MIX <u>for the sauce recipe</u>.

♣Combine with beans in a large mixing bowl and add

1/4 CUP SHERRY	1/4 teasp. THYME
1 SMALL CAN SLICED WATER CHESTNUTS	1 teasp. SWEET HOT MUSTARD
1/2 teasp. ZEST SEASONING SALT or herb salt	1/2 CUP GRATED CHEDDAR
1/4 teasp. LEMON PEPPER	1/4 CUP KEFIR CHEESE

♣Turn into a shallow casserole. Sprinkle with MORE CHEDDAR to cover and scatter with CRUNCHY CHINESE NOODLES. Bake for 30 minutes to heat through and crisp.

※

755   BUTTERED BEANS WITH PINE NUTS

For 4 servings:

♣Blanch a 20-OZ. PACKAGE ITALIAN GREEN BEANS in boiling water until bright green. Drain.

♣Heat butter sauce in a small pan until golden and sizzling

3 TBS. BUTTER	1 teasp. SESAME SALT
1/4 CUP CHOPPED PARSLEY	1/2 teasp. GROUND PEPPER
1 CUP PINE NUTS	PINCH THYME

♣Toss with beans and serve hot.

Nutritional analysis: per serving; 125 calories; 3gm. protein; 15gm. carbohydrate; 4gm. fiber; 9mg. fats; 23mg. cholesterol; 66mg. calcium; 2mg. iron; 39mg. magnesium; 326mg. potassium; 181mg. sodium; 1mg. zinc.

※

756   CREAMY SESAME BEANS

For 4 servings: Preheat oven to 350°.

♣Toast 1/4 CUP SESAME SEEDS in the oven until golden. Leave oven on.

♣Blanch in 1 CUP VEGETABLE STOCK for 8 minutes	♣Drain and mix in
1 CUP SLICED CELERY	2 TBS. WHOLE WHEAT FLOUR
3 CUPS FROZEN FRENCH CUT GREEN BEANS	1 teasp. SESAME SALT
1/2 ONION SLICED IN RINGS	1 CUP PLAIN LOW-FAT YOGURT

♣Turn into a deep casserole. Mix together and spread over

1/2 CUP LOW-FAT COTTAGE CHEESE	1/2 teasp. PEPPER
1/4 teasp. GARLIC LEMON SEASONING	1/2 teasp. OREGANO

♣Sprinkle with sesame seeds and 1/2 CUP BREAD CRUMBS and bake for 30 minutes.

※

757   HOT CINNAMON LEMON LENTILS

For 4 to 6 servings:

♣Sauté 1 LARGE SLICED ONION and 1 CLOVE CHOPPED GARLIC in 2 TBS. OIL until transparent.

♣Add and sauté until fragrant
1 TB. FRESH GRATED GINGER ROOT
1 LB. WASHED LENTILS
1/4 teasp. HOT PEPPER SAUCE

2 BAY LEAVES
2 BROKEN CINNAMON STICKS
1/4 teasp. PAPRIKA

♣Add 3 1/2 CUPS CHICKEN or VEGETABLE BROTH. Lower heat, cover and cook for 15 to 20 minutes until lentils are tender. Add the JUICE of 1 LEMON and 1 teasp. LEMON PEPPER.
♣Remove bay leaves and cinnamon sticks. Serve hot.

Nurritional analysis: per serving; 318 calories; 22gm. protein; 49gm. carbohydrates; 10gm. fiber; 5gm. fats; 0 cholesterol; 56mg. calcium; 7mg. iron; 89mg. magnesium; 779mg. potassium; 97mg. sodium; 3mg. zinc.

758   PASTITSIO

This is a favorite Italian dish - first tried at a little restaurant near Assisi, and many times at home since then.
For 8 people: Preheat oven to 400°.

♣Cover 3/4 CUP LENTILS with 3 CUPS WATER in a kettle and let soak for a few hours. Add 1 teasp. SEA SALT and 1 TB. OLIVE OIL and let cook til water is almost evaporated, about 30 minutes.

♣Sauté in a large skillet until aromatic
3 TBS. OLIVE OIL
2 TBS. BUTTER
2 CLOVES CHOPPED GARLIC
2 LARGE CHOPPED ONIONS
1 LARGE CHOPPED PEELED EGGPLANT

1/2 teasp. CINNAMON
1/2 teasp. OREGANO
1 teasp. SEA SALT
1/2 teasp. PEPPER
PINCH ANISE SEED

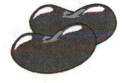

♣Cover and cook for 10 minutes
♣Add 8 CHOPPED TOMATOES, THE COOKED LENTILS and any remaining liquid. Cook until very thick, stirring occasionally. Add 1 SMALL CAN TOMATO PASTE and stir in to blend.

♣Meanwhile, bring salted water to a boil for SESAME or VEGETABLE PASTA. Cook for 10 minutes to *al dente*. Toss with a little oil to separate.
♣Butter a large casserole and cover the bottom with a layer of noodles. Sprinkle with PARMESAN CHEESE to cover.
♣Top with a layer of lentil mixture. Repeat until all ingredients are used, ending with the lentils.

♣Make the sauce. Melt 3 TBS. BUTTER in a small pan. Add 3 TBS. WHOLE WHEAT FLOUR and stir until bubbly. Whisk in 1 1/2 CUPS PLAIN YOGURT, 1 CUP WATER, and 1/2 CUP WHITE WINE.
♣Remove from heat and whisk in 3 EGGS. Pour them over casserole.
♣Sprinkle with PARMESAN and ROMANO CHEESES and bake for 1 hour. Serve very hot.

Italian Lessons:
Complex Carbohydrates From Whole Grain Pasta

The renaissance of authentic Italian food in America is an excellent avenue for healthy cooking. You would have to be almost dead not to have your mouth water over some of the delicious pasta recipes. Whole grain and vegetable pastas are rich in complex carbohydrates, low in fats with plenty of vitamins, minerals and fiber. And they aren't just made from wheat any more. Buckwheat, corn, artichoke, spinach, rice and spelt all have an up and coming place in the popularity of pasta. (See page 225 for PASTA PREP information.)

759   WHOLE GRAIN PASTA SALAD
Pasta and fresh vegetables for the taste of an Italian summer.
For 6 servings:

♣Bring 2-qts. salted water to a boil, and cook 1 LB. WHOLE GRAIN PASTA to *al dente*. Drain, toss with 1 teasp. OIL to keep separated, and place in a large mixing bowl.

♣Mix the salad together

1 CHOPPED RED BELL PEPPER	1 CHOPPED TOMATO
1 PEELED CHOPPED CUCUMBER	3 CHOPPED GREEN ONIONS
$1/4$ CUP FRESH CHOPPED PARSLEY	1 SLICED AVOCADO
1 SMALL CAN SLICED BLACK OLIVES	3 TBS. CHOPPED FRESH BASIL

♣Toss with the pasta. Top with GRATED PARMESAN CHEESE to cover and serve with a **MUSH-ROOM LEMON VINAIGRETTE**.

For $1^1/4$ cups:
♣Sauté $1/2$ CUP SLICED MUSHROOMS in 2 teasp, OLIVE OIL for 6 minutes. Add 1 CUP WATER and simmer for 10 minutes to extract the mushroom flavor. Strain and discard mushrooms. Boil liquid over high heat for 3 minutes until reduced to 3 TBS. Set aside.
♣Whisk 2 TBS. TAMARI, 2 TBS. LEMON JUICE, and $2/3$ CUP OLIVE OIL together with $1/2$ teasp. SESAME SALT and $1/4$ teasp. LEMON PEPPER. Chill and serve with the pasta salad.

760   HONEY OF A PASTA SALAD

For 4 to 6 servings:

♣Bring 2 qts. salted water to a boil, and cook 2 CUPS VEGETABLE ROTELLI SPIRALS for 9 minutes to *al dente*. Rinse in cold water and drain. Toss with 1 teasp. oil to separate. Set aside.
♣Sauté 3 TBS. SOY BACON BITS and 2 TBS. SLICED ALMONDS in 2 teasp. OIL for 6 minutes until aromatic and brown. Add to pasta and set aside.
♣Mix the sauce together in a bowl

$1/2$ CUP CHOPPED CELERY	$1/3$ CUP LIGHT MAYONNAISE
$1/2$ CUP SHREDDED CARROT	1 TB. HONEY
1 SLICED GREEN ONION	$1/2$ teasp. BLACK PEPPER

♣Add to pasta and toss together. Serve on lettuce cups.

761   LOW FAT SPINACH & MUSHROOM LASAGNA

One 8 x 8" pan for 6 people: Preheat oven to 400°.

♣Stem, rinse and chop 1 LARGE BUNCH SPINACH.

♣Bring 2 qts. salted water to a rapid boil. Toss in 9 SPINACH LASAGNA NOODLES and cook for 8 minutes. Drain, rinse in cold water and toss with 1 teasp. OIL to separate. Set aside.

♣Make the filling. Cook in a saucepan until fragrant

1 LB. CHOPPED ROMA TOMATOES	1 TB. TOMATO PASTE
4-OZ. SLICED MUSHROOMS	$1^1/_2$ teasp. LEMON PEPPER
$^1/_4$ CUP FRESH CHOPPED BASIL	$^1/_2$ teasp. OREGANO

♣Make the sauce. Cook in another saucepan until thickened

1 CUP PLAIN LOW-FAT YOGURT	3 TBS. WHOLE WHEAT FLOUR
$^1/_2$ CUP WATER	$^1/_2$ teasp. NUTMEG
1 MINCED SHALLOT	$^1/_4$ teasp. GROUND ROSEMARY

♣Remove from heat and add 1 BEATEN EGG. Mix in RESERVED SPINACH and 2 TBS. PARMESAN CHEESE.

♣Assemble the lasagna. Spread some of the filling on the bottom of the 8 x 8" pan. Top with 3 lasagna noodles. Top with a layer of the sauce, and chunks of LOW-FAT MOZARRELLA or SOY CREAM CHEESE. Repeat two more times til all ingredients are used, ending with your cheese choice.
♣Bake until browned and bubbly for 30 minutes. Let stand for 15 minutes to blend and set. Sprinkle with 2 TBS. PARMESAN CHEESE and serve hot.

Nutritional analysis: per serving; 334 calories; 19gm. protein; 49gm. carbohydrates; 6gm. fiber; 8gm. fats; 50mg. cholesterol; 328mg. calcium; 3mg. iron; 139mg. magnesium; 762mg. potassium; 260mg. sodium; 3mg. zinc.

762   PASTA WITH ONION SAUCE
This dish has a subtle flavor that goes well with herb and vegetable-flavored pastas.
For 4 to 6 servings:

♣Bring a large pot of salted water to boil for the pasta.

♣Sauté 6 CUPS THIN-SLICED SWEET ONIONS in 2 TBS. BUTTER and 2 TBS. OIL in a large covered pot until they melt, about 30 minutes. Stir occasionally so they won't burn.

♣Dissolve 2 TBS. TOMATO PASTE in 2 TBS. SHERRY and add with 1 CUP WATER to the onions. Simmer uncovered for 10 minutes. Season with SEA SALT and PEPPER. Cover and remove from heat. Let cool slightly and stir in 2 BEATEN EGGS.

♣Cook $^3/_4$ LB. of your PASTA CHOICE in the boiling water to *al dente*. Drain, place in a serving bowl. Top with the onion sauce and sprinkle with $^2/_3$ CUP PARMESAN CHEESE.

763   PASTA WITH FRESH TUNA

This is a fast, low-fat version of a traditional Sicilian dish that melts in your mouth.
For 6 to 8 servings:

♣Bring a large pot of salted water to boil with 3 CLOVES PEELED GARLIC for the pasta.

♣Sauté 1 LARGE DICED ONION in 4 TBS OLIVE OIL until soft, about 10 minutes.

♣Add 1 LARGE (35-OZ.) CAN ITALIAN TOMATOES, drained and coarsely chopped. Season with ³/₄ teasp. SEA SALT and ¹/₂ teasp. CRACKED PEPPER. Cook, partially covered until juices thicken to form a sauce, about 5 minutes. Remove vegetables from the skillet and set aside in a bowl.

♣Add 2 TBS. more OLIVE OIL to the skillet and heat. Season a 1 LB. FRESH TUNA STEAK on both sides with ¹/₂ teasp. LEMON PEPPER. Dice and sauté in the hot skillet, tossing for <u>4 minutes only.</u>
♣Add the tomato sauce back to the skillet with ¹/₂ CUP CHOPPED FRESH MINT and 3 CHOPPED SCALLIONS.
♣Cook for 2 or 3 minutes until tuna is just opaque.
♣Toss 1 LB. SPAGHETTI in the boiling water and cook to *al dente,* about 9 minutes. Drain, and transfer to a shallow serving bowl. Pour on the hot tun/tomato sauce and toss quickly to mix.

Nutritional analysis: per serving; 402 calories; 22gm. protein; 51gm. carbohydrate; 5gm. fiber; 12gm. fats; 21mg. cholesterol; 45mg. calcium; 4mg. iron; 69mg. magnesium; 592mg. potassium; 211mg. sodium; 1mg. zinc.

764   WHOLE GRAIN MACARONI BEST

This has been one of our favorites for years. Serve hot or cold. The flavor comes through.
For 6 servings:

♣Cook 2 CUPS VEGETABLE MACARONI ELBOWS just to al dente, toss with 1 teasp. OIL. Put in a large casserole and set aside.

♣Add 2 LARGE CHOPPED TOMATOES and mix together.
♣Blanch 1 BUNCH CHOPPED BROCCOLI FLORETS and 1 CUP CHOPPED YELLOW ZUCCHINI or CROOKNECK SQUASH in boiling salted water until color changes.

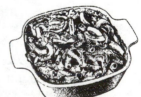

♣Make the dressing in a cup and pour over
¹/₄ CUP LIGHT MAYONNAISE
¹/₂ CUP PLAIN LOW FAT YOGURT
2 TBS. SNIPPED CHIVES
PINCHES SESAME SALT and BLACK PEPPER to taste

♣Serve as is, or if you like it hot, sprinkle with GRATED CHEDDAR or CORN BREAD STUFFING MIX to cover and heat til bubbly, about 15 minutes at 350∞.

Nutritional analysis: per serving; 229 calories; 8gm. protein; 33gm. carbohydrate; 4gm. fiber; 4gm. fats; 5mg. cholesterol; 77mg. calcium; 2mg. iron; 45mg. magnesium; 439mg. potassium; 71mg. sodium; 1mg. zinc.

Complex Carbohydrates From Vegetables

765 QUICK HOMEMADE VEGETABLE STEW

For 6 people:

♣Sauté 4 TBS. SOY BACON BITS and 3 CLOVES CHOPPED GARLIC in 2 teasp. OIL until aromatic.

♣Add 1 LB. CHUNKED POTATOES and 2 SLICED CARROTS and toss for 5 minutes.

♣Bring 4 CUPS SALTED WATER to a boil in a large pot. Add 1 SMALL PACKAGE FROZEN BABY LIMA BEANS, and 1 LARGE PACKAGE FROZEN FRENCH CUT or ITALIAN GREEN BEANS.

♣When water returns to a boil, add the sauté, and simmer for 15 minutes.

♣Add 1 HEAD SLICED GREEN CABBAGE, and simmer until potatoes are tender, usually about 10 more minutes. Add 1 TB. TAMARI, 1/2 teasp. BLACK PEPPER, and 1 teasp. SEASONING SALT.

♣Turn into a large dish and sprinkle with CHOPPED PARSLEY.

Nutritional analysis: per serving; 167 calories; 8gm. protein; 31gm. carbohydrate; 11gm. fiber; 2gm. fats; 0 cholesterol; 126mg. calcium; 7mg. iron; 84mg. magnesium; 780mg. potassium; 149mg. sodium; 1mg. zinc.

766 SPAGHETTI SQUASH WITH TOMATO BASIL SAUCE

For 6 servings: Preheat oven to 375°.

♣Cut a large SPAGHETTI SQUASH in half, and bake face down on a buttered sheet for 30 minutes. Remove from oven and scoop out "spaghetti strands" with a fork into a serving bowl. Set aside.

♣Sauté 2 CHOPPED ONIONS and 1 CLOVE MINCED GARLIC in 3 TBS. OIL until transparent. Add ONE 28-OZ. CANNED TOMATOES, chopped (or 2 LBS. FRESH), 2 TBS. DRY BASIL (or 1/4 CUP FRESH), and 1/2 teasp. DRY OREGANO. Simmer for 5 minutes. Add 1 teasp. FRUCTOSE, SEA SALT and PEPPER.

♣Spoon over squash in the bowl and serve.

767 MIXED VEGETABLES WITH CHEESE

This is a very simple recipe that we like better every time we have it. I change the vegetable mix and the sauce every once in a while, but it never fails to be delicious.
For about 4 servings: Preheat oven to 350°.

♣Chop and slice 6 CUPS of MIXED VEGETABLES. Use BELL PEPPERS, CAULIFLOWER, BROCCOLI FLORETS, CARROTS, MUSHROOMS, and WATER CHESTNUTS.

♣Bring 2-qts. salted water to a boil in a large pot. Add vegetables and blanch until color changes, about 5 to 7 minutes. Place in a lecithin-sprayed casserole.

♣Make up 1 PACKAGE of MAYACAMAS MUSHROOM SOUP MIX for the sauce directions. Add 3 TBS. BUTTER, 2 TBS. NATURAL BOTTLED BARBECUE or HICKORY SAUCE, and 1 TB. TAMARI.

♣Pour over veggies and cover with GRATED CHEDDAR. Bake until brown and bubbly.

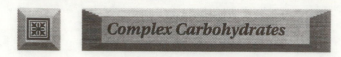

768 RAINBOW VEGGIE MOLDS

These are best made in individual serving-size casseroles. Oil them well, so you can unmold easily.
For 6 servings: Preheat oven to 350°

♣Sauté in 1 TB. BUTTER for 3 minutes until aromatic
2 SMALL SLICED LEEKS (white parts with a little green)
1 teasp. LEMON/GARLIC SEASONING   ¹/₄ teasp. THYME
PINCH LEMON PEEL   ¹/₄ teasp. DRY CHIVES
♣Add 1 SLICED CARROT, 1 teasp. SESAME SALT and ¹/₄ teasp. PEPPER and sauté for 1 minute.

♣Add 3 CUPS MIXED DICED VEGETABLES of your choice - Make a rainbow selection so that the mold
will reflect the different colors: CAULIFLOWER, GREEN PEAS, BROCCOLI, RED BELL PEPPER, and
GOLDEN ZUCCHINI, for instance. Sauté for 1 more minute.
♣Add 2 CUPS CHOPPED MIXED GREENS of your choice - such as CHARD, SPINACH and ROMAINE;
with ¹/₄ CUP CHOPPED FRESH PARSLEY. Remove skillet from heat, and cover immediately to let them
wilt. Toss to coat.

♣Make the sauce in the blender
¹/₄ CUP WHITE WINE or WATER   5 EGGS
¹/₂ CUP DICED FARMER CHEESE   ¹/₂ CUP PLAIN YOGURT
♣Mix with vegetables, and ladle the whole blend into buttered ramekins that have been dusted with
PARMESAN CHEESE. Divide sauce over each. Set in a shallow baking pan with sides touching.
♣Place on oven rack and pour in water to halfway up the sides. Bake for 1 hour until golden. Remove
and let sit for 10 minutes while you make the **QUICK FRESH TOMATO SAUCE** to spoon over top.

♣For 2 cups: Blend in the blender
1 LB. FRESH CHOPPED TOMATOES   1 teasp. HONEY
1 teasp. DRY BASIL (or 1 TB. FRESH)   1 teasp. TARRAGON
♣Run a knife around each ramekin and unmold onto individual salad plated.
♣Spoon sauce over and top with SPRINKLES of PARMESAN CHEESE.

❋

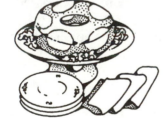

769 PUFFY POSH SQUASH

For 6 servings: Preheat oven to 375°.

♣Slice 2 LBS. YELLOW CROOKNECK or GOLDEN ZUCCHINI in rounds. Blanch in boiling salted water
for 3 to 4 minutes until color intensifies. Drain.

♣Blend in the blender with
¹/₂ CUP LIGHT MAYONNAISE   2 BEATEN EGGS
¹/₂ CUP PLAIN YOGURT   ¹/₂ teasp. SEA SALT
1 SMALL CHOPPED RED ONION   ¹/₄ teasp. DRY THYME
¹/₄ CHOPPED GREEN PEPPER   ¹/₄ teasp. LEMON PEPPER
♣Spread in a shallow baking dish and sprinkle with PARMESAN CHEESE. Bake for 25 minutes until
browned and puffy.

❋

770   EGGPLANT MOUSSAKA

A vegetable Italian version of the Greek favorite.
For 6 servings: Preheat oven to 375°. Oil a 9 x 13" baking dish.

♣Peel and slice 1 EGGPLANT into rounds. Salt lightly, and let drain in a colander to remove bitterness for 1 hour. Lay in a single layer in an oiled baking sheet. Cover with foil and bake for 1 hour.

♣Make the sauce in a skillet. Sauté 2 CLOVES CHOPPED GARLIC and 2 CUPS CHOPPED ONION in 3 TBS. OLIVE OIL until aromatic. Add

4 or 5 CHOPPED ROMA TOMATOES	2 TBS. MINCED PARSLEY
1 CHOPPED GREEN BELL PEPPER	1/2 teasp. DILL WEED
PINCHES SESAME SALT and PEPPER	1/4 teasp. NUTMEG

♣Remove to a bowl.
♣Add 1 TB. OLIVE OIL to the skillet and sauté 2 SMALL SLICED ZUCCHINI briefly. Set aside.

♣Make the WHITE SAUCE in a small pan. Melt 3 TBS. BUTTER and 3 TBS. OIL. Stir in 6 TBS. WHOLE WHEAT FLOUR until bubbly. Add 1 CUP PLAIN YOGURT and 1 CUP VEGETABLE BROTH. Whisk smooth. Remove from heat and whisk in 2 EGGS.

♣Assemble the moussaka. Layer half the tomato sauce on the bottom of the oiled dish. Cover with all the eggplant. Sprinkle on 1/2 CUP CRUMBLED FETA CHEESE. Sprinkle on 1/2 CUP CHOPPED WAL-NUTS. Top with rest of sauce. Cover with all of the ZUCCHINI. Sprinkle with 1/2 CUP FETA CHEESE.
♣Sprinkle on 1/2 CUP CHOPPED WALNUTS.
♣Pour WHITE SAUCE over top. Scatter with minced PARSLEY and a little PARMESAN. Bake for 50 minutes until bubbly.

♣Make a FRESH ITALIAN BASIL SAUCE if desired. Blend in the blender right after you put the moussaka in the oven, and let it sit for an hour, for the best flavor. Spoon over at serving time.

3 LARGE RIPE ROMA TOMATOES	1 CHOPPED GREEN ONION
12 FRESH BASIL LEAVES	2 TBS. OLIVE OIL
1 teasp. BLACK PEPPER	1/2 teasp. SESAME SALT

771   SUNDAY SQUASH

This was a Sunday dinner favorite growing up. There were four kids and we all liked this.
For 6 side servings: Preheat oven to 350°.

♣Slice ONE or MORE POUNDS YELLOW SQUASH in rounds. Sauté in 1 TB. BUTTER with 1/2 SLICED SWEET ONION until fragrant, about 5 minutes.

♣Blend in the blender with	♣Pour in a mixing bowl and add
4 TBS. BUTTER	1 CUP GRATED LOW-FAT CHEDDAR
4 TBS. PLAIN LOW-FAT YOGURT	1/2 CUP CRUMBLED CORNBREAD
1 EGG	1/2 teasp. SEA SALT

♣Turn into a shallow casserole and top with MORE GRATED CHEDDAR and MORE CORN BREAD (or cornbread stuffing mix) CRUMBLES. Bake for 20 minutes until steaming.

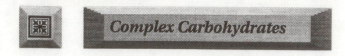

772 BROCCOLI PLUS

For 6 to 8 servings: Preheat oven to 350°.

♣Lecithin-spray a 9 x 13" pan and lay BUTTERED BREAD SLICES to fit in one layer. Have ready the same amount to fit on top and set aside.

♣Sauté 1 LARGE CHOPPED ONION and 8-OZ. SLICED MUSHROOMS in 4 TBS. OIL for 5 minutes.

♣Blanch 3 CUPS CHOPPED BROCCOLI in a large pot of boiling salted water until color changes to bright green. Drain and mix with the onions, mushrooms, 2 TBS. DRY BASIL, and 1 teasp. PEPPER.

♣Shred 16-OZ. LOW-FAT CHEDDAR and set aside.

♣Mix 1 1/2 CUPS PLAIN YOGURT and 1 1/2 CUPS WATER with 6 EGGS for the custard. Set aside.

♣Assemble the casserole. Layer half the vegetable mix over the bread. Top with half the cheese to cover and the rest of the bread layer. Repeat with the vegetables and cheese. Pour custard mix over. Cover with plastic wrap and chill. Bake uncovered about 45 minutes, until edges are light brown and the center is firm when jiggled. Let set for 15 minutes before cutting in serving rectangles.

Nutritional analysis: per serving; 433 calories; 27gm. protein; 24gm. carbohydrates; 4gm. fiber; 26gm. fats; 201gm. cholesterol; 578 calcium; 3mg. iron; 71mg. magnesium; 538mg. potassium; 520mg. sodium; 4mg. zinc.

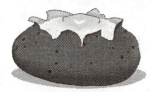

Potato Profits:
Potatoes Are Hot Properties For Complex Carbos

Potatoes could be a perfect food. They are rich in fiber and complex carbohydrates and have virtually no fat, no cholesterol, and just a trace of salt. They are a fine source of vitamin B6 for nerve stability, have measureable potassium, and contain over 40% of the RDA of vitamin C. Boil 'em, bake 'em, chill 'em, fill 'em, broil 'em, or sauce 'em. Any way you make them, potatoes are a delicious, nutritious, low-fat, vegetable.

773 VEGETABLE STUFFED BAKED POTATOES

For 4 servings: Preheat oven to 375°.

♣Rub 4 LARGE BAKING POTATOES with oil and bake for 60 minutes until tender. Halve potatoes lengthwise. Scoop out meat. Leave shell intact for filling. Arrange in a baking dish for stuffing.

♣Steam 1 CUP CHOPPED BROCCOLI til color changes to bright green. Drain and set aside.

♣Mix the filling in a bowl

1 CUP COTTAGE CHEESE	3 CHOPPED SCALLIONS
1/2 CUP PLAIN LOW FAT YOGURT	1 TB. TARRAGON VINEGAR
1 STALK DICED CELERY	2 PINCHES PAPRIKA
THE POTATO MEAT	

♣Fill potato shells. Top with broccoli and LOW-FAT FARMER CHEESE CHUNKS. Sprinkle with SEA SALT and PEPPER. Bake for 15 minutes until hot through and cheese is melted.

❈

774   POTATOES ALFREDO

This Alfredo sauce is also good with pastas and as a cracker spread.
For 4 servings:

♣Mix the sauce in the blender until smooth

1 SMALL CARTON LOW-FAT CREME FRAICHE
1 teasp. GARLIC/LEMON SEAONING
2 teasp. BALSAMIC VINEGAR

1/4 teasp. DRY BASIL
1/4 teasp. DILL WEED
1/4 teasp. OREGANO

♣Add 1 to 2 teasp. WATER or SHERRY if necessary to make very smooth and sauce consistency. Cover and chill to blend flavors.
♣Serve over baked potatoes. Garnish with MINCED CHIVES.

775   GREEK POTATOES

This recipe will become a solid favorite if you just like to throw things all together in a dish, leave them alone, and have them come out delicious.
For 6 servings: Preheat oven to 425°.

Mix all ingredients right in the 8 x 12" baking dish

Cube in 6 SCRUBBED POTATOES
1/2 CUP LEMON JUICE
1/3 CUP OLIVE OIL
2 CLOVES MINCED GARLIC
3 CUPS HOT WATER

2 teasp SEA SALT
1/2 teasp. BLACK PEPPER
1 1/2 teasp. OREGANO
1/2 teasp. THYME
PINCH NUTMEG

♣Stir around in the pan to mix. Bake uncovered for 1 1/2 hours. Check occasionally to make sure there is enough liquid. Add more water if necessary, until the last 20 minutes of cooking. Then let liquid evaporate until only oil is left.
♣Garnish with 2 TBS. CHOPPED FRESH PARSLEY and FETA CHEESE or HARD BOILED EGG CRUMBLES.

Nutritional analysis: per serving; 363 calories; 7gm. protein; 55gm. carbohydrate; 5gm. fiber; 14gm. fats; 71mg. cholesterol; 47mg. calcium; 4mg. iron; 65mg. magnesium; 914mg. potassium; 270mg. sodium; 1mg. zinc.

776   STEAMED BABY POTATOES WITH MUSTARD BUTTER

For 4 servings:

♣Steam 8 to 12 SMALL BABY POTATOES until tender, about 25 to 30 minutes.

♣Sauté 3 TBS. CHOPPED PEELED SHALLOTS, 1 1/2 teasp. DIJON MUSTARD, SEA SALT and PEPPER in 4 TBS. BUTTER until fragrant.
♣Add potatoes and toss to coat. Serve hot.

777 ROASTED POTATOES WITH GINGER VINAIGRETTE

For 12 servings: Preheat oven to 475°.

♣Heat 4 TBS. BUTTER, 4 TBS. OLIVE OIL and 3 WHOLE GARLIC CLOVES in a 12 x 15" baking pan.
♣Peel 2 LBS. WHITE POTATOES and 2 LBS. SWEET POTATOES and cut in chunks. Roll chunks in garlic butter to coat. Bake on the bottom rack of the oven for 30 minutes until tender. Stir frequently.
♣Remove and let stand to absorb flavors. Sprinkle with 1/2 CUP CHOPPED HAZELNUTS and return to the oven for 15 more minutes.

♣Mix the **GINGER VINAIGRETTE** and pour over to serve.

1/4 CUP TARRAGON VINEGAR	1/2 teasp. FRESH GRATED GINGER
1/2 teasp. GARLIC/LEMON SEASONING	1 1/2 TBS. LIME JUICE
1/2 teasp. TAMARI	1 CUP OIL

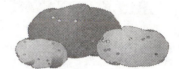

778 TWICE BAKED POTATOES #1

For 4 halves: Preheat oven to 375°.

♣Bake 2 LARGE RUSSET POTATOES. Slice in half lengthwise and scoop out flesh into a bowl.
♣Mix potato meat with

1/2 CUP LOW-FAT COTTAGE CHEESE	2 MINCED GREEN ONIONS
2 TBS. FRESH CHOPPED PARSLEY	3 TBS. PLAIN LOW-FAT YOGURT
1 SMALL GRATED CARROT	1/2 teasp. DRY THYME

♣Refill potato shells. Sprinkle with PARMESAN CHEESE and PAPRIKA and bake for 35 minutes until browned on top.

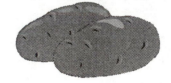

779 TWICE BAKED POTATOES #2

For 4 halves: Preheat oven to 375°.

♣Bake 2 LARGE RUSSET POTATOES. Slice in half lengthwise and scoop out flesh into a bowl.

♣Mix potato meat with

3 TBS. LIGHT MAYONNAISE	1/2 teasp. SEA SALT
1/2 CUP LOW-FAT COTTAGE CHEESE	1/2 teasp. PEPPER
1 CHOPPED HARD BOILED EGG	1/2 teasp. DILL WEED
2 teasp. YELLOW MUSTARD	1/4 teasp. PAPRIKA
1/2 CUP GRATED LOW-FAT CHEDDAR	

♣Divide filling between the shells. Top with FRESH TOMATO SLICES and MORE GRATED CHEDDAR CHEESE. Sprinkle with PAPRIKA and bake for 35 minutes until browned.

Complex Carbohydrates From Baked Goodies

780   ZUCCHINI BREAD

This is a sweet bread from the Rainbow Kitchen. I have also used grated carrots and other squashes in place of the zucchini. They all worked. Be creative. This is a good, easy, healthy basic recipe.
For 2 loaves: Preheat oven to 350°.

♣Combine all ingredients in a big mixing bowl

2 CUPS GRATED ZUCCHINI
2$^1/_2$ CUPS UNBLEACHED FLOUR
$^1/_2$ CUP WHEAT GERM
1 CUP HONEY
$^1/_4$ CUP MAPLE SYRUP
2 TBS. FRUCTOSE
1 teasp. BAKING SODA

$^3/_4$ CUP OIL
$^1/_2$ teasp. BAKING POWDER
1 teasp. SESAME SALT
3 teasp. CINNAMON
1 teasp. NUTMEG
1 CUP CHOPPED WALNUTS

♣Turn into 2 lecithin-sprayed loaf pans. Bake for 1 hour or more, until springy when touched. Cool and cut in thick slices.

Nutritional analysis: per serving; 591 calories; 9gm. prtoein; 79gm. carbohydrates; 7gm. fiber; 31gm. fats; 0 cholesterol; 72mg. calcium; 3mg. iron; 104mg. magnesium; 466mg. potassium; 148mg. sodium; 2mg. zinc.

781   ORANGE GINGERBREAD

For 12 pieces: Preheat oven to 350°.

♣Combine the wet ingredients

$^3/_4$ CUP WATER
$^1/_4$ CUP ORANGE JUICE
$^1/_2$ CUP UNSULPHURED MOLASSES
$^1/_2$ CUP MAPLE SYRUP

1 EGG
1 TB. ORANGE PEEL
$^1/_3$ CUP MELTED BUTTER
$^1/_3$ CUP OIL

♣Mix the dry ingredients

2$^1/_2$ CUPS WHOLE WHEAT PASTRY FLOUR
1$^1/_2$ teasp. GINGER POWDER

1 teasp. BAKING SODA
1 teasp. CINNAMON

♣Combine the two mixtures together just enough to moisten. Turn into a greased 9 x 9" square baking pan, and bake for 35 to 40 minutes until a toothpick inserted in the center comes out clean.
♣Center should still be moist. Serve warm or cool.

Nutritional analysis: per servimg; 251 calories; 4gm. protein; 36gm. carbohydrates; 3gm. fiber; 12gm. fats; 31mg. cholesterol; 121mg. calcium; 5mg. iron; 74mg. magnesium; 537mg. potassium; 55mg. sodium; 1mg. zinc.

782   MOLASSES CORN MUFFINS

For 12 muffins: Preheat oven to 400°.

♣Mix all ingredients together gently

1 CUP YELLOW CORNMEAL
1 1/2 CUPS UNBLEACHED FLOUR
1 CUP PLAIN LOW FAT YOGURT
1/2 CUP SPARKLING WATER
4 TBS. UNSULPHURED MOLASSES
1/2 teasp. CINNAMON

1/2 teasp. BAKING SODA
2 teasp. BAKING POWDER
PINCH SEA SALT
1 EGG
2 TBS. OIL

♣Bake for 25 minutes until a toothpick inserted in a muffin comes out clean.

❊

783   DEEP SOUTH CORN AND RICE MUFFINS

For 12 muffins: Preheat oven to 400°.

♣Combine all ingredients in a bowl just to moisten

1 CUP YELLOW CORNMEAL
1 TB. BAKING POWDER
1 CUP <u>COOKED</u> BROWN RICE
3 TBS. MELTED BUTTER or OIL
1/2 CUP PLAIN LOW-FAT YOGURT

2 EGGS
1 TB. MAPLE SYRUP
2 TBS. HONEY
1 teasp. SESAME SALT
1/3 CUP WATER

♣Bake for 20 minutes til a toothpick inserted in a muffin comes out clean.

Nutritional analysis: per serving; 115 calories; 3gm. protein; 16gm. carbohydrates; 1gm. fiber; 4gm. fats; 43mg. cholesterol; 80mg. calcium; 1mg. iron; 24mg. magnesium; 299mg. potassium; 77mg. sodium; 1mg. zinc.

❊

784   SESAME RAISIN OATMEAL COOKIES

These are delicious little morsels. Make them very small because they are very rich.
For 36 cookies: Preheat oven to 350°.

♣Toast 1/4 CUP SESAME SEEDS in the oven until golden. Remove and set aside.

♣Mix dry ingredients together

1/2 CUP WHOLE WHEAT PASTRY FLOUR
1/2 CUP UNBLEACHED FLOUR
3/4 teasp. SESAME SALT
1/4 teasp. NUTMEG
1 teasp. CINNAMON
THE TOASTED SESAME SEEDS

♣Mix wet ingredients together

2 EGGS
1 STICK BUTTER
4 TBS. OIL
3/4 CUP FRUCTOSE
1/4 CUP MAPLE SYRUP
1 teasp. VANILLA

♣Combine both ingredients and stir in 1 CUP RAISINS and 1 CUP ROLLED OATS.

♣Drop onto lecithin-sprayed baking sheets and bake for 10 to 12 minutes, until browned on the edges.

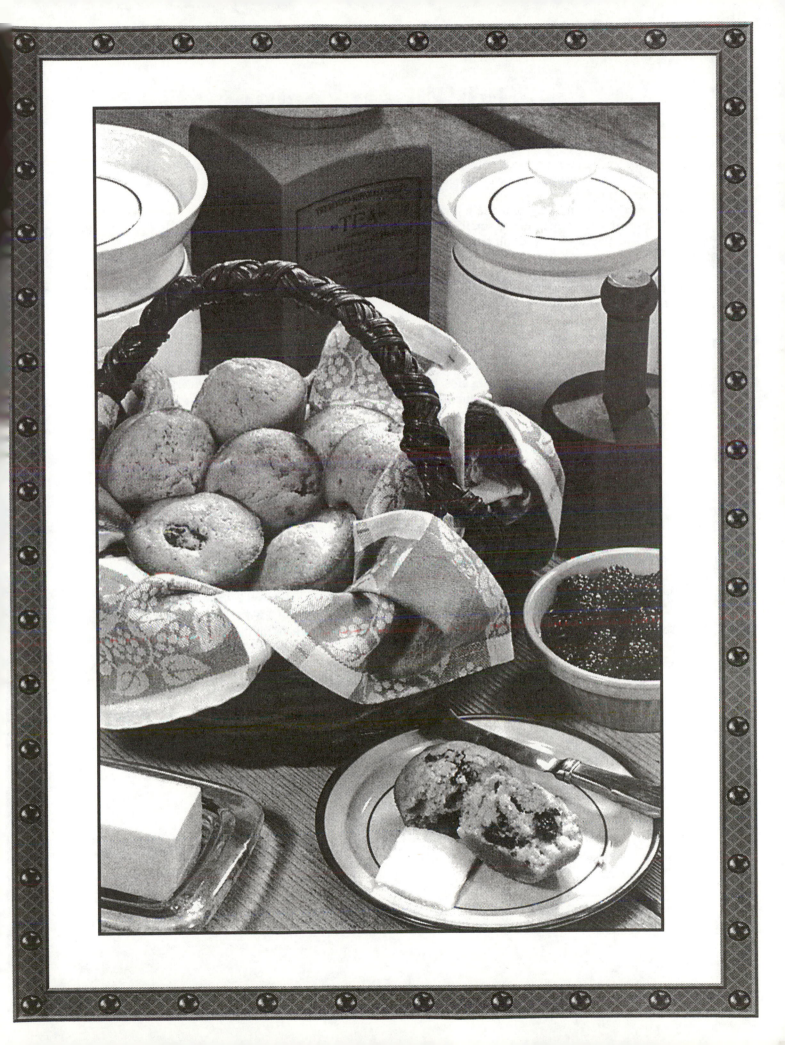

High Fiber Recipes

Dietary fiber in whole foods is the metabolic companion to good complex carbohydrates. Soluble fiber promotes the growth of healthy bacteria in the colon and enhances body functions to help lower cholesterol and fat levels. High fiber foods slow down calorie absorption. Since much plant fiber is not digested by the human system at all, high fiber foods take up space in the stomach, and make you feel full. They absorb water in the small intestine and pass along through the colon acting as a fibrous "sweep," to help the body eliminate wastes more easily.

A diet rich in high fiber foods is one of the few things in this world that gives you something for nothing. Without adding calories or bulk of its own, it helps control your weight, eases and regulates elimination, helps prevent cardiovascular problems, and acts as a colon and fat cleanser.

On a healing and health maintenance level, a diet high in soluble fiber has proven effective in the prevention of major, life threatening diseases. Cancer, heart and circulatory diseases, gout, gallstones, high blood pressure, diabetes, pernicious anemia, digestive/elimination problems such as Crohn's disease, colitis, diverticulitis, varicose veins, hemorrhoids, ulcers, chronic constipation and irritable bowel syndrome have all responded to an increase in dietary fiber.

Fiber is a valuable aid in lowering triglycerides, cholesterol, and blood sugar fluctuations. So inclusion of high fiber foods in the diet can help control the moods swings, irritability and energy drops from these problems, and build a feeling of well being in the body.

Soluble fiber comes in several forms in food: cellulose, hemicellulose and lignin from brans and cereal grains; pectin from fruits and vegetables; gums from legumes and some herbs; mucilages from seeds.

☞Vegetable fiber sources include spinach, corn, peas, sweet potatoes, cucumbers, squashes, broccoli, cabbage, carrots, celery, potatoes and onions.
☞Fruit fiber sources include strawberries, bananas, raisins, figs, pears, prunes, apples and avocados.
☞Whole grain fiber sources include brown rice, oats, barley, and wild rice.
☞Bean and legume fiber sources include lentils, split peas, pinto beans, and green beans.

Healthy dietary fiber is easy to get when you are eating whole natural foods. This chapter includes representative examples in each area to get you started in the right direction.

❧HIGH FIBER SALADS ❧WHOLE GRAIN MUFFINS and BAKED TREATS ❧VEGETABLES FOR CLEANSING FIBER ❧HIGH FIBER FROM WHOLE GRAINS ❧HIGH FIBER FROM BEANS and LEGUMES ❧HIGH FIBER FRUITS and BREAKFAST FOODS ❧

For a health maintenance diet, a high fiber portion contains 2 or more grams of soluble fiber. Add fiber to your diet gradually, to allow your body to adapt to more "roughage" easily.

For more information and recipes, see the following chapters:
☛COMPLEX CARBOHYDRATES FOR ENERGY - page 571.
☛HIGH PROTEIN WITHOUT MEAT - page 548.
☛HIGH MINERAL FOODS - page 523.
☛LOW CHOLESTEROL RECIPES - page 376.
☛BREAKFAST & BRUNCH FOODS - page 264.
☛WHEAT FREE BAKING - page 410.

High Fiber Salads

785   BROCCOLI WALNUT SALAD

For 6 servings:

♣Pan roast ²/₃ cup LARGE WALNUT PIECES in 2 TBS. OLIVE OIL until brown and aromatic.

♣Make the dressing. Whisk
1/4 CUP OLIVE OIL
2 TBS. BASMATI VINEGAR
1/2 teasp. LEMON/GARLIC SEASONING
DROPS of HOT PEPPER SAUCE
♣Chill while rest of salad is being prepared.

1/2 teasp. DRY BASIL
1/2 teasp. DRY MUSTARD
1/2 teasp. SESAME SALT

♣Blanch 2 BUNCHES of BROCCOLI FLORETS and CHOPPED STEMS, and 2 CUPS SLICED ZUCCHINI ROUNDS in boiling water or light stock until color changes to bright green. Drain and chill.
♣Toss vegetables with dressing and top with walnuts. Serve in lettuce cups.

Nutritional analysis: per serving; 206 calories; 6gm. protein; 10gm. carbohydrates; 5gm. fiber; 17gm. fats; 0 cholesterol; 82mg. calcium; 63mg. magnesium; 2mg. iron; 575mg. potassium; 113mg. sodium; 1mg. zinc.

786   HOT CRUNCHY TOP TOFU SALAD

For 6 people:

♣Blanch 2 CAKES of CUBED TOFU in boiling salted water for 10 minutes. Drain. Add 1/2 CUP BOTTLED NATURAL TOMATO FRENCH DRESSING. Chill in the fridge to marinate for 30 minutes.

♣Assemble the rest of the salad in a baking dish.
Mix
1/2 CUP LIGHT MAYONNAISE
1/2 CUP PLAIN YOGURT or YOGURT CHEESE or KEFIR CHEESE
1¹/₂ CUPS DICED CELERY
1/2 CUP TOASTED SLICED ALMONDS
1 CUP CRISP CHINESE NOODLES

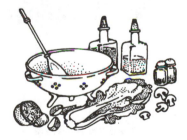

♣Add the marinated tofu and dressing. Mix all together. Sprinkle with 1 MORE CUP CRISP CHINESE NOODLES and 1 CUP LOW-FAT CHEDDAR CHEESE.
♣Serve cold as is **or** run under the broiler for 30 seconds until the top is browned and crunchy, **or** bake for 15 minutes to heat through and melt cheese.

Nutritional analysis: per serving; 361 calories; 12gm. protein; 20gm. carbohydrates; 4gm. fiber; 20mg. fats; 19mg. cholesterol; 229mg. calcium; 3mg. iron; 89mg. magnesium; 312mg. potassium; 285mg. sodium; 2mg. zinc.

787 POLENTA SPINACH SALAD WITH FETA CHEESE

For 4 servings: Preheat oven to 325°.

♣Bring 2 CUPS WATER to a boil. Add 3/4 CUP POLENTA. Cook for 5 minutes until water is absorbed.
♣Spoon into a lecithin-sprayed square pan. Chill and slice into 4 squares. Bake for 5 minutes until edges are crisp.

♣Toast 3 TBS. PINE NUTS in the oven until golden and aromatic.

♣Cover individual salad plates with SHREDDED LETTUCE GREENS and place one polenta square on each plate.
♣Top each with a SLICE of FETA CHEESE.

Wash and tear 4 CUPS SPINACH LEAVES. Toss with 3 TBS. SHARP VINAIGRETTE, CAESAR DRESS-ING, or a LEMON/OIL DRESSING. Divide between salad plates. Sprinkle with the pine nuts.

※

788 LIGHT POTATO SALAD

For 4 people:

♣Boil 6 RED POTATOES in boiling salted water until soft. CUBE and mix together with

1/2 CUP LIGHT MAYONNAISE	1/2 CUP PLAIN YOGURT
2 SLICED HARD BOILED EGGS	1/2 CUP CHOPPED CELERY
1/2 CUP CHOPPED GREEN ONION	1/2 CUP SWEET PICKLE RELISH

♣Serve in lettuce cups.

※

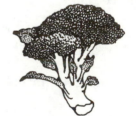

789 HOT BROCCOLI SALAD

For 4 people:

♣Blanch 1 LARGE BUNCH CHOPPED BROCCOLI FLORETS and STEMS in boiling salted water until color changes to bright green, about 5 minutes. Drain and set aside while you make the dressing.

♣Make the dressing. Whisk in a bowl

1 TB. FRESH LEMON JUICE	1/2 teasp. SESAME SALT
1/4 teasp. DRY MUSTARD	1/4 teasp. BLACK PEPPER
DASHES of HOT PEPPER SAUCE	

♣Sauté 1/4 CUP MINCED RED ONION and 1/4 CUP CASHEWS in 2 TBS. OIL until aromatic. Add to broccoli and toss all with dressing.

Nutritional analysis: per serving; 139 calories; 4gm. protein; 9gm. carbohydrates; 4gm. fiber; 11gm. fats; 0 cholesterol; 50mg. calcium; 1mg. iron; 46mg. magnesium; 351mg. potassium; 121mg. sodium; 1mg. zinc.

※

790   SUCCOTASH BROWN RICE SALAD

For 4 servings:

♣Have ready 3 CUPS COOKED BROWN RICE.
♣Toss in a bowl with

3/4 CUP ITALIAN VINAIGRETTE
THE KERNELS from 3 EARS of STEAMED CORN
1 CUP STEAMED BABY LIMA BEANS
1 PEELED CUBED CUCUMBER

2 TBS. CHOPPED PARSLEY
2 SLICED RED RADISHES
3/4 CUP CRUMBLED FETA CHEESE
1/2 teasp. ITALIAN HERBS

♣Serve in lettuce cups.

※

791   BEAN SALAD WITH FRESH BASIL VINAIGRETTE

For 8 small salads:

♣Marinate 2 LARGE SLICED SHALLOTS in 1/4 CUP WINE VINEGAR for 1 hour.
♣Blanch ONE LARGE PKG. (24 OZ.) FRENCH CUT GREEN BEANS in boiling salted water until just tender and bright green. Drain, rinse under cold water and chill while you make the dressing.
♣Whisk together 1 TB. DIJON MUSTARD, 1 teasp. PEPPER, and 1/2 CUP OLIVE OIL. Add shallots and vinegar, 1/2 CUP FRESH CHOPPED BASIL and 3 CUPS HALVED CHERRY TOMATOES.
♣Divide beans between salad plates and spoon on dressing.

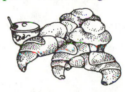

Whole Grain Muffins & Baked Treats

High fiber was almost synonymous with bran muffins in the early days of "fiber consciousness," and muffins are still a tasty way to get good whole grain fiber. Here are a few variations to keep you interested.

792   SWEET CORN MUFFINS

For 12 muffins: Preheat oven to 350°.

♣Mix the dry ingredients
2 CUPS GOURMET FLOUR MIX (pg. 647)
1 TB. BAKING POWDER
1 teasp. CINNAMON
1/2 teasp. GROUND CLOVES
1/2 teasp. NUTMEG

♣Combine the wet ingredients
2 EGGS
1/2 CUP PLAIN YOGURT
1/2 CUP OIL
1/4 CUP MAPLE SYRUP
2 CUPS CORN KERNALS

♣Mix both together until just lumpy. Spoon into greased or paper muffin cups, and bake until toothpick comes out clean when inserted in the center.

793   RAISIN GRAPENUTS MUFFINS

♣For 6 big deli-style Sunday breakfast muffins: Preheat oven to 375°. Use oiled pyrex custard cups.

♣For 8 regular-size muffins: Preheat oven to 400°. Use paper-lined muffin cups in a muffin tin.

♣Mix the dry ingredients
1 CUP UNBLEACHED FLOUR
1/2 CUP WHOLE WHEAT PASTRY FLOUR
1 CUP GRAPENUTS
1 CUP ROLLED OATS
1 1/2 teasp. BAKING SODA

♣Form a well in the center and pour in
1 CUP PLAIN YOGURT
1/2 CUP HONEY
1 EGG
1/4 CUP OIL
1/2 CUP RAISINS

♣Stir until lumpy and bake for 30 minutes until springy when touched.

Nutritional analysis: per serving; 340 calories; 9gm. protein; 60gm. carbohydrates; 6gm. fiber; 9gm. fats; 28mg. cholesterol; 83mg. calcium; 6mg. iron; 66mg. magnesium; 386mg. potassium; 157mg. sodium; 2mg. zinc.

794   ZUCCHINI NUT MUFFINS

These muffins can be made the same way as the RAISIN OAT BRAN MUFFINS - either very large deli-style or regular size. See baking instructions above.

♣Mix the dry ingredients
1 1/2 CUPS UNBLEACHED FLOUR
3/4 CUP WHOLE WHEAT FLOUR
2 1/2 teasp. BAKING POWDER
1 teasp. NUTMEG or SWEET TOOTH BAKING MIX
1/2 teasp. ALLSPICE
1/2 teasp. BAKING SODA
3/4 CUP TOASTED WALNUTS

♣Mix the wet ingredients
1/2 CUP HONEY
1 CUP GRATED ZUCCHINI
1/2 CUP PLAIN YOGURT
1/4 CUP WATER
1 EGG
1/4 CUP OIL
1/4 teasp. SEA SALT

♣Mix both together gently, just to moisten. Bake for 30 minutes until springy when touched.

795   PIÑA COLADA MUFFINS

For 8 muffins: Preheat oven to 375°. Use paper-lined muffin cups.

♣Combine all ingredients together just to moisten in a bowl
1 1/2 CUPS WHOLE WHEAT FLOUR
2 teasp. BAKING POWDER
1/2 CUP OAT BRAN
1/2 CUP PLAIN YOGURT
1 1/4 CUP PINEAPPLE/COCONUT JUICE

1/4 CUP SHREDDED COCONUT
1 EGG
1/4 CUP OIL
1 CUP PINEAPPLE PIECES

♣Spoon into muffin cups and bake for 20 minutes until a toothpick inserted in the center comes out clean.

♣Sprinkle with COCONUT SHREDS and press in to muffin top.

796   CARROT OAT BRAN MUFFINS

For 12 big muffins: Preheat oven to 325°.

♣Mix dry ingredients

1/2 CUP WHOLE WHEAT PASTRY FLOUR   1 teasp. BAKING SODA
1/2 CUP UNBLEACHED FLOUR   1 teasp. BAKING POWDER
1/2 CUP OAT BRAN   1/2 teasp. SEA SALT
1 teasp. ALLSPICE POWDER or SWEET TOOTH BAKING MIX

♣Mix wet ingredients

2/3 CUP LIGHT OIL   2 TBS. MAPLE SYRUP
2/3 CUP HONEY   2 EGGS
11/2 CUPS GRATED CARROTS

♣Mix all gently just to moisten, spoon into paper muffin cups or greased muffin tins, and bake for about 30 minutes until springy when touched.

Nutritional analysis: per serving; 235 calories; 3gm. protein; 29gm. carbohydrates; 3gm. fiber; 13gm. fats; 35mg. cholesterol; 38mg. calcium; 1mg. iron; 18mg. magnesium; 194mg. potassium; 167mg. sodium; 1mg. zinc.

797   PRUNE WALNUT MUFFINS

For 16 to 18 muffins: Preheat oven to 350°.

♣Mix the dry ingredients large bowl   ♣Mix the fruits, nuts and spices
1 CUP WHOLE WHEAT PASTRY FLOUR   1 CUP CHOPPED PRUNES
1/2 CUP WHEAT GERM   11/2 teasp. CINNAMON
1/2 CUP BRAN FLAKES   1/2 CUP CHOPPED WALNUTS
1 TB. BAKING POWDER   1/4 teasp. NUTMEG
1/4 teasp. BAKING SODA   1/4 teasp. GINGER
♣Combine both mixtures together.

♣Heat together til syrupy
1 CUP BUTTERMILK
2 EGGS
2 TBS. FROZEN ORANGE JUICE CONCENTRATE
3 TBS. BUTTER
3 TBS. HONEY

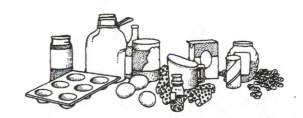

♣Add to ingredients in the bowl and combine until just gently moistened. Pour into oiled or paper-lined muffin cups and bake for 20 to 25 minutes until a toohpick inserted in the center comes out clean.

Nutritional analysis: per serving; 152 calories; 4gm. protein; 23gm. carbohydrates; 4gm. fiber; 5gm. fats; 33mg. cholesterol; 80mg. calcium; 2mg. iron; 37mg. magnesium; 410mg. potassium; 41mg. sodium; 1mg. zinc.

Vegetables For Cleansing Fiber

798   LIGHT ITALIAN VEGETABLE STRATA

For 6 servings: Preheat oven to 400°.

♣Oil a 9 x 13" baking pan and sprinkle some of the bread crumbs on bottom and sides.
♣Peel 1 LARGE EGGPLANT and 1 POTATO. Slice into rounds, and place on separate baking sheets drizzled with olive oil. Bake for 45 minutes until tender. Set aside.
♣Slice 1 ZUCCHINI and 4 TOMATOES separately and set aside.
♣Mix 3 EGGS, 1/2 teasp. ITALIAN SEASONING, and 1/4 teasp. LEMON PEPPER. Set aside.
♣Mix 1 CUP WHOLE GRAIN BREAD CRUMBS, 2 TBS. FRESH CHOPPED BASIL, and 3 TBS. FRESH CHOPPED PARSLEY.

Assemble the vegetable strata.
♣Lay all eggplant in a single layer. Drizzle with olive oil. Sprinkle on some crumb mix.
♣Layer on a few slices of MOZARRELLA CHEESE. Sprinkle with 1 TB. PARMESAN CHEESE.
♣Spoon on 1/4 of the egg mixture.
♣Lay the potato slices in a single layer. Drizzle with olive oil. Sprinkle with more of the crumbs.
♣Top with a few more slices of MOZARRELLA and 1 TB. PARMESAN CHEESE.
♣Pour on 1/4 more of the egg.
♣Lay all the zucchini slices in a single layer. Drizzle with olive oil. Sprinkle with more of the crumbs.
♣Top with a few more MOZARRELLA SLICES and 1 TB. PARMESAN CHEESE.
♣Pour on 1/4 of the egg mixture.
♣Lay all tomatoes in a single layer. Drizzle with olive oil. Sprinkle with last of the crumbs.
♣Top with last of the MOZARRELLA SLICES.
♣Combine the last of the EGG MIX and PARMESAN CHEESE and spread over the top.
♣Cover and bake for 40 minutes until flavors are blended. Let sit for 10 minutes to concentrate texture and cut in large squares to serve.

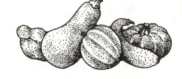

799   ACORN SQUASH WITH TOFU RICE STUFFING

For 8 servings: Preheat oven to 375°.

♣Have ready 2 1/2 CUPS COOKED BROWN RICE or GOURMET GRAIN BLEND (pg. 647).
♣Halve and seed 4 ACORN SQUASH. Place face down on a lecithin-sprayed baking sheet, and bake until tender and shell gives when pressed. Scoop out flesh into a bowl to leave a shell. Set shells with sides touching in a shallow baking dish.

♣Sauté in 2 TBS BUTTER until golden
1 SMALL GRATED ZUCCHINI
1 GRATED YELLOW SQUASH
1/4 CUP CHOPPED SHALLOTS

♣Mix with squash meat and add
1/4 CUP MINCED PARSLEY
1/2 teasp. GREAT 28 SEASONING
2 CUBES CRUMBLED TOFU

♣Fill acorn squash shells and re-bake for 15 minutes until hot and browned.

800 TUSCAN ONIONS

We love Italian and mediterranean cooking for its simplicity and of-the-earth quality. One feels as if a garden is just around the corner with the sun smiling on it - probably why eating al fresco became an Italian treat.
For 6 servings: Preheat oven to 350°.

♣Sauté 4 SLICED WHITE ONIONS in 2 TBS. BUTTER and 2 TBS. OIL until golden.
♣Add 4 SLICED HARD BOILED EGGS and toss together. Put in a shallow oiled baking dish.

♣Make 1 CUP of WHITE WINE SAUCE in a small pan. Stir 2 TBS. BUTTER and 2 TBS. UNBLEACHED FLOUR together until bubbly and golden.
♣Add 1/2 CUP PLAIN LOW-FAT YOGURT, 1/2 CUP WHITE WINE, and 1/2 teasp. DRY MUSTARD.
♣Cook until smooth and thickened. Pour over onions. Top with 1 CUP LOW-FAT COTTAGE CHEESE or POT CHEESE and 2 TBS. MINCED FRESH ITALIAN PARSLEY.

♣Sprinkle with 1/2 CUP WHOLE WHEAT BREAD CRUMBS or TOASTED CORN BREAD.
♣Bake for 25 to 30 minutes. Let rest a few minutes before serving.

Nutritional analysis: per serving; 260 calories; 13gm. protein; 17gm. carbos; 3gm. fiber; 14gm. fats; 71mg. cholesterol; 183mg. calcium; 2mg. iron; 55mg. magnesium; 355mg. potassium; 136mg. sodium; 3mg. zinc.

801 POTLUCK VEGETABLE BAKE

Almost any vegetable can go in this recipe. Use your favorite compatibles. The combination here is rather like a baked Scandinavian stew.
For 6 people: Preheat oven to 350°.

♣Sauté 2 SLICED YELLOW ONIONS in 2 TBS. OIL in a large skillet until aromatic, about 3 minutes.

♣Add and stir briefly

2 CARROTS SLICED in thin julienne	1 TB. LOW SALT TAMARI
1/2 HEAD GREEN CABBAGE	1/4 CUP WHITE WINE
2 CAKES CUBED TOFU	1/4 CUP WATER

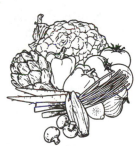

♣Reduce heat to simmer. Cover and let bubble about 5 minutes. Remove from heat.

♣Add 1 SMALL HEAD CHOPPED SWISS CHARD or KALE and toss to coat.

♣Mix the topping in a bowl

1 CUP WHOLE GRAIN BREAD CRUMBS	1 TB. DRY BASIL
1/2 CUP GRATED PARMESAN	1/2 teasp. DRY OREGANO
1/4 CUP OIL	1 teasp. PAPARIKA
1/2 teasp. PEPPER	

♣Spoon veggies into a 9 x 13" shallow baking dish. Sprinkle with topping, and bake for 15 to 20 minutes until brown and bubbly.

Nutritional analysis: per serving; 280 calories; 10gm. protein; 25gm. carbohydtrates; 5gm. fiber; 16gm. fats; 6mg. cholesterol; 222mg. calcium; 4mg. iron; 86mg. magnesium; 483mg. potassium; 249mg. sodium; 1mg. zinc.

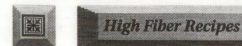

802   SWEET CARROT CRUNCH

For 4 servings:

♣Cut 6 to 8 medium CARROTS in julienne slivers. Cook <u>covered</u> in a small amount of salted water until just barely tender. Drain, remove from pan and set aside.
♣Melt 1¹/₂ TBS. BUTTER in the pan. Add 1¹/₂ TBS. MAPLE SYRUP, 1¹/₂ TBS. GRATED ORANGE PEEL, and 4 TBS. SLIVERED ALMONDS or CHOPPED WALNUTS.
♣Simmer until a nice sauce is formed. Return carrots to pan and toss to heat through, about 3 minutes.

Nutritional analysis: per serving; 161 calories; 3gm. protein; 19gm. carbohydrates; 5gm. fiber; 8gm. fats; 11mg. cholesterol; 68mg. calcium; 1mg. iron; 45mg. magnesium; 487mg. potassium; 46mg. sodium; 1mg. zinc.

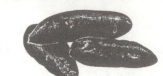

803   SWEET ANNA YAMS

A very simple, but very rich recipe. This is one of my husband's favorites.
For 6 people: Preheat oven to 425°.

♣Cut 2 LBS. YAMS in paper thin slices. Melt 4 TBS. BUTTER and 4 TBS. OIL with 1 teasp. NUTMEG, ¹/₂ teasp. SEA SALT and ¹/₄ teasp. BLACK PEPPER. Drizzle some on the bottom of a 9" cake pan.

♣Arrange ¹/₆ of the yam slices in overlapping rounds to cover bottom. Drizzle with a little more butter mix, and sprinkle with 1 TB. PARMESAN CHEESE.
♣Repeat layers until all ingredients are used. Cover pan with foil, and press down to compress layers.

♣Bake on the lowest oven rack for 30 minutes. <u>Uncover</u> and bake 45 minutes longer, until edges are crisp and brown. Let stand for a few minutes to concentrate texture. Drain off butter.
♣Loosen yams around the edges. Place a round plate on top of the pan, invert and remove pan. Cut in wedges to serve.

Nutritional analysis: per serving; 299 calories; 4gm. protein; 42gm. carbohydrates; 5gm. fiber; 13gm. fats; 22mg. cholesterol; 87mg. calcium; 1mg. iron; 33mg. magnesium; 595mg. potassium; 218mg. sodium; trace zinc.

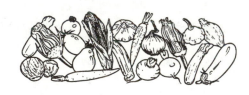

804   BUBBLE TOP ZUCCHINI

For 4 servings: Preheat broiler.

♣Melt 2 TBS. OIL and 2 TBS. BUTTER, and DASHES of SEA SALT and LEMON PEPPER in a flat dish for broiling.
♣Cut 1 LB. ZUCCHINI in rounds and roll in the butter and seasonings to coat. Arrange in one layer. Broil for 30 seconds. Turn and broil for 30 more seconds. Remove from oven.

♣Top with TOMATO SLICES and LOW-FAT MOZZARELLA CHEESE SLICES to cover. Broil again until everything bubbles.

High Fiber From Whole Grains

805 SOUTHERN CORN & RICE SPOONBREAD

Coming from the South, I love light spoonbreads. There are several from my collection of these savory dishes in this book. They satisfy healthy criteria - light, low-fat, high fiber and whole grain - bread without density.
For 6 servings: Preheat oven to 375°.

♣Combine 1 CUP YELLOW CORNMEAL and 1 CUP BOILING WATER and let stand for an hour.

♣Separate 2 EGGS. Combine yolks with

1/2 CUP PLAIN YOGURT	1 teasp. HONEY
1/2 CUP WATER	1/2 teasp. SEA SALT
3 TBS. OIL	

♣Pour over cornmeal meal and mix well. Add and mix in 2 CUPS COOKED BROWN RICE.

♣Beat EGG WHITES to stiff peaks and fold in gently until just barely blended. (This is very important for lightness).

♣Pour into a 9" square pan and bake for 40 to 45 minutes until puffed and golden, and shrinking slightly from the sides of the pan. Let cool for 5 minutes.

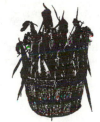

806 COUNTRY CORN BREAD STUFFING

We never use this as a stuffing for anything, always as a hearty whole meal casserole; but it has that "Thanksgiving reminder" flavor.
For 8 servings: Preheat oven to 350°.

♣Heat 1 CUP FRESH CRANBERRIES in a pan until they begin to pop.

♣Sauté 1 LARGE CHOPPED ONION in 2 TB. OIL until translucent, about 10 minutes.
♣Add 8-OZ. SLICED TOFU HOT DOGS and sauté for 5 more minutes. Remove to a large open baking bowl. Add 1 MORE TB. BUTTER and let sizzle a minute.

♣Sauté briefly and toss to coat

3 CUPS CRUMBLED WHOLE GRAIN BREAD	2 TART APPLES CHOPPED
1 teasp. POULTRY SEASONING or SAGE, crumbled	THE COOKED CRANBERRIES
1/4 CUP CHOPPED FRESH PARSLEY	1 1/2 CUPS CRUMBLED CORN BREAD
3/4 CUP CHOPPED TOASTED WALNUTS	

♣Mix with onions in the baking bowl. Pour over 1/2 CUP ONION or CHICKEN STOCK, 1/4 CUP WHITE WINE or SHERRY, and 1/4 CUP PLAIN YOGURT.
♣Bake for 30 minutes until golden and aromatic.

Nutritional analysis: per serving; 270 calories; 8gm. protein; 29gm. carbohydrates; 5gm. fiber; 15gm. fats; 24mg. cho;lesterol; 91mg. calcium; 3mg. iron; 74mg. magnesium; 248mg. potassium; 240mg. sodium; 1mg. zinc.

807   GOURMET GRAINS WITH ZUCCHINI

We have a kitchen garden. Small tender gold and green zucchini are favorite veggies that we grow every year.
For 6 to 8 people: Preheat oven to 425°.

♣Slice 6 SMALL ZUCCHINI in rounds. Salt and place in a colander to drain.

♣Bring 2 CUPS WATER or VEGETABLE BROTH to a boil. Add 1 CUP GOURMET GRAIN BLEND.
♣Cover, reduce heat and steam for 25 minutes until water is absorbed.

♣Toss with 2 TBS. PARMESAN CHEESE and 2 TBS. FRESH CHOPPED PARSLEY. Set aside.

♣Sauté 1 CLOVE CHOPPED GARLIC and 1 CHOPPED ONION in a skillet with 2 TBS. BUTTER AND 2
TBS. OIL until aromatic and light brown.

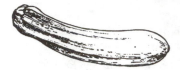

♣Add
1/2 CHOPPED BELL PEPPER
1 LB. CHOPPED TOMATOES
THE ZUCCHINI ROUNDS

♣Sauté for 2 minutes to blend. Reduce heat, and simmer until most of the tomato juice is evaporated. Mix
with the cooked grains, and put in a buttered baking dish.
♣Sprinkle with WHOLE GRAIN BREAD CRUMBS, a little more PARMESAN CHEESE, and 1/4 teasp.
BLACK PEPPER. Bake for 30 minutes. Cool slightly to set and serve.

Nutritional analysis: per serving; 177 calories; 5mg. protein; 29mg. carbohydrates; 4mg. fiber; 5gm. fats; 10mg. cholesterol; 72mg. calcium; 66mg. magnesium; 1mg. iron; 456mg. potassium; 192mg. sodium; 1mg. zinc.

808   QUICK COUSCOUS & BROCCOLI FRITTATA

This is perfect for left-overs, or a quick busy week night meal.
For 4 people: Preheat oven to 350°.

♣Have ready 2 CUPS COOKED COUSCOUS.

♣Blanch 1 CUP DICED BROCCOLI PIECES in boiling salted water until color changes to bright green.
♣Sauté 4 TBS. DICED ONION in 2 teasp. OIL until aromatic.

♣Mix COUSCOUS, BROCCOLI and ONION together in a bowl with
3 TBS. PARMESAN CHEESE
1/2 teasp. SEA SALT
2 BEATEN EGGS
1/4 teasp. PEPPER
2 TBS. LIGHT MAYONNAISE
2 TBS. PLAIN YOGURT

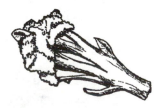

♣Turn into a lecithin-sprayed casserole. Sprinkle with 1/3 CUP GRATED LOW-FAT MOZARRELLA
CHEESE and bake for 25 minutes until set.

809   PUNGENT WOK- FRIED RICE

For 4 servings:

♣Toast 1/2 CUP CASHEWS in the oven until golden brown. Remove and set aside.
♣Cook 2 CUPS BASMATI RICE in 3 CUPS WATER or LIGHT ONION BROTH for 25 to 30 minutes until water is absorbed. Fluff, and set aside to cool.

♣Cube 2 CAKES TOFU and add to the following marinade while rice is cooking
8 MINCED SCALLIONS (1 BUNCH)   1/4 CUP BROWN RICE VINEGAR
4 SLICES FRESH MINCED GINGER ROOT   1/4 CUP TAMARI

♣Dice the following vegetables and have them ready on a plate
1 STALK CELERY   1 STALK BROCCOLI
1 CARROT   1/2 GREEN BELL PEPPER

♣Heat a large wok for 2 minutes over medium high heat. Add and sauté until aromatic
1 TB. PEANUT OIL   1 CLOVE CHOPPED GARLIC
1 teasp. CHOPPED FRESH GINGER   1 TB. TOASTED SESAME OIL

♣Add prepared vegetables and sauté for 5 minutes. Add 1/4 CUP WHITE WINE and 2 TBS. MIRIN or SHERRY.
♣Add rice and stir-fry, tossing to coat well.
♣Add tofu mixture and toss.
♣Add 2 BEATEN EGGS. Toss and stir all until eggs are set, about 3 more minutes.
♣Remove to a large serving platter, and sprinkle on DROPS of CHILI OIL.
♣Top with the toasted cashews and serve.

810   ONION LAYERS WITH RICE

I have made this with broccoli and zucchini in place of the onion layers, and they are both good. Try mushrooms or cooked turkey slices. There are lots of possibilities with a layered dish.
For 6 people: Preheat the oven to 350°.

♣Mix and toss 3 CUPS COOKED BROWN or BASMATI RICE with 1 teasp. TAMARI, 1 teasp. DRY BASIL, 1/2 CUP MINCED FRESH PARSLEY LEAVES, and 1/4 CUP CHOPPED ALMONDS.
♣Sauté 3 LARGE CHOPPED ONIONS and 1 CLOVE CHOPPED GARLIC or 2 TBS. CHOPPED SHALLOTS in 2 TBS. OLIVE OIL until translucent and aromatic.
♣Add 1 LARGE RED BELL PEPPER in thin strips and sauté for 3 minutes.

♣Assemble the layers in an oiled 8 x 8" square pan. Spoon a layer of rice over the bottom.
♣Top with a layer of CRUMBLED FETA CHEESE or LIGHT RICOTTA CHEESE to lightly cover.
♣Top with a layer of the onions and peppers.
♣Repeat layers. Top all with 2 TBS. GRATED PARMESAN.
♣Bake for 20 to 25 minutes to warm through, and run under the broiler for 30 seconds to brown.

High Fiber From Lean Beans & Legumes

Remember that a 3" piece of any sea vegetable added to bean and legume cooking water increases digestibility.

811 SPANISH RICE & BEANS

For 8 servings: Preheat oven to 350°.

♣Have ready 3 CUPS COOKED BROWN RICE and 1 1/2 CUPS COOKED PINTO BEANS.
♣Sauté 1 SMALL CHOPPED ONION and 2 CLOVES CHOPPED GARLIC in a large skillet in 1 TB. OLIVE OIL for 5 minutes.
♣Add 1 SMALL CAN CHOPPED GREEN CHILIES and sauté for 3 minutes until aromatic.
♣Add beans and rice and toss to coat for 2 minutes.

♣Assemble the layers. Add half the rice mixture to a large oiled casserole dish.
♣Spread with 4-OZ. LOW-FAT COTTAGE CHEESE, 1/2 CUP GRATED JACK CHEESE, and 1/2 CUP LIGHT SALSA. Sprinkle on 2 TBS. ROSÉ WINE.
♣Spoon on rest of beans and rice.
♣Top with 1/2 CUP GRATED JACK CHEESE.
♣Bake for 25 minutes to heat and melt cheese. Remove, top with 3 MINCED SCALLIONS. Serve hot.

Nutritional analysis: per serving; 204 calories; 10gm. protein; 30gm. carbohydrate; 6gm. fiber; 5gm. fats; 7mg. cholesterol; 141mg. calcium; 2mg. iron; 62mg. magnesium; 321mg. potassium; 131mg. sodium; 1mg. zinc.

812 CASHEW FRENCH BEANS IN SHERRY BUTTER

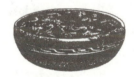

This doesn't even begin to be as rich as it sounds; and it's easy and fiber-rich.
For 4 servings: Preheat oven to 350°.

♣Toast 2 HANDFULS CASHEWS in the oven until golden. Set aside.
♣Cook ONE 10-OZ. PKG. FROZEN FRENCH CUT GREEN BEANS in salted water until color changes to bright green and beans are tender crisp.
♣Melt 3 TBS. BUTTER in a small saucepan. Add 4 TBS. SHERRY, and 1 teasp. LEMON JUICE. Boil until reduced by half, about 3 minutes. Pour over beans and sprinkle with the cashews. Serve hot.

813 EASY GREEN BEANS WITH LEMON & CHEESE

For 6 servings:

♣Steam 1 LB. TRIMMED ITALIAN STYLE GREEN BEANS until color changes and beans are tender.
♣Sauté 1/2 CUP CHOPPED GREEN ONION in 2 teasp. OLIVE OIL until color changes to bright green.
♣Mix beans and onions together and toss with 2 TBS. LEMON JUICE, SESAME SALT and PEPPER.
♣Sprinkle with 2 TBS. GRATED PARMESAN and GRATED LOW-FAT CHEDDAR. Serve hot.

814   DELUXE FRENCH BEANS

For 6 people: Preheat oven to 350°.

♣Make the MUSHROOM SAUCE. Use MAYACAMAS MUSHROOM SOUP & SAUCE MIX or your favorite mushroom sauce from scratch. You will need about 2 CUPS of sauce.
♣Put 3 to 4 CUPS FROZEN FRENCH CUT GREEN BEANS in a large casserole.

♣Sauté 1 CUP SLICED MUSHROOMS in 2 teasp. BUTTER until aromatic, and add to beans.
♣Add $1/2$ teasp. OREGANO, $1/2$ teasp. BASMATI VINEGAR, and 1 teasp. TAMARI and toss to coat.

♣Beat 2 EGGS well and pour over bean/mushroom mix. Pour on mushroom sauce.
♣Chop 1 YELLOW ONION IN RINGS, and soak them in ANOTHER BEATEN EGG. Remove one by one and roll in a mixture of $1/4$ CUP TOASTED SESAME SEEDS, $1/4$ CUP TOASTED WHEAT GERM, and $1/4$ CUP GRATED ROMANO CHEESE.
♣Place in a single overlapping layer on top of the casserole. Bake 45 minutes until browned.

Nutritional analysis: per serving; 221 calories; 12gm. protein; 17gm. carbos; 4gm. fiber; 12gm. fats; 122mg. cholesterol; 180mg. calcium; 3mg. iron; 73mg. magnesium; 463mg. potassium; 411mg. sodium; 2mg. zinc.

815   BAKED BEANS WITH VEGETABLES

For 8 servings:

♣Put 2 CUPS DRY NAVY BEANS in a pot with 6 CUPS WATER and 1 teasp. SEA SALT. Simmer covered, until tender, about two hours. Drain and mix with

1 CHOPPED GREEN BELL PEPPER	$3/4$ CUP MOLASSES
2 TBS. STONEGROUND MUSTARD	2 CHOPPED RED ONIONS
$1/2$ teasp. GARLIC POWDER	$1/2$ teasp. CINNAMON

♣Turn into a 3-qt. baking dish and bake covered, at 375° for 1 hour.

816   WESTERN SUCCOTASH

For 4 people: Preheat oven to 350°.

♣Combine in an oiled dish

1 CUP FRESH CORN KERNALS	$1/2$ CUP CHOPPED ONION
1 CUP FRESH OR FROZEN LIMA BEANS	$1/2$ teasp. SEA SALT
1 CUP CHOPPED TOMATOES	$1/2$ teasp. PAPRIKA
$1/4$ teasp. LIQUID SMOKE or HICKORY SAUCE	1 teasp. HONEY
DASHES of HOT CHILI SAUCE	

♣Stick in about 12 to 16 NACHO TORTILLA CHIPS or BLACK BEAN CHIPS points down, and bake for 35 minutes.

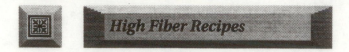

817   BEANS AND WATER CHESTNUTS

This dish sounds ordinary, but it is very very good. A definite request at our house, where there is hardly ever time for a recipe request.
For 4 servings:

♣Steam 1 LB. FRENCH CUT FROZEN GREEN BEANS until tender and bright green. Rinse in cold water to set color, and set aside.

♣Toast 1/4 CUP SLIVERED ALMONDS in the oven and set aside.

♣Sauté 1 1/2 CUPS SLICED MUSHROOMS briefly in 1 TB. OIL until aromatic.
♣Add and toss 2 CHOPPED GREEN ONIONS and 1/4 teasp. PEPPER.
♣Add 1 CUP CHICKEN STOCK.
♣Add 2 TBS. ARROWROOT mixed in 2 TBS. TAMARI.
♣Cook and bubble until thickened. Lower heat and add 1 can SLICED WATER CHESTNUTS.

♣Mix with beans. Toss to coat, and top with the cashews. Serve right away.

Nutritional analysis: per serving; 165 calories; 6gm. protein; 21gm. carbohydrates; 6gm. fiber; 8gm. fats; 0 cholesterol; 78mg. calcium; 3mg. iron; 69mg. magnesium; 505mg. potassium; 137mg. sodium; 1mg. zinc.

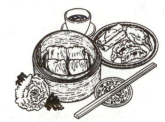

818   ORIENTAL BEAN BURGERS

Adzukis are small red beans native to the Orient and available in most health food stores. They are very digestible with a delicate sweet flavor and light texture.
For 10 patties: Preheat oven to 350°.

♣Have ready 1 1/2 CUPS COOKED BROWN RICE.

♣Soak 1 CUP DRY ADZUKI BEANS overnight in water, to cover. Drain and add 3 CUPS WATER in a large pot. Cook for about 1 hour until tender.

♣Mix cooked beans with the cooked rice in a bowl and add
1 TBS. CHINESE FIVE SPICE POWDER   1/2 CUP MINCED SCALLIONS
1 teasp. MINCED GINGER   1/2 CUP WHOLE WHT. BREAD CRUMBS
2 TBS. TAMARI   1 DICED RED BELL PEPPER
1/4 teasp. HOT PEPPER SAUCE   1/2 teasp. SESAME SALT
♣Form into 10 patties. Roll in TOASTED SESAME SEEDS, and put on lecithin-sprayed baking sheets.
♣Bake until piping hot in the center, about 15 to 20 minutes. Serve on toasted rice cakes with a **QUICK HOT & SOUR SAUCE** and SUNFLOWER SPROUTS.

QUICK HOT & SOUR SAUCE:
♣Combine all together and let stand to blend flavors.
1 1/2 TBS. CHICKEN BROTH   1 TB. TOASTED SESAME OIL
2 TBS. TAMARI   1/2 teasp. HOT PEPPER SAUCE
1 TB. RICE VINEGAR   1 TB. THIN SLICE SCALLION

High Fiber Fruits & Breakfast Foods

*Many fruits, such as prunes, apples, figs, dates, papaya and mangos, are well-known for their beneficial fiber and enzyme precursers. Check out the **BREAKFAST & BRUNCH chapter** in this book for more high fiber morning foods. The recipes in this section are good at any meal.*

819   CARROT & RAISIN OATMEAL

For 4 servings:

♣Shred 2 CARROTS in a grater or salad shooter. Toss with $1/2$ teasp. SEA SALT. Add to 4 CUPS WATER.
♣Bring to a rapid boil. Reduce heat to a simmer and cook for 4 minutes.
♣Add $1/2$ CUP of RAISINS and cook for 3 minutes.
♣Stir in $2/3$ CUP OAT BRAN, $11/3$ CUPS ROLLED OATS, and $1/2$ teasp. CINNAMON. Cook stirring until thickened, about 5 minutes. Serve at once.

820   HONEY APPLE PANCAKES

These are dairy-free, but sweet, rich and high in fiber.
For 8 pancakes: Preheat a griddle to hot.

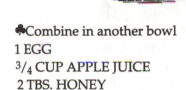

♣Mix in a bowl
1$1/4$ CUPS WHOLE WHEAT PASTRY FLOUR
2 teasp. BAKING POWDER
$1/4$ teasp. APPLE PIE SPICE
$1/4$ teasp. SEA SALT
$1/4$ teasp. BAKING POWDER

♣Combine in another bowl
1 EGG
$3/4$ CUP APPLE JUICE
2 TBS. HONEY
1 TB. OIL

♣Combine the two mixtures together, blending until slightly lumpy. Ladle onto hot oiled griddle, turn when bubbles appear and cook for 1 more minute.

821   ORANGE KIWI POLENTA CAKES

For 6 servings:

♣Toast 3 TBS. SHREDDED COCONUT in the oven until golden. Set aside.
♣Mix 1 SLICED KIWI and 1 CUP ORANGE SECTIONS with 1 CUP PLAIN YOGURT. Set aside.

♣Bring 2$1/2$ CUPS ORANGE JUICE, $1/2$ teasp. GRATED ORANGE PEEL, and $1/2$ teasp. SEA SALT to a boil in a pan. Add 1 CUP POLENTA and stir to blend for 3 to 5 minutes. Add $1/4$ CUP HONEY and 2 TBS. BUTTER. Divide between 6 oiled custard cups and press in.
♣Let cool for 10 minutes. Run a knife around to loosen and invert on serving plates.
♣Sprinkle with TOASTED COCONUT and top with the yogurt and fruit mix.

822 PRUNE BREAD

For 2 loaves: Preheat oven to 350°.

♣Put prunes in a saucepan with 1 CUP WATER. Bring to a boil and simmer for 1 minute until plumped.
♣Drain and reserve ½ CUP of the liquid. Set aside.

♣Mix dry ingredients together
1 CUP WHOLE WHEAT PASTRY FLOUR
1½ CUPS UNBLEACHED FLOUR
1½ teasp. BAKING POWDER
1 teasp. BAKING SODA

♣Mix wet ingredients together
¼ CUP BUTTER
½ CUP DATE SUGAR
½ CUP FRUCTOSE
1 EGG

♣Combine both mixtures just to moisten. Blend in the RESERVED PRUNE LIQUID, ½ CUP PLAIN YO-GURT and ½ CUP WATER. Add PRUNES and pour into the prepared loaf pans.
♣Bake for 50 to 55 minute until golden. Cool 15 minutes before slicing.

823 MINCE MEAT DESSERT

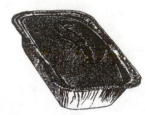

For about 2 cup, or 6 servingss:

♣Combine into a saucepan
2 CUPS CHOPPED TART APPLES
1 CUP RAISINS or CURRANTS
¼ CUP CHOPPED PECANS
¼ CUP CHOPPED WALNUTS
½ CUP APPLE JUICE
¼ CUP ORANGE JUICE

2 TBS. MAPLE SYRUP
⅓ CUP HONEY
2 teasp. GRATED LEMON PEEL
2 teasp. GRATED ORANGE PEEL
2 teasp. APPLE PIE SPICE

♣Bring to a boil, and simmer until thickened, about 30 minutes. Let cool slightly. Serve in a small open bowl like a rice bowl for a light dessert.

Nutritional analysis: per serving; 268 calories; 2gm. protein; 55gm. carbohydrates; 4gm. fiber; 7gm. fats; 0 cholesterol; 46mg. calcium; 2mg. iron; 32mg. magnesium; 383mg. potassium; 6mg. sodium; 1mg. zinc.

824 TRAIL MIX BARS

For 12 cookies: Preheat oven to 350°.

♣Combine all ingredients in a bowl
½ CUP DATE SUGAR
½ CUP MOLASSES
¼ CUP HONEY
1 CUP CHOPPED WALNUTS
½ CUP WHOLE WHEAT PASTRY FLOUR

3 EGGS
¼ CUP TOASTED OATS
1 CUP CHOPPED DATES
1 CUP COCONUT SHREDS
½ CUP TOASTED WHEAT GERM

♣Press into an oiled square baking pan and bake for 20 minutes. Cut in squares.
Nutritional analysis: per serving; 45 gm.; 157 calories; 19 gm. carbohydrate; 7 gm. protein; 4 mg. iron;.058 gm. choles-terol; 2 gm. fiber; .008 mg. sodium; 3 gm. PUFA; 9 gm. fat; 33 mg.calcium

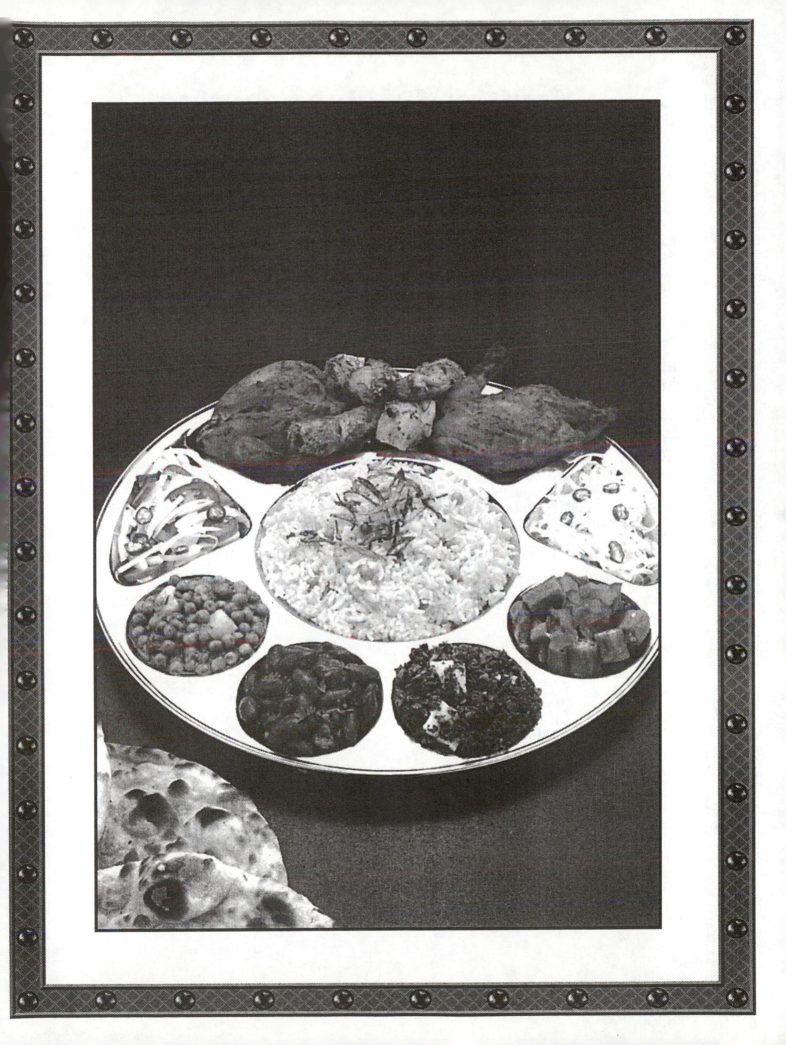

Healthy Holiday Feasting & EntertaininG

You can have both health and tradition. The holidays can be a genuine harvest celebration.

The great American excuse for going off a healthy diet because of holidays and celebrations doesn't have to be yours. This section has some great low-fat menus and recipes for parties and gatherings. Everybody will enjoy them, so you can keep your friends and family happy, partake of traditional holiday foods, and still stay reasonably close to your diet program. It just takes a small effort and change from conventional cooking methods and ingredients.

The recipes in this section are among the few in this book that use sugar as a sweetener. For occasional treats at holiday times, a small amount of sugar can be handled by most people. A little sugar can clearly add to the pleasure of special festive foods, and won't jeopardize your healing program for long. A small sweet treat every now and then is better for social and emotional balance than weeks of feeling deprived, and a possible "sugar orgy" later.

HEALTHY TIPS FOR HOLIDAY & CELEBRATION TIMES:
1) Take only small portions of anything.
2) Keep fats and calories as low as possible in whatever you fix.
3) Make only 3 or 4 recipes, including breads and desserts, for each meal. A "groaning board" will only have everybody overstuffed and groaning later.
4) Keep up your exercise and fitness program during the holidays.
5) Continue with your diet for all meals except the special ones. When the holiday gatherings are over, return to the total program right away.

These recipes will help keep you leaner, cleaner and healthier at a time of year when it's easy to forget a good diet.

❧GREAT BEGINNINGS - HEALTHY APPETIZERS, SNACKS and HORS D'OEUVRES ❧FANCY, NO-EXCUSES HEALTHY HOLIDAY ENTREES ❧HEALTHY HOLIDAY COOKIES ❧HEALTHY HOLIDAYS PIES and DESSERTS ❧SPECIAL BAKED TREATS FOR FEASTING ❧

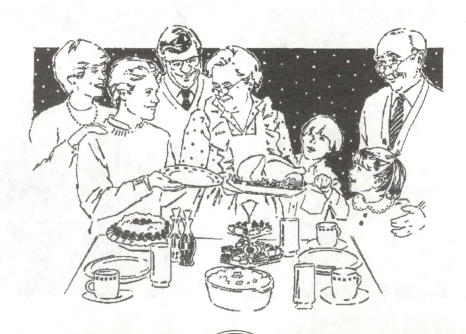

Great Beginnings - Healthy Appetizers

Holiday and celebration times are party times. Giving a "healthy food" party can seem almost impossible at first.
Most of us are so used to appetizers, hors d'oeuvres, and cocktails that are loaded with fat calories, sugar and salt.
It doesn't have to be that way. With just a little thought and the recipes in this chapter,
*you can stay on your healthy healing diet, celebrate, have a good time, **and** please your guests.*
The foods offered here are particularly appropriate for winter holiday parties.

826   VEGETABLE PATÉ WITH SWEET & SOUR GLOSS

This paté can be made in different sizes and shapes. It looks very festive, like a big, shiny glazed jewel sitting on a
bed of ruffles greens. Surround with apple slices and/or little pumpernickle toasts.

For about 8 to 10 people: Preheat oven to 375°.

♣Mix the paté in the blender
3 CAKES MASHED TOFU
2 TBS. PEANUT BUTTER
3 TBS. TAMARI
8 GREEN CHOPPED ONIONS
1 1/2 CUPS CHOPPED MUSHROOMS

♣Turn into a bowl and add
 1 CHOPPED RED BELL PEPPER
 1 CAN DICED WATER CHESTNUTS
 1/4 CUP CHOPPED PARSLEY
 1/2 teasp. PEPPER

♣Oil a decorative mold. Line with waxed paper, and oil the paper. Pack in paté. Bake for 45 minutes. Remove and cool in the mold. Chill until ready to serve.

♣Make the **SWEET & SOUR GLOSS** at serving time. Combine in a saucepan
1 1/2 CUPS PINEAPPLE/ORANGE JUICE   1/4 CUP TAMARI
1/4 CUP HONEY or MAPLE SYRUP   1/4 teasp. GARLIC POWDER
1/3 to 1/2 CUP BROWN RICE VINEGAR
♣Bring to a boil and let simmer for 5 minutes while you unmold the paté on a greens-covered plate.

♣Stir in 2 TBS. ARROWROOT dissolved in 2 TBS. WATER. Simmer until thickened and glossy.
♣Spoon over paté and serve.

Nutritional analysis: per serving; 109 calories; 5gm. protein; 17gm. carbohydrate; 2gm. fiber; 3gm. fats; 0 cholesterol; 54mg. calcium; 3mg. iron; 54mg. magnesium; 265mg. potassium; 130mg. sodium; 1mg. zinc.

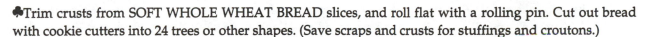

827   EASY CHEESE TREES

The kids can help with these. They like to eat 'em, too.
For 24 trees: Preheat oven to 400°.

♣Trim crusts from SOFT WHOLE WHEAT BREAD slices, and roll flat with a rolling pin. Cut out bread with cookie cutters into 24 trees or other shapes. (Save scraps and crusts for stuffings and croutons.)

♣Make the sauce. Combine 3/4 CUP GRATED PARMESAN or LOW-FAT CHEDDAR CHEESE, 1/2 CUP LIGHT MAYONNAISE, 2 TBS. MINCED GREEN ONION, and 1/4 teasp WHITE PEPPER.
♣Spread on sauce mix and bake on lecithin-sprayed baking sheets until golden and bubbly.

828 LOBSTER CHUNKS IN ROSEMARY MARINADE

I know lobster is expensive, but this is such a lovely hors d'oeuvre to present in a silver chafing dish on your party table. Nothing else works as well as lobster tails.
For 25 to 30 pieces:

♣Bring enough salted water to a boil for EIGHT 4-OZ. LOBSTER TAILS. Boil the tails until just pink, about 6 minutes. Cool, remove shell and cut meat into 1" chunks. Chill and marinate in the following sauce for several hours, turning occasionally

1 CUP WHITE WINE	2 teasp. FRUCTOSE
1/2 CUP OIL	2 TBS. MINCED SHALLOTS
1 teasp. ROSEMARY	1/2 teasp. LEMON PEPPER

♣Reserve 1/2 cup of the marinade and place lobster chunks in the chafing dish.
♣Combine 1 STICK UNSALTED BUTTER, THE RESERVED MARINADE and 2 TBS. LEMON JUICE in a small saucepan. Heat gently and pour over lobster. Light chafing dish candle. Serve with picks.

829 EVERYTHING CHEESEBALL

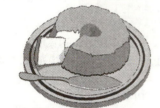

For 1 big ball:

♣Have cheeses at room temperature for best results. Mix 2 CUPS SHREDDED SWISS, 2 CUPS, SHREDDED LOW-FAT CHEDDAR, 8-OZ. NEUFCHATEL CHEESE and 1/2 CARTON CREME FRAICHE together in a large bowl. Set aside.
♣Sauté 1/2 CUP DICED ONIONS, 3 TBS. SOY BACON BITS, ONE 2-OZ. JAR PIMIENTOS, 2 TBS. SWEET PICKLE RELISH, 1/4 teasp. LEMON PEPPER and 1/4 CUP CHOPPED NUTS until fragrant.
♣Add to cheese blend. Cover and chill overnight. When ready to serve, make a coating mix of 1/4 CUP CHOPPED NUTS, 3 to 4 TBS. SOY BACON BITS, 1/2 teasp. SESAME SALT, 1/4 CUP SNIPPED PARSLEY and 1 TB. POPPY SEEDS. Unwrap chilled cheese ball, roll in the coating mix.
♣Press onto ball to adhere. Let stand 30 minutes to blend flavors and serve.

830 MACAROON JAM SLICES

For 24 slices: Preheat oven to 350°. Butter a baking sheet. Sprinkle with flour and tip to coat.

♣Combine 1 1/2 CUPS DICED WALNUTS and 2/3 CUP TURBINADO SUGAR in a bowl.
♣Whip 2 EGG WHITES stiff with a PINCH CREAM OF TARTER, and add to nuts to form a kneadable paste. Shape into 2 rolls 10" long. Make a 1/2" deep channel down the center of each with your finger, leaving 1/4" at each end. Place rolls on the prepared sheet and bake until lightly browned. Remove and cool.
♣Heat ONE 12-OZ. JAR RASPBERRY JAM in a small saucepan until runny.
♣Fill channels in the rolls. Cool and slice.

Nutritional analysis: per slice; 109 calories; 1gm. protein; 17gm. carbohydrates; 1gm. fiber; 5gm. fats; 0 cholesterol; 10mg. calcium; trace iron; 14mg. magnesium; 55mg. potassium; 7mg. sodium; trace zinc.

831   TINY CHICKEN KEBABS WITH ORANGE GLAZE

For 36 nuggets: Preheat broiler.

♣Rinse, skin and bone 6 CHICKEN BREAST HALVES. Cut each into 6 lengthwise slices. Weave each onto a small wooden skewer *that has been soaked in water for 30 minutes or more.* Lay on a lecithin-sprayed 10 x 15" baking sheet. Cover and chill while you make the sauce.
♣Combine the glaze in a saucepan
2 TBS. PREPARED HORSERADISH or PINCHES WASABI POWDER
1 CUP SUGARLESS ORANGE or APRICOT JAM
2 TBS. HONEY
2 TBS. GRATED ORANGE PEEL
2 TBS. MINCED FRESH GINGER
1/4 CUP ORANGE JUICE
♣Stir over med. heat until jam melts. Brush chicken with sauce and broil for 4 minutes basting twice.
♣Turn skewers and broil for 4 more minutes, basting again. Put skewered chicken on greens-covered serving platter.

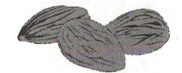

832   ROMAN ALMONDS
This is an authentic ancient recipe. They are delicious and easy to make.

Preheat oven to *300°*.

♣Beat 1 EGG WHITE until frothy. Stir in 1 LB. WHOLE ALMONDS and toss to coat. Spread on a greased baking sheet, and sprinkle with *COARSE* SALT. Bake until shiny, crisp and golden, stirring frequently.

Nutritional analysis: per 1 oz. serving; 168 calories; 6gm. protein; 6gm. carbohydrates; 3gm. fiber; 15gm. fats; 0 cholesterol; 77mg. calcium; 1mg. iron; 85mg. magnmesium; 209mg. potassium; 270mg. sodium; 1mg. zinc.

833   FRESH HOMEMADE CRANBERRY CANDY

For 24 pieces:

♣Combine 2 CUPS CRANBERRIES, 1 1/2 teasp. GRATED ORANGE PEEL, 2 teasp. FRESH GRATED GINGER and 3/4 CUP ORANGE JUICE in a pan. Heat until berries begin to pop. Remove from heat to cool slightly, and purée in the blender until smooth. Add back to the saucepan with 3/4 CUP BROWN SUGAR and 3 TBS. UNFLAVORED GELATIN.
♣Cook over medium heat for 15 minutes, stirring constantly until you can see the bottom of the pan when a spoon is drawn across it. Stir in 1/3 CUP CHOPPED WALNUTS, and spread mixture in an oiled loaf pan. Let stand uncovered overnight. Cut in squares.

Nutritional analysis: per 1 oz. serving; 46 calories; 1gm. protein; 8gm. carbohydrates; 1gm. fiber; 1gm. fats; 0 cholesterol; 4mg. calcium; trace iron; 5mg. magnesium; 33mg. potassium; 1mg. sodium; trace zinc.

834   HOMEMADE HONEY CRACKED TOFFEE

For 24 pieces: Have ready oiled flat pans.

♣Boil together in a heavy pot with a candy thermometer until it reaches 285°.
1/2 CUP HONEY
1/4 CUP FRUCTOSE
1/2 teasp. SEA SALT
1/2 CUP BUTTER
♣Add 1/2 CUP WALNUTS and turn onto oiled pans. Spread out to cool.

♣Melt 12-OZ. CAROB CHIPS in the pot, and spread over the cooled toffee. Sprinkle with 1/2 CUP MORE WALNUTS. Cool again. Crack with a hammer into pieces. Serve in a small candy dish.

Nutritional analysis: per piece; 150 calories; 1gm. protein; 17gm. carbohydrates; 1gm. fiber; 10gm. fats; 5mg. cholesterol; 10mg. calcium; 1mg. iron; 28mg. magnesium; 46mg. sodium; trace zinc.

835   SPICY APPLE DIP

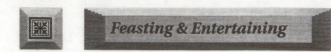

For about 2 cups:

♣Mix all together in the blender
1/4 CUP LIGHT MAYONNAISE
1 LARGE GOLDEN DELICIOUS APPLE
1/2 CUP COTTAGE CHEESE
1 TB. PREPARED HORSERADISH

1 teasp. VINEGAR
1/2 teasp. GROUND ALLSPICE
11/2 teasp. HONEY
1/4 teasp. WHITE PEPPER

♣Turn into a bowl and mix in 1 CHOPPED GREEN ONION, 1/4 CUP CHOPPED PARSLEY, and 1/4 CUP CURRANTS or RAISINS.
♣Turn into a serving bowl. Snip green onions over for garnish, and serve with raw vegetable dippers.

Nutritional analysis: per 2 oz. serving; 96 calories; 2gm. protein; 13gm. carbohydrates; 1gm. fiber; 2gm. fats; 4mg. cholesterol; 21mg. calcium; trace iron; 6mg. magnesium; 108mg. potassium; 75mg. sodium; 1mg. zinc.

836   CHEESE & NUT CRISPS

For 15 to 20 crisps: Preheat oven to 350°.

♣Mix and toss together in a bowl, 1 CUP SHREDDED SWISS or JARLSBERG CHEESE, 1/2 CUP SLIVERED ALMONDS, 1/2 teasp. CUMIN, and a PINCH PAPRIKA. Drop in 1 TB. mounds on a lecithin-sprayed baking sheet. Bake for 12 to 15 minutes until golden brown. Remove and cool.
♣Arrange on a serving plate around a small bowl of salsa for dipping.

837   RICH PARTY FRUIT CAKE

This is a very rich, no-sugar cake, Serve in thin sliver pieces.
For 12 servings: Preheat oven to 350∞. Have ready a buttered 9 x 12" baking pan.

♣Combine the cake ingredients

1/2 CUP HONEY	2 EGGS
1/2 CUP OIL	1/4 CUP RICE FLOUR
1 1/2 CUPS WHOLE WHEAT PASTRY FLOUR	1/4 teasp. ORANGE EXTRACT

♣Spread into prepared pan, and bake for 15 minutes. Cool slightly while you make the topping.

♣Mix together

3/4 CUP MAPLE SYRUP	1/2 CUP RAISINS
1/4 CUP WHOLE WHEAT FLOUR	1/4 CUP TOASTED COCONUT
1/2 CUP TOASTED SESAME SEEDS	1/4 CUP CHOPPED WALNUTS
1/2 CUP CHOPPED DRY PINEAPPLE	1/2 teasp. NUTMEG
1/4 CUP CHOPPED DRY APRICOTS	1/4 teasp. SEA SALT
1 teasp. VANILLA	1/2 teasp. CINNAMON

♣Spread on cake and return to the oven for 20 more minutes until light brown. Cool, cut and serve.

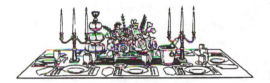

Fancy, No-Excuses, Healthy Holiday Recipes

Pick from the dishes in this section to put together a delicious, healthy holiday feast.

A WORD ABOUT TURKEY

Naturally-raised, free-run turkeys, such as those from the Diestel and Shelton farms, are good high grade sources of protein, free of hormone injections and anti-biotics. Not only are these turkeys more ecologically responsible as they run and scratch for their food, but they are allowed a longer life span, which develops the meat with much more flavor. Turkey meat in general is leaner, lower in saturated fat and cholesterol, with more available vitamins and minerals, than chicken. In fact, one serving of cooked skinless white meat is approximately 180 calories, with **less total fat than any other meat.** Turkey is a very practical diet, as well as feasting, food all year round. For even lower fat calories, roast turkey with the skin *on* to keep the meat from drying out, but remove the skin before you eat it. Remember that the back, giblets and wings are mostly fat. Either discard these pieces, or use them in a strained stock for gravy.

HOLIDAY TURKEY BASTE

This baste lends a lovely, fragrant scent and a nice crust to the turkey.

♣Heat in a small pan

6 TBS. BUTTER	1 TB. LEMON JUICE
2 TBS. SHERRY or MADEIRA	1/2 teasp. ALLSPICE

♣Spread on turkey to cover before roasting

VERY LIGHT TURKEY GRAVY

♣When the turkey roast is tender, simply remove it to the serving platter, and put the roasting pan on medium-low heat on the stove. You should have about $1/2$ CUP DRIPPINGS. When they are hot, deglaze with 1 CUP WHITE WINE. Whisk and stir until all the stuck-on bits are free. Mix $1/2$ CUP ARROWROOT with 1 CUP CHICKEN or TURKEY BROTH until smooth and dissolved. Add to the gravy, season with SEA SALT and PEPPER and whisk until boiling. Serve hot.

❦

AROMATIC ONION GRAVY FOR TURKEY

♣After roasting, pour off 2 TBS. drippings into a skillet. Add 2 SLICED ONIONS, add 2 TBS. WHOLE WHEAT FLOUR and stir over high heat for 3 minutes. Add 1 CUP WATER and 1 CUP ROSÉ WINE and stir until gravy comes to a boil and thickens smooth. Stir in 1 teasp. CIDER VINEGAR, $1/2$ teasp. SEA SALT and $1/4$ teasp. PEPPER. Serve hot over turkey slices.

❦

MUSHROOM GRAVY FOR TURKEY

♣After roasting, pour 4 TBS. drippings from the roasting pan into a skillet. Add 3 TBS. WHOLE GRAIN FLOUR and stir for 2 minutes over medium heat until browned and bubbly. Whisk in 3 CUPS CHICKEN or TURKEY BROTH (from boiled giblets).
♣Bring to a boil and whisk until thick and smooth, about 4 minutes.
♣Sauté 8 OZ. SLICED MUSHROOMS in $1^1/_2$ TBS. butter until tender. Add to gravy with $1/2$ teasp. SEA SALT and $1/4$ teasp. PEPPER. Heat briefly to blend flavors.

838   FANCY UN-STUFFING
If you are using a small turkey roast, make the "stuffing" as a separate dish, and cook right along with the turkey. Enough for 4 people: Preheat oven to 325°.

♣Mix 8 CUPS WHOLE GRAIN BREAD CUBES or DICED CORN BREAD in a large bowl.
♣Sauté in a large skillet for about 5 minutes til fragrant
1 LARGE CHOPPED ONION
1 CHOPPED RED BELL PEPPER
2 STALKS CELERY chopped with leaves
$1/2$ teasp. GROUND SAGE

1 teasp. SESAME SALT
1 teasp. LEMON PEPPER
$1/4$ teasp. POWDERED ROSEMARY
$1/4$ teasp. NUTMEG

♣Add **either** 1 PINT OYSTERS, **or** 1 CAN WATER CHESTNUTS **or** 1 CUP SLICED MUSHROOMS.
♣Add $1/2$ CUP TURKEY or CHICKEN STOCK, and $1/2$ cup WHISKEY OR SHERRY. Toss to coat and heat. Mix with bread cubes and toss.
♣Turn into an oiled 3-qt. casserole. Cover and bake for 30 minutes until crusty at the edges.

Nutritional analysis: per serving; 281 calories; 11gm. protein; 46gm. carbohydrates; 8gm. fiber; 4gm fats; 0 cholesterol; 91mg. calcium; 4mg. iron; 95mg. magnesium; 410mg. potassium; 486mg. sodium; 2mg. zinc.

839   SOUTHERN SPOONBREAD DRESSING

For 8 servings: Preheat oven to 350°.

♣Have ready a large lecithin-sprayed straight-sided casserole dish.
♣Bring 2 CUPS CHICKEN BROTH and 1 CUP PLAIN YOGURT to a boil in a large saucepan.
♣Add 1¼ CUPS CORNMEAL. Stir until thick. Remove from heat. Add 6 BEATEN EGGS and set aside.

♣Sauté for 10 minutes until translucent
4 TBS. BUTTER
2 CHOPPED ONIONS
1 STALK CHOPPED CELERY with leaves

♣Add and stir in
1 teasp. SESAME SALT
1 teasp. SAGE POWDER
1 TBS. CHOPPED PARSLEY

♣Add to egg mixture, and stir in 2 teasp. BAKING POWDER.
♣Beat vigorously about 5 minutes til everything is smooth, well blended and light. Turn into a buttered casserole and bake for 35 to 40 minutes til puffy and golden brown.
♣Serve right away with spoonfuls of a light gravy. (See previous page.)

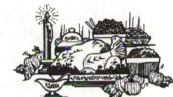

840   CORNMEAL BATTY CAKES

This simple grain recipe is probably as old as the first Thanksgiving. That's called standing the test of time.
For 24 batty cakes: Preheat a griddle to hot and a drop of water skitter on the surface. Oil with a little butter on a paper napkin.

♣Combine ³⁄₄ CUP YELLOW CORNMEAL, ¹⁄₂ teasp. BAKING POWDER, ¹⁄₂ teasp. SEA SALT, and ¹⁄₂ teasp. BAKING SODA with 1 EGG and 1 CUP BUTTERMILK until smooth.
♣Ladle 1 TB. BATTER on the griddle for each cake. Cook for 2 to 3 minutes on each side until brown.
♣Keep batter stirred and finished cakes hot. Serve with honey to accompany roast turkey.

841   PUFFY LAYERED STUFFING CASSEROLE

Even though this is technically a stuffing, we like it all winter as a nice hearty dish.
For 4 servings: Preheat oven to 350°.

♣Sauté 1 teasp. GARLIC/LEMON SEASONING and 1 CHOPPED YELLOW ONION in 2 TBS. BUTTER in a skillet for 5 minutes. Add 1 CUP CHOPPED CELERY and sauté for 5 minutes more.

♣Mix in a large bowl and let stand for 20 minutes to blend flavors
1¹⁄₂ cups WHOLE GRAIN BREAD CUBES or CORN BREAD, crumbled
2 CUPS SPARKLING WHITE WINE or SPARKLING WATER
1 teasp. SESAME SALT   3 EGGS
1 TB. WORCESTERSHIRE SAUCE   1 teasp. POULTRY SEASONING
¹⁄₄ teasp. HOT PEPPER SAUCE   ¹⁄₂ teasp. PEPPER

♣Layer half of the bread mix in a 2-qt. buttered casserole. Cover with half of the onion sauté. Cover with ³⁄₄ cup GRATED FARMER CHEESE. Repeat layers and bake for 35 to 40 minutes. Serve hot.

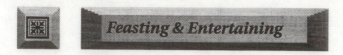

*T**hanksgiving is such a uniquely American holiday. Part of its charm are the native American harvest foods that we traditionally enjoy at this time: squashes, corn, potatoes, yams, berries, nuts, cranberries and maple syrup. It's so hard to decide which to have. But since they all taste wonderful at the same meal, you can make anything you want - like a wild potluck. It will be great. Here are some healthy recipes to choose from.*

842   SHERRY, NUTS & WILD RICE on the side

For 6 servings:

♣Heat 1 CUP RAISINS and $^1/_2$ CUP SHERRY in a small saucepan to boiling. Reduce heat, simmer for 5 minutes, remove from heat and set aside.

♣Toast 1 CUP SLIVERED ALMONDS in the oven until golden. Remove and set aside.

♣Put 1 CUP WILD RICE in a pot with 2 CUPS CHICKEN or TURKEY STOCK and 1 TB. BUTTER. Cook over <u>low heat</u> for 1 hour.

♣Bring $2^2/_3$ CUPS CHICKEN or TURKEY STOCK to a boil in another pot and add 1 CUP BROWN RICE and 1 TB. BUTTER. Reduce heat and cook until liquid is absorbed, about 45 minutes.

♣Combine all ingredients in a serving dish. Season with SEA SALT and PEPPER, and snip $^1/_2$ CUP FRESH PARSLEY over top.

Nutritional analysis: per serving; 404 calories; 10gm. protein; 65gm. carbohydrates; 7gm. fiber; 11gm. fats; 5mg. cholesterol; 79mg. calcium; 2mg. iron; 128mg. magnesium; 520mg. potassium; 176mg. sodium; 2mg. zinc.

❈

843   SWEET POTATO SOUFFLÉ
This recipe is also good using cup for cup of pumpkin, carrots, or golden zucchini instead of the sweet potatoes, and it's so easy.
For 6 servings: Preheat oven to 450°.

♣Separate 4 EGGS. Put the whites in a large mixing bowl and set aside.

♣Mix all ingredients in the blender and whirl until smooth

4 EGG YOLKS	$^1/_2$ teasp. LEMON EXTRACT
$^1/_2$ CUP MAPLE SYRUP	$^1/_2$ teasp. SESAME SALT
1 CUP PLAIN YOGURT	1 teasp. LEMON PEEL
$^1/_2$ teasp. SWEET TOOTH BAKING MIX (pg. 645)	2 CUPS CHICKEN BROTH
2 CUPS GRATED SWEET POTATOES without the skin	

♣Beat the EGG WHITES to stiff peaks with 1 teasp. HONEY and fold into squash mix.
♣Turn into a buttered casserole, and bake for 10 minutes. Lower heat to 325°. and bake for 45 minutes until sweet potatoes are tender and a toothpick comes out clean.

Nutritional analysis: per serving; 235 calories; 8gm. protein; 42gm. carbohydrates; 2gm. fiber; 4gm. fats; 140mg. cholesterol; 148mg. calcium; 2mg. iron; 39mg. magnesium; 376mg. potassium; 225mg. sodium; 1mg. zinc.

❈

844   SWEET & SOUR ROASTED ONIONS

For 4 servings: Preheat oven to 375°.

♣Peel and chunk 2 LARGE RED ONIONS. Arrange them in a baking dish cut side down. Brush on a mixture of 2 TBS. RED WINE VINEGAR and 2 teasp. HONEY. Roast until onions are brown and tender, about 1 1/4 hours. Baste often. They should be very brown and very aromatic when ready.

845   EASY SHERRY SWEET POTATOES

For 8 people: Preheat oven to 350°.

♣Cover 8 SWEET POTATOES with water in a large pot. Bring to a boil and simmer until tender, about 20 minutes. Peel and cut in half. Arrange in a baking dish and sprinkle with

1/4 CUP HONEY	4 TBS. BUTTER
1/3 CUP SHERRY	1/4 teasp. SEA SALT

♣Bake until brown and bubbling, about 35 minutes, basting often.

846   CAROB YAMS

♣Pan or oven roast 1/3 CUP PECANS. Set aside.
♣Peel and slice 2 LBS. YAMS. Sauté in 3 TBS. BUTTER in one layer in a large skillet until light brown, about 5 to 7 minutes. Turn slices and cook until brown again. Transfer to a large bowl, and repeat until all yams are done. Toss yams in the bowl to coat with

1/4 CUP ORANGE JUICE CONCENTRATE	1 1/2 TBS. CAROB POWDER
1/4 CUP ORANGE LIQUEUR	1 teasp LEMON PEEL
1/4 CUP HONEY	1/2 teasp. CINNAMON
2 TBS. LEMON JUICE	1/4 teasp. NUTMEG

♣Return to the skillet and simmer covered until tender, about 15 minutes. Uncover and cook until sauce thickens. Turn onto a serving platter and sprinkle with the toasted pecans.

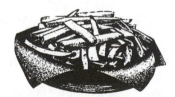

847   BRANDY POTATO STICKS

For 4 people:

♣Cut 1 1/2 LBS. THIN SKIN WHITE POTATOES in matchsticks. Sauté quickly in 2 TBS. BUTTER in a skillet for 10 minutes. Add 1/2 CUP BRANDY and 1/2 CUP CHICKEN BROTH. Cover and simmer until tender, about 15 minutes. Add 3/4 CUP PLAIN LOW-FAT YOGURT and 1/4 CUP WATER. Cook over high heat quickly for 5 minutes. Season with SEA SALT, PEPPER and NUTMEG.

848   PUFFY MASHED POTATOES

For 4 to 6 people: Preheat oven to 450°.

♣Separate 2 EGGS. Put the whites in a bowl and set aside.
♣Cook 3 LARGE POTATOES in boiling water until tender. Drain, peel and mash in a bowl. Add

THE EGG YOLKS	3 TBS. BUTTER
1/4 CUP PLAIN YOGURT	1 teasp. SEA SALT
1/2 CUP LOW-FAT COTTAGE CHEESE	PINCH WHITE PEPPER

♣Beat the egg whites to stiff and fold into potato mixture. Turn into a lecithin-sprayed baking dish, and bake for 25 minutes until puffy and brown on top. Serve hot with **BUTTER MUSTARD SAUCE**.

BUTTER MUSTARD SAUCE
♣Combine in a small saucepan

4 TBS. BUTTER	1/2 teasp. CIDER VINEGAR
1 TB. OIL	1/2 teasp. SWEET MUSTARD
1 teasp. HONEY	1/4 teasp. SALAD HERBS
1 TB. WHITE WINE	1 teasp. TAMARI

♣Simmer for 5 minutes to blend flavors, and pass with mashed potatoes.

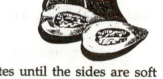

849   STUFFED SPAGHETTI SQUASH

For 4 to 6 people: Preheat oven to 375°.

♣Cut 1 LARGE SPAGHETTI SQUASH in half lengthwise. Bake for 30 minutes until the sides are soft when pressed but meat is still crunchy on the inside. Pull out strands into a large bowl. Put hollow shells in a baking dish for stuffing.
♣Peel and cube 1 EGGPLANT. Salt and let drain in a colander for 30 minutes to remove bitterness.
♣Sauté 1 teasp. LEMON/GARLIC SEASONING in 2 TBS. OLIVE OIL until fragrant. Add eggplant and squash strands and toss until coated. Add 1/4 CUP SNIPPED PARSLEY. Pile into squash shells and top with PARMESAN CHEESE if desired. Serve hot.

850   KID TESTED GINGERBREAD

For 9 squares: Preheat oven to 350°.

♣Combine in a saucepan 1/2 CUP MOLASSES, 11/2 teasp. GROUND GINGER, 11/2 teasp. CINNAMON, 1/4 teasp. NUTMEG, 1 teasp. SODA, and 1/2 teasp. SEA SALT. Heat until bubbly. Add 1 STICK BUTTER, 1/2 CUP BROWN SUGAR, 1/4 CUP WATER. When butter is melted remove from heat and add 3 EGGS, beating each one in until blended. Beat in 2 CUPS WHOLE WHEAT PASTRY FLOUR.
♣Pour into a lecithin-sprayed square pan and bake for 45 to 50 minutes until a toothpick inserted in the center comes out clean.

Holiday Turkey Leftovers

It really can be better the second time around. With these recipes you can look forward to leftovers.

851   HOT TURKEY SALAD WITH CHEESE

For 4 servings: Preheat oven to 350°.

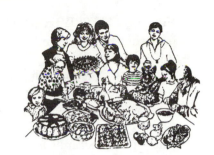

♣Have ready four individual lecithin-sprayed baking dishes.
♣Have ready ¹/₄ CUP LEFTOVER TURKEY GRAVY.
♣Have ready 2 CUPS CHOPPED COOKED TURKEY.
♣Have ready 2 CUPS LEFTOVER STUFFING.
♣Have ready 2 CUPS WASHED TORN SPINACH.
♣Layer in each baking dish; ¹/₄ of the stuffing, ¹/₄ of the turkey, ¹/₄ of the spinach, and 1 SLICE of SWISS CHEESE. Top with 1 TB. gravy, PAPRIKA, SALT and PEPPER. Bake until hot and bubbly.

852   TURKEY SANDWICH IN A DIP

For 3 cups:

♣Mix everything in the blender
16-OZ. LOW-FAT COTTAGE CHEESE
¹/₄ CUP LIGHT MAYONNAISE
¹/₄ CUP SHERRY
1 TB. SOY BACON BITS
¹/₂ teasp. WORCESTERSHIRE SAUCE

2 CUPS DICED COOKED TURKEY
4 CHOPPED GREEN ONIONS
1 teasp. DIJON MUSTARD
1 teasp. CRACKED PEPPER
1 teasp. SEA SALT

♣Serve with celery sticks or rye rounds, or bake until brown on top in a 350° oven and use like a hot paté.

853   BABY TURKEY CALZONES

Absolutely everybody likes these.
For 24 calzones: Preheat oven to 400°.

♣Sauté 1 CLOVE MINCED GARLIC and 1 CHOPPED onion in 2 TBS. BUTTER until brown and aromatic in a large skillet. Add 4-OZ. SLICED MUSHROOMS, cover pan and sauté for 2 more minutes over high heat. Uncover and cook for 5 minutes.

♣Mix the rest of the filling in a bowl
1 CARTON (16 OZ.) LIGHT RICOTTA
6-OZ. GRATED MOZARRELLA
1 teasp. OREGANO

2 CUPS DICED COOKED TURKEY
¹/₄ CUP MINCED PARSLEY
1 teasp. LEMON PEPPER

♣Mix with the onions and mushrooms.
♣Split BABY SESAME PITAS. Fill with filling, and bake for 12 to 15 minutes until cheese is melted.

854   PUMPKIN ALMOND TART WITH LEMON HONEY GLAZE

For 8 to 10 people: Preheat oven to 325°. Oil a 9" springform pan and dust with flour.

♣Whirl 1/2 CUP SLIVERED ALMONDS in the blender. Set aside.

♣Separate 4 EGGS into mixing bowls. Set whites aside.

♣Mix the cake

2/3 CUP TURBINADO SUGAR	1 1/2 teasp. LEMON PEEL
1 CUP CANNED or COOKED PUMPKIN	1 teasp. NUTMEG
1 1/2 teasp. APPLE PIE SPICE	6 TBS. WHOLE WHEAT PASTRY FLOUR
THE EGG YOLKS	

♣Beat egg whites until foamy. Add 2 TBS. FRUCTOSE and beat until stiff. Fold into yolk mixture and turn into prepared pan. Bake for 45 minutes until a toothpick inserted in the center comes out clean. Remove from oven. Cool slightly. Remove pan rim. Cool completely. Spoon on **LEMON GLAZE**.

LEMON GLAZE:

♣Heat 1/4 CUP HONEY, 1 TB. LEMON JUICE, and 1/4 teasp. LEMON PEEL in a small saucepan until syrupy.

❋

855   CHRISTMAS FRUIT CAKE WITH HONEY GLAZED FRUITS

This has no sugar and no candied fruits.
For 24 small rich slices: Preheat oven to 325°.

♣Boil together in a large pot for about 15 minutes

1/2 CUP WATER	♣Cool and add
1/2 CUP ANY FRUIT JUICE	2 CUPS WH. WH. PASTRY FLOUR
1/2 CUP DATE SUGAR	1/2 CUP CHOPPED DATES
1/2 CUP HONEY	1/2 CUP CHOPPED WALNUTS
1/2 CUP BUTTER	1 teasp. BAKING SODA
1 TB. MAPLE SYRUP	1 CUP RAISINS
1 teasp. SWEET TOOTH BAKING SPICE (pg. 645)	2 TBS. BOURBON or PORT WINE

♣Turn into a greased loaf pan or 9 x 13" pan, and bake until firm. Remove, cool, invert onto a serving plate and spoon over **HONEY GLAZE**.

HONEY GLAZED FRUITS

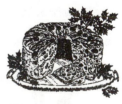

♣Bring 1 CUP HONEY and 1/2 CUP WATER or BOURBON to a boil until syruyp.

♣Add and cook in syrup until tender

4 1/2 CUPS your choice of CUT UP DRIED MIXED FRUITS

1/2 CUP SHREDDED OR SHAVED COCONUT CURLS

1/2 CUP WALNUT HALVES

♣Remove the fruits and nuts with a slotted spoon and top the cake. **Or** cut the cake in half lengthwise. Fill it, and then top it. Pour honey syrup over if desired and chill before slicing.

Nutritional analysis: per 4 oz. serving; 356 calories; 2gm. protein; 80gm. carbohydrates; 9gm. fiber; 7gm. fats; 0 cholesterol; 18mg. calcium; 1mg. iron; 26mg. magnesium; 367mg. potassium; 60mg. sodium; trace zinc.

❋

856   CRANBERRY PUDDING CAKE

For one 9" square pan: Preheat oven to 325°.

♣Sprinkle the bottom of a 9" buttered baking pan with ¹/₂ CUP TURBINADO SUGAR, 2 CUPS CHOPPED CRANBERRIES and ¹/₂ CUP WALNUT PIECES. Put in the oven to melt for 10 minutes.
♣Remove and cool for filling.
♣Beat together

| 2 EGGS | ¹/₂ CUP WH. WH. PASTRY FLOUR |
| 3 TBS. MELTED BUTTER | ¹/₂ CUP HONEY |

♣Pour over berries and shake to settle. Bake in a lecithin-sprayed 9" pan until top is golden and springs back when touched, about 45 minutes to 1 hour. Serve hot or cold.

Nutritional analysis: per serving; 226 calories; 3gm. protein; 35gm. carbohydrates; 2gm. fiber; 9gm. fats; 57mg. cholesterol; 18mg. calcium; 1mg. iron; 23mg. magnesium; 100mg. potassium; 17mg. sodium; 1mg. zinc.

857   CRANBERRY DATE NUT BREAD

For one loaf: Preheat oven to 350°.

♣Cream in a bowl

♣Mix in another bowl

1 STICK BUTTER	2 CUPS WH. WH. PASTRY FLOUR
²/₃ CUP HONEY	1¹/₄ teasp. BAKING POWDER
1 EGG	³/₄ teasp. SEA SALT
¹/₂ CUP ORANGE JUICE	¹/₂ teasp. BAKING SODA
1 teasp. GRATED ORANGE PEEL	

♣Mix the two sets of ingredients gently together. Fold in 1 CUP FRESH CRANBERRIES, ¹/₂ CUP CHOPPED DATES, and ¹/₂ CUP WALNUT PIECES. Turn into a lecithin-sprayed/floured loaf pan.
♣Bake for 1 hour. Cool. Turn out and serve.

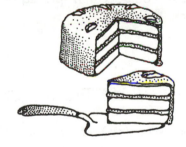

858   BASIL BLACK WALNUT CAKE

Preheat oven to 325°.

♣Mix all ingredients together in a bowl

¹/₄ CUP BUTTER	1¹/₂ teasp. VANILLA
¹/₄ CUP OIL	2¹/₂ CUPS WH. WH. PASTRY FLOUR
¹/₂ CUP BROWN SUGAR	3 teasp. BAKING POWDER
¹/₂ CUP MAPLE SYRUP	¹/₄ CUP FRESH CHOPPED BASIL
4 EGGS	¹/₄ CUP PLAIN YOGURT
¹/₂ CUP BLACK WALNUT PIECES	¹/₄ CUP WATER

♣Drizzle with ¹/₂ CUP HONEY or BROWN SUGAR and ¹/₄ CUP FRESH BASIL, chopped. Bake 25 min.

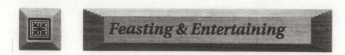

Healthier Holiday Cookies

859   NATURAL TOLL HOUSE COOKIES

For about 100 cookies: Preheat oven to 375°.

♣Combine the dry ingredients in a large bowl
1¹/₂ CUPS WHOLE WHEAT PASTRY FLOUR
1¹/₂ teasp. BAKING SODA
1 teasp. SEA SALT
³/₄ CUP BROWN SUGAR
¹/₄ CUP TURBINADO SUGAR

♣Combine the wet ingredients until creamy
1 CUP BUTTER
¹/₄ CUP MAPLE SYRUP
1¹/₂ teasp. VANILLA
¹/₂ teasp. WATER
 2 EGGS

♣Combine mixtures together to form a dough.

♣Add 12-OZ. CAROB CHIPS, ³/₄ CUP CHOPPED NUTS, ¹/₂ CUP RAISINS just to mix. Drop spoonfuls onto greased sheets and bake for 10 to 12 minutes until edges are crispy.

Nutritional analysis: per 3 cookie serving;173 calories; 3gm. protein; 20gm. carbos; 2gm. fiber; 10gm. fats; 28mg. cholesterol; 54mg. calcium; 1mg. iron; 19mg. magnesium; 139mg. potassium; 94mg. sodium; trace zinc.

860   MOLASSES CRUNCH COOKIES

These taste like old fashioned holiday country cooking.
For 4 dozen cookies: Preheat oven to 350°.

♣Beat with a mixer at high speed for 4 minutes
1 STICK SOFT UNSALTED BUTTER
6 TBS. MOLASSES
6 TBS. BROWN SUGAR
1 EGG

♣Add and mix in
1 CUP WHOLE WHEAT PASTRY FLOUR
¹/₂ teasp. BAKING SODA
¹/₂ CUP CHOPPED WALNUTS
¹/₂ teasp. VANILLA

♣Drop onto lecithin-sprayed sheets and bake for 8 to 10 minutes til dark brown on the edges. Cool on racks to crisp.

861   EASY FARMER'S COOKIES

For 36 cookies: Preheat oven to 400°.

♣Mix in a bowl until a dough is formed
1 CUP + 2 TBS. WHOLE WHEAT PASTRY FLOUR
¹/₄ CUP + 2 TBS. BROWN SUGAR
¹/₂ teasp. BAKING POWDER
1¹/₂ teasp. MOLASSES

6 TBS. BUTTER
2 TBS. CHOPPED WALNUTS
1¹/₂ teasp. WATER

♣Roll into a log. Cover and chill for 1 hour. Slice in ¹/₈" slices. Place on lecithin-sprayed baking sheets. Bake for 12 minutes.

862 CAROB CHIP BARS

For 24 bars: Preheat oven to 375°.

♣Mix in a bowl
1¼ cup WH. WH. PASTRY FLOUR
1 teasp. BAKING SODA
1½ CUPS COCONUT ALMOND GRANOLA
1½ CUPS CAROB CHIPS
1 CUP CHOPPED NUTS

♣Cream together in another bowl
1 CUP BUTTER
1 CUP BROWN SUGAR
1½ teasp. VANILLA

♣Spread on a lecithin-sprayed baking pan and bake for 20 minutes until golden. Cool and cut in bars.

Nutritional analysis: per serving; 254 calories; 4gm. protein; 27gm. carbohydrates; 3gm. fiber; 16gm. fats; 21mg. cholesterol; 71mg. calcium; 1mg. iron; 33mg. magnesium; 181mg. potassium; 27mg. sodium; 1mg. zinc.

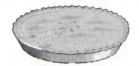

Healthy Holiday Pies

863 APPLE BRANDY PIE
This recipe is a statement for rich autumn harvests - perfect for Thanksgiving.

Preheat oven to 375°.

♣Make the flaky crust with light measures. Mix together gently, 1 CUP SIFTED WHOLE WHEAT PASTRY FLOUR or GOURMET BAKING FLOUR MIX, ½ teasp. SEA SALT, ¼ CUP OIL and 2 TBS. ICE WATER. Press into a ball. Wrap in wax paper and chill. Press out into greased pie plate.
♣Sprinkle crust with CHOPPED WALNUTS, and bake for 15 minutes. Cool and fill.

♣Make the topping first. Bring to boil in a saucepan
1 CUP ROSÉ WINE
½ CUP BRANDY or APPLE JACK
3 LARGE SLICED TART APPLES
½ teasp. NUTMEG
♣Cook for 10 minutes until apples are just tender but still firm. Remove the apples with a slotted spoon, and set aside for garnish.
♣Add ⅓ CUP HONEY, 1 teasp. LEMON JUICE, and ½ teasp. LEMON PEEL to the pan. Stir and cook on very low heat while you make the filling.

♣Mix the filling in a bowl
8-OZ. KEFIR CHEESE or YOGURT CHEESE
1 teasp VANILLA
1 TB. FRUCTOSE
¼ CUP of the TOPPING LIQUID
♣Spread on the crust. Top with reserved apple slices in a concentric circle arrangement.
♣Mix 2 teasp. of the topping liquid with 3 TBS. ARROWROOT POWDER until dissolved. Add back to topping and whisk until thickened and glossy, about 5 to 8 minutes. Pour over apple slices and chill.

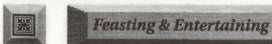

864   PIÑA COLADA PIE

The crust for this pie is really dreamy. You can use it for any fruit or frozen creamy filling.
For 12 slices: Preheat oven to 350°.

♣Make the CHEWY MACAROON CRUST. Mix 4 CUPS SHREDDED COCONUT, 4 TBS. MAPLE SYR-UP, and 1 teasp. VANILLA.

♣Fold in 2 EGG WHITES beaten to stiff peaks with a PINCH CREAM of TARTER. Beat until mixture is thick and shiny. Turn into an oiled pie pan and bake for 15 minutes, until coconut begins to brown at the tips. Let cool and fill.

♣Make the filling in a mixing bowl. Soften 2 pints of HONEY VANILLA ICE CREAM or RICE DREAM just to the point where you can stick a spoon in it. Add 1 teasp. VANILLA and 1/2 CUP CRUSHED PINE-APPLE.

♣Turn into crust and top with CUBES or HALF RINGS of FRESH PINEAPPLE. Return to the freezer. Crust will become chewy like a macaroon.

Nutritional analysis: per serving; 265 calories; 4gm. protein; 27gm. carbohydrates; 2gm. fiber; 17gm. fats; 33mg. cholesterol; 112mg. calcium; 1mg. iron; 26mg. magnesium; 251mg. potassium; 80mg. sodium; 1mg. zinc.

865   MAPLE HARVEST PIE

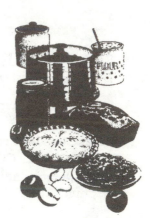

For 8 slices: Preheat oven to 450°.

♣Have ready 1 1/2 CUPS ANY SWEET COOKED WINTER SQUASH or CARROTS.

♣Make the POPPY SEED CRUST. Mix and cut in together to form a dough
3/4 CUP WHOLE WHEAT PASTRY FLOUR	1/2 teasp. SEA SALT
1/2 CUP CORNMEAL	2 TBS. BUTTER
2 TBS. POPPY SEEDS	3 TBS. ICE WATER

♣Roll out or press into a pie plate. Cover. <u>Freeze</u> for 15 minutes while you make the filling.

♣Blend the filling in the blender
THE COOKED SQUASH	1/2 teasp. GINGER
3/4 CUP MAPLE SYRUP	1 teasp. CINNAMON
3/4 CUP PLAIN YOGURT	1/2 teasp. ALLSPICE
3 EGGS	1/4 teasp. SEA SALT

♣Pour into the poppy seed shell and bake in the lower third of the oven for 10 minutes. Reduce heat to 325°, and bake for 45 minutes until center is almost set, but still wobbly.
♣Remove and cool.

Nutritional analysis: per serving; 232 calories; 6gm. protein; 39gm. carbohydrates; 3gm. fiber; 6gm. fats; 89mg. cholesterol; 131mg. calcium; 2mg. iron; 50mg. magnesium; 282mg. potassium; 240mg. sodium; 1mg. zinc.

Special Baked Treats For Feasting

These recipes are goodies for the celebrations and parties in your life. All are rich, satisfying, proven treats, with very little sugar or fat per serving.

866   MARVELOUS MUFFINS

These are party muffins - worth every minute of your time. I have used this recipe so much that I can hardly read it. The description is true. I have never found anybody who didn't like these muffins.
For 18 melt-in-your-mouth muffins: Preheat oven to 375°.

♣Use a salad shooter, and grate into a large bowl
1¹/₂ CUPS CARROTS (2)
1¹/₂ CUPS TART APPLES (1)
¹/₂ CUP PECANS
¹/₂ CUP CHOPPED DATES

♣Add and mix in
³/₄ CUP SHREDDED COCONUT
3 EGGS
³/₄ CUP + 2 TBS. LIGHT OIL
¹/₂ teasp. VANILLA

♣Add dry ingredients, and mix gently after each addition
2 CUPS WHOLE WHEAT PASTRY FLOUR
1¹/₄ CUP BROWN or TURBINADO SUGAR
1 teasp. BAKING SODA

1 teasp. BAKING POWDER
1 teasp. CINNAMON
1 teasp. NUTMEG

♣Spoon into lecithin-sprayed muffin tins or paper lined muffin cups, and bake for 18-20 minutes until a toothpick comes out clean. Cool.

Nutritional analysis: per serving; 240 calories; 3gm. protein; 29gm. carbohydrates; 3gm. fiber; 14gm. fats; 35mg. cholesterol; 30mg. calcium; 1mg. iron; 29mg. magnesium; 209mg. potassium; 47mg. sodium; 1mg. zinc.

867   LIGHTEST EVER POPOVERS

These taste decadent, but aren't. They make very showy little cups for your best gourmet efforts, and can be used with many different fillings, from vegetables to cheeses, to seafoods. You can also eat them hot and plain with a little butter or kefir cheese.
For 6 popovers: Preheat oven to 400°.

♣Butter 6 POPOVER CUPS or PYREX CUSTARD CUPS. Set them in a shallow pan in a <u>400∞. oven to heat while you make the batter.</u>

♣Beat with electric beaters until light and smooth
3 EGGS
1 CUP CALISTOGA SPARKLING WATER
1 CUP SIFTED UNBLEACHED FLOUR

2 TBS. MELTED BUTTER
¹/₂ teasp SEA SALT
¹/₂ teasp. FRUCTOSE

♣Turn into hot cups and bake for 60 minutes until brown and puffy. Remove, cool slightly, and cut a slit in the top to let out steam so the popovers won't get soggy. Cut off top and fill, or eat plain.

Nutritional analysis: per serving; 143 calories; 5gm. protein; 15gm. carbohydrates; 1gm. fiber; 6gm. fats; 117mg. cholesterol; 18mg. calcium; 1mg. iron; 7mg. magnesium; 52mg. potassium; 208mg. sodium; trace zinc.

868 GINGER CHEESECAKE

For 8 to 10 people: Preheat oven to 350°. Butter a 9" springform pan.

♣Beat the filling with a mixer until very smooth
16-OZ. NEUFCHATEL CHEESE
1/2 CUP + 2 TBS. TURBINADO SUGAR

1 teasp. VANILLA
4 EGGS

♣Make the gingerbread in a bowl. Mix
4 TBS. BUTTER
1/4 CUP MOLASSES
1/4 teasp. NUTMEG
1/2 CUP PACKED BROWN SUGAR
1 CUP WHOLE WHEAT FLOUR

1 teasp. CINNAMON
1 teasp. GROUND GINGER
PINCH CLOVES
1/4 teasp. SEA SALT
1 1/2 teasp. BAKING SODA

♣Drop half the gingerbread in dollops in one layer into the prepared pan. Drop in cheese mixture to fill spaces. Repeat. Swirl with a knife to marbelize top. Smooth over with rest of cheese filling. Bake in the middle of the oven for 50 minutes until top of cake begins to crack. Let cool in the oven with the door open. ♣Remove side of pan and serve.

Nutritional analysis: per serving; 327 calories; 6gm. protein; 35gm. carbos; 2gm. fiber; 18gm. fats; 130mg. cholesterol; 111mg. calcium; 3mg. iron; 44mg. magnesium; 367mg. potassium; 320mg. sodium; 1mg. zinc.

869   VERY BEST CARROT CAKE

This recipe was a daily treat from the Rainbow Kitchen. It is very versatile. Make it as a whole cake, or in muffin cups. Make it with grated carrots, or carrots and apples, or carrots and zucchini, or carrot pulp from the juicer.

For 12 servings: Preheat oven to 325°.

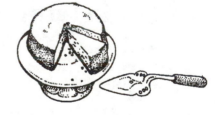

♣Mix the wet ingredients in the blender
2/3 CUP OIL
3/4 CUP HONEY
2 TBS. FRUCTOSE
2 EGGS
2 CUPS GRATED CARROTS, or 1 1/2 CUPS CARROTS and 1/2 CUP GRATED APPLE (1 small)

♣Mix the dry ingredients in a bowl
1 1/2 CUPS WHOLE WHEAT PASTRY FLOUR
1 teasp. BAKING SODA
1 1/2 teasp. BAKING POWDER
1 teasp. SEA SALT

1/2 teasp. ORANGE PEEL
1 teasp. CINNAMON
1/2 teasp. ALLSPICE
1/4 teasp. NUTMEG

♣Combine both mixtures together just to moisten, and turn into a greased loaf pan or 9 x 9" square pan. Bake for 1 hour til *just* firm. Or spoon into paper-lined muffin cups and bake for 35 minutes.

Nutritional analysis: per serving; 250 calories; 3gm. protein; 33gm. carbohydrates; 3gm. fiber; 13gm. fats; 35mg. cholesterol; 47mg. calcium; 1mg. iron; 26mg. magnesium; 256mg. potassium; 230mg. sodium; 1mg. zinc.

870   WALNUT RAISIN BAKLAVA PACKETS

Making baklava sounds long and intimidating, but it's really easy, and is a treat that's worth the trouble. This recipe substantially reduces the fat and sugar of traditional baklava, but it is still rich. One piece is usually enough.
For about 30 pieces: Preheat oven to 325°.

♣Thaw according to directions, and have ready <u>half of a package</u> of WHOLE WHEAT FILO PASTRY.

♣Have ready 1/2 STICK MELTED BUTTER and 3/4 CUP LIGHT CANOLA OIL in a warm saucepan.

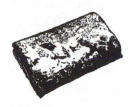

♣Make the filling in a bowl

1 1/2 CUPS CHOPPED WALNUTS	3/4 CUP RAISINS
3/4 CUP TURBINADO SUGAR	1/2 CUP FRUCTOSE
1 teasp. SWEET TOOTH BAKING SPICE	

♣Assemble the pastry packets on a cutting board.

♣Be sure to keep filo sheets covered with a moist towel as you work so they won't dry out.

♣Lay out 1 sheet and <u>lightly</u> brush with butter mix. Top with another sheet and brush. Spoon 1 TB. filling on the lower half of the sheet and make a packet, by folding both sides into the center, and rolling up from bottom to top. Brush with more butter mix and place with sides touching on a large 11 x 15" baking sheet until all sheets are used. You should have 30 packets. Bake for 20 to 25 minutes until golden. Remove and pour hot syrup over immediately to absorb into the pastry.

♣Make the syrup while pastry is baking. Bring to boil in a saucepan

2 CUPS WATER	1 CINNAMON STICK
1/2 CUP TURBINADO SUGAR	2 teasp. LEMON JUICE
1 1/2 CUPS ORANGE HONEY	1/4 teasp. NUTMEG
2 PIECES FRESH LEMON PEEL	1/4 teasp. ALLSPICE
2 PIECES FRESH ORANGE PEEL	

♣Cook for 10 minutes until syrupy. Remove cinnamon stick and peels, and pour over hot pastry.

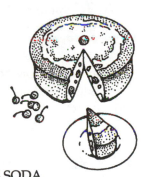

871   EASY, NO-SUGAR FRUIT CAKE

For 12 pieces: Preheat oven to 325°. Lecithin-spray a 9 x 9" baking pan.

♣Mix together in a large bowl

2 CUPS WH. WH. GOURMET FLOUR BLEND (pg. 647)	3 TBS. BUTTER
1/2 CUP HONEY	2 EGGS
1/2 CUP WHOLE PITTED DATES	1 1/2 teasp. BAKING SODA
1/2 CUP RAISINS	1 1/2 teasp. VANILLA
1/2 CUP SHREDDED COCONUT	2 TBS. MAPLE SYRUP
1/2 CUP PECAN HALVES	1 teasp. BAKING POWDER

♣Spoon into prepared pan, and bake for 45 to 50 minutes until firm and springy when pressed.

Nutritional analysis: per piece; 250 calories; 5gm. protein; 43gm. carbohydrates; 4gm. fiber; 8gm. fats; 43mg. cholesterol; 43mg. calcium; 1mg. iron; 42mg. magnesium; 311mg. potassium; 75mg. sodium; 1mg. zinc.

872 ZUCCHINI CAKE WITH PECAN FROSTING

For one 9 x 12" pan: Preheat oven to 350°.

♣Mix the dry ingredients
2 CUPS WHOLE WHEAT PASTRY FLOUR
1 teasp. BAKING SODA
1/2 teasp. SEA SALT
2 teasp. BAKING POWDER
3 teasp. CINNAMON
2 teasp. ORANGE PEEL
1/4 CUP FRUCTOSE

♣Blender blend the wet ingredients
3 EGGS
3/4 CUP + 2 TBS. OIL
3/4 CUP BROWN SUGAR
4 TBS. HONEY
2 TBS. MAPLE SYRUP
2 teasp. VANILLA

♣Combine the two ingredients together just to moisten, and stir in 1 CUP RAISINS and 1 CUP CHOPPED NUTS. Turn into a greased 9 x 12" pan and bake for 40 minutes until springy when pressed in the center.

♣Make the SOUTHERN PECAN FROSTING in the blender, and spread on the hot cake.
1 CUP CHOPPED PECANS
1/2 CUP MAPLE SUGAR GRANULES
5 TBS. MELTED BUTTER
2 TBS. PLAIN YOGURT
♣Run the cake under the broiler for 1 minute. Remove and let sit for 30 minutes to absorb topping.

Nutritional analysis for cake and frosting; per serving; 420 calories; 5gm. protein; 48gm. carbos; 4gm. fiber; 25gm. fats; 49mg. cholest.; 71mg. calcium; 2mg. iron; 51mg. mag.; 354mg. potass.; 108mg. sodium; 1mg. zinc.

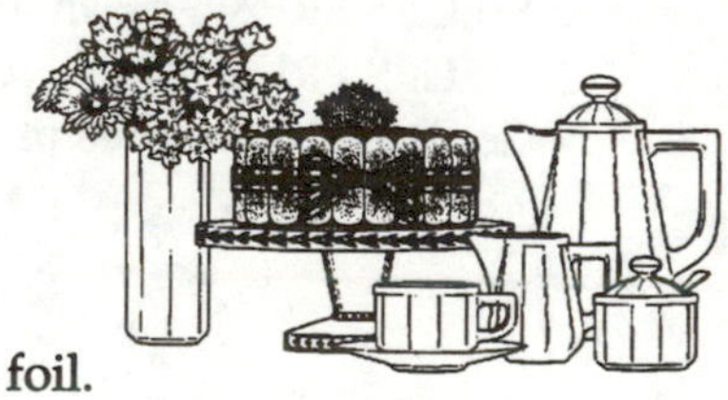

873 VICTORIAN FRUIT AND NUT CAKE

This is an everything cake, definitely in the opulent holiday spirit.

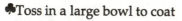

For 1 cake: Preheat oven to 325°. Butter a loaf pan. Line with foil, and butter the foil.

♣Toss in a large bowl to coat
1 LB. WHOLE PITTED DATES
3 TBS. WHOLE WHEAT PASTRY FLOUR
1/3 CUP CANDIED CHERRIES
21/2 CUPS WALNUT HALVES
♣Separate 2 EGGS. Put the whites in a beating bowl.

♣Beat til light and fluffy in another bowl
1/2 CUP WHOLE WHEAT PASTRY FLOUR
11/2 TBS. PLAIN YOGURT
1/2 CUP BROWN SUGAR
1 teasp. LEMON PEEL
1/2 teasp. ALMOND, RUM or BRANDY EXTRACT
4 TBS. BUTTER
2 teasp. VANILLA
11/2 teasp. BAKING POWDER
1 teasp. ORANGE PEEL
THE EGG YOLKS

♣Beat WHITES to stiff peaks, and fold into batter to lighten it. Pour over fruit mix to coat. Spoon into pan, mounding batter slightly. Cover with more buttered foil. Bake for 15 minutes until firm. Cool on wire rack. Wrap and store for several weeks before serving for the most concentrated flavor.

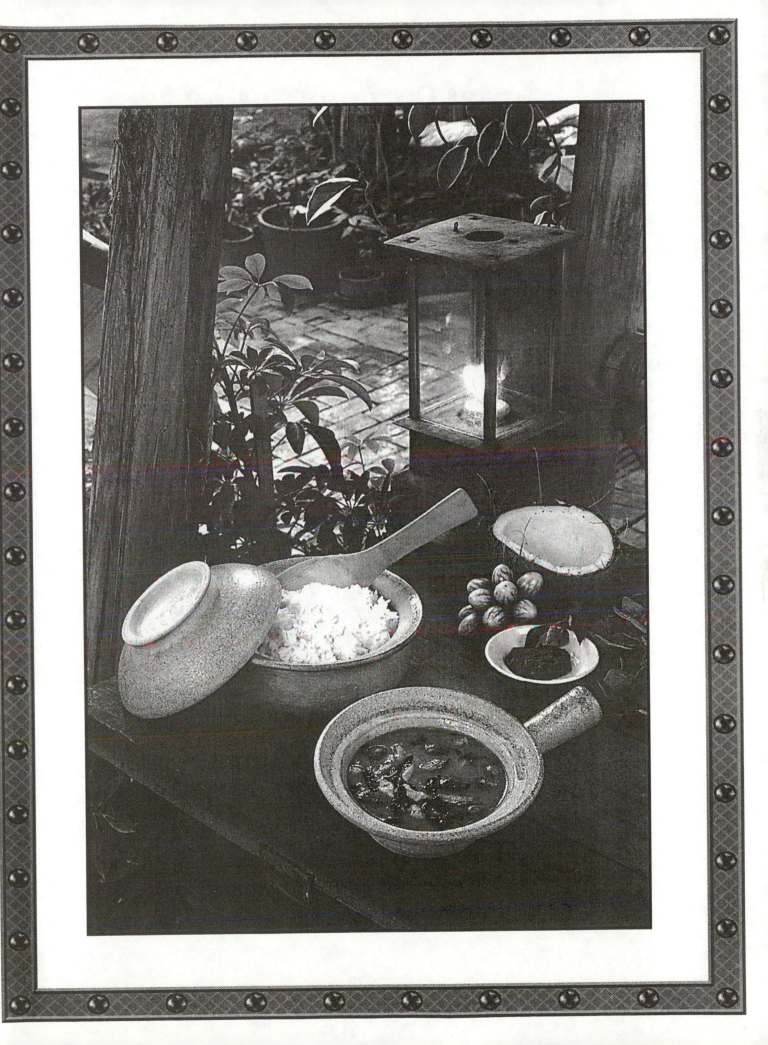

Great Outdoor Eating

There's something about eating out of doors. Maybe it's the sunshine, the fresh air, or the surrounding green. Our appetites and metabolisms increase to a healthy level. We breathe deeper, relax more, and somehow feel better about almost everything. When your ego needs a boost, have an outdoor barbeque. Since the Stone Age, foods have tasted great on the grill - and almost everything is better barbecued, from fruits to vegetables to tofu to grains. Make a barbecue a family affair. You won't have any trouble getting everybody to show up with bells on. Outdoor cooking is easy. Kids can help with everything.

This chapter offers some inspiration recipes, but don't worry, there's hardly any way to cook a bad meal out of doors. Enjoy!

❧FISH and SEAFOOD ON THE GRILL ❧TURKEY and CHICKEN ON THE GRILL and ON THE PICNIC TABLE ❧VEGETABLES, PIZZAS and GRAINS ON THE GRILL ❧GREAT GRILLING MARINADES ❧HEALTHY FINGER FOODS FOR PICNICS ❧

Remember to remove foods from the grill when they are golden, before they become charred, to avoid denaturing amino acids and DNA damage. Grill low-fat foods and discard any charred portions to avoid dangerous hydro-carbons.

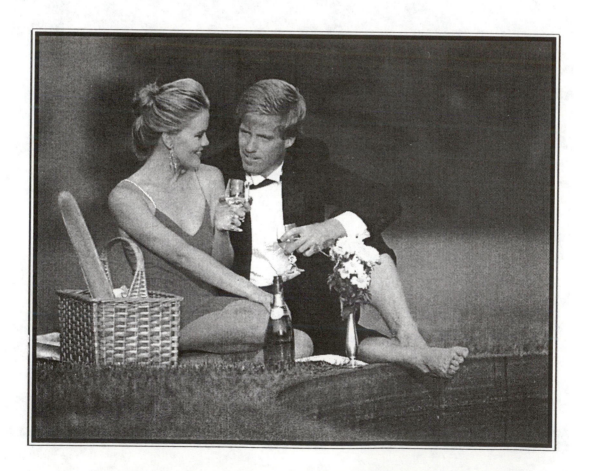

Fish & Seafood On The Grill

Fish and outside cooking just seem to go together, right from the old tradition of cooking your catch over a campfire 20 minutes after reeling it in. I used to wonder why grilling fish smelled so good outside, but not inside the house. I never found out the answer, but the recipes in this outdoor section are definitely a delicious way to eat fish.

874   SALMON WITH GINGER MUSHROOM STUFFING

For about 6 to 8 people:

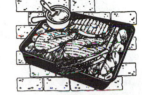

♣Use about a 3 to 4 LBS. SALMON, cleaned, rinsed and patted dry. Put in a shallow pan to marinate.
♣Make the marinade in the blender

1 CHOPPED JALAPEÑO CHILI
1-OZ. FRESH GINGER, peeled and chopped
3 SHALLOTS, chopped
3 to 4 CLOVES CHOPPED GARLIC

3 TBS. SHERRY
3 TBS. TAMARI
2 TBS. SESAME OIL
1 TB. LEMON JUICE

♣Pour over salmon, cover and chill for 1 hour.

♣Make the stuffing.
In a small skillet, sauté 1 CHOPPED ONION in 3 TBS. OIL until translucent. Add 12-OZ. MIXED MUSH-ROOMS (BUTTON, PORCINI, OYSTER, or SHIITAKE), 1 teasp. GINGER POWDER, 1 TB. TAMARI, and 2 TBS. marinade from the salmon.
♣Stir together to blend and spoon into chilled salmon cavities.
♣Grill on silver foil sheets folded up to make a lip. Cover and cook for about 1$^1/_4$ hours. Test for done-ness in one hour.

Nutritional analysis: per serving; 330 calories; 36gm. protein; 6gm. carbohydrates; 1gm. fiber; 17gm. fats; 93mg. cho-lesterol; 33mg. calcium; 2mg. iron; 61mg. magnesium; 1090mg. potassium; 167mg. sodium; 2mg. zinc.

875   GRILLED FRESH TUNA STEAKS WITH HERBS

For 4 people:

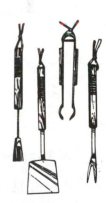

♣Use 4 FRESH YELLOW FIN AHI TUNA STEAKS, 1" THICK (about 1$^1/_2$ LBS.).

♣Make the marinade. Pour over swordfish, cover and marinate for 2 hours.
4 SAGE LEAVES, crushed
2 CLOVES GARLIC, minced
2 SPRIGS ROSEMARY, crushed
1/2 CUP OLIVE OIL

1/4 teasp. HERB SALT
1/4 teasp. LEMON PEPPER
1 TB. LEMON JUICE

♣Reserve marinade for the sauce.
♣Grill steaks for 6 to 8 minutes, turning once, until barely cooked. Keep warm while you make the sauce.
♣Mince herbs from the marinade. Put in a hot saucepan and add 1/2 CUP SLICED BLACK OLIVES.
♣Heat briefly until bubbly and add 4 TBS. CAPERS.
♣Pour over swordfish.

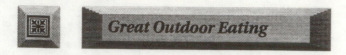
876   FAST FIRE SWORDFISH STEAKS

For 6 to 8 people: Heat the grill to hot. Brush the grill with oil.

♣Have ready 6 TO 8 rinsed SWORDFISH STEAKS (about 1$^1/_2$ lbs.)
♣Make the marinade in a large flat pan. Mix

$^1/_4$ CUP OLIVE OIL	1$^1/_2$ teasp. DRY MUSTARD
2 TBS. LEMON JUICE	1$^1/_2$ teasp. COARSE MUSTARD
1 teasp. LEMON/GARLIC SEASONING	1 teasp. DIJON MUSTARD
2 teasp. SHERRY	

♣Marinate fish covered for 1 hour. Place swordfish in the center of the hot oiled grill and cover. Cook for 7 minutes. Uncover, slide a spatula under the fish and rotate for cross grilling marks. Cover again and cook 8 minutes. Turn fish and repeat the process. Check for doneness by removing fish with spatula and pressing with your fingers. Fish will be firm when done. Cover and cook for 3 minutes more if not firm.
♣Remove and let rest for 5 minutes before slicing against the grain to serve.

877   SKEWERED SHRIMP WITH LEMON PESTO

For 32 skewers: Heat the grill to hot. Brush the grill with oil.

♣Have ready 32 LARGE PEELED SHRIMP. Thread onto wooden skewers, <u>into but not through the wide end of the shrimp</u>.
♣Make the pesto in the blender and pour into a large flat pan.

$^1/_4$ CUP OLIVE OIL	2 TBS. GRATED PARMESAN
2 TBS. FRESH GRATED LEMON PEEL	1 TB. PINE NUTS
1 teasp. GARLIC/LEMON SEASONING	1 teasp. FRUCTOSE

♣Roll skewered shrimp in the marinade. Cover and chill. Cook on the hot oiled grill for 5 to 6 minutes, basting often.

878   BARBECUED PRAWNS

I make these in an old skillet that we just heat right on the grill, or you can make a shallow "pan" out of several layers of foil folded up on the edges to form a lip, and let the prawns bubble in the sauce.

For 4 servings:

♣Heat 1 TB. BUTTER and 1 TB. OIL in a skillet. Add 1 CLOVE of MINCED GARLIC and let it bubble until aromatic. Add 16 to 20 PEELED PRAWNS and let them sizzle until they are just pink. Watch so that they don't overcook.
♣Add 2 minced green ONIONS, $^1/_4$ CUP TAMARI, $^1/_4$ HONEY KETCHUP and DASHES HOT PEPPER SAUCE. Let bubble just a minute to blend flavors.

Nutritional analysis: per serving; 176 calories; 24gm. protein; 8gm. carbohydrates; 1gm. fiber; 5gm. fats; 170mg. cholesterol; 68mg. calcium; 3mg. iron; 48mg. magnesium; 269mg. potassium; 300mg. sodium; 1mg. zinc.

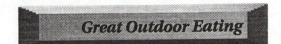

Kebabs are classic outdoor grill food. I have included 2 different marinades and 2 different skewer combinations. Each is enough for 6 people.

879   KEBABS # 1

♣For a mix of SCALLOPS, SHRIMP or PRAWNS, BROCCOLI FLORETS, RED BELL PEPPER CHUNKS, GREEN ONION PIECES and ORANGE SECTIONS.
♣Make the **PEPPER MARINADE:** Mix together until well blended

1 to 2 teasp. FRESH CRACKED BLACK PEPPER

1/4 CUP OIL

2 TBS. TARRAGON VINEGAR

1 teasp. HONEY MUSTARD

1/2 teasp. SEA SALT

1 TB. WHITE WINE

♣Pour over all kebab ingredients and marinate for 1 hour. Thread on skewers and grill.

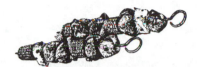

880   KEBABS # 2

♣For a mix of SHRIMP and SCALLOPS, WHOLE CHERRY TOMATOES, GREEN PEPPER CHUNKS, FRESH PINEAPPLE CUBES and RED ONION CHUNKS.

♣Make the **SHERRY MARINADE:** Mix all together until well blended

1/2 CUP DRY SHERRY

2 TBS. TOASTED SESAME OIL

1 CLOVE MINCED GARLIC

1 TB. SESAME SEEDS

1/4 teasp. BLACK PEPPER

2 teasp. FRESH GRATED GINGER

♣Marinate all kebab ingredients for 1 hour. Thread on skewers and grill.

Nutritional analysis: per serving; 217 calories; 22gm. protein; 15gm. carbohydrate; 2gm. fiber; 6gm. fats; 101mg. cholesterol; 61mg. calcium; 2mg. iron; 75mg. magnesium; 522mg. potassium; 181mg. sodium; 1mg. zinc.

881   MANGO SCALLOP & SHRIMP KEBABS

For 4 people: Preheat grill and brush with oil.

♣Rinse 3/4 LB. LARGE FRESH SCALLOPS and PEEL 1/2 LB. LARGE PRAWNS. Lay in a shallow baking pan and marinate in 2 TBS. OLIVE OIL and 3 TBS. LIME JUICE for one hour.
♣Cut 1 LARGE PEELED MANGO into 1" chunks.

♣Bring salted water to a boil and blanch 24 TRIMMED SNOW PEAS until color changes to bright green.
♣Drain and rinse in cold water to set color.
♣Thread snow peas, seafood and mango chunks onto skewers. Grill 4 " from heat until seafood is opaque, about 1 1/2 minutes on each side, basting frequently.
♣Serve with a small dish of the lime oil for dipping.

Nutritional analysis: per serving; 208 calories; 27gm. protein; 13gm. carbohydrates; 2gm. fiber; 5gm. fats; 114mg. cholesterol; 65mg. calcium; 3mg. iron; 79mg. magnesium; 506mg. potassium; 223mg. sodium; 2mg. zinc.

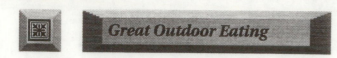

882   SWEET & SOUR PRAWNS

For 6 servings: Preheat grill and brush with oil.

♣Leave tail on for a handle. Slit 1¹/₂ LBS. down the back, spread open and marinate in 2 TBS. DIJON MUSTARD, 2 TBS. RICE VINEGAR, 2 TBS. OIL, and 2 TBS. HONEY.
♣Grill until just pink, squeezing with lime juice frequently while grilling.

✽

Ahi is yellow fin tuna from Hawaiian waters. The steaks are meaty and delicious with very little fat.

883   FRESH AHI WITH ROSEMARY & THYME

For 4 servings: Preheat grill and brush with oil.

♣Marinate 1 LB. THICK FRESH AHI STEAKS for 1 hour in
2 TB. LEMON JUICE
2 teasp. FRESH THYME LEAVES
¹/₂ teasp. SESAME SALT
2 teasp. ROSEMARY SPRIGS
3 TBS. OLIVE OIL
¹/₂ teasp. CRACKED PEPPER
♣Grill AHI for 4 minutes on each side until just pink in the center, squeezing with lemon juice during grilling. Garnish with LEMON QUARTERS and ROSEMARY SPRIGS.

✽

884   GRILLED AHI WITH SHIITAKE MUSHROOMS

For 4 servings: Preheat grill and brush with oil.

♣Roast 6 to 8 PEELED SHALLOTS in a 300∞ oven for 30 minutes until soft. Mash in a large pan. Add ¹/₂ CUP LIGHT MAYONNAISE, 1 TB. DIJON MUSTARD, 1 teasp. LEMON JUICE, ¹/₂ teasp. SESAME SEED, and ¹/₂ teasp. LEMON PEPPER. Spread on toasted French bread slices.

♣Brush 1 LB. FRESH THICK AHI STEAKS with OLIVE OIL. Soak dried SHIITAKE MUSHROOMS in water until soft, and remove woody stems. Or use fresh or canned OYSTER MUSHROOMS. Brush with OLIVE OIL.
♣Grill AHI for 4 minutes on each side until just pink in the center, squeezing with lemon juice during grilling. Arrange mushrooms on foil folded up to make a lip, and cook for 5 to 7 minutes.
♣Divide fish and mushrooms on toast. Top with TART LETTUCE LEAVES and serve open face.

✽

885   ISLAND AHI SEVICHE
We first had this on a remote south pacific island of 500 residents, where the people fish every day for their evening meal. The citrus cold cooks the fish without drying it. There is no way to describe the unusual taste. Low calories, low-fat, and solid delicious protein.

♣Cut very fresh yellow fin Ahi or Mahi Mahi in 1" chunks. Cover in LIME JUICE, 1 teasp. FRESH CHOPPED GINGER and 1 teasp. PEPPERCORNS. Let sit for 24 hours.

✽

886   SEAFOOD MEAL-IN-A-POUCH ON THE GRILL

For 4 people: Preheat grill to hot.

♣Tear off and have ready 4 <u>two-foot long</u> sheets of heavy foil. Lay out and place some of each of the following ingredients in the center of each:

4 THIN-SLICED SHALLOTS
1 LARGE TOMATO in eight slices
4 TBS. BUTTER
16 to 20 BAY SCALLOPS

1 teasp. SEA SALT
1/2 CUP WHITE WINE
1/4 teasp. CRACKED PEPPER
1 LEMON in eight wedges

♣Bring long ends of the foil together and roll down tightly over ingredients. Roll up short ends and roll up to form packets. Place on the grill and steam for 10 minutes. Turn over and cook for 15 more minutes.
♣Empty each packet into an individual bowl to serve.

Nutritional analysis: per serving; 240 calories; 20gm. protein; 10gm. carbohydrates; 1gm. fiber; 12gm. fats; 68mg. cholesterol; 51mg. calcium; 1mg. iron; 76mg. magnesium; 552mg. potassium; 324mg. sodium; 1mg. zinc.

887   MAHI MAHI BURGERS

For 6 burgers: Preheat the grill and brush with oil.

♣Have ready 1 1/2 LBS. MAHI MAHI in 6 pieces. Grill on silver foil sheets folded up to make a lip.
♣Mix the sauce

1/2 CUP LIGHT MAYONNAISE
1/4 CUP RED BELL PEPPER
1 TB. LEMON JUICE
1 TB. MINCED PARSLEY

2 TBS. SWEET RELISH
1 TB. DRAINED CAPERS
1/2 teasp. LEMON PEPPER
5 to 8 DROPS LIQUID SMOKE

♣Grill on silver foil sheets folded up to make a lip. Broil burgers 3" from heat for 5 minutes, turning once. Check frequently.
♣Toast split burger buns on the grill while fish is cooking. Spread with sauce. Top with lettuce and tomato slices. Fill each with a fish piece and top with a bun half.

888   GINGER GRILL SWORDFISH

For 4 people: Preheat and oil grill.

♣Have ready 4 RINSED SWORDFISH STEAKS, about 1" thick. Marinate for 1 hour in

2/3 CUP TAMARI
1/4 CUP SHERRY 1
1 DICED CARROT
1 teasp. GARLIC/LEMON SEASONING

1 TB. MINCED BELL PEPPER
1/2 teasp. MINCED FRESH GINGER
2 CHOPPED SCALLIONS
1 teasp. LEMON PEEL

♣Brush fish with oil and grill 4" from heat turning once, and basting until opaque, about 5 minutes.

Turkey & Chicken On The Grill

A whole turkey or chicken becomes an indescribable gourmet delight when it's roasted out doors over a charcoal fire. With just a little attention and a few instructions, your barbecued poultry can be perfect.

◆Pick your favorite marinade or basting sauce, and cover the whole bird. Place in a large plastic bag and chill in the fridge for 4 hours or overnight. Turn bag several times to marinate well.

◆On the firegrate in a covered barbecue, ignite 50 charcoal briquets. When coals are covered with grey ash, bank them equally on opposite sides of the grate; put a drip pan in the middle. Add 10 briquets to the coals. Add 10 more every 30 minutes while the bird is roasting to maintain heat. Place grill 6" above coals. Place turkey or chicken breast-side down with wings akimbo, directly above the drip pan.

◆Reserve marinade for basting. Cover barbecue, open dampers, and roast for 45 minutes. Turn bird breast up and continue to cook until meat at bone in thickest part of breast registers 160°. Baste bird often. Set bird on a platter, drape loosely with foil, and let stand for 20 minutes before carving.

889   STUFFED TURKEY BURGER

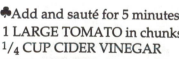

For 8 wedges:

♣Mix the burger
1¼ CUP WHOLE GRAIN or CORN BREAD STUFFING MIX
1 SMALL CAN DRAINED MUSHROOM PIECES or ⅓ CUP CHOPPED FRESH
1 teasp. LIQUID SMOKE or 1 TB. HICKORY SAUCE
¼ CUP CHOPPED GREEN ONION   1 EGG
¼ CUP CHOPPED ALMONDS   2 TBS. BUTTER
⅓ CUP CHICKEN BROTH   1 teasp. LEMON JUICE
¼ CUP CHOPPED FRESH PARSLEY

♣Mix 2 LBS. GROUND TURKEY with 1½ teasp. SEA SALT. Divide in half, and pat into two 8" circles on waxed paper. Spoon stuffing mix onto 1 circle. Top with other circle and seal the edges.
♣Cook on foil or in a grill basket on an outside grill for 10 to 15 minutes.
♣Serve with **GOURMET BARBECUE SAUCE**.

Nutritional analysis: per serving; 319 calories; 37gm. protein; 14gm. carbohydrates; 1gm. fiber; 12gm. fats; 120mg. cholesterol; 73mg. calcium; 3mg. iron; 51mg. magnesium; 459mg. potassium; 344mg. sodium; 4mg. zinc.

GOURMET BARBECUE SAUCE

♣Sauté in a saucepan until very fragrant   ♣Add and sauté for 5 minutes
2 TBS. OIL   1 LARGE TOMATO in chunks
1 SLICED ONION   ¼ CUP CIDER VINEGAR
½ RED BELL PEPPER in chunks   3 TBS. HONEY
½ teasp. HOT PEPPER SAUCE
♣Remove from heat, cool slightly and put the sauce in the blender with 6 RIPE ROMA OR PLUM TOMA-TOES. Whirl briefly so sauce is still chunky.

890   GRILLED TURKEY TENDERLOIN IN ROMAINE WRAPS

For 4 people: Preheat and oil the grill.

♣Have ready 1 LB. BONED, SKINNED TURKEY TENDERLOIN cut in 4 equal pieces.
♣Have ready 4 LARGE THIN SLICES LOX (smoked salmon).
♣Blender blend the dressing

1/3 CUP OLIVE OIL	1 TB. MINCED PARSLEY
1/4 CUP TARRAGON VINEGAR	3/4 teasp. GROUND SAGE
2 TBS. MINCED GREEN ONION	3/4 teasp. THYME

♣Plunge 4 LARGE ROMAINE LETTUCE LEAVES in boiling water to wilt. Wrap each turkey piece in lox, then in the romaine leaf. Grill 4 to 6" above coals for 20 to 25 minutes. Cut in 1" slices and arrange on plates cut side up. Season with SEA SALT and CRACKED PEPPER and top with dressing.

891   CHICKEN OR TURKEY SALAD FOR A PICNIC CROWD

Use some of that wonderful leftover barbecued turkey for this spicy, crowd pleasing salad.
For 25 to 30 people:

♣Have ready 8 LBS. SKINLESS, BONELESS CHICKEN or TURKEY BREAST, cooked and diced.
♣Pan toast 3/4 CUP YELLOW MUSTARD SEEDS in 1/4 CUP OLIVE OIL over medium heat. Cover pan, and shake until seeds pop, about 1 to 2 minutes.
♣Remove from heat and shake again until all are popped and fragrant.
♣Combine the sauce ingredients

2 CUPS LIGHT MAYONNAISE	THE POPPED MUSTARD SEEDS
1/4 CUP SWEET/HOT MUSTARD	1/2 CUP LEMON JUICE
1/2 CUP SHARP DIJON MUSTARD	1 teasp. LEMON PEPPER

♣

Place the diced poultry in a large bowl and toss with 12 STALKS DICED CELERY and the triple mustard sauce. Spoon into a serving bowl lined with lettuce leaves.

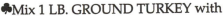

892   MEXICAN TURKEY BURGERS ON THE GRILL

For 6 burgers: Preheat and oil the grill.

♣Mix 1 LB. GROUND TURKEY with

2 TBS. CORNMEAL	2 teasp. CHILI POWDER
1 TB. LIME JUICE	1 EGG
1 JALAPEÑO PEPPER, seeded and minced	1/4 teasp. PEPPER
2 teasp. CUMIN POWDER	

♣Form into patties, and grill until no longer pink. Serve on grilled buns with salsa and a squeeze of lime.

Vegetables, Pizzas & Grains On The Grill

The sweet flavors of fresh garden vegetables are intensified on the grill.
The idea is to keep the subtle taste of the vegetable and add the smoky taste of the barbecue.
Aromatic wood chips, herb stems and leaves, or herb teas can be sprinkled over the hot coals
to impart unique, complex flavors. To use vegetable pieces larger than 1/4" thick, such as broccoli, cauliflower,
and potato chunks, blanch them first in boiling water, then plunge them into cold water to stop cooking,
before bringing them to the grill. Sliced vegetables such as onions, bell pepper, tomatoes or eggplant,
do not need to be pre-cooked. Used closed, wire-mesh baskets or flat skewers for the best results with vegetables.

893   BASIC GRILLED VEGGIES

Good vegetables for this basic recipe include yams, broccoli, cauliflower, fennel, leeks and zucchini.
For 2 to 4 people: Preheat the charcoal grill and brush with oil.

♣Have ready 3 SMALL SUMMER SQUASH, sliced lengthwise in quarters. Blanch if necessary in boiling water for a few minutes, 12 FRESH ASPARAGUS SPEARS, trimmed, 1 RED BELL and 1 GREEN ot YEL-LOW BELL PEPPER, sliced lengthwise into eight slices each, and 1 RED ONION, sliced in 1/4" rounds.
♣Brush all vegetables lightly with olive oil, place in a closed wire-mesh basket and grill to dark golden brown. Divide on plates and pass TAMARI SAUCE and LEMON JUICE.

♣Serve with this easy no-cook **SWEET & SAVORY SAUCE:**
♣Mix togehter in a bowl
1¹/₂ CUPS THICK TOMATO SAUCE   1 TB. OLIVE OIL
3 TBS. HONEY   2 TBS. TAMARI
1 TB. MOLASSES   2 TBS. MUSTARD
and 1 teasp. EACH: PAPRIKA, CHILI POWDER, GARLIC POWDER, OREGANO, and BASIL.

894   GRILLED ORIENTAL VEGETABLES WITH SESAME SAUCE

For 4 people: Preheat the charcoal grill and brush with oil.

♣Mix the grilling marinade
¹/₂ CUP MIRIN or SHERRY   1 TB. TOASTED SESAME OIL
2 TBS. TAMARI   2 teasp. MAPLE SYRUP
♣Marinate the following vegetables for 2 hours
8 SLICED GREEN ONIONS   8 DRY SHIITAKE MUSHROOMS
4 PEELED, SLICED ORIENTAL EGGPLANT 4 SLICED CROOKNECK SQUASH
♣Grill and baste for 10 to 15 minutes until vegetables are tender.

♣Whirl the **SESAME SAUCE** in the blender until smooth
¹/₂ CUP TOASTED SESAME SEEDS   2 TBS. LEMON JUICE
3 TBS. OLIVE OIL   2 TBS. MINCED GINGER
¹/₄ CUP WATER   1 TB. FRUCTOSE
¹/₄ TEASP. GARLIC POWDER   PINCH PAPRIKA

895   HERB ROASTED POTATO FANS

For 8 people: Preheat and oil grill.

♣Heat together in a sauce pan for 3 minutes
6 TBS. BUTTER   1/2 teasp. PEPPER
1 1/2 teasp. GARLIC SALT   1/2 teasp. BASIL
4 teasp. MINCED PARSLEY   1 teasp. OREGANO
♣Make deep diagonal cuts in 8 WASHED POTATOES to within 3/4" of the bottom. Place in foil jackets with the top left open to hasten cooking. Roast over the coals until tender, basting frequently with the herb butter. Test for doneness after 25 minutes. Top with PARMESAN CHEESE and serve hot.

896   GRILLED ONION & RADICCHIO

A favorite dish that shows off the essence of grilled vegetables.

For 4 people: Preheat and oil grill.

♣Carefully remove peel from 4 NAVEL ORANGES. Squeeze out as much juice as possible into a small bowl. Set aside orange segments.
♣Mix the small amount of juice with 4 teasp. SHERRY, 2 teasp. OLIVE OIL, 1/2 teasp. SEA SALT and 1/2 teasp. PEPPER. Toss half with 1 LARGE HEAD SEPARATED RADICCHIO LEAVES. Toss half with the orange segments and arrange them on a serving platter.
♣Brush slices of 1 LARGE RED ONION with 1 teasp. OLIVE OIL, and sprinkle with SEA SALT and PEPPER. Roast about 4" from coals until soft and just beginning to blacken. Arrange onion on serving platter.
♣Grill radicchio leaves from 2 to 4 minutes until softened, just beginning to brown, and fragrant. Arrange on platter with the rest and serve hot.

Nutritional analysis: per serving; 117 calories; 2gm. protein; 21gm. carbohydrates; 4gm. fiber; 3gm. fats; 0 cholesterol; 72mg. calcium; 1mg. iron; 21mg. magnesium; 356mg. potassium; 269mg. sodium; trace zinc.

Pizza on the grill is deliciously special, and a totally different experience from the oven-baked variety. Here are three to start you off.

897   GRILLED TOMATO & MOZARRELLA PIZZA

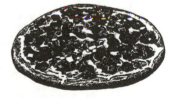

For 2 big pizzas: Preheat and oil grill.

♣Have ready 2 LARGE WHOLE WHEAT CHAPATIS. Top each with
CRUMBLED FETA CHEESE   DICED PLUM TOMATOES
FRESH CHOPPED BASIL LEAVES   SLICED BLACK OLIVES
STRIPS OF BELL PEPPER   PINCHES ITALIAN HERBS
DOLLOPS of TOMATO SAUCE   TOASTED WALNUT PIECES
♣Cover and cook for 6 to 8 minutes until heated through and cheese is melted. Watch carefully so that the bottom doesn't burn.

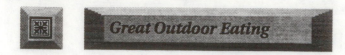

898   PIZZA WITH SHRIMP & SUN-DRIED TOMATOES

Enough for 2 large pizzas: Preheat the grill to hot.

♣Place ready made pizza dough on foil and freeze for 10 minutes. Pinch up rims to be thicker than middle, so pizzas can hold sauce. Brush each with 1¹/₂ teasp. CHILI OIL.
♣Oven roast 10 LARGE CHOPPED SHALLOTS AND 1 RED ONION in slices until aromatic. Divide between pizzas. Distribute ¹/₂ LB. TINY SHRIMP between pizzas.
♣Sprinkle on ¹/₄ CUP FRESH MINCED BASIL. Cover *each* with ¹/₂ CUP GRATED FONTINA CHEESE, and 1 CUP CHUNKED LOW-FAT MOZARRELLA CHEESE.
♣Top with 12 SUN DRIED, OIL-PACKED TOMATOES in slivers.
♣Cover and cook for 6 to 8 minutes until heated through and cheese is melted. Watch carefully so that the bottom doesn't burn.

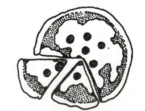

899   GRILLED GOURMET PIZZA

For 1 large pizza:

♣Place ready made pizza dough on foil and freeze for 10 minutes. Then invert on the hot grill. Peel off foil and grill for 3 minutes until bottom is light brown.
♣Make the simple tomato sauce in the blender. Puree a few oil-packed dried tomatoes with a little garlic powder and enough oil from the jar to make a smooth paste. Make just enough to paint on the grilled side of the crust.
♣Arrange SLICED MOZZARELLA, SLICED RED ONION, SLICED BLACK OLIVES AND CHERRY TOMATO HALVES on top of the sauce. Sprinkle with GRATED ROMANO or PROVOLONE CHEESE and return to the grill. Cover and cook for 6 to 8 minutes until heated through and cheese is melted. Watch carefully so that the bottom doesn't burn.

Nutritional analysis: per slice; 238 calories; 13gm. protein; 17gm. carbohydrates; 3gm. fiber; 14gm. fats; 29mg. cholesterol; 310mg. calcium; 1mg. iron; 44mg. magnesium; 288mg. potassium; 280mg. sodium; 2mg. zinc.

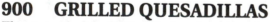

900   GRILLED QUESADILLAS
The same principle, for the Mexican lover in you.

For 4 flour tortillas: Preheat grill to hot and brush with oil.

♣Make the CHILI SAUCE. Mix ¹/₄ CUP LIGHT MAYONNAISE, 2 teasp. RED WINE VINEGAR, 1 teasp. CHILI POWDER, ¹/₂ teasp. SESAME SALT and ¹/₄ teasp. CUMIN POWDER.
♣Spread each tortilla with some of the sauce and top with
CHOPPED TOMATO SLIVERS   SHREDDED JACK CHEESE
CHOPPED RED ONION   CHOPPED FRESH CILANTRO
♣Grill, covered on foil until cheese melts and veggies are fragrant. Fold in half and grill for 1 minute.

Great Grilling Marinades

These sauces and marinades are robust and tangy. They lend themselves well to any foods you want to grill.

901 HERB & SPICE

This is excellent for very moist, tender poultry.
For 2 cups:

1/2 CUP TAMARI
1/2 CUP SHERRY
1/2 CUP CHICKEN BROTH
1/4 CUP LEMON JUICE
1/2 teasp. LEMON/GARLIC SEASONING

3/4 teasp. GROUND GINGER
1/2 teasp. PEPPER
1/4 teasp. NUTMEG
1/4 teasp. POULTRY SEASONING
1/4 teasp. ROSEMARY

Nutritional analysis: per 1 oz. serving; 17 calories; 1gm. protein; 2gm. carbohydrate; trace fiber; trace fats; 0 cholesterol; 6mg. calcium; trace iron; 5mg. magnesium; 36mg. potassium; 96mg. sodium; trace zinc.

902 SWEET WINE BUTTER

This marinade is particularly good for thick fish steaks such as salmon.
For 1 cup:

♣Combine and heat briefly in a saucepan
1/2 CUP GEWERTZTRAMINER or SAUTERNE
1 MINCED SHALLOT
2 TBS. BUTTER

1/2 teasp. CHAMPAGNE VINEGAR
2 TBS. MINCED FRESH HERBS
1/4 teasp. LEMON PEPPER

♣Add and stir until glossy 1/8 teasp. ARROWROOT POWDER mixed in 1 teasp. WATER

903 TROPICAL FRUIT GRILLING SAUCE for CHICKEN

Enough for 8 people:

♣Toss together
1 CUP FRESH PINEAPPLE CUBES
4 PEACHES or NECTARINES in cubes
1 PEELED PAPAYA in cubes
2 TBS. LEMON JUICE
6 TBS. CHAMPAGNE VINEGAR

2 DICED PEELED TOMATOES
1 BU. CHOPPED SCALLIONS
1 TB. CHOPPED JALAPEÑOS
3/4 CUP OLIVE OIL
1 TB. HONEY

Nutritional analysis: per serving; 234 calories; 1gm. protein; 17gm. carbohydrate; 3gm. fiber; 21gm. fats; 0 cholesterol; 24mg. caicium; 1mg. iron; 16mg. magnesium; 339mg. potassium; 6mg. sodium; trace zinc.

Healthy Finger Foods For Picnics

You can put these tasty snacks together quickly whenever the mood for a picnic strikes.
They hold and keep well, and are sized for passing around. Just make'em and take'em.

904   SALMON STUFFED EGGS

For 20 halves:

♣Hard boil 10 EGGS. Scoop out yolks into a bowl, and mix with ONE 7-OZ. CAN SALMON (or leftover cooked salmon), 6 TBS. TOMATO SAUCE, 2 TBS. MINCED PARSLEY, 1/2 teasp. SESAME SALT, and 1/2 teasp. LEMON PEPPER. Stuff whites, cover and chill.

Nutritional analysis: per stuffed egg; 53 calories; 5gm. protein; 1gm. carbohydrate; trace fiber; 3gm. fats; 110mg. cholesterol; 15mg. calcium; trace iron; 6mg. magnesium; 99mg. potassium; 56mg. sodium; trace zinc.

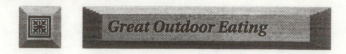

905   CHEESE FILLED APRICOT HALVES

For 32 halves:

♣Toast 32 PECAN or WALNUT HALVES in the oven until fragrant. Remove and cool.

♣Blender blend the filling
3-OZ. NEUFCHATEL CHEESE   1 1/2 teasp. WHITE PEPPER
5-OZ. BRIE CHEESE   1/4 teasp. NUTMEG
♣Fill 32 DRIED APRICOT HALVES. Press a nut half on top of each.
♣Place 3 to 4 TBS. FRESH MINCED MINT on a dish. Press apricots cheese side down into mint to coat. Cover and chill.

906   CHEESE & HERB MUFFINS

For 12 muffins: Preheat oven to 375°.

♣Sauté 1/4 CUP MINCED ONION and 1/2 CUP MINCED BELL PEPPER in 1 TB. OIL until limp. Mix together with
3/4 CUP GRATED CHEDDAR   2 TBS. OIL
1 1/2 CUPS WHOLE WHEAT PASTRY FLOUR 2 TBS. HONEY
1/2 CUP CORNMEAL   1 TB. DIJON MUSTARD
1/2 CUP PLAIN YOGURT   2 teasp. BAKING POWDER
1/2 CUP WATER   1/2 teasp. THYME
2 EGGS   1/2 teasp. TARRAGON
1/2 teasp. SEA SALT   PINCH WHITE PEPPER
♣Spoon into paper-lined muffin cups and bake until well browned, about 25 to 30 minutes.

907 GOURMET BLACK BEAN PESTO

For 4 cups:

♣Combine 1²/₃ CUPS DRY BLACK BEANS in a pot with 6 CUPS CHICKEN BROTH and 1¹/₂ teasp. CUMIN POWDER. Bring to a boil. Cover and simmer until tender, about 2 hours. Drain. Mash 1 cup of the beans and mix it with the rest of the whole beans. Set aside.
♣Mince ONE JAR ROASTED RED PEPPERS rinsed and patted dry. Set aside.
♣Have ready 4 OZ. CRUMBLED FETA CHEESE.
♣Make the CILANTRO PESTO in the blender

3 CUPS PACKED FRESH CILANTRO LEAVES   4 teasp. OLIVE OIL
1 teasp. GARLIC/LEMON SEASONING   1/3 CUP TOASTED PINE NUTS
♣Assemble the pesto layers. Line a loaf pan with plastic wrap, with lots of excess drape over the sides.
♣Spoon in 1/3 of the bean mix. Press down and smooth. Top with cilantro pesto. Top with all but 2 TBS. roasted peppers. Top with feta cheese. Top cheese with remaining beans. Press down and smooth. Fold over the draped plastic wrap and chill until firm.
♣Invert on a plate or shallow dish. Top with the reserved minced peppers and serve with rye toasts.

908 ZUCCHINI BISCUIT SQUARES

For 48 squares: Preheat oven to 350°.

♣Mix all ingredients together and spread in a lecithin-sprayed 9 x 13" baking pan.

3 CUPS GRATED ZUCCHINI   1/2 teasp. GARLIC SALT
1 CUP WHOLE GRAIN BISCUIT MIX   1/2 teasp. OREGANO
1/3 CUP CHOPPED ONION   1/2 teasp. BASIL
1/2 CUP GRATED PARMESAN   1/2 CUP OIL
2 teasp. CHOPPED PARSLEY   4 EGGS
♣Bake for 45 minutes until brown. Cool and cut in squares.

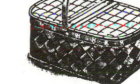

909 TINY CHICKEN ALMOND PITA SANDWICHES

For 24 pita halves: Preheat oven to 400°.

♣Have ready 12 APPETIZER SIZE SESAME PITA BREADS, split in half. Warm slightly in the oven.
♣Have ready 4 CHICKEN BREAST HALVES, cooked and diced.
♣Mix the filling in a bowl and set aside to blend flavors

1 CUP ALMOND BUTTER   1 TB. WHITE WINE VINEGAR
3 TBS. SOY BACON BITS   1 TB. SWEET HOT MUSTARD
2 teasp. GARLIC/LEMON SEASONING 1 CUP WATER
3 TBS. TAMARI   1/4 teasp. HOT PEPPER SAUCE
♣Stuff pitas with bits of THIN SLICED RED ONIONS, ALFALFA SPROUTS, TOMATO SLIVERS, SHREDDED LETTUCE, and CHICKEN. Stand upright in a shallow dish with sides touching. Spoon on sauce. Cover and chill to set stuffing before transporting.

*L*aughter
is the most beautiful
and
beneficial therapy
God ever granted humanity.

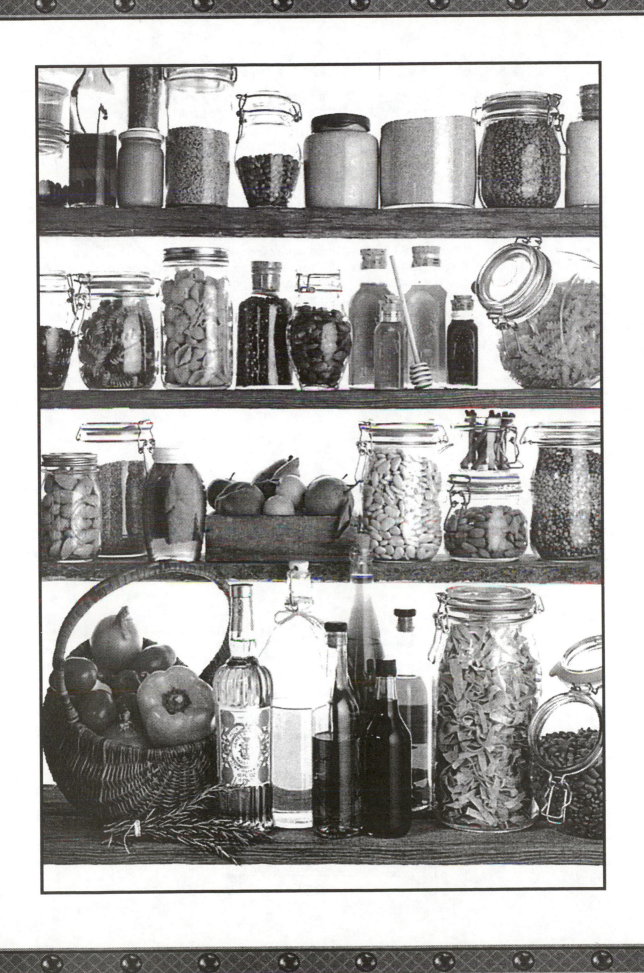

Making Your Own Salts, Seasonings, & Cooking Mixes

The seasoning of a recipe really defines its character. When we remember a delicious dish from childhood or a foreign country, we remember the *flavor* instead of the contents.
Blending your own salts, seasonings, condiments and stocks assures you of the highest quality ingredients, tailored to your healthy diet, with no "hidden" additives.

In the past generation, because of our super-busy lives, restaurant food habit, and processed convenience foods that must have a long shelf life, Americans have generally consumed too much salt for good body balance. We all know that excessive salt causes heart problems, high blood pressure and hypertension. Circulation is restricted, excess water is retained, migraines occur. A salt-free diet is very desirable for someone who has these problems in order to normalize body fluid salinity.
Once these fluids are back in balance, some salts are needed for intesinal tone, strong blood, and healthy glands and organs. *Low salt,* not *no salt,* is best for a permanent diet.

Good salts can be obtained through foods that have enzyme and alkalizing properties which make the salts usable and absorbable. These foods include tamari, shoyu, misos, umeboshi plums, sauerkraut and other fermented foods. Herbal salts and seasonings can play a very healthy part in an ongoing balanced diet.

Most of the combinations in this section come from the Rainbow Kitchen restaurant. They are all easy, food <u>enhancing</u> rather than overpowering blends.

Use them as they are here, or experiment and create your own, starting with these recipes as a basis. There is a great variety and they will definitely make a difference to your cooking.

❧SEASONING SALTS and SPICE BLENDS ❧CUSTOM FLOUR and GRAIN MIXES ❧RELISHES and CONDIMENTS ❧SOUP STOCKS and BROTH POWDERS ❧PESTOS and BUTTERS ❧VINEGARS ❧

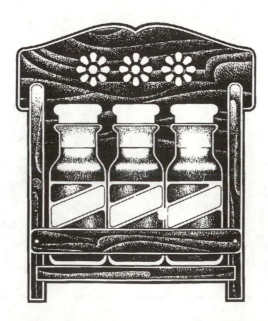

Seasoning Salts & Spice Blends

The recipe amounts given here are small enough for a container that you can handle easily in the kitchen, but large enough so that you don't have to make them up very often.

LEMON PEPPER

This mixture is one of the first and best we have made. There is a noticeable difference in taste between this and other lemon pepper you may have used. When our staff has been too busy to make this up for the Country Store, and we buy a stop-gap pound or two from another company, customers complain immediately. The secret is in the lemon oil. Just use a few drops from a small bottle of essential pharmaceutical grade lemon oil. It is inexpensive and well worth the investment.

1-OZ. SEA SALT
2½ OZ. BLACK COARSE GRIND PEPPER
½ teasp. GARLIC POWDER
2 teasp. DRY PARSLEY FLAKES
DROPS of LEMON OIL to taste

2 teasp. LEMON PEEL POWDER
2 TBS. SESAME SEEDS
½ teasp. ONION POWDER
½ teasp. FRUCTOSE
2 TBS. TVP or SOY GRITS

♣Whirl all ingredients in the blender <u>briefly</u> for consistency and flavor. Store tightly covered.

ZEST SEASONING SALT

This is a fairly bold salt with a slight smoky bacon flavor. Very good in soups, with hearty entrees or potatoes.

¼ CUP SEA SALT
1 TB. SOY BACON BITS
1 TB. SOVEX SMOKED YEAST
1 TB. ONION GRANULES
1 TB. DRY CHOPPED CHIVES
1 TB. DRY PARSLEY FLAKES
1 TB. CHOPPED DRIED TOMATO
½ teasp. LEMON PEEL GRANULES

2 teasp. DRY BASIL
½ teasp. OREGANO
½ teasp. SAVORY
1 teasp. GARLIC GRANULES
½ teasp. HORSERADISH POWDER
½ teasp. BLACK PEPPER
½ teasp. PAPRIKA

♣Whirl all ingredients in the blender to granular consistency.

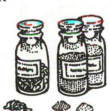

ORIENTAL COOKING SPICE

This seasoning is good as the base for stir-fry sauces, in spicy baking, and as a sprinkle over steamed vegetables.

♣Measure and whirl in the blender til fine

2 TBS. CHOPPED DRIED GINGER
1 TB. STAR ANISE
1 teasp. FENNEL SEED
½ teasp. CINNAMON
½ teasp. HOT ORIENTAL MUSTARD POWDER
¼ teasp. PAPRIKA or CAYENNE

½ teasp. GROUND CARDAMOM
¼ teasp. BLACK PEPPER
¼ teasp. FRUCTOSE
¼ teasp. ORANGE PEEL POWDER
¼ teasp. CLOVES

DONA'S SESAME SALT DELIGHT

Everybody used to beg Dona for this, so she has finally started making and selling it. This mix is a wonderful way to wean yourself away from salt, and never miss the salty taste.

♣Stir 2 CUPS BROWN SESAME SEED in a heavy dry skillet on low heat until seeds pop.

♣Add 1 OZ. CHOPPED DRIED DULSE LEAVES, 4 to 6 teasp. SEA SALT, and 2 teasp. GRANULATED KELP. Stir, heating until aromatic.

♣Turn into a blender or seed mill and grind until fine. Store covered in the fridge. Very high in nutrients.

GARLIC LEMON SEASONING

This is a very popular seasoning, because its uses are so many. It is excellent in a sauté in place of chopped garlic for aroma, and adds a more complex flavor to Italian and European cooking without all the work.

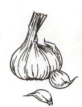

8-OZ. TOASTED SESAME SEEDS
1/4 CUP DRIED PARSLEY FLAKES
2 teasp. GARLIC GRANULES
2-OZ. DRY CHOPPED ONION PIECES
2 TBS. DRY BASIL
DROPS of LEMON OIL to taste

1 teasp. GINGER POWDER
1 teasp. PAPRIKA
1/2 teasp. TARRAGON
1/2 teasp. CELERY SEED
2 teasp. LEMON PEEL GRANULES
PINCH STEVIA SWEET HERB

♣Whirl all ingredients in the blender until aromatic.

SALTERNATIVE HERB SALT

This mixture is completely without salt. It relies instead on dried sea vegetables for its "saltiness." It is delicious, and is particularly tasty with macrobiotic foods and recipes.

2 TBS. KELP GRANULES
2 TBS. DRIED WAKAME FLAKES
2 TBS. DRIED DULSE FLAKES
1 TBS. GARLIC GRANULES
2 TBS. ONION GRANULES
2 TBS. BASIL

1 teasp. DILLWEED
1/2 teasp. THYME
1/2 teasp. MARJORAM
1/2 teasp. CELERY SEED
1/2 teasp. PAPAYA LEAF
1/2 teasp. DRIED COMFREY LEAF

♣Whirl all in the blender to sprinkling consistency.

SPICY ITALIAN HERBS

♣Stir together in a bowl, and store airtight.

1 1/2 TBS. OREGANO LEAF
3 TBS. DRIED BASIL
1 TBS. DRUSHED ROSEMARY LEAVES
1 TB. MINCED DRIED GARLIC

1 TB. PARSLEY FLAKES
1/2 teasp. FENNEL SEED
1/2 teasp. RUBBED SAGE
1/2 teasp. MARJORAM

GREAT 28 MIX

*This is probably the mix we use the most. It seems to have everything **in** it, with a wonderful versatility. It is a delicious seasoning by itself, or you can mix it with kefir cheese, sour cream or other medium as a dip, sauté it in butter for the base of a soup or sauce, or use as a flavoring stock for cooking grains. Mix it with mayonnaise for a sandwich spread, with yogurt, or oil and vinegar for a salad dressing. The list could go on and on.*

♣Measure and whirl all in the blender

1 TB. KELP GRANULES	1 teasp. CELERY SEED
1 TB. DULSE GRANULES	1 teasp. BLACK PEPPER
1 TB. CHILI POWDER	1/2 teasp. GARLIC POWDER
3 TBS. DRIED ONION GRANULES	1/2 teasp. OREGANO
2 TBS. DRIED CHOPPED TOMATOES	1/2 teasp. PAPRIKA
1 TB. SOY BACON BITS	1/2 teasp. DILLWEED
2 TBS. TOASTED SESAME SEEDS	1/2 teasp. SAGE
2 TBS. CHOPPED TOASTED WALNUTS	1/2 teasp. LEMON PEEL POWDER
1 TB. DRY BASIL	1/2 teasp. FRUCTOSE
1 TB. DRY CHOPPED CHIVES	1/2 teasp. ORANGE PEEL
2 TBS. CHOPPED DRIED MUSHROOMS	1/2 teasp. ROSE HIPS
1 TB. DRY TAMARI GRANULES	1/2 teasp. TARRAGON
1 TB. BREWER'S YEAST FLAKES	1/2 teasp. CURRY POWDER
1 TB. DRIED PARSLEY FLAKES	1/2 teasp. SAVORY

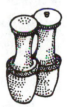

SWEET TOOTH BAKING MIX

When I was baking for the restaurant, this recipe became a "convenience mix" to save time and proportion measuring. It is just right for spicing sweet baked things.

4 TBS. CINNAMON	1 teasp. GINGER POWDER
2 TBS. NUTMEG	1 teasp. ORANGE PEEL POWDER
2 teasp. GROUND CLOVES	1 teasp. LEMON PEEL POWDER
1 teasp. GROUND ALLSPICE	1 teasp. MACE POWDER

♣Measure into jar. Cover and shake.

SALAD HERBS

The mint is the secret, and really makes a difference to the flavor. Use the most aromatic mint you can find.

♣Mix together in a small bowl and store in a jar

2 TBS. DRY BASIL LEAVES	1 teasp. MARJORAM
1 TB. DRY PARSLEY FLAKES	1/2 teasp. TARRAGON
1 TB. DRY DILL WEED	1/2 teasp. CHERVIL
1 TB. DRY THYME LEAVES	1/2 teasp. CELERY SEED
2 teasp. DRY SPEARMINT LEAVES	

GREEK SEASONING

I refine this mixture every time we come back from Greece. It brings you memories of the islands and pungent Greek cooking. Try it on fresh Mediterranean produce, such as roma tomatoes, dark green salads, and sautéed zucchini.

3 TBS. SEA SALT
2 TBS. TOASTED SESAME SEEDS
2 TBS. TOASTED TVP or SOY GRIT
1 TB. ONION POWDER
DROPS of LEMON OIL to taste

½ teasp. GARLIC POWDER
1 TB. OREGANO LEAF
½ teasp. FRUCTOSE
½ teasp. PAPRIKA
1 TB. LEMON PEEL POWDER

♣Measure into a jar. Cover and shake to blend.

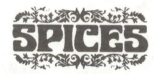

TEX-MEX MIX

This chili spice was also developed as a "convenience mix" for the Rainbow Kitchen. We fixed lots of spicy Mexican dishes, and the proportions are just right.

♣Measure and whirl in the blender til fragrant
3 TBS. CORNMEAL
3 TBS. CHILI PEPPER FLAKES
1 TB. DRIED CHOPPED BELL PEPPER
3 TBS. CHILI POWDER
2 TBS. ONION POWDER

1 teasp. SEA SALT
1 teasp. CUMIN POWDER
½ teasp. MINCED GARLIC
½ teasp. CAYENNE
½ teasp. OREGANO

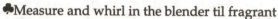

Other Seasoning Tips For Enhancing Your Cooking

I have learned much about healthy flavorings over the years of cooking professionally and personally for other people. The following tips are included so you won't have to "re-invent the wheel" when you season for a healing diet.

✹Toast nuts, seeds and grains to bring out their full flavor. Dry roast grains in the cooking pot before adding water or stock. Toast nuts and seeds in a 400∞ oven on baking sheets until golden brown.

✹Use fresh lemon or lime zest to bring out the flavor of food. Just rub the peel against a hand grater, or remove strips with a vegetable peeler, and sliver. Squeeze a little fresh lemon juice (or cider vinegar) over a dish just before serving to heighten flavor.

✹Use fresh herbs when you can. Chop and stir them in at the last minute for the most intense taste.

✹Use a mortar and pestle when pounding herbs and spices for the most flavor.

✹Begin a sauté with the strong spices or seasonings of a recipe. Add them to a dry heated pan, or with the oil, and sauté for a few minutes until their fragrance is released. Then continue with your recipe. This one little change will make a big difference in the robustness of a recipe's flavor.

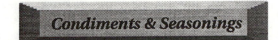

Custom Flour & Grain Mixes

A mix of grains lends lightness, taste interest, and more health benefits to a recipe.
We make up three different grain and flour mixes and keep them on hand in big covered cannisters for easy use.

GOURMET WHOLE GRAIN BLEND

This mix is a versatile, healthy, non-fattening, fiber cereal, pilaf, rice, pasta, or salad blend.

♣Mix in a large bowl

2 CUPS LONG GRAIN BROWN RICE	1 CUP MILLET
1 CUP OAT GROATS (uncut oats)	1 CUP BUCKWHEAT BERRIES
1½ CUPS WINTER WHEAT BERRIES	1 CUP TRITICALE
1¼ CUPS WHOLE RYE	1 CUP PEARL BARLEY
1 CUP HULLED SESAME SEEDS	

♣To cook: dry roast 1 cup of the grains in a pot over medium heat until aromatic, about 5 minutes. Add 2 cups boiling water. Let bubble for a minute. Cover and reduce heat. Steam for about 25 minutes until water is absorbed.

❈

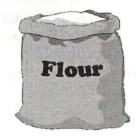

GOURMET FLOUR & BAKING MIX

This mix can be used wherever flour is called for. It is very light and has a slightly nutty flavor.

♣Mix

3 CUPS UNBLEACHED FLOUR	½ CUP OAT FLOUR
1½ CUPS WHOLE WHEAT PASTRY FLOUR	½ CUP BARLEY FLOUR

❈

BREAD & BAKING MIX

This mix can also be used where regular flours are called for, but it has a higher gluten content for elasticity and shape. It is good for breads and many pastries.

♣Mix

3 CUPS UNBLEACHED FLOUR	½ CUP OAT FLOUR
½ CUP RYE FLOUR	½ CUP BUCKWHEAT FLOUR

❈

CUSTOM BEAN MIX

This combination has become a staple for most of our bean cooking, and lends a nice complexity of taste with all the health advantages of beans and legumes.

♣Just shake in a big jar and store until ready for use

2 PARTS GREEN SPLIT PEAS	2 PARTS PINTOS
2 PARTS BLACK BEANS	1 PART KIDNEY BEANS
1 PART SMALL WHITE BEANS	1 PART GARBANZOS

❈

Relishes & Condiments

*This food area often includes the worst offenders for adding chemicals, preservatives and colorings.
It's easy to make your own fresh condiments, and they will keep beautifully in your fridge.*

GOURMET KETCHUP

Make this in a large pot and cook slowly; all day if necessary, until ketchup consistency is reached. It is a sweet, spicy, complex condiment, and needs the long cooking time for flavors to blend just right. I make this about every six months when the tomato harvest is in, and freeze in pint jars for later use. The recipe makes 5 pints.

♣Sauté in 4 TBS. OIL until very brown
1 LB. ONIONS
1/2 CUP MAPLE SUGAR GRANULES
2 teasp. DRY MUSTARD
1/2 teasp. CAYENNE or HOT PEPPER SAUCE

♣Add and bring to a simmer
1 CORED CHOPPED APPLE
2 CHOPPED RED BELL PEPPERS
2 CHOPPED RIBS CELERY
7 LBS. PEELED CHOPPED
PLUM TOMATOES

♣Add
1/4 CUP UNSULPHURED MOLASSES
1/2 CUP RASPBERRY VINEGAR
1/2 CUP ROSÉ WINE
4 teasp. SEA SALT

♣Add the seasonings
1 teasp. CINNAMON
1/2 teasp. GROUND CLOVES
1/4 teasp. GROUND ALLSPICE
1/4 teasp. NUTMEG

♣Simmer slowly, partially covered until thick. Store in glass jars. Freeze whatever you won't use in a month.

QUICK HONEY KETCHUP

This doesn't have the complex flavors or slow-cook quality, but it is easy to make, with a fresh no-salt taste.

♣Measure and whirl in the blender until smooth and thick
1 CUP PUREED ROMA TOMATOES
1/4 CUP OIL
2 TBS. HONEY
PINCHES of BASIL, OREGANO, TARRAGON, THYME to taste

1 CHOPPED GREEN ONION
1 TB. CHOPPED ONION
1 TB. LEMON JUICE

HOMEMADE MAYONNAISE

It only takes a minute to make, and the taste difference from the store-bought kind is amazing. Add your own variations, like an AVOCADO, or a GREEN ONION, or 2 TBS. of PARMESAN CHEESE.

♣Make it all in the blender
1 EGG
1 TB. LEMON JUICE
1 TB. TARRAGON VINEGAR

1 teasp. DIJON MUSTARD
1/2 teasp. SEA SALT
1 TB. HONEY

♣Whirl briefly, and with the motor running, add 1 CUP SALAD or CANOLA OIL in a thin steady stream until mayonnaise thickens to good consistency.

DONA'S HIGH SIERRA RANCH DRESSING MIX

This mix is a good natural convenience food for fresh-made dressing whenever you want it. Dona served it in her own restaurant for years to great raves.

♣Make up the mix

3/4 CUP ONION FLAKES
1/4 CUP PARSLEY FLAKES
2 TBS. CHIA SEEDS
2 TBS. GARLIC POWDER
2 TBS. ONION POWDER

2 TBS. SEA SALT
2 TBS. LEMON PEPPER
2 TBS. POPPY SEEDS
1/8 teasp. CAYENNE

♣To make the ranch style dressing. Mix well in a bowl
1 CUP LIGHT MAYONNAISE
1 CUP BUTTERMILK
2 TBS. LEMON JUICE
1/4 CUP HIGH SIERRA MIX

   OR
♣To make up the vinaigrette style dressing. Whisk in a bowl.
1/2 CUP SALAD OIL
1/4 CUP LEMON JUICE
1/4 CUP HIGH SIERRA MIX
♣Chill. This is very good for pasta salads as well as greens. Store either dressing in a jar.

QUICK HOT SALSA

*This is very easy to make for all of you who want your tacos **fast**.*

♣Whirl in the blender
4 TOMATOES
1 SMALL CAN GREEN DICED CHILIES
4 to 6 GREEN ONIONS, chopped

2 teasp. MINCED GARLIC
1/2 teasp. CHILI POWDER

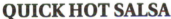

PEACH & MINT CHUTNEY

This is excellent with grain dishes or curries.
For 8 to 10 servings:

♣Blanch 4 RIPE PEACHES in boiling water for 1 minutes. Drain and peel. Chop flesh and set aside.
♣Sauté 1 CHOPPED ONION in 1 TB. OIL in a saucepan until golden. Add THE PEACHES, 1 HOT FRESH CHOPPED CHILI PEPPER, 1/4 CUP APPLE JUICE. 1 TB. HONEY, 3 TBS. CIDER VINEGAR, and 1 teasp. CHOPPED GINGER.
♣Cover and cook over low heat for 20 minutes, until liquid is absorbed. Stir in 1/2 CUP PACKED CHOPPED MINT LEAVES and simmer for 5 minutes. Cool and store in a jar.

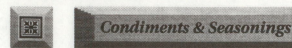

SWEET HOT MUSTARD

For about 4 cups:

♣Mix and let stand for 1 hour
1¹/₃ CUPS CHAMPAGNE VINEGAR
1¹/₃ CUPS DRY MUSTARD (4-OZ.)

♣Add 6 EGGS, 1 CUP HONEY and 1 CUP TURBINADO SUGAR and whisk in til smooth. Pour into a heavy pan and stir over medium heat until thickened and beginning to bubble, about 10 minutes. Remove from heat and pour into jars. Cool and chill.

HOT PINEAPPLE DAIKON RELISH

For about 1¹/₂ cups:

♣Mix ingredients together in a bowl
1/₂ CUP CHOPPED FRESH PINEAPPLE   2 TBS. LIME
1 TB. DRY MUSTARD in 1 TB. WATER   1 TB. FRESH MINCED GINGER
2 teasp. HORSERADISH   1/₂ teasp. SESAME SALT
♣Add 1/₄ LB. FRESH DAIKON RADISH, peeled and shredded. Cover and chill.

LEMON PEEL RELISH
This is so delicious with poultry and fish, hot or cold.
For about 2 cups:

♣Peel the yellow skin and a little of the white pith from 6 LEMONS. Mince peel and cut remaining pith off the lemons. Cut 2 of the LEMONS in chunks and remove seeds. (Save other 4 lemons for another use.)

♣Sauté 1/₂ CUP FINE CHOPPED ONION in 1 TB. OIL until limp but not brown, about 7 minutes.
♣Add the lemon and the lemon peel, 1/₂ CUP WHITE WINE, 4 TBS. FRUCTOSE and 1 teasp. WHITE PEPPER. ♣Stir until most of the liquid is evaporated and mixture is syrupy, about 15 minutes. Let cool. Cover and chill.

CRANBERRY GINGER RELISH
This relish can be a delicious change from the ordinary at Thanksgiving meals.

For about 3 cups:

♣Cut 2 KARGE TANGERINES, TANGELOS or MANDARIN ORANGES in 1" chunks. Chop into fine mince in the blender with 1/₄ CUP CRYSTALLIZED GINGER, 12 OZ. CRANBERRIES, and 1/₃ CUP FRUCTOSE. Stir and chill.

NATURAL APPLESAUCE WITH RAISINS

For about 6 cups:

♣Core and chop 6 APPLES. Put in a heavy pan on the lowest possible heat. Add enough water so the apples don't burn. Partially cover and simmer slowly until apples begin to soften.
♣Add 1 CUP HONEY or ¹/₂ CUP FRUCTOSE, and 2 teasp. SWEET TOOTH BAKING MIX. Cook until soft and fragrant. Remove from heat and puree in the blender. Add 2 TBS. LEMON JUICE to intensify flavor. Add 1 CUP RAISINS.

✳

APRICOT PINEAPPLE HONEY BUTTER

For about 4 cups:

♣Puree 2 LBS. FRESH APRICOTS in the blender. Add 12-OZ. FRESH CUBED PINEAPPLE. Turn into a bowl and mix with ¹/₂ teasp. GRATED ORANGE PEEL, 2 TBS. LEMON JUICE, ³/₄ CUP HONEY and ¹/₂ CUP MAPLE SYRUP.
♣Simmer uncovered, stirring until thick, about 2 hours.

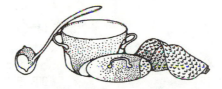

Soup Stocks & Broth Powders

The stock is the essence of a soup. Fresh homemade stocks inevitably have the best flavor; in many cases, canned products are over-salted, or full of MSG and other chemical enhancers. Like most condensed flavor foods, broths freeze nicely - even in ice cube trays, so you can make up a large batch, and use a little or a lot at a time. Remember, when making a purifying soup for a healing diet, shred the greens and veggies beforehand, and heat the broth only long enough for the vegetables to become tender crisp.

SPICY VEGETABLE BROTH MIX
This is a convenience dry soup mix. Just make it up and store it . Use as much as you want any time.

♣Blend briefly in the blender so that there are still recognizable chunks

¹/₄ CUP DRIED ONION FLAKES	1 TB. SOY BACON BITS
4 TBS. CHOPPED DRIED TOMATOES	1 TB. TAMARI POWDER
3 TBS. SOY GRITS or TVP	¹/₂ teasp. CELERY SEED
3 TBS. CHOPPED DRIED CARROTS	¹/₂ teasp. CHILI POWDER
2 TBS. CHOPPED DRIED MUSHROOMS	¹/₂ teasp. MIXED SALAD HERBS
¹/₂ teasp. GARLIC/LEMON SEASONING	2 TBS. BREWER'S YEAST FLAKES

♣For a quick delicious broth, sauté 2 teasp. MIX in 2 teasp. BUTTER til fragrant. Add 1¹/₂ to 2 cups water and simmer for 10 minutes.

✳

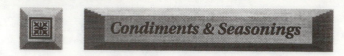

BASIC HERB & ONION STOCK

For about 6 cups:

♣Sauté in a large soup pot until aromatic and translucent
2 TBS. OIL
4 CUPS CHOPPED YELLOW ONIONS   1 TB. MIXED SALAD HERBS
1/2 teasp. PEPPER   1 TB. SEA SALT
♣Add 1 CUP MIXED CHOPPED VEGETABLES, such as CELERY, CARROTS, or GREENS, and 1/4 CUP FRESH CHOPPED PARSLEY and toss until green. Add 1-QT. WATER. Cover, and simmer for 30 minutes. ♣Strain if using as a stock.

✖

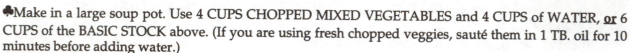

BASIC HERB & VEGETABLE BROTH

For about 8 cups of broth:

♣Make in a large soup pot. Use 4 CUPS CHOPPED MIXED VEGETABLES and 4 CUPS of WATER, **or** 6 CUPS of the BASIC STOCK above. (If you are using fresh chopped veggies, sauté them in 1 TB. oil for 10 minutes before adding water.)
♣Add and bring to a boil
3/4 CUP TOMATO JUICE   1 teasp. SESAME SALT
2 TBS. CHOPPED GREEN ONION   1/2 teasp. SAVORY
2 TBS. FRESH BASIL or 1 teasp. DRIED   1/2 teasp. OREGANO
11/2 CUPS TAMARI or MISO SOUP   1 TB. BREWER'S YEAST FLAKES
♣Partially cover and let simmer until aromatic, about 30 minutes.

✖

RICH BROWN STOCK
This stock is for very hearty soups and broths, and can also be taken as a soup on its own.
For about 8 cups:

♣Sauté 4 SLICED RED ONIONS in 4 TBS. BUTTER in a large soup pot until very brown and aromatic.
♣Add 1 CUP RED or ROSÉ WINE, 6 CUPS WATER, and 6 teasp. VEGEX YEAST PASTE and bring to a boil. Simmer to concentrate flavors, and add FRESH CHOPPED PARSLEY and SNIPPED CHIVES.
♣Strain if using as a stock.

✖

BEST FISH STOCK

♣Sauté 2 CHOPPED LEEKS and 2 CHOPPED ONIONS in 2 TBS. OLIVE OIL until aromatic.
♣Add 2 LBS. FISH PARTS and sauté for 10 minutes.
♣Add 2-QTS. SALTED WATER, 1 RIB CHOPPED CELERY, and 1 teasp. THYME.
♣Simmer for 25 minutes until flavor concentrates. Strain and discard solids.

✖

MISO MARINADE

This is a basic healthy sauce to marinate and baste fish, vegetables, tofu, potatoes, or chicken. It keeps beautifully. A little goes a long way.

♣Shake in a jar and chill

1/2 CUP MISO
1/2 CUP SHERRY
1/3 CUP TAMARI

1 1/2 TBS. HONEY
1 TB. FRESH GRATED GINGER
1/4 teasp. GARLIC POWDER

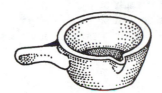

Pestos & Herb Butters

BASIC PESTO

This is a wonderful condiment to keep on hand in the freezer. Just pour into ice cube trays, freeze and pop one cube out any time you need pesto.

For 1 1/2 cups:

♣Whirl all ingredients in the blender
2 CUPS FRESH PACKED BASIL or CILANTRO LEAVES
1 CUP GRATED PARMESAN CHEESE
1/2 to 2/3 CUPS OLIVE OIL
1 CLOVE MINCED GARLIC

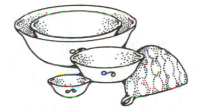

BASIL BUTTER

This is particularly good on steamed vegetables.
For about 16 ounces:

Cream 2 STICKS SOFT BUTTER with 1/4 CUP + 2 TBS. MINCED FRESH BASIL, 1 teasp. LEMON/ GARLIC SEASONING, and 1 TB. LEMON JUICE. Store in a crock and use as needed.

ROSEMARY BUTTER

For about 16 ounces:

♣Cream 2 STICKS SOFT BUTTER with 1 TB. FRESH ROSEMARY LEAVES, 1 MINCED SHALLOT, 1 CLOVE MINCED GARLIC, and 2 TBS. FRESH MINCED PARSLEY.
♣Store in a crock and use as needed.

Vinegars

Why settle for plain when you can make your favorite flavors? Easy homemade vinegars really make a dressing or marinade sing. When you make them yourself, you know there are no preservers, alum or enhancers to affect a healing diet. If you are consciously lowering fat in your diet, vinegars can spark a recipe with piquancy that used to belong to butter and cream sauces.

The simple vinegars on this page are just to get you started. It's so easy. Each recipe makes about 1-quart. Start with white wine vinegar for each of the flavors. The will vinegars keep up to 4 mionths at room temperature. The fruit in the bottle will slowly fall apart, but that isn't harmful to the vinegar. If you don't like the look of the aged fruit, simply pour though a strainer and discard the fruit. Then add more fresh fruit. Buon Appetito!

RASPBERRY VINEGAR

♣Rinse and drain 4 CUPS FRESH RASPBERRIES, or use ONE 16-OZ. FROZEN PKG. Set aside 8 of the berries. Combine the rest of the berries in a saucepan with 3 CUPS WHITE WINE VINEGAR, and 2 TBS. HONEY. Cover and bring to a boil over high heat. Remove and let stand, covered, until cool. Then pour liquid into a bottle through a fine strainer. Discard residue. Add reserved berries to the bottle and seal.

LEMON VINEGAR

♣Pare off 3 to 4 long peel parings for the bottle. Shred 1/4 CUP LEMON PEEL. Combine with 3 CUPS WHITE WINE VINEGAR, and 2 TBS. HONEY. Cover and bring to a boil over high heat. Remove and let stand, covered, until cool. Then pour liquid into a bottle through a fine strainer. Discard residue. Add reserved peel to the bottle and seal.

CIDER VINEGAR

♣Pare and core 4 LARGE TART APPLES. Combine with 3 CUPS WHITE WINE VINEGAR, and 2 TBS. HONEY. Cover and bring to a boil over high heat. Remove and let stand, covered, until cool. Then pour liquid into a bottle through a fine strainer. Discard residue.

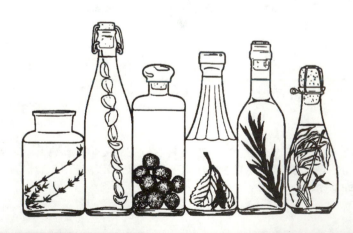

Index for the Diets and Healing Programs

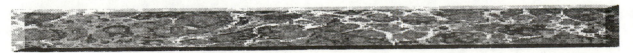

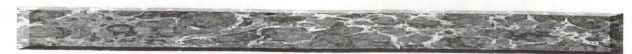

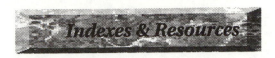
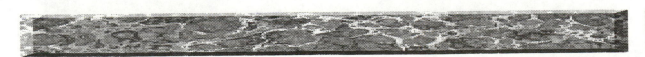

Index by Recipe Type
Indexed By Recipe Number or Page Number

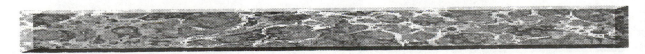

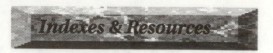
❋Breakfast & Brunch:
HIGH PROTEIN, LOW-FAT, HIGH FIBER FOODS, EGGS, CEREALS & GRAINS, BREAK-FAST BREADS, DRINKS

 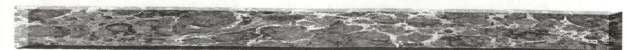

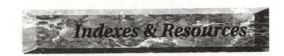

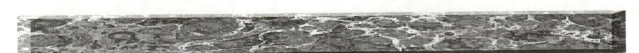

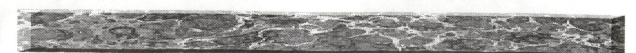

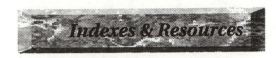

❈Salads:

**CLEANSING, MACROBIOTIC, LOW CHOLES-
TEROL, HIGH PROTEIN, HIGH FIBER, LOW-
FAT, COMPLEX CARBOHYDRATE, HIGH MIN-
ERAL,TOFU, WHOLE MEAL & ENTREE, FAN-
CY, HEALTHY DRESSINGS**

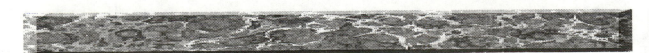

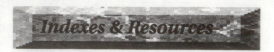
♣ LOW CHOLESTEROL SALADS:

♣ HIGH PROTEIN SALADS:

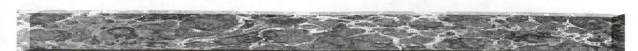

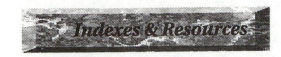

♣HIGH FIBER SALADS:

♣HIGH COMPLEX CARBO. SALADS:

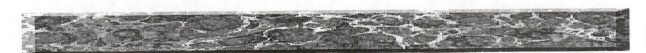

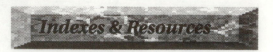
♣HIGH MINERAL SALADS:

♣SALADS WITH TOFU:

♣WHOLE MEAL SALADS:

♣FANCY COMPANY SALADS:

 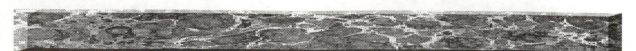

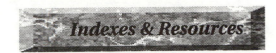
♣HEALTHY DRESSINGS & SAUCES:

❈Soups:

CLEANSING, MACROBIOTIC, DAIRY FREE, LOW-FAT, LOW CHOLESTEROL, HIGH PROTEIN, FANCY & EXOTIC

♣CLEANSING SOUPS & BROTHS:

♣MACROBIOTIC SOUPS:

♣LOW-FAT SOUPS:

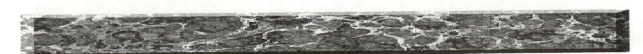

♣LOW CHOLESTEROL SOUPS:

♣DAIRY FREE SOUPS:

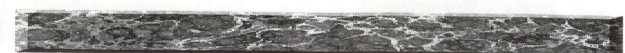

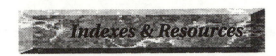

✹Sandwiches & Pizzas:
**MACROBIOTIC, LOW-FAT, WHEAT FREE,
HIGH PROTEIN, LOW CHOLESTEROL, TOFU,
SEAFOOD, CHICKEN & TURKEY**

♣MACROBIOTIC SANDWICHES:

♣LOW FAT SANDWICHES:

♣LOW CHOLESTEROL SANDWICHES:

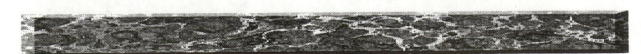

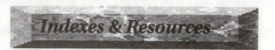

※ Breads & Baked Goodies:
LOW-FAT, WHEAT FREE, HIGH PROTEIN, HIGH FIBER, HIGH COMPLEX CARBOHYDRATE

 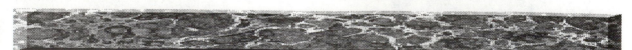

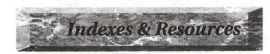

♣HIGH FIBER BAKING:

♣HIGH COMPLEX CARBOHYDRATE BAKED GOODIES:

✺Fish & Seafood:

APPETIZERS, LOW -AT, LOW CHOLESTEROL, HIGH PROTEIN, HIGH MINERAL, OUTDOOR GRILL

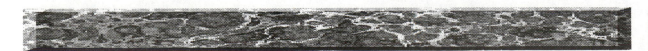

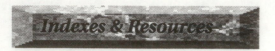
 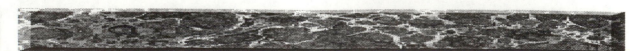

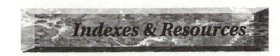
♣HIGH PROTEIN SEAFOOD:

♣HIGH MINERAL SEAFOOD:

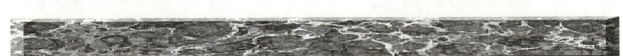

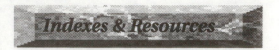

❋Eggs & Cheese:
LOW-FAT, LOW CHOLESTEROL, HIGH PROTEIN, APPETIZERS

❋Turkey & Chicken:
LOW-FAT, LOW CHOLESTEROL, HIGH PROTEIN, APPETIZERS, FESTIVE & FEASTING, OUTDOOR GRILL

 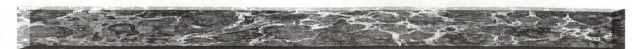

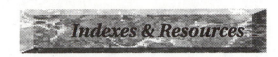

✷ Tofu & Soy Foods:

TOFU SAUCES, MACROBIOTIC, LOW-FAT, HIGH PROTEIN, HIGH MINERAL, HIGH FIBER, ENTREE, DESSERT

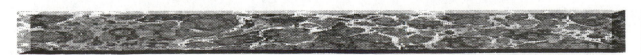

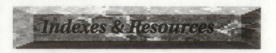
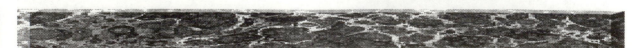

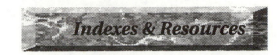
▓Pasta & Rice:
MACROBIOTIC, LOW-FAT, HIGH PROTEIN, HIGH COMPLEX CARBOHYDRATE, HIGH MINERAL, HIGH FIBER, WHEAT FREE, WHOLE MEAL & ENTREE

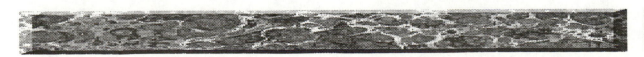

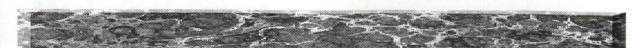

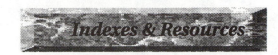
♣WHEAT FREE PASTA:

♣WHOLE MEAL PASTA RECIPES:

⚒Vegetables:

CLEANSING, MACROBIOTIC, LOW-FAT, HIGH FIBER, HIGH PROTEIN, HIGH COMPLEX CARBOHYDRATE, WHOLE MEAL & ENTREE RECIPES, OUTDOOR GRILL

♣CLEANSING VEGETABLE RECIPES:

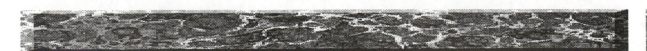

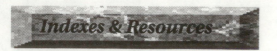

♣MACROBIOTIC VEGETABLE RECIPES:

♣LOW-FAT VEGETABLES:

♣HIGH FIBER VEGETABLES:

 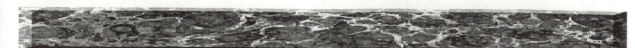

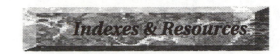
✦HIGH PROTEIN VEGETABLES:

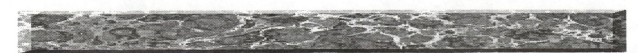

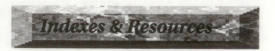

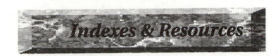
♣OUTDOOR GRILL:

✹Desserts:

SUGAR FREE, DAIRY FREE, LOW FAT, LOW CHOLESTEROL, WHEAT FREE, FANCY & FEASTIVE

♣SUGAR FREE DESSERTS:

♣LOW-FAT DESSERTS:

♣LOW CHOLESTEROL DESSERTS:

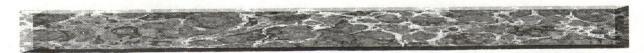

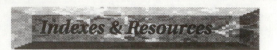
 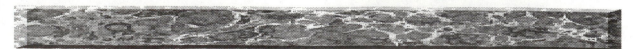

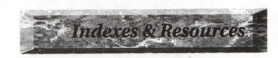

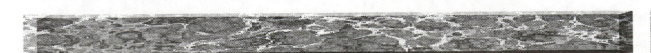

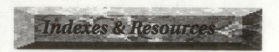
 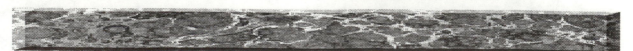

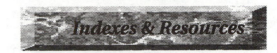

Index by Recipe Name and Page Number

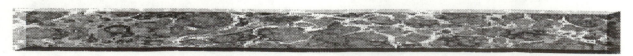

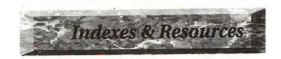

D

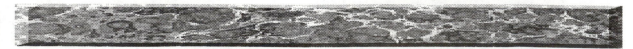

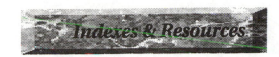

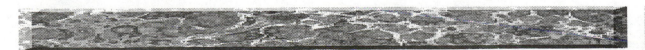

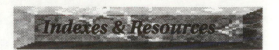

 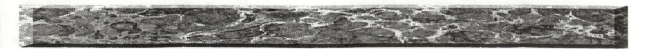

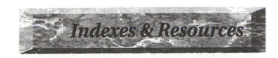

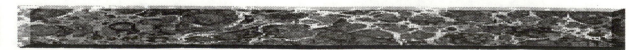

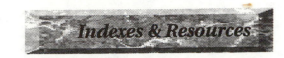
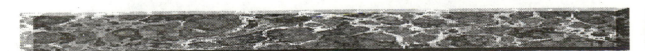

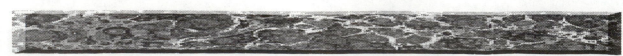

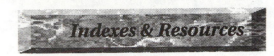

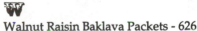

Resources & Contributors

* Healthy Healing, 8th Edition - Dr. Linda Rector-Page, N.D., Ph.D.

* Better Health Through Natural Healing - Dr. Ross Trattler

* Jane Brody's Good Food Cookbook - Jane Brody

* Food & Healing - Anne-Marie Colbin

* The Natural Healing Cookbook - Mark Bricklin & Sharon Claessens

* The New Laurel's Kitchen - Roberts, Flinders & Ruppenthal

* Diet & Disease - Cheraskin, Ringsdorf & Clark

* Enzymatic Therapy - Nutritional Formulas for the Right Body Chemistry

* Experiencing Quality: A Shopper's Guide to Whole Foods - M. Wittenberg

* The Healing Foods - Hausman & Hurley

* Nutritional Influences on Illness - Werbach

* The Food Pharmacy - Jean Carper

* Nutritional Herbology - Mark Pedersen

* How To Get Rid of the Poisons in Your Body - Gary Null

* The Underburner's Diet - Edelstein

* Nutrition Almanac - Dunne

* Raw Vegetable Juices - Walker

* How to Get Well - Airola

* Vegetarian Times Magazine - 1988, 1989, 1990, 1991.

* Whole Foods Magazine - 1989, 1990, 1991.